AF412249

RHEUMATOID ARTHRITIS

RHEUMATOID ARTHRITIS

PATHOGENESIS, ASSESSMENT, OUTCOME, AND TREATMENT

EDITED BY

FREDERICK WOLFE
University of Kansas School of Medicine
Wichita, Kansas

THEODORE PINCUS
Vanderbilt University School of Medicine
Nashville, Tennessee

Marcel Dekker, Inc.   **New York • Basel • Hong Kong**

Library of Congress Cataloging-in-Publication Data

Rheumatoid arthritis : pathogenesis, assessment, outcome, and
    treatment / edited by Frederick Wolfe, Theodore Pincus.
        p.   cm.
    Includes bibliographical references and index.
    ISBN 0-8247-8878-8 (alk. paper)
    1. Rheumatoid arthritis · I. Wolfe, Frederick.
II. Pincus, T. (Theodore).
    [DNLM: 1. Arthritis, Rheumatoid.   WE 346 R47305 1994]
RC933.R4287   1994
616.7'227--dc20
DNLM/DLC
for Library of Congress   94-20078
                                                                      CIP

The publisher offers discounts on this book when ordered in bulk quantities. For more information, write to Special Sales/Professional Marketing at the address below.

Marcel Dekker, Inc.
270 Madison Avenue, New York, New York 10016

Current printing (last digit):
10 9 8 7 6 5 4 3 2 1

PRINTED IN THE UNITED STATES OF AMERICA

Preface

These are exciting times for clinicians and investigators concerned with rheumatoid arthritis (RA). As recently as 1985, textbooks of rheumatology suggested that treatment of patients with RA using aspirin or nonsteroidal anti-inflammatory drugs (NSAIDs) was appropriate for the first 2–3 years of observation, followed by gold salts at three years, and immunosuppressives after nine years of disease. During the early 1990s, however, rheumatologists proposed that treatment of RA should be begun early in disease, with consideration of multiple drugs in combination, as well as new biotechnology reagents—a dramatic difference over just a few years.

The new approaches to treatment of RA are based in part on observations from long-term studies that indicate that most patients with RA have radiographic abnormalities within the first two years of disease. These abnormalities generally progress to deformities over the next decade, and often are not ameliorated by available drugs in most studies. Most patients experience substantial declines in their ability to perform activities of daily living and in other measures of functional status. Work disability is seen in more than 60% of patients with RA who are seen in rheumatology clinical care settings. Increased mortality rates have been observed in patients with RA from all treatment centers, with a shortening of life span by 8–15 years.

Recognition of the serious consequences of RA to individual patients provides a rationale for new approaches, including the "step-down bridge," "sawtooth," and "target" approaches, and the routine use of combination therapies as well as emerging biotechnology therapies. Studies of these new approaches include randomized controlled clinical trials, as well as new approaches to data collection in routine care, to overcome limitations in standard clinical trials.

To capture the excitement of current studies, a panel of 32 experts has been assembled to review critical issues concerning RA in the 1990s. The book is divided into four sections: pathogenesis, assessment, outcome, and treatment.

The pathogenesis section includes up-to-date reviews of pathogenetic mechanisms by Dr. Gabriel Panayi of Guy's and St. Thomas's Hospitals in London; a review of rheumatoid factors by Drs. Nancy Olsen of Vanderbilt University and Pojen Chen of the University of California, San Diego, in La Jolla; the major histocompatibility (HLA) locus by Dr. Gerald Nepom of the Virginia Mason Research Center in Seattle, Washington; and a section on epidemiology by Drs. Deborah Symmons and Alan Silman of the University of Manchester, in Manchester, England.

The section concerning assessment includes reviews of the joint count as an assessment tool by Drs. Howard Fuchs of Vanderbilt University and Jennifer Anderson of Boston University; radiographic assessment by Dr. John Sharp of Emory University and Tifton Medical Clinic; and questionnaire measurement of functional status by Dr. Robert Meenan of Boston University.

The section on outcome includes reviews of morbidity by Drs. Simon Donnelly of Whipps Cross Hospital and David Scott of King's College Hospital in London; mortality by Dr. Heikki Isomäki of Rheumatism Foundation Hospital, Heinola, Finland; economic consequences by Dr. Deborah Lubeck of Stanford University; work disability by Dr. Edward Yelin of the University of California at San Francisco; psychological issues by Dr. Larry Bradley of the University of Alabama at Birmingham; and socioeconomic status and outcome by Dr. Leigh Callahan of Vanderbilt University.

The section on treatment includes reviews of first-line nonsteroidal anti-inflammatory drug therapies by Drs. Steven Abramson and Elizabeth Kitsis of New York University and Hospital for Joint Diseases; second-line antirheumatic drugs by Dr. David Felson of Boston University; combination therapy by Dr. Peter Tugwell of University of Ottawa in Ontario and Maarten Boers of University Hospital Maastricht, The Netherlands; biotechnology in treatment of RA by Drs. Arthur Kavanaugh and Peter Lipsky of the University of Texas Southwestern Medical Center at Dallas; analysis of toxicities of antirheumatic therapy by Dr. James Fries of Stanford University; physical therapy by Drs. Antoine Helewa of University of Western Ontario and Hugh A. Smythe of the University of Toronto and Wellesley Hospital; surgery by Drs. Matthew Liang and Gerold Stucki of Harvard Medical School and Brigham and Women's Hospital; and patient education by Dr. Kate Lorig of Stanford University. In the final chapter, Dr. Wolfe provides a methodology of data collection and utilization in the setting of clinical practice and research.

The authors have summarized the ''state of the art'' and commented on controversial areas and directions for future investigation and research. We are very grateful to the contributors for their excellent and timely work. We hope the readers will find the material as interesting and clinically relevant as we have.

Frederick Wolfe
Theodore Pincus

Contents

II. Assessment

III. Course and Outcome

IV. Treatment

Contributors

Steven B. Abramson, M.D. Department of Rheumatology, New York University Medical Center, and Hospital for Joint Diseases, New York, New York

Jennifer J. Anderson, Ph.D. Associate Research Professor of Medicine (Biostatistics), The Arthritis Center, Boston University School of Medicine, Boston, Massachusetts

Maarten Boers, M.D., Ph.D., M.Sc. Associate Professor, Department of Internal Medicine, University Hospital Maastricht, The Netherlands

Laurence A. Bradley, Ph.D. Professor, Departments of Psychology and Medicine, University of Alabama at Birmingham, Birmingham, Alabama

Leigh F. Callahan, Ph.D. Epidemiologist, Aging Studies Branch, Division of Chronic Disease Control and Community Intervention, National Center for Chronic Disease Prevention and Health Promotion, Centers for Disease Control and Prevention, Atlanta, Georgia

Pojen P. Chen, Ph.D. Associate Professor of Medicine, Department of Medicine, University of California, San Diego, La Jolla, California

Simon Donnelly, M.R.C.P. Senior Registrar, Department of Rheumatology, Whipps Cross Hospital, London, England

David T. Felson, M.D., M.P.H. Professor of Medicine, Boston University School of Medicine, Boston, Massachusetts

James F. Fries, M.D.   Professor of Medicine, Division of Immunology and Rheumatology, Stanford University School of Medicine, Palo Alto, California

Howard A. Fuchs, M.D.   Associate Professor of Medicine, Division of Rheumatology, Vanderbilt University School of Medicine, Nashville, Tennessee

Antoine Helewa, P.T., M.Sc.   Professor and Chair, Department of Physical Therapy, University of Western Ontario, London, Ontario, Canada

Heikki A. Isomäki, M.D.   Professor of Rheumatology, Rheumatism Foundation Hospital, Heinola, Finland

Arthur F. Kavanaugh, M.D.   Assistant Professor of Internal Medicine, The University of Texas Southwestern Medical Center at Dallas, and Chief of Rheumatology, Department of Veterans Affairs Medical Center at Dallas, Dallas, Texas

Elizabeth A. Kitsis, M.D.   Department of Rheumatology, New York University Medical Center, and Hospital for Joint Diseases, New York, New York

Matthew H. Liang, M.D., M.P.H.   Associate Professor, Departments of Medicine and Rheumatology/Immunology, Harvard Medical School, and Robert B. Brigham Multipurpose Arthritis and Musculoskeletal Diseases Center, Brigham and Women's Hospital, Boston, Massachusetts

Peter E. Lipsky, M.D.   Professor of Internal Medicine, Director, Harold C. Simmons Arthritis Research Center, Department of Internal Medicine, The University of Texas Southwestern Medical Center at Dallas, Dallas, Texas

Kate R. Lorig, RN, Ph.D.   Director, Stanford Patient Education Research Center, Stanford University School of Medicine, Palo Alto, California

Deborah P. Lubeck, Ph.D.   Senior Research Scientist, Department of Medicine, Stanford University, Stanford, California

Robert F. Meenan, M.D., M.P.H., M.B.A.   Director, Boston University School of Public Health, Boston, Massachusetts

Gerald T. Nepom, M.D., Ph.D.   Scientific Director, Diabetes and Immunology Programs, Virginia Mason Research Center, Seattle, Washington

Nancy J. Olsen, M.D.   Associate Professor, Department of Medicine, Vanderbilt University, Nashville, Tennessee

Gabriel S. Panayi, M.D.   Arthritis and Rheumatism Council, Professor of Rheumatology, Rheumatology Unit, United Medical and Dental Schools of Guy's and St. Thomas's Hospitals, London, England

Theodore Pincus, M.D.   Professor of Medicine, Division of Rheumatology, Department of Medicine, Vanderbilt University School of Medicine, Nashville, Tennessee

David L. Scott, M.D., F.R.C.P.   Reader in Rheumatology, Department of Rheumatology, King's College Hospital, London, England

John T. Sharp, M.D., F.A.C.P., M.A.C.R.   Clinical Professor of Medicine, Department of Medicine, Rheumatology Division, Emory University School of Medicine, Atlanta, and Staff Rheumatologist, Tifton Medical Clinic, Tifton, Georgia

Alan J. Silman, M.D., F.R.C.P., F.F.P.H.M.   Director, ARC Epidemiology Research Unit, University of Manchester, Manchester, England

Hugh A. Smythe, M.D., F.R.C.P.C.   Professor, Department of Medicine, University of Toronto and Wellesley Hospital, Toronto, Ontario, Canada

Gerold Stucki, M.D.   Departments of Medicine and Rheumatology/Immunology, Harvard Medical School, and Robert B. Brigham Multipurpose Arthritis and Musculoskeletal Diseases Center, Brigham and Women's Hospital, Boston, Massachusetts

Deborah P. M. Symmons, M.D., M.R.C.P.   Senior Scientist, ARC Epidemiology Research Unit, University of Manchester, Manchester, England

Peter Tugwell, M.D.   Chairman, Department of Medicine, University of Ottawa, Ontario, Canada

Frederick Wolfe, M.D.   Clinical Professor of Internal Medicine and Family and Community Medicine, University of Kansas School of Medicine, Wichita, Kansas

Edward H. Yelin, Ph.D.   The Rosalind Russell Arthritis Center and Institute for Health Policy Studies, University of California, San Francisco, California

RHEUMATOID ARTHRITIS

Introduction: Updating a Reassessment of Traditional Paradigms Concerning Rheumatoid Arthritis

Theodore Pincus

Vanderbilt University School of Medicine
Nashville, Tennessee

Frederick Wolfe

University of Kansas School of Medicine
Wichita, Kansas

Leigh F. Callahan

National Center for Chronic Disease Prevention and Health Promotion
Centers for Disease Control and Prevention
Atlanta, Georgia

I. RATIONALE FOR REASSESSMENT OF PARADIGMS

Rheumatoid arthritis (RA) was regarded traditionally in the 1970s and 1980s as a disease that could be managed effectively by most physicians in most patients. In the 1981 edition of the Kelley textbook (Fig. 1), it was suggested that 70–80% of patients with RA were ''controlled'' with a first-line nonsteroidal anti-inflammatory drug, 95% were controlled with a second-line drug, such as gold, penicillamine, or antimalarials, and third-line drugs, such as corticosteroids and cytotoxic drugs, were ''highly toxic'' with ''little evidence of benefit upon the underlying disease process'' (1). In the 1985 edition of the McCarty textbook

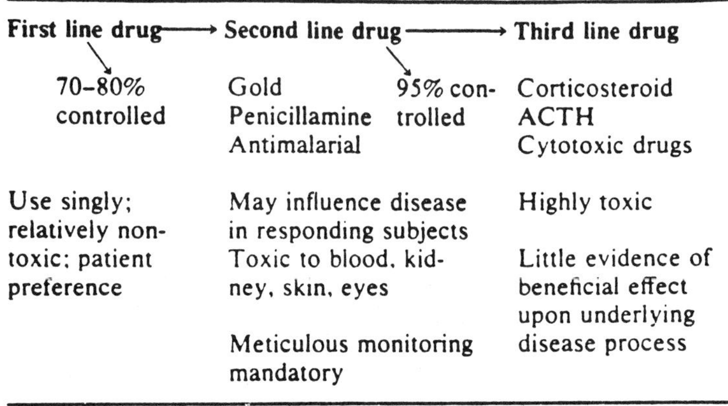

Fig. 1   Schema from 1981 edition of Kelley textbook presenting a proposed approach to drug treatment of rheumatoid arthritis. (From Ref. 1.)

(Fig. 2), "management choices in a hypothetical patient" with RA were nonsteroidal anti-inflammatory drugs (NSAIDs), including aspirin, for 2 years, other NSAIDs after 2 years, gold after 2.5 years, antimalarial drugs after 4.5 years, and immunosuppressive drugs after about 8.5 years of treatment (2).

A reassessment of this traditional approach emerged from many clinical centers during the 1980s, with evidence that adequate disease control for patients with RA was not provided, as summarized in a 1988 review entitled, *Reassessment of twelve traditional paradigms concerning rheumatoid arthritis (RA)* (3). *Paradigms* have been defined by Kuhn (4) as "universally recognized scientific achievements that for a time provided model problems and solutions to a community of practitioners," including "the entire constellation of beliefs, values, and techniques shared by members of a given community, employed as models or examples," which "replace explicit rules as a basis for solution of the remaining puzzles" (4). Kuhn has pointed out that progress in science often results from a "paradigm shift," in which new "models or examples" become available toward "solution of the remaining puzzles," e.g., Copernicus' recognition that the sun was the center of the universe, rather than the earth, or Semmelweis' recognition that infection was the primary basis of postpartum mortality, which could be prevented by washing the hands.

Although control of RA does not present a scientific puzzle of generalized importance compared with the foregoing examples, to patients and to health professionals who provide their care, effective management of RA is at least as important a problem as any in the universe. If the efforts of health professionals to control RA are based on incorrect paradigms, these efforts may be limited. It

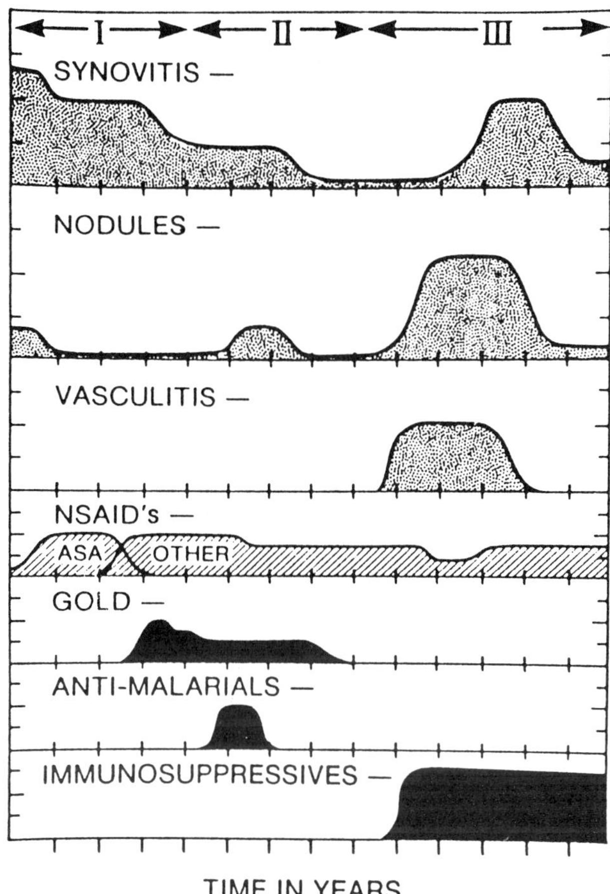

Fig. 2 Schema from 1985 edition of McCarty textbook entitled *Management Choices in a Hypothetical [RA] Patient Over Several Years*. Note that initiation of gold is not projected until after 2 1/2 years, antimalarial drugs until after 4 1/2 years, and immunosuppressive drugs until after 8 1/2 years. (From Ref. 2.)

is often more valuable to define a correct paradigm to solve a problem, than to work hard within an incorrect paradigm; if a paradigm is incorrect, further steps may lead in the wrong direction, no matter how well-conceived and executed.

A recurrent theme in an ongoing paradigm shift concerning RA in the late 1980s and 1990s involves a reassessment of the traditional biomedical model (5) (Table 1), which has governed the approach to solution of medical

Table 1   Reassessment of the Traditional Biomedical Model

Traditional model	Proposed reassessment
Pathogenesis	
There is a single "cause" for each disease involving a single identifiable physiologic mechanism.	The pathogenesis of most chronic diseases is multifactorial, including genetic, environmental, and possibly internal dysregulatory components.
Assessment	
Patients should be assessed primarily according to laboratory, radiographs, scan, and other high-technology data.	The assessment of disease should include emphasis on functional and psychological status, as well as on constructs, such as pain and fatigue, which are not measured by any laboratory tests, scans, or radiographs.
Outcome	
Outcome is determined primarily according to the physician and other health care providers, drugs, and the health care system, regardless of actions of the patient.	The outcome of chronic diseases, such as RA, depends in large part on actions of the patients as well as the actions of health care providers and the health care system.
Treatment	
The treatment involves a single drug as a "cure" based on laboratory discoveries and scientific data.	Treatment may require multiple drugs, as well as other approaches, including patient education, physical and occupational therapies.

problems during the 20th century. The principles of this model include that the pathogenesis of disease involves a single identifiable physiologic "cause," which may be assessed in clinical settings through the laboratory, a radiograph, or other high-technology source. The results of this assessment lead to a "cure" based on high-technology data, in the form of a "wonder drug," surgery, or other high-technology intervention. The outcome appears to be determined exclusively by the actions of health professionals and the medical care system through correct diagnostic and therapeutic procedures, regardless of the patient's actions.

The biomedical model has been extraordinarily effective in advancing care of many diseases, notably infectious diseases and trauma, but has proved limited in advancing management of chronic noninfectious diseases. Some limitations in the approach to chronic diseases were reviewed almost two decades ago by Engel (5), Holman (6), and others, and are summarized briefly in Table 1. The pathogenesis of most chronic diseases is now recognized to result from multiple factors. Assessment of clinical status requires attention to the functional and psychological status of the patient, as well as laboratory and imaging data. Treatment depends on multiple approaches rather than on a single "cure" ("wonder drug" or "silver bullet"), as a single therapy is unlikely to result in optimal control or cure. Outcomes of chronic diseases are increasingly recognized to depend, in large part, on patients' actions, as well as on those of health professionals, drugs, and medical care system.

In this chapter, we update (3,7) evidence for various paradigm shifts in the approach to RA, based on previous review articles (3,7–13) and original reports noted within the chapter.

II.   REASSESSMENT OF SPECIFIC PARADIGMS

A.   Pathogenesis of Rheumatoid Arthritis

A1.   Traditional Paradigm.   The pathogenesis of RA can be defined by a single cause external to the host, amenable to analysis according to Koch's Postulates.

Paradigm Shift.   The pathogenesis of RA is multifactorial, including host genetic predispositions and internal dysregulations, and may not require any external antigen or pathogen.

Comment.   The paradigm of Koch's Postulates was developed in the late 1800s to include the following principles:

1.   The organism is found regularly in the lesions of the disease.
2.   The organism can be isolated in pure culture on an artificial medium.
3.   Inoculation of this culture produces a similar disease in experimental animals.
4.   The organism can be recovered from the lesions in these animals.

These Postulates have proven invaluable in the description of acute and chronic infectious diseases, providing a foundation for spectacular advances in the treatment of such diseases, based on the biomedical model, as discussed above. However, limitations have been recognized in application of Koch's Postulates to most diseases, particularly to noninfectious chronic diseases.

Koch's Postulates are limited, even to understand fully the pathogenesis of acute infectious diseases, as they are focused exclusively on the pathogen, without recognition of the importance of host genetic and comorbid contribution to pathogenetic regulatory mechanisms and comorbid conditions, which may affect interactions of the pathogen with the host. Exposure of a host to an infectious agent does *not* invariably result in disease, as host genetic control mechanisms will result in no pathogenetic consequences of exposure in many, if not most, instances. Furthermore, various host characteristics, including age, presence of other diseases, drugs taken, and others, may affect susceptibility to pathogens and outcome of infectious diseases. Indeed, if host resistance to infectious agents in some members of a given species were not present, that species would be rendered extinct by an infectious agent, which probably has occurred many times in history.

Earlier in the 20th century, RA was known as ''chronic infectious arthritis'' (14), thought to have a pathogenesis similar to tuberculosis, involving a mycobacterium or other infectious agent. Indeed, the introduction of gold salts into therapy for RA was based on recognition that gold appeared to be effective in the treatment of tuberculosis (15–17). However, a search for an infectious agent in RA has been unsuccessful, and Koch's Postulates have not been met to describe the pathogenesis of this disease. Indeed, application of the paradigm of Koch's Postulates may focus too narrowly on possible pathogenetic mechanisms. More recently, interest in pathogenesis of RA has turned away from external events toward understanding of internal host dysregulations involving cytokine production and growth factors (see Chapter 1), host immune regulation (see Chapter 2), and host immunogenetic control mechanisms (see Chapter 3).

These considerations suggest that the pathogenesis of RA is not likely to be understood according to Koch's Postulates. Rheumatoid arthritis may be viewed primarily as a disease of the host, and it is possible that no external antigen or pathogen is needed to initiate pathogenetic events. Although it appears reasonable that footprints of an infectious agent in RA be sought using newly developed techniques, even if an infectious agent were identified, the contribution of the host genetic background, including histocompatibility and other genes, as well as demographic and environmental variables such as age, other diseases, and socioeconomic status, may be important determinants of pathogenetic mechanisms in RA.

A2. Traditional Paradigm. All individuals identified as having RA according to American Rheumatism Association (ARA) Criteria (18,19) have a similar pathogenesis and prognosis.

Paradigm Shift. Individuals identified as meeting Criteria for RA in population-based studies usually have a self-limited process, whereas patients who meet Criteria for RA in clinical settings usually have a progressive disease.

Comment. The 1958 ARA Criteria (18) were used in studies of RA over more than 29 years, until their revision in 1987 (19). Establishment of these Criteria led to an assumption that all people who meet them were homogeneous in pathogenesis and prognosis. However, emerging evidence suggests that most individuals identified in population-based studies as meeting ARA Criteria for RA appear to have a self-limited process, whereas most patients identified in clinical settings as meeting ARA Criteria for RA appear to have a severe progressive disease.

Evidence that RA identified in populations is a self-limited process, rather than a progressive disease, is derived from two sources:

1. *Rheumatoid factor prevalence in individuals who meet ARA Criteria for RA in population-based studies:* Five studies have been conducted in which individuals were analyzed both for whether they met the 1958 ARA Criteria for RA and whether they had rheumatoid factor (Table 2) (20). These studies, from diverse locations including Tecumseh, Michgan (21), Wensleydale, England (22), Jerusalem, Israel (23), and Arizona (24), indicated that rheumatoid factor was seen in only about 25% of individuals who met ARA Criteria for RA (20).

2. *Reevaluation of individuals who met ARA Criteria for RA 3–5 years later:* Only two studies are available in which almost all individuals in a population were examined to identify those who met ARA Criteria from RA, and then were reexamined 3–5 years later. In both of these population-based studies, fewer than 30% of those who met Criteria at baseline also met Criteria at later review (25,26). In Sudbury, Massachusetts (Table 3), 118 of 4522 persons (2.6%) examined at baseline met the 1958 ARA Criteria for definite or probable RA. When 109 of these 118 people were reexamined 3–5 years later, only 30 (27.5%) still met the Criteria for definite or probable RA (25) (see Table 3). In Tecumseh, Michigan, only 109 of 402 (26.6%) individuals who met ARA Criteria for RA at baseline met the Criteria 4 years later (26), remarkably similar to the Sudbury data.

In contrast to data from population-based studies, about 75–80% of patients who meet ARA Criteria for RA in clinical settings have rheumatoid factor in their serum (27,28), and more than 60% (possibly up to 90%) show evidence of disease 3–5 years later, generally with substantial progression (29–42) (see Paradigms C1 and C2 and Chapters 8–13).

These observations suggest that the 1958 ARA Criteria for RA identify persons with at least two types of pathogenetic processes:

1. Persons identified in the general population as meeting ARA Criteria for RA most likely will *not* have evidence of disease 3–5 years later. Only about 25% have rheumatoid factor in their sera. Many of these individuals may never see a physician for their symptoms, but may be overrepresented in certain clinical trials (see Paradigm D3 (43)).

2. Persons identified in clinical rheumatology settings as meeting ARA Criteria for RA are likely to show disease progression over periods longer than 3 years. At least 75% have rheumatoid factor in their sera, most will likely have evidence of disease 3–5 years later.

It is not known how the 1987 Criteria for RA (19), with a requirement for joint swelling, rather than tenderness alone, might function in population-based

Table 2 Prevalence of Rheumatoid Factor (RF) in Individuals Identified in Entire Populations Who Met 1958 American Rheumatism Association (ARA) Criteria for Rheumatoid Arthritis

Population RF test	Wensleydale, England (1960; 21) Latex fixation	Tecumseh, Michigan (1959–60; 20) Latex fixation	Study population Jerusalem, Israel (1962–64; 22) Latex fixation[a]	Blackfeet Indians, Montana (1961; 23) Bentonite flocculation	Pima Indians, Arizona (1961; 23) Bentonite flocculation
RF titer	>1:80	>1:20	>1:320	>1:128	>1:128
No. tested	870	6590	1602	1046	959
ARA criteria	Definite and probable	Definite, probable, and possible	Definite and probable	3–7 criteria	3–7 criteria
RA prevalence by criteria (%)	4.9	6.1	2.4	3.6	4.5
Prevalence of positive RF test in individuals who met ARA criteria for RA (sensitivity) (%)	24	19	25	24	33
Percentage of individuals who had positive RF test who met ARA criteria for RA (specificity) (%)	92	98	96	98	93

[a]Data also available for Rose-Waaler RF tests, in which only 12% of individuals meeting ARA criteria for RA had positive tests, whereas specificity was 99% (25).
Source: Adapted from Ref. 20.

Table 3 Follow-up Evaluation of Individuals Who Met 1958 ARA Criteria for Rheumatoid Arthritis[a]

	Initial evalua- tion	Number reexam- ined	Evaluation 3–5 years after initial evaluation			
Category			Probable RA	Definite RA	Total RA	No evidence of RA
Definite RA	40(0.9%)	36	7(19.4%)	12(33.3%)	19(52.8%	17(47.2%)
Probable RA	79(1.7%)	73	7(9.6%)	4(5.7%)	11(15.1%)	2(84.9%)
Total	118(2.6%)	109	14(12.8%)	16(14.7%)	30(27.5%)	79(72.5%)

[a]Evaluations were performed in 4552 individuals at baseline. The 1958 ARA criteria were met by 118 individuals (2.6%). A review 3–5 years later was performed on 109 of the 118 individuals who met ARA criteria for RA according to 1958 ARA criteria.
Source: Adapted from Ref. 25.

studies, and costs might not allow such studies. This question has been answered in part in a clinical study of 532 patients with early undifferentiated polyarthritis (Table 4) (44). In patients who met 1987 criteria for RA and had symptoms for less than 6 months at evaluation, 46% were completely free of symptoms at follow-up, while 31% had evidence of disease. In patients whose symptoms have been present for less than 2 years, 36% were completely resolved at follow-up,

Table 4 Proportion of Patients with Undifferentiated Polyarthritis, Who Met 1958 or 1987 American Rheumatism Association (ARA) Criteria for Classification of Rheumatoid Arthritis (RA) at First Evaluation Who Developed RA or Resolved by the Time of Follow-up Evaluation[a]

Criteria	RA at follow-up (N = 47)	Resolved at follow-up (N = 198)	RA at follow-up (N = 89)	Resolved at follow-up (N = 287)
	0–6 Months		0–24 Months	
ARA 1958 Negative	8.0%	59.8%	10.2%	58.5%
ARA 1958 Possible	13.3%	60.0%	13.2%	55.7%
ARA 1958 Probable	13.8%	59.8%	14.1%	57.0%
ARA 1958 Definite	30.6%	46.9%	38.5%	38.5%
ACR 1987 Negative	11.6%	59.6%	12.6%	57.3%
ACR 1987 Positive	30.8%	46.1%	41.6%	35.6%
Rheumatoid Factor				
Positive	41.7%	25.0%	43.1%	29.2%

[a]At 6 months 342 patients were studied for each criteria grouping (ACR 1987 (+/−), ARC 1958 (+/−), and R.F. (Latex) (+)). At >6–24 months 190 were studied, and at 0–24 months 532 were studied. Percentages in the table are the percent meeting the criterion in column 1 who resolved or had RA at follow-up for the 3 time periods. *Source:* Adapted from Ref. 44.

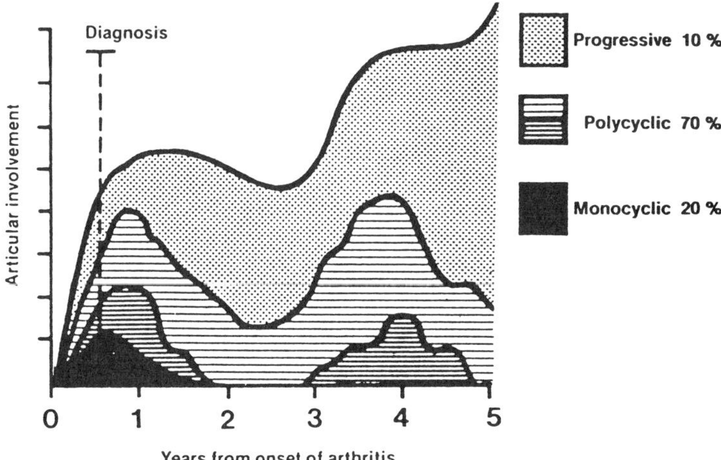

Fig. 3 Articular course patterns over 5 years in young adult patients with early-diagnosed rheumatoid arthritis. (From Ref. 45.)

while 42% had evidence of disease (44). These results would appear intermediate between those found using the 1958 Criteria and those in patients with established RA from clinical settings.

In the only long-term "inception cohort" study of 50 patients who met ARA Criteria for definite or probable RA for less than six months at the time of evaluation (Fig. 3), most patients did not show evidence of a progressive disease (45). However, these patients were recruited over 5 years from a busy clinic, and probably represent fewer than 5% of patients with RA seen in this clinical setting over a 5-year period.

The ARA Criteria for RA have been quite effective in distinguishing RA from other rheumatic diseases such as osteoarthritis, systemic lupus erythematosus, and other musculoskeletal diseases. However, both the 1958 and 1987 ARA Criteria were established from observations of individuals seen in rheumatology office settings, and not in the general population, and are only partially effective to distinguish a self-limited polyarthritis from progressive RA. The likelihood of a progressive disease, rather than a self-limited process, appears substantially greater when symptoms have been present for longer than six months, although some patients may experience an indolent course over many years. Recognition that ARA Criteria for RA may identify a heterogeneous group of individuals with very different outcomes would appear to clarify some apparently contradictory statements concerning disease course in the rheumatology literature.

A3. Traditional Paradigm. The prevalence of RA and other chronic diseases is similar in all persons of the same age and sex, regardless of socioeconomic status.

Paradigm Shift. Rheumatoid arthritis and most chronic diseases are much more common in persons of lower socioeconomic status, most notably persons who have not completed high school, adjusted for age, sex, and race.

Comment. In epidemiologic studies of the prevalence of diseases, the most common demographic variables included as possible modifiers are age, race, and gender. However, over the last two decades, it has been recognized that the prevalence of many diseases is associated significantly with socioeconomic status. In the 1978 US population aged 18–64, differences in disease prevalence according to formal education level are seen for most conditions (Table 5), including 17 of the 20 conditions found in more than 1% of the population (46). All common cardiovascular, musculoskeletal, gastrointestinal, pulmonary and renal diseases (other than asthma) occur two to three times more commonly in people less than age 65 who have not completed high school than in those who have completed 12 years of formal education, not explained by age, sex, race, or smoking (46). Thyroid disease, allergies, and asthma are not associated significantly with education level, and most associations with cancer are explained by smoking and age. An inverse pattern, with higher prevalence in more educated individuals, is seen for only one condition—multiple sclerosis (46). Therefore, a low formal education level is associated with a high prevalence of many chronic diseases.

Formal education level is a surrogate for socioeconomic status, which is more easily measured and less likely to be influenced by chronic disease than other indicators of socioeconomic status such as income and occupation. Associations between socioeconomic status and disease have been described in cardiovascular (47–56), pulmonary (57,58), neoplastic (59–64), central nervous system (65–67), and musculoskeletal (68–75) diseases. These associations have been observed in surveys in the United States (46–48,76–80), United Kingdom (49,51,81–85), Spain (86), Italy (87), the Netherlands (88), Belgium (89), Norway (90,91), Sweden (92,93), Finland (94–97), Russia (98), Japan (99,100), Australia (101), and New Zealand (102), and in studies of aging (103–105). Many differences in health status observed according to race appear to be explained by associations of race with education level (60,106–109).

Indicators of socioeconomic status are not included in most clinical investigations, as most physicians are unaware of associations between health and socioeconomic status, or believe that these associations are explained by recognized biomedical risk factors and limited access to medical care for individuals of lower socioeconomic status. However, several recent studies indicate that medical services are utilized as much or more by individuals of lower socioeconomic status than as by those of upper socioeconomic status (110). Furthermore, several lines of evidence strongly indicate that associations between education level and health are, in general, only minimally explained by recognized biomedical risk factors or limited access to medical care.

Table 5 Percentage of Individuals in the 1978 United States Population Aged 18–64 Reporting Various Selected Health Conditions According to Level of Formal Education

Condition	Total number × 10⁻³ (% of total population) aged 18–64 reporting condition (%)	Percentage of individuals reporting condition according to years of formal education				Odds ratios according to years of formal education*			
		1–8	9–11	12	>12	1–8	9–11	12	>12
Arthritis	14,215 (11.3)	26.4	13.1	11.0	6.8	5.0	2.1	1.7	1.0
Symmetric polyarthritis	2,366 (1.9)	8.9	4.4	3.1	1.7	6.5	2.9	1.9	1.0
Asymmetric oligoarthritis	4,261 (3.4)	14.2	9.7	7.0	4.3	4.0	2.5	1.7	1.0
Hypertension	14,015 (11.1)	26.1	15.1	9.5	7.2	4.6	2.3	1.4	1.0
Allergies	5,313 (4.2)	3.6	3.3	4.6	4.4	0.8	0.8	1.1	1.0
Stomach ulcer	4,568 (3.6)	6.9	5.7	3.4	2.1	3.4	2.8	1.6	1.0
Diabetes	3,205 (2.5)	5.2	3.6	2.5	1.4	3.9	2.6	1.8	1.0
Thyroid disease	3,015 (2.4)	1.9	2.5	3.0	1.9	1.0	1.3	1.6	1.0
Kidney disease	2,354 (1.9)	5.1	2.4	1.4	1.3	4.2	1.9	1.1	1.0
Chronic bronchitis	2,033 (1.6)	4.0	2.3	1.6	0.7	5.6	3.2	2.2	1.0
Heart attack	1,805 (1.4)	4.9	2.0	1.2	0.6	8.8	3.4	2.0	1.0
Cancer	837 (0.7)	1.5	0.6	0.6	0.5	2.7	1.1	1.1	1.0
Tuberculosis	261 (0.2)	0.3	0.4	0.1	0.2	1.8	2.2	0.6	1.0
Multiple sclerosis	148 (0.1)	0.0	0.1	0.1	0.2	0.2	0.4	0.7	1.0

*Data depicted are unadjusted odds ratios; all trends are statistically significant adjusted for age, race, gender and smoking, other than for allergies, thyroid disease, while multiple sclerosis trends are significant inversely (higher prevalence in individuals with higher formal education).
Source: Adapted from Ref. 46.

In the Whitehall study of 15,730 London civil servants, Marmot, Rose, and colleagues (49,51,111) observed that cardiovascular mortality was four times greater in unskilled workers, and three times greater in secretarial personnel, than in administrators, those with the highest socioeconomic status (Fig. 4). In these studies, all subjects were working, and only about one-third of the differences could be explained by recognized risk factors of blood pressure, smoking and cholesterol (Fig. 5). In a clinical trial in which propranolol versus placebo was tested to prevent a second myocardial infarction (54), mortality over three

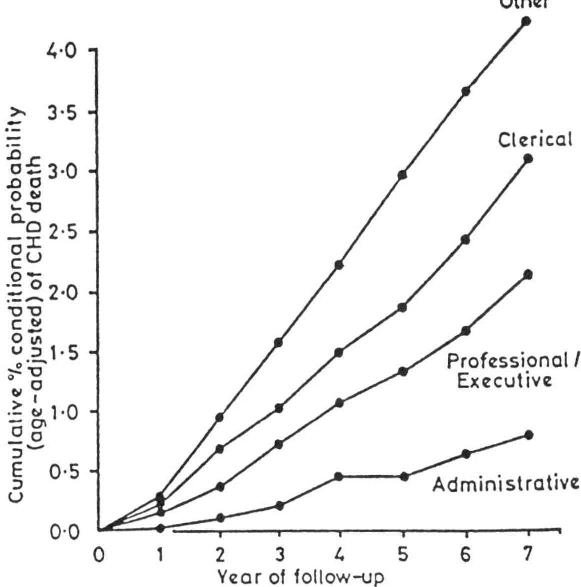

Fig. 4 Seven and a half year CHD mortality according to employee grade. (From Ref. 51.)

years differed more according to level of education than according to whether patients were treated with propranolol or placebo.

In the United Kingdom, higher mortality was observed in manual than in nonmanual workers for lung cancer, coronary artery disease, and cerebral vascular diseases. Disparities in mortality according to job classification *increased* further between the 1970s and 1980s, despite availability of baseline national health service care to all people (112,113). In studies of RA at Vanderbilt University (see Paradigm C4 and Chapter 13), formal education level predicted significant differences in morbidity and mortality over 9 years (38,40,68), and significant differences in clinical status (69), not explained by age, duration of disease, race, gender, treatments, functional status, laboratory, or radiographic data.

A hypothesis has been proposed that low formal education level is a composite or surrogate variable that identifies behavioral risk factors predisposing to the etiology and poor outcomes of most chronic diseases (114,115). Some of these behaviors include diet, smoking, compliance, efficiency in using medical services, problem-solving capacity, sense of personal responsibility, capacity to cope with stress, life stress (54), social isolation (54), health locus of control (116), and learned helplessness (115,117) (Table 6). The data strongly suggest

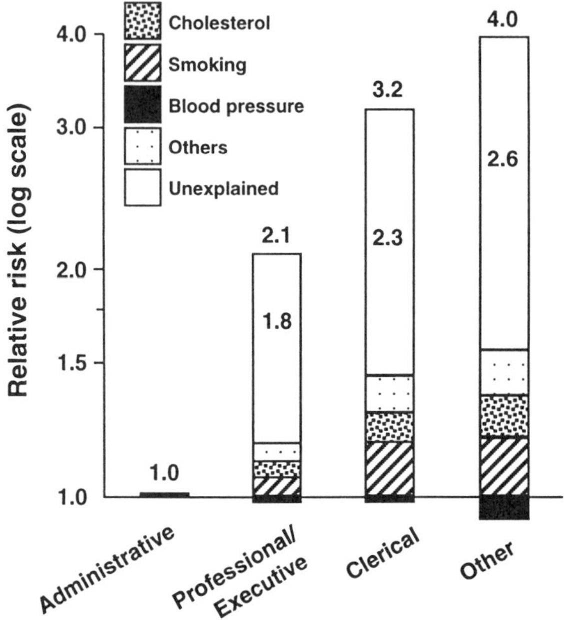

Fig. 5 Relative risk of CHD death according to employment grade "explained" by risk factors (age-standardized) at entry. The figures on top of the histograms are the relative risk of CHD death (age-standardized), taking the administrative grade as 1.0. The figures in the histograms are the relative risk of CHD death in the different grades after the effect of the other risk factors has been taken into account (From Ref. 51).

Table 6 Socioeconomic Status and Health—Possible Variables Mediating the Associations Based on Personal Health Behaviors and Psychological and Cognitive Constructs

Personal health behaviors	Psychological and cognitive constructs
Diet and nutrition	Social support
Exercise	Anxiety
Smoking	Depression
Seat belt use	Health locus of control
Life stresses	Learned helplessness
Efficiency in use of medical services	Sense of coherence
Health insurance status	Self-efficacy
Use of preventive medical services	Optimism
Coping skills	Time preference
Problem-solving skills	Health knowledge

Source: From Ref. 115.

that associations between poor outcomes and low formal education levels are not likely to be explained simply on the basis of biomedical risk factors or limited access to medical care. Further studies of these associations might lead to new understanding of disease prevention and improved outcomes.

A4. Traditional Paradigm. Pathogenetic mechanisms in RA affect primarily joints, and associated comorbid conditions such as cardiovascular, pulmonary, and renal diseases, are not related to pathogenetic mechanisms in RA.

Paradigm Shift. Comorbid conditions are increased in patients with RA relative to the general population, and RA itself may be a marker for increased risk of comorbid conditions.

Comment. Although RA is recognized to be a systemic disease, the prominence of joint symptoms and signs have appropriately directed most investigations of pathogenesis and evaluation of treatments to be focused on joints. However, most patients with RA have other diseases as well, and many diseases appear more likely to occur in patients with RA than in the general population, adjusted for age, sex, race, and education. Among 256 consecutive patients with RA studied at the Vanderbilt Clinic, fewer than 20% had no other disease (Table 7). By contrast, hypertension was seen in 36%, allergies in 22%, peptic ulcer disease in 21%, diabetes in 5%, and chronic bronchitis in 13% of these patients (see Table 7a), levels which are considerably higher than those reported in the US population (see Table 7b).

In analyses of the prevalence of comorbidities in RA, it is necessary to consider potential confounding variables such as age, education level, and ''Berkson's bias'' (118), which recognizes that diseases are more likely to be identified in individuals seen in medical settings than in the general population. These possibilities cannot be analyzed using clinical data, in which small numbers of patients are selected for inclusion, but require studies using population-based data designed to be representative of the US population. The Health Interview Survey, a national population-based survey, includes data concerning pain or swelling of specific joints. This information allowed creation of a variable entitled ''symmetric polyarthritis,'' in which pain or swelling was seen in more than four joints, including at least two symmetric joints, which serves as a surrogate for RA (70).

Prevalences of comorbidities in population-based data for persons with symmetric polyarthritis (see Table 7c) were remarkably similar to those seen in Nashville clinical RA patients (see Table 7a), and considerably higher than in individuals with no arthritis (119) (see Table 7d). These findings are explained only slightly by the higher age and lower formal education level of individuals with symmetric polyarthritis (38), as well as in clinical patients with RA (46,68), compared with the general population. Nonetheless, odds ratios indicate that various comorbidities are significantly more common in individuals with symmetric polyarthritis than in individuals with no arthritis, adjusted for age, formal

Table 7 Percentage of Individuals Reporting Various Conditions in Different Populations

Health condition	(a) 256 Vanderbilt University potential patients with RA (%)	(b) Survey: total US population[a] (%)	(c) Survey: people with symmetric polyarthritis[a] (%)	(d) Survey: people with no arthritis[a] (%)	(e) Odds ratio: symmetric polyarthritis vs no arthritis[b]
Hypertension	36	11.1	41.2	7.8	3.4:1
Allerties	22	4.2	15.0	3.2	5.1:1
Stomach ulcer	21	3.6	6.5	2.7	2.9:1
Diabetes	5	2.5	11.3	1.8	3.0:1
Kidney disease	5	1.9	4.6	1.1	4.7:1
Chronic bronchitis	13	1.6	6.9	0.9	4.3:1
Heart attack	8	1.4	6.6	0.7	4.3:1
Cancer	4	0.7	1.3	0.5	2.4:1
No other disease	18	57	—	—	—

[a]Data from the 1978 Health Interview Survey for United States population aged 18–64.
[b]Adjusted for age, sex, race, and formal education level.
Source: Adapted from Ref. 3.

education level, sex, and race (see Table 7, column (e)). Therefore, RA may be viewed as a marker for development of many comorbid chronic conditions, partially explaining higher mortality rates in patients with RA.

B. Assessment of Rheumatoid Arthritis

B1. Traditional Paradigm. "Clinical rheumatology can advance only in relation to laboratory science" (120).

Paradigm Shift. *At this time,* data obtained from patient self-report of status appear more effective than traditional laboratory or radiographic data to predict and monitor the course of physician-diagnosed RA.

Comment. Assessment of rheumatic diseases traditionally has emphasized laboratory investigation, and many clinicians decide whether or not a patient has RA almost entirely on the basis of a rheumatoid factor test, rather than on data from the history and physical examination. However, studies over the last decade suggest that nonlaboratory measures, particularly self-report questionnaires, provide an optimal measure for assessment of status and outcomes in patients with RA, based on several findings:

1. Questionnaire data are at least as effective or more effective than radiographs or laboratory tests to predict functional and work disability, as well as mortality, in patients with RA (3,32,37,40,121–123).
2. Self-report questionnaire data are correlated strongly with data from traditional joint counts, with other measures of physical and functional status, and with radiographs and laboratory tests at lower levels (Table 8) (124).
3. Changes in status in clinical trials in RA may be detected as effectively with questionnaire data as with traditional physical, radiographic, or laboratory data (125–127).
4. Data from self-report questionnaires may not only be the *optimal,* but also the *only,* data to document long-term functional declines in patients with RA (128). In analyses of patient status over 5–10 years (Fig. 6), self-report data in the Health Assessment Questionnaire (HAQ) Disability Index (DI) indicated severe disease progression, whereas data from joint counts and the laboratory were essentially unchanged. Therefore, long-term progression of RA in these patients would not be recognized in the absence of self-report questionnaire data.

The most commonly used questionnaires in clinical rheumatology include the Health Assessment Questionnaire (HAQ) (Fig. 7) (129), Arthritis Impact Measurement Scales (AIMS) (130), a Modified Health Assessment Questionnaire (MHAQ) (131), and McMaster Patient Preference Disability (MACTAR) questionnaire (132). Data from these various questionnaires appear to provide relatively similar information (133).

Table 8 Percentage of 259 Patients with Rheumatoid Arthritis Who Had Different Levels of Clinical Status According to Various Measures in Relation to Their Scores on the Self-Report Modified Health Assessment Questionnaire in Different Questionnaire Score Groups[a]

| | Range of questionnaire scores | | | | | | | |
Variable	1.00 ($n=16$)[b]	1.01–1.50 ($n=51$)	1.51–2.00 ($n=84$)	2.01–3.00 ($n=86$)	3.01–4.00 ($n=22$)	% of Total ($n=259$)[c]	Trend[d]	P value
% of Patients	6%	20%	32%	33%	9%			
Clinical status measure								
Joint count score > 10	11%	37%	67%	79%	100%	65	−7.10	<0.001
Radiographic score > 1.0	57%	73%	66%	75%	82%	85	−1.99	<0.05
Erythrocyte sedimentation rate > 20 mm/hour	29%	49%	64%	74%	85%	64	−4.21	<0.05
Rheumatoid factor positive	87%	84%	88%	84%	94%	86	−0.42	>0.05
Grip strength < 100 mmHg	19%	29%	57%	83%	100%	61	−8.02	<0.001
Walking time > 8 seconds	6%	29%	42%	69%	100%	48	−6.31	<0.001
Button test > 40 seconds	31%	53%	71%	88%	100%	73	−6.44	<0.001

[a]Patients answered a modified health assessment questionnaire (MHAQ) (Ref 131). Cutoff points for indicators of poor clinical status were determined according to previous data.
[b]Numbers in parentheses indicate the number of patients.
[c]% of total number of patients whose clinical status met criterion for inclusion in group, e.g. joint count score >10.
[d]Trend according to χ^2 statistic.   *Source:* Ref. 124.

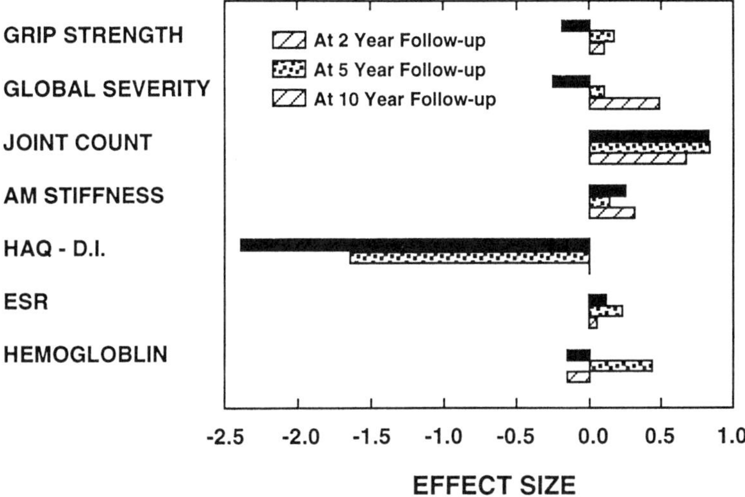

Fig. 6 Changes in clinical status assessment (effect sizes) according to various clinical variables in patients with rheumatoid arthritis followed over 10 years, compared at 2, 5, and 10 years. Effect sizes are calculated at each time, using values from the initial visit (From Ref. 128).

While patient questionnaires were designed initially for use in research studies as adjuncts to traditional measures of clinical status, such as radiographs and laboratory tests, with experience in their use, self-report questionnaires have been introduced into routine patient care by ourselves and others (9,134). Adaptation of research questionnaires to shorter clinical versions, such as the Clinical HAQ (CLINHAQ) and MHAQ, may be considered analogous to adaptation of rheumatoid factor measures from analytical ultracentrifugation to latex fixation test kits for use in physicians' offices today. The compromises of measurement in use of simpler measures such as a 1 to 2 page questionnaire or laboratory kit to measure rheumatoid factor are comparable to provide useful information in a pragmatic manner for routine clinical care.

Current management of individual patients with RA remains based primarily on empirical dialogue between patients and health professionals. Such dialogues are clearly essential to patient care, but introduction of simple functional status questionnaires provides quantitative cost-effective data to document and monitor the course of RA and other rheumatic diseases (72). Routine use of questionnaires facilitates quantitative comparisons of individual patients from one visit to the next and comparisons of patients seen in different rheumatology clinical settings according to the same data. Standardized data collection in

HEALTH ASSESSMENT QUESTIONNAIRE

Name ______________ TOR NO: ____

Date ______________

In this section we are interested in learning how your illness affects your ability to function in daily life. Please feel free to add any comments on the back of this page.

·Please check the one response which best describes your usual abilities OVER THE PAST WEEK:

	Without ANY Difficulty	With SOME Difficulty	With MUCH Difficulty	UNABLE To Do	
DRESSING & GROOMING					
Are you able to — Dress yourself, including tying shoelaces and doing buttons?	____	____	____	____	
— Shampoo your hair?	____	____	____	____	(184) ____
ARISING					
Are you able to: — Stand up from an armless straight chair?	____	____	____	____	
— Get in and out of bed?	____	____	____	____	(175) ____
EATING					
Are you able to — Cut your meat?	____	____	____	____	
— Lift a full cup or glass to your mouth?	____	____	____	____	(183) ____
— Open a new milk carton?	____	____	____	____	
WALKING					
Are you able to — Walk outdoors on flat ground?	____	____	____	____	
— Climb up five steps?	____	____	____	____	(174) ____

·Please check any AIDS OR DEVICES that you usually use for any of these activities:

____ Cane ____ Devices Used for Dressing (button hook, zipper pull, long-handled shoe horn, etc.)

____ Walker ____ Built Up or Special Utensils

____ Crutches ____ Special or Built Up Chair

____ Wheelchair ____ Other (Specify ______________)

·Please check any categories for which you usually need HELP FROM ANOTHER PERSON:

____ Dressing and Grooming ____ Eating

____ Arising ____ Walking

WICHITA ARTHRITIS CENTER DISABILITY AND DISCOMFORT SCALE. 1985

·Please check the one response which best describes your usual abilities OVER THE PAST WEEK:

	Without ANY Difficulty	With SOME Difficulty	With MUCH Difficulty	UNABLE To Do	
HYGIENE					
Are you able to: — Wash and dry your entire body?	____	____	____	____	
— Take a tub bath?	____	____	____	____	(185) ____
— Get on and off the toilet?	____	____	____	____	
REACH					
Are you able to: — Reach and get down a 5 pound object (such as a bag of sugar) from just above your head?	____	____	____	____	(172) ____
— Bend down to pick up clothing from the floor?	____	____	____	____	
GRIP					
Are you able to — Open car doors?	____	____	____	____	
— Open jars which have been previously opened?	____	____	____	____	(584) ____
— Turn faucets on and off?	____	____	____	____	
ACTIVITIES					
Are you able to: — Run errands and shop?	____	____	____	____	
— Get in and out of a car?	____	____	____	____	(583) ____
— Do chores such as vacuuming or yardwork?	____	____	____	____	

·Please check any AIDS OR DEVICES that you usually use for any of these activities:

____ Raised Toilet Seat ____ Bathtub Bar Other ______________

____ Bathtub Seat ____ Long-Handled Appliances for Reach

____ Jar Opener (for jars previously opened) ____ Long-Handled Appliances in Bathroom

·Please check any categories for which you usually need HELP FROM ANOTHER PERSON:

____ Hygiene ____ Gripping and Opening Things

____ Reach ____ Errands and Chores

We are also interested in learning whether or not you are affected by pain because of your illness.

·How much pain have you had because of your illness IN THE PAST WEEK?

PLACE A MARK ON THE LINE TO INDICATE THE SEVERITY OF THE PAIN

NO PAIN — VERY SEVERE PAIN

0 ———————————————— 100 (446) ____

·Considering ALL THE WAYS THAT YOUR ILLNESS AFFECTS YOU, RATE HOW YOU ARE DOING on the following scale by placing a mark on the line.

0 very well — 20 well — 40 — fair — 60 — 80 poor — 100 very poor (156) ____

Fig. 7 Stanford Health Assessment Questionnaire (HAQ) (From Ref. 129).

patients with RA could promote comparison of patient status according to quantitative data (9,126), leading to clinical staging procedures.

Although research in rheumatic diseases may someday identify laboratory or imaging markers that may be clinically invaluable in predicting the course of RA, the inclusion of questionnaire data in clinical care appears of considerable value, regardless of future availability of prognostic laboratory data. These considerations suggest that questionnaires might be used in routine clinical care of patients with RA, as well as other rheumatic diseases.

B2.　Traditional Paradigm.　Measures of functional status are "subjective" and poorly reproducible, in contrast to "objective" radiographic and laboratory measures.

Paradigm Shift.　Measures of functional status are among the most reproducible in clinical medicine, and are as free of measurement error as laboratory and radiographic measures.

Comment.　Health professionals commonly distinguish "objective" data, i.e., information perceptible to persons external to the affected individual, from "subjecive" data, i.e., information provided by a person about themselves. The term "objective" is also defined as without bias or prejudice, and therefore more reproducible than "subjective" data. These two definitions of "objective" are often regarded as synonymous, with an inference that external information is without bias or prejudice, which has better reproducibility than "subjective" data provided by a person. Conversely, "subjective" data are regarded as more likely to include bias or prejudice and be poorly reproducible.

Recent studies indicate that reproducibility of "subjective" data to access functional status through self-report questionnaires and physical measures to analyze functional status is generally as great or greater than data from "objective" physical examination, radiographs, scans, and laboratory tests. An example of reproducibility of "subjective" data is found in studies of grip strength, walk time, and button test, three physical measures of functional status. When these measures are performed according to a standard set of instructions, analogous to a laboratory test (Fig. 8) (135), data from two observers indicate excellent reproducibility (Fig. 9), with highly significant correlations (135), comparable with analyses of readings of radiographs by two radiologists (136). Furthermore, patient self-report questionnaires show similar levels of reproducibility on scales for activities of daily living (ADL), pain, fatigue, and global status (Table 9). Studies of serologic tests indicate a range of measurement error as great or greater than has been observed for physical and questionnaire measures of functional status (137).

Measurement error is seen in any effort to quantitate a physical or functional phenomenon, even in the physical sciences in which it is considerably less than in medical or clinical sciences. Measurement error in assessment of functional status is as low as has been described for any measure in clinical medicine

<u>Physical measures of functional status</u>

ASK: "Are you right-handed or left-handed?"   R ___, L ___

SAY: "Let's begin with your R ___, L ___ hand."

<u>BUTTON TEST--READ:</u>   "When I tell you to do so, using one hand only, please unbutton and then button the 5 buttons on this board. You may use your other hand to steady the frame. I will time you while you do this."

R (secs)____, L (secs)____,   Unable to do ___.

<u>GRIP STRENGTH</u> (Inflate cuff encased in black fabric container to 20 mm)-- READ: "When I tell you to do so, please squeeze the cuff as hard as you can." (Measure grip strength for each hand three times and record each measurement)

R (mmHg) ____ ____ ____

L (mmHg) ____ ____ ____   Unable to do ___

<u>WALKING TIME--READ:</u>   "When I tell you to do so, please walk from here to me. (show patient starting and stopping points for 25-foot course). Walk as though you are going somewhere. I will time you while you do this."

________ (secs),   Unable to do ___

Fig. 8 Standard instructions to perform and record measurements of grip strength, walking time, and button test. (From Ref. 135.)

(9,138). This phenomenon, along with the usefulness in prognosis of functional status measures discussed in the last section, suggests that such "subjective" measures be used routinely in clinical rheumatology practice along with "objective" laboratory and radiographic measures.

Every encounter between a patient with a rheumatic disease and a health professional may be viewed as an encounter with the unknown. If the encounters include assessment of clinical status according to empirical impressions only, as is the case in more than 99% of the time, an opportunity for scientific data collection and analysis is lost, and misleading long-term impressions may emerge. If *any* quantitative data, whether "subjective" data from questionnaires or physical measures of functional status, or "objective" radiographs and laboratory tests, are recorded for organized retrieval at a later date, an opportunity for a scientific study is initiated. The "scientific" collection of data is optimal if the most valuable prognostic data, i.e., data regarding functional status, are included. Thus, "subjective" data can improve the "scientific" basis of clinical medicine, enhancing accurate prognosis and description of results of treatment, to improve control of RA.

B3. Traditional Paradigm. Different types of measures of clinical status in RA, including radiographs, joint counts, laboratory tests, functional

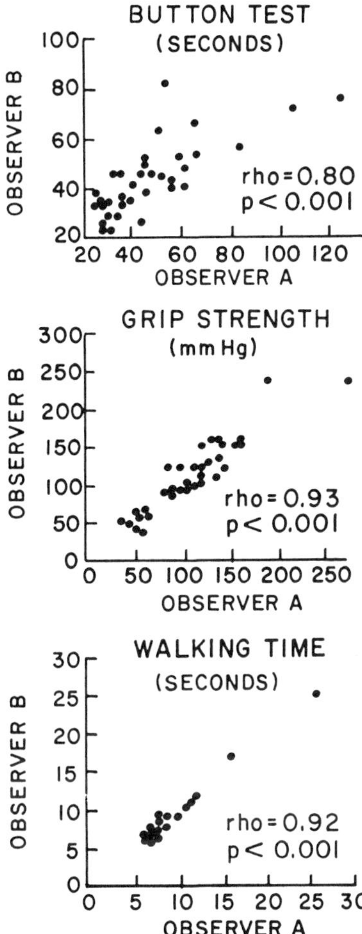

Fig. 9 Interobserver reliability of button test, grip strength, and walking time measures in 40 patients with rheumatoid arthritis assessed by two observers using standard instruction. Evidence of excellent interobserver reliability is seen. (From Ref. 135.)

status questionnaires, and physical measures, may be used relatively interchangeably to describe clinical severity and outcome.

Paradigm Shift. Different types of measures of clinical status may detect different components of pathogenetic mechanisms and disease progression in patients with RA.

Comment. Clinical severity of RA is assessed according to many types of measures, including laboratory, radiographic, physical examination (joint count), questionnaire, and physical measures of functional status, psychological

Table 9 Correlations of Six Self-Report Questionnaire Scores in 232 Patients When Completed Twice by the Same Patient and Compared to an Observer[a]

Self-report questionnaire scale	Patient completed twice	Patient compared to observer
Number of patients	132	100
Activities of daily living (ADL)	0.97	0.91
Global self-assessment	0.89	0.85
Global satisfaction	0.84	0.79
Pain (visual analog scale)	0.91	0.74
Fatigue (visual analog scale)	0.91	0.85
Gastrointestinal symptoms (visual analog scale)	0.94	0.87

[a]Numbers shown are Pearson r values; all are statistically significant $p < 0.001$.

scales, evidence of extra-articular disease, comorbidity, and others. An important consideration in interpreting studies of clinical status and outcomes in RA is that different studies may include different measures to describe patient status and outcome, reaching different conclusions on the basis of the measurement used.

An example of this phenomenon can be seen in studies of whether the HLA-DR4 gene, which is recognized to be associated with a sixfold increase in the relative risk to develop RA (see Chapter 3) is also associated with the severity of RA. In certain studies, HLA-DR4 was reported to be associated with more severe clinical disease, whereas in other studies no association was seen between HLA-DR4 and clinical severity (139). The apparent contradictions between the two types of conclusions may be explained on the basis of different outcome measures used in different studies. The HLA-DR4 gene is associated with a higher likelihood of rheumatoid factor positivity and higher radiographic scores (Table 10), but is not associated with greater joint tenderness or functional status declines according to questionnaire and physical measures (139). Therefore, in studies that were based on radiographic outcomes, HLA-DR4 appeared to predict more severe outcomes, but in studies which were based on functional status outcomes, HLA-DR4 was not associated with more severe disease.

The data indicate that various clinical measures of status and outcomes in patients with RA are not interchangeable. One important example of the absence of interchangeability of measures to assess RA is seen in studies of articular involvement based on either a physical examination or a radiograph (140). Radiographic scores are correlated significantly with joint examination scores for limited motion and deformity of joints (Fig. 10), and at lower levels with scores for number of swollen joints. However, radiographic scores are not correlated significantly with scores for joint tenderness, as in the Ritchie Index (Fig. 10).

Table 10　Relative Frequencies (Odds Ratios) for Disease Status Variables in HLA-DR4 Putative Homozygous, HLA-DR4 Heterozygous, and Non–HLA-DR4 Patients with Rheumatoid Arthritis[a]

	Patient HLA-DR4 status		
	Putative homozygous HLA-DR4	Heterozygous HLA-DR4	Non– HLA-DR4
Number of patients	24	76	54
Demographic variables			
Age	0.67	0.45	1.0
Duration of disease	1.07	0.75	1.0
Formal educational level	1.44	0.84	1.0
Laboratory measures			
Erythrocyte sedimentation rate	1.58	1.01	1.0
Rheumatoid factor titer	1.86	1.86	1.0[b]
Rheumatoid factor positivity	8.10	2.61	1.0[b]
Radiographic scores			
Joint space narrowing	1.47	2.16	1.0[b]
Erosions	2.10	1.17	1.0[b]
Malalignment	4.00	3.05	1.0[b]
Total radiographic score	3.45	2.34	1.0[b]
Joint count scores			
Swelling	1.21	0.58	1.0
Deformity	1.67	2.99	1.0
Pain on motion	0.43	0.63	1.0
Limited motion	2.24	2.78	1.0
Tenderness	1.04	0.79	1.0
Total joint count score	1.05	0.80	1.0
Functional status measures			
ARA functional class	0.98	0.82	1.0
Patient self-assessment	1.32	1.03	1.0
ADL difficulty score	1.58	0.91	1.0
Button test	0.68	0.81	1.0
Grip strength	1.92	1.15	1.0
Walking time	0.80	0.77	1.0

ARA, American Rheumatism Association; ADL, difficulty in activities of daily living assessed using self-report questionnaire.

[a]One hundred fifty-four patients with rheumatoid arthritis were dichotomized into two groups, the most severely affected quartile and the other patients. Odds ratios for individuals with more severe disease who are HLA-DR4 homozygous or heterozygous relative to the referent non–HLA-DR4 patients are presented.

[b]Differences between patients who are and are not HLA-DR4 are statistically significant.

Source: Adapted from Ref. 139.

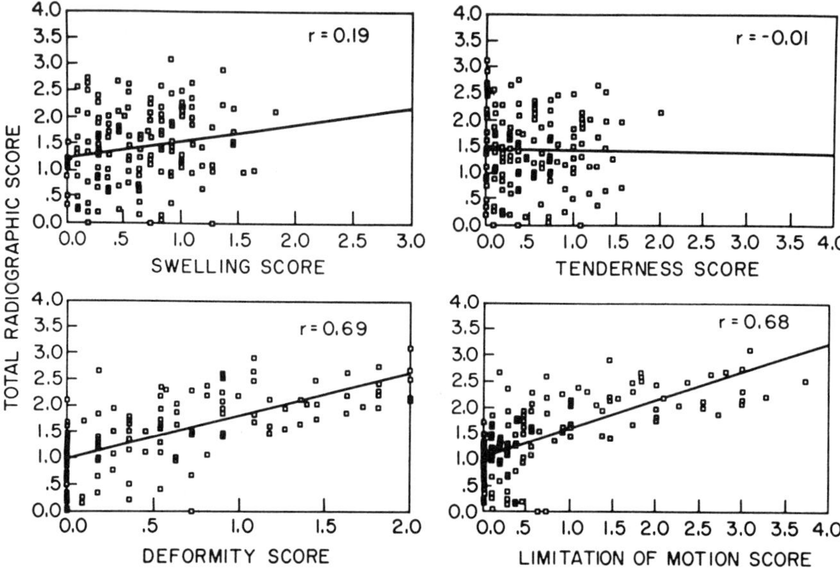

Fig. 10 Correlations between total radiographic score and subtotals of joint count scores for swelling, tenderness, deformity, and limitation of motion in 154 patients with rheumatoid arthritis. (From Ref. 140).

Therefore, long-term assessment of RA according to a Ritchie Index may suggest that patient clinical status is unchanged or even improved, while radiographic scores may show substantial progression.

These observations suggest that at least two types of measures of disease progression may be seen in RA. One group of measures includes rheumatoid factor, radiographic severity, duration of disease, joint deformity, and limited motion, which appear more correlated with one another than with the second group of measures, which includes joint tenderness, functional status, disability, and pain. Each group of measures is correlated with measures within the group at higher levels than with measures of the other group, although some correlation is seen between the two groups of measures, as expected.

Traditionally, measures such as radiographs or laboratory tests have been regarded as the more important ''hard'' clinical data, in contrast to ''soft'' data from questionnaires and functional status measures. However, pertinent outcomes in RA, such as work disability, functional declines, and mortality, appear to be predicted and monitored more effectively according to the ''soft'' measures of functional status and joint tenderness, than to the ''hard'' measures of radiographic and laboratory findings (13,44). These observations suggest that monitoring of disease might include measures from each category to describe optimally clinical outcomes in RA.

B4. Traditional Paradigm. "Our belief in disease as a direct reflection of mental state is largely folklore" (141).

Paradigm Shift. Assessment of the psychological constructs of learned helplessness, sense of coherence, or self-efficacy adds meaningful information to assessment of individual patients with RA and other rheumatic diseases.

Comment. Although most clinicians would acknowledge the importance of psychological status in rheumatic and other diseases, analysis of diseases according to the biomedical model (see Section I, Rationale) (5) over the second half of the 20th century has virtually ignored the potential contribution of psychological status to disease pathogenesis and course. One explanation may be that psychological measures traditionally have not provided useful tools for prognosis or monitoring of clinical status. Indeed, early explanations of RA as a "psychosomatic disease" with a "rheumatoid personality" were not supported by data (142). Further efforts to analyze depression in patients with RA have been hindered by "criterion contamination" (143), in which responses on depression

Table 11 Items in Widely Used Depression Scales Affected by "Criterion Contamination" that Would Be Interpreted as Indicating Depression in a Person Who Does Not Have a Chronic Disease, but that May Reflect Activity of a Chronic Disease[a]

Minnesota Multiphasic Personality Inventory (MMPI)
- 9. I am about as able to work as I ever was.
- 51. I am in just as good physical health as most of my friends.
- 153. During the past years I have been well most of the time.
- 163. I do not tire quickly.
- 243. I have few or no pains.

Beck Depression Inventory
- 15. I can work about as well as before.
- 16. I can sleep as well as usual.
- 17. I don't get more tired than usual.
- 18. My appetite is no worse than usual.
- 20. I am no more worried about my health than usual.
- 21. I have not noticed any recent change in my interest in sex.

Center for Epidemiologic Studies Depression Index (CES-D)
- 2. I did not feel like eating; my appetite was poor.
- 7. I felt that everything I did was an effort.
- 11. My sleep was restless.
- 20. I could not "get going."

[a]See text and references for definition of "disease-related" items.
Source: Refs. 143, 144, 147.

scales were interpreted as indicating depression, but actually indicated the presence of a chronic disease (Table 11).

The problem of "criterion contamination" in interpretation of psychological scales in patients with rheumatic disease is of considerable importance. For example, several early reports (144) suggested that patients with RA had high levels of depression, hypochondriasis, and hysteria, based on high scores for these constructs on the Minnesota Multiphasic Personality Inventory (MMPI). These conclusions were based on responses of "false" to statements such as "I am about as able to work as I ever was," "I am in just as good physical health as most of my friends," or "I have few or no pains." Responses of "false" to these statements in individuals who do not have a somatic disease may indicate tendencies to depression, hysteria, and hypochondriasis, but in patients with RA and other somatic diseases, such responses may be appropriate statements of fact (144).

Further studies have suggested that "criterion contamination" is seen to some degree in all self-report depression scales (143), including the Beck Depression Inventory (BDI) (145), Centers for Epidemiologic Studies Depression scale (CESD) (146), and General Well-Being scale (GWB) (147). In these scales, items including "I am no more worried about my health than usual," "I felt I could not get going," and "I felt like everything I did was an effort," would evoke stereotypic responses in patients with RA that would not indicate depression. Patients with RA may have higher levels of depression than expected (145,146,148), but these levels may be exaggerated by widely-used self-report depression scales.

Recognition of problems with "criterion contamination" in use of depression scales in patients with RA has been accompanied by recognition that several psychological constructs, including learned helplessness, sense of coherence, and self-efficacy, appear to provide meaningful data in assessment of clinical status in RA.

Learned helplessness is a psychological construct which describes feeling that an individual cannot cope with a stressful situation. Studies of this construct according to a "rheumatology attitudes index" (RAI) (116,117,149) have indicated that scores are related to functional status scores, and changes over one year in functional status were associated with changes in RAI scores (116). The scale has now been revised to include only five items (150) (Table 12). A sense of coherence scale appears to identify patients with good or poor outcomes in RA (151,152). In the arthritis self-help course, changes in self-efficacy have been documented to be more explanatory of effective responses than knowledge gained or changes in behavior that may be associated with the self-help course (153,154).

These considerations would suggest that assessment of psychological status might be of considerable value in assessment of RA, possibly as valuable as laboratory tests and radiographs. Furthermore, current research is directed toward

Table 12 A Five-Item Rheumatology Attitudes Index to Assess Learned Helplessness in Patients with Rheumatic Diseases

The Statements below concern your personal beliefs. Please circle the number beside each statement that best describes how you feel about the statement. There are no right or wrong answers.

	Strongly disagree	Disagree	Do not agree or disagree	Agree	Strongly agree
1. My condition is controlling my life.	1	2	3	4	5
2. I would feel helpless if I couldn't rely on other people for help with my condition.	1	2	3	4	5
3. No matter what I do, or how hard I try, I just can't seem to get relief from my pain.	1	2	3	4	5
4. I am coping effectively with my condition.	1	2	3	4	5
5. It seems as though fate and other factors beyond my control affect my condition.	1	2	3	4	5

Sources: Refs. 116, 117, 149, 150.

the extent which these constructs may be modifiable by treatment in a way that might contribute to improved outcomes in patients with RA.

C. Outcome Of Rheumatoid Arthritis

C1. Traditional Paradigm. "RA is, in the majority of instances, a disease with a good prognosis" (155).

Paradigm Shift. "RA is a chronic and progressive disease, and it is likely that once it is active and chronic in a given individual it will become progressively worse" (156).

Comment. The above paradigm quoted from the 1985 edition of the Kelley textbook, may have emerged in large part from the observation that many individuals who meet ARA Criteria for RA have a self-limited process (see Paradigm A2), and from favorable results in clinical trials (see Paradigm D3). However, most individuals who present in rheumatology settings have experienced disease for longer than 2 years. In general, these patients do not have a self-limited process, but rather a progressive disease characterized by substantial declines in radiographic (29–31) and functional (32–34) status, work disability (32,35,36), and increased mortality rates (38–41), as summarized in the following:

1. Among 50 RA patients monitored over 20 years by Scott and colleagues (30) (Fig. 11), 48 showed evidence of radiographic progression according to a quantitative scoring system.

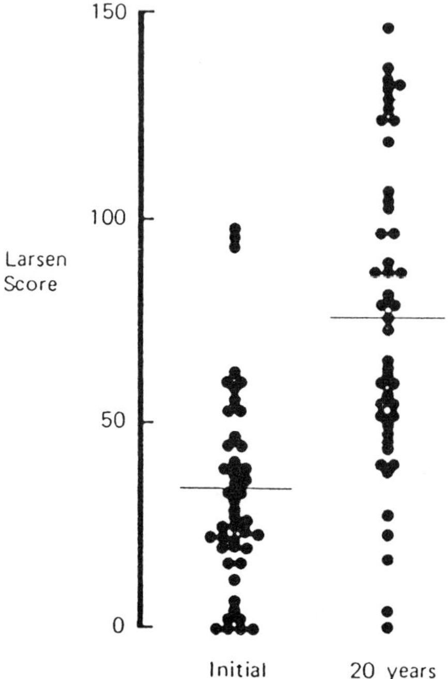

Fig. 11   Radiological changes in the hands and wrists of 50 rheumatoid arthritis patients over 20 years. Note evidence of substantial radiographic progression in mean level and in most individual patients. (From Ref. 30.)

2.   When functional capacity was compared 9 years apart in 75 RA patients (32, 138), most showed severe declines in capacities to perform physical measures, such as grip strength and the button test, as well as according to questions concerning activities of daily living (Fig. 12). Many patients showed improvement in morning stiffness over 9 years, suggesting that the disease process may "burn out" over time, but leave an individual patient with significant losses in functional capacity.

Functional capacity declines measured according to the Health Assessment Questionnaire (HAQ) were monitored in 1274 patients with RA over periods up to 12 years (37). The rate of functional loss was found to be sharply increased after the first clinic visit. HAQ scores of 1 (indicating *some* difficulty in performance of usual activities of daily living) were seen in 50% of RA patients within 2 years, and scores of 2 (indicating *much* difficulty in performance of usual activities of daily living) were seen in 50% of RA patients within 6 years after the first clinic visit. Functional

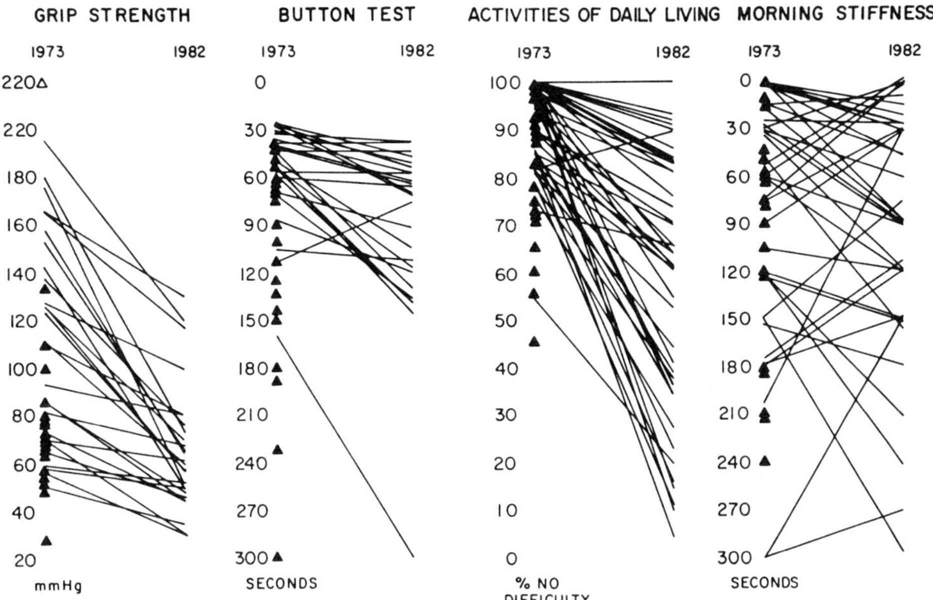

Fig. 12 Changes over 9 years in patients with RA for grip strength, button test, responses to questions about activities of daily living, and morning stiffness. Patients who had died over the 9 years are depicted by ▲. Note that only one patient shows improvement and a few have maintained functional capacity over the 9-year interval, while most patients show significant functional declines. Morning stiffness had improved in half of the patients, suggesting that the disease process may "burnout" over time, but leaving an individual severely dysfunctional. (From Ref. 138.)

disability appears to progress more rapidly in most patients during the first few years than later in the course of disease (37).

3. Work disability has been seen after 5 years of RA in 60–70% of patients younger than 65 years who had been working at onset of disease (32,35,36). Work disability was only weakly associated with radiographic stage, and appeared as effectively explained by demographic variables as by disease variables (38).

The foregoing studies involve only patients seen in rheumatology settings, who may have more severe clinical status among all RA patients. However, data that are representative of the entire United States population, found in a subset of the 1978 US Health Interview Survey, also indicate substantial work disability in individuals with symmetric polyarthritis, a surrogate for RA (noted in Paradigm A3) (70), in which pain or swelling was found in at least four joints, including at least two symmetric joints.

Table 13 Work, Disability Status, and Earnings of Working-Aged (18–64 yr) Persons in 1978 US Populations

	Females		Males	
	No arthritis	Symmetric polyarthritis[a]	No arthritis	Symmetric polyarthritis[a]
Number ($\times 10^{-3}$)	51,520	1,511	54,033	855
Disability status				
None (%)	90.1	22.2	90.6	29.7
Moderate (%)	5.4	26.8	5.8	23.3
Severe (%)	4.5	51.0	3.7	47.0
% working	61.6	31.0	89.4	56.1
US$ earned per person[b]	8,006	2,182	19,360	9,198
Earnings gap (US$)[c]		5,884 (73.5%)		10,162 (52.5%)
Total earnings losses (US$)[b]		8.9 billion		8.7 billion

[a]Derived variable to simulate rheumatoid arthritis—individuals who responded "yes" to the category of "arthritis or rheumatism" when asked, "Which of the following conditions or illnesses do you have now that a doctor told you about?" and who reported pain or swelling in four or more joints, at least two of which were symmetric, in response to the question, "Does pain (or swelling) in any part of your body bother you enough to be a problem?" See Mitchell *et al.* for additional information.
[b]Expressed in 1986 dollars.
[c]Earnings of individuals with symmetric polyarthritis vs earnings of individuals with no arthritis.
Source: Adapted from Ref. 70.

Among men aged 18–64 in 1978, 87% were working, including 89% of those with no arthritis, versus only 56% of those with symmetric polyarthritis. Similar findings were seen for women; although fewer women were working, more were affected by symmetric polyarthritis. Earnings were considerably lower for women with symmetric polyarthritis than for those with no arthritis (Table 13). In econometric analyses, women with symmetric polyarthritis (2.4% of all women) had only 26.5% of the earnings of women with no arthritis, and men with symmetic polyarthritis had only about half of the earnings of men with no arthritis. The 1.9% of the working-aged population with symmetric polyarthritis experienced earnings losses of 17.6 billion dollars, indicating major economic consequences of RA in the general population, in addition to the substantial direct and indirect costs of disease and its treatment (70).

Therefore, many individuals in the population who develop symmetric polyarthritis, including those who meet ARA Criteria for RA, may have a good prognosis. However, most people with sustained symmetic polyarthritis, even in populations, experience severe functional declines, work disability, radiographic progression, and premature mortality.

C2. Traditional Paradigm. "RA rarely kills patients, but therapies for RA have the capacity to kill patients" (157).

Table 14 Attributed Causes of Death in 2262 Patients With RA in 13 Series

	Cobb et al. (1953)	Van Dam et al. (1961)	Duthie et al. (1964)	Uddin et al. (1970)	Monson and Hall (1976)	Lewis et al. (1980)	Allebeck et al. (1981)	Rasker and Cosh (1981)	Vandenbroucke et al. (1984)	Pincus et al. (1984)	Prior et al. (1984)	Mutru et al. (1985)	Mitchell et al. (1986)	Cumulative Total	1977 US Population
Number of deaths	130	229	75	94	570	46	84	43	165	20	199	356	251	2,262	
Attributed cause of death (%)															
Cardiovascular disease	25	39	36	51[a]	43	41	49	42	43	40	31	47	43	42	41
Cancer	12	15	13	7	13	28	24	12	20	25	15	12	13	14	20
Infection	25	13	15	19	NL	13	2	19	2	20	2	2	14	9[b]	1
Renal disease	13	8	17	4	4	NL	0	9	6	0	3	21	3	8	1
Respiratory disease	3	NL	4	4	10	7	1	NL	12	5	15	8	5	7	4
RA	NL	NL	NL	NL	7	2	5	NL	10	5	17	NL	10	5	NL
Gastrointestinal disease	6	7	8	2	4	2	6	NL	6	5	6	NL	6	4	2
CNS disease	9	NL	5	NL	11	NL	6	19	NL	0	0	NL	1	4	10
Accidents	0	NL	1	NL	NL	NL	NL	NL	1	0	0	4	4	1	5
Miscellaneous	8	17	NL	3	8	6	7	NL	1	0	4	8	2	6	15
Unknown	NL	2	NL	9	NL	NL	NL	NL	0	0	0	0	0	1	NL

Abbreviations: NL, not listed as a cause of death in this series; CNS, central nervous system.

[a]Pulmonary embolus classified as "cardiovascular disease."

[b]Percentage calculation does not include Monson and Hall's 570 cases because infection was not listed as a cause of death.

Source: Refs. 3, 38.

Paradigm Shift.   Mortality rates in RA are increased over the general population matched for age and sex, with a natural history involving a shortening of life span by 10–15 years.

Comment.   Patients with RA appear to die with acute attributed causes of death similar to those in the general United States population (Table 14). Among 2262 deaths of patients with RA from 13 locations in North America and Europe (38), cardiovascular disease was the major attributed cause of death in about 40%, similar to the general US population. Patients with RA are more likely to have their acute cause of death attributed to infection, renal disease, respiratory disease, or gastrointestinal disease than are persons in the general population. However, the overall frequency patterns of various attributable causes of death in patients with RA are not recognized to differ meaningfully from those in the general population when patients are viewed one at a time. Rheumatoid arthritis is not listed anywhere on the death certificate in more than one-half of the patients who die with this disease (38,158).

Although death in patients with RA appears to result from immediate causes substantially similar to the general population, all of 13 studies from rheumatology clinical settings indicate that patients with RA die at an earlier age than would be expected for persons of similar age and sex in the general population (see Ref. (41)). Ten studies from such diverse locations as Massachusetts (159,160), Canada (39,161), Sweden (158), England (162), the Netherlands (163), Finland (164), Minnesota (165), and Tennessee (40) include actuarial life table analyses to examine survival and mortality (Fig. 13). All of these studies indicate accelerated mortality rates in patients with RA compared with the general population (one study incorporates comparisons with osteoarthritis patients rather than with the general population; see Fig 13C).

Recent analyses of mortality in RA have been conducted at four centers monitored by the Arthritis Rheumatism and Aging Medical Information System (ARAMIS) (166). Among 3501 patients from four centers in Saskatoon, Wichita, Stanford, and Santa Clara County, 922 patients died, indicating a standard mortality ratio (observed versus expected mortality, adjusted for age and sex) of 2.26 (Table 15). Standard mortality ratios were 2.24 in Saskatoon, 1.98 in Wichita, 3.08 in Stanford, and 2.18 in Santa Clara, indicating rates of 1.98 or more in all centers. These data underscore the fact that in large community-based databases, patients with RA treated according to the methodologies of the 1970s and 1980s experienced mortality rate considerably higher than expected (166).

The data concerning mortality in RA from many locales indicate several similarities, including a need to monitor patients for at least 2–3 years—periods longer than those found in clinical trials and most clinical studies—and higher life expectancies for women than for men in both the general population and patients with RA. Mortality rates of patients with RA have remained higher than those in the general population over the last 35 years, although mortality rates in both groups are considerably lower today than 35 years ago (41).

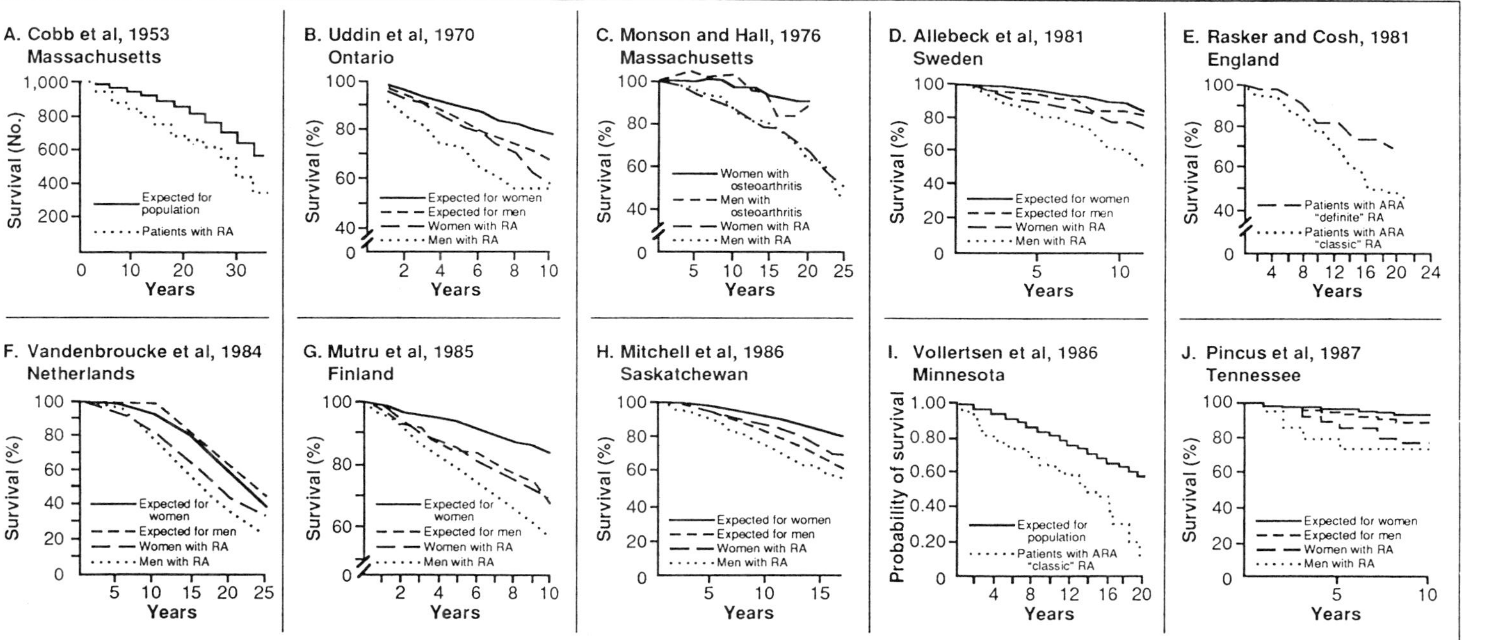

Fig. 13 Analyses of actuarial survival in patients with RA compared to the general population (Exceptions: in C, patients with RA are compared with patients with osteoarthritis; in E, two different groups of patients with RA are compared). Note increased mortality rates in patients with RA over more than 35 years of studies from ten diverse locales in North America and Europe, including the United States (Boston, MA, A and C; Rochester, MN, I; Nashville, TN, J), Canada (Ontario, B; Saskatchewan, H), Scandinavia (Sweden, D; Finland, G), England (E), and the Netherlands (F). (From Refs. 3, 41.)

Table 15 Standardized Mortality Ratio (SMR)[a] for 3501 Rheumatoid Arthritis Patients at 4 ARAMIS Centers Monitored over 30 Years

Center	Deaths	Combined SMR (S.E.)	Female SMR (S.E.)	Male SMR (S.E.)
Saskatoon	459	2.24 (.07)	2.44 (.09)	2.04 (.09)
Wichita	228	1.98 (.11)	1.94 (.14)	2.05 (.17)
Stanford	175	3.08 (.16)	3.29 (.23)	2.77 (.22)
Santa Clara	60	2.18 (.24)	1.98 (.28)	2.83 (.46)
All Centers	922	2.26 (.05)	2.36 (.07)	2.14 (.07)

[a]The standardized mortality ratio (SMR) is the ratio of observed deaths in the group under study to expected deaths in the general population.
Source: Adapted from Ref. 166.

C3. Traditional Paradigm. The outcome of RA is unpredictable.

Paradigm Shift. A prognostic estimate of morbidity and mortality in RA can be made according to quantitative data, analogous to other chronic diseases, including cardiovascular and neoplastic diseases.

Comment. The outcome of RA in an individual patient has often been regarded as entirely unpredictable. However, recent studies suggest that morbidity and mortality in RA can be predicted according to quantitative data. In analyses of functional status declines over nine years, significant correlations were seen between values for four measures of functional status, questionnaire responses regarding activities of daily living, grip strength, walking time, and button test (138) (Fig. 14). These observations indicate that a result at baseline predicts results nine years later, indicating that quantitative measures are useful not only to monitor clinical status but to predict them in the future. Further studies using the HAQ indicated not only progression in most patients, but that progression occurred at predictable rates early and late in disease (37).

The clinical severity of RA predicts not only future morbidity but functional capacity as well. The classical early studies of Duthie and colleagues (167), Rasker and Cosh (168), and others, indicated that poor baseline global functional status was predictive of earlier mortality. Gordon et al. (169) found that RA patients with rheumatoid factor and extra-articular disease (excluding nodules only) had a 5-year mortality of about 40%, compared to a 5-year mortality of about 12% in the subgroup with no rheumatoid factor or extra-articular disease (170) (Fig. 15).

Analyses of quantitative functional and articular measures as potential markers of subsequent mortality in RA were conducted over 9 years (40,41) (Fig. 16). Age was an important predictive marker, as expected (Fig. 16A), whereas duration of disease was not discriminatory to predict increased risk of mortality (Fig. 16B). The number of involved joints (Fig. 16C), presence of comorbid

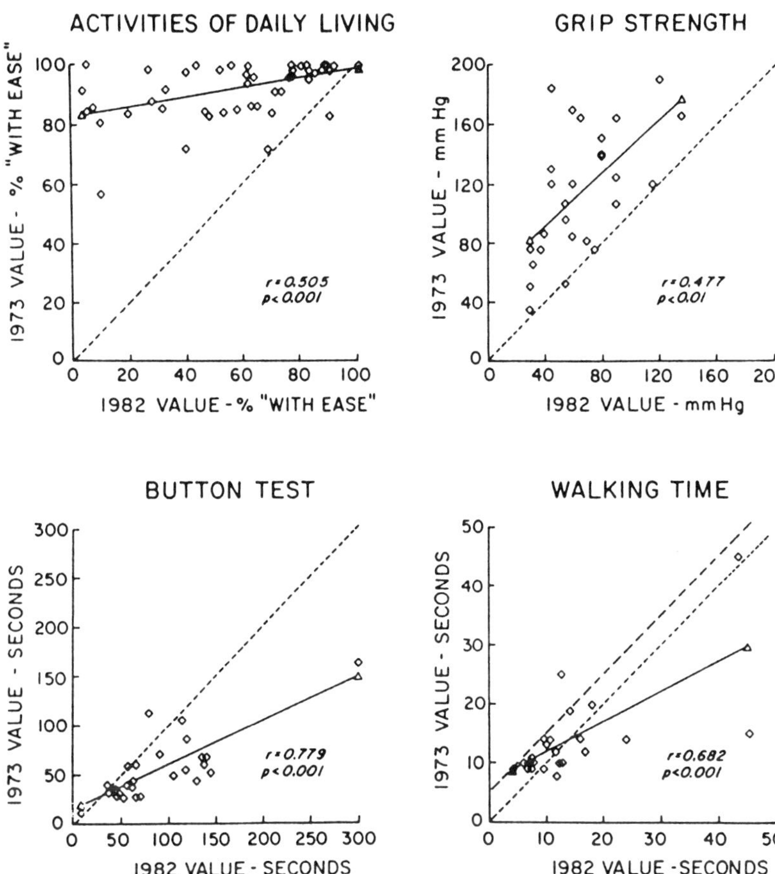

Fig. 14 Comparison of values for 4 measures of functional status measured 9 years apart in patients with RA. The 45-degree dotted lines show projected values, assuming no change in clinical status. Values above this line for ADL and grip strength and below this line for button test and walking time show declines in functional status. Two dashed lines show walking time, as the methods used in 1973 and 1982 differed, with the 1973 method requiring 52% longer in direct comparisons. Seconds recorded are shown. A second dashed line shows projected values, assuming no change in walking time over the 9-year period and a 9-year result 52% higher than the actual value due to the change in method. Data indicate significant correlations between values 9 years apart, with severe decline in functional status in most patients (From Ref. 138).

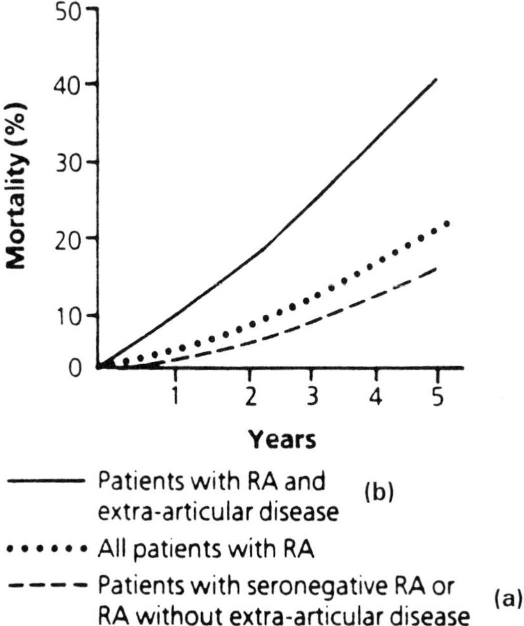

Fig. 15 Analyses of mortality over 5 years in 116 patients with rheumatoid arthritis. Two subgroups were identified: (a) patients with no rheumatoid factor and no extra-articular disease, for whom mortality was 14% at 5 years; (b) patients with extra-articular disease, for whom mortality was 40% at 5 years. (From Ref. 169.)

Fig. 16 Analyses of survival in 75 patients with rheumatoid arthritis based on various quantitative measures available at baseline. Note significant differences according to age (A), joint count (C), cardiovascular disease (D), questionnaire scores for activities of daily living (E), modified walking time score (F), button test (G), and formal education level (I). The only variable depicted that does not significantly predict differences in mortality rates is duration of disease (B). The most explanatory variable in these analyses was questionnaire scores for activities of daily living. Although different measures of functional capacity were correlated, there was evidence of dose–response relations for mortality rates and the presence of none, one, two, or three measures of severe dysfunction (H) for activities of daily living questionnaire responses, modified walking time, and button test. (Data from Refs. 40, 68.)

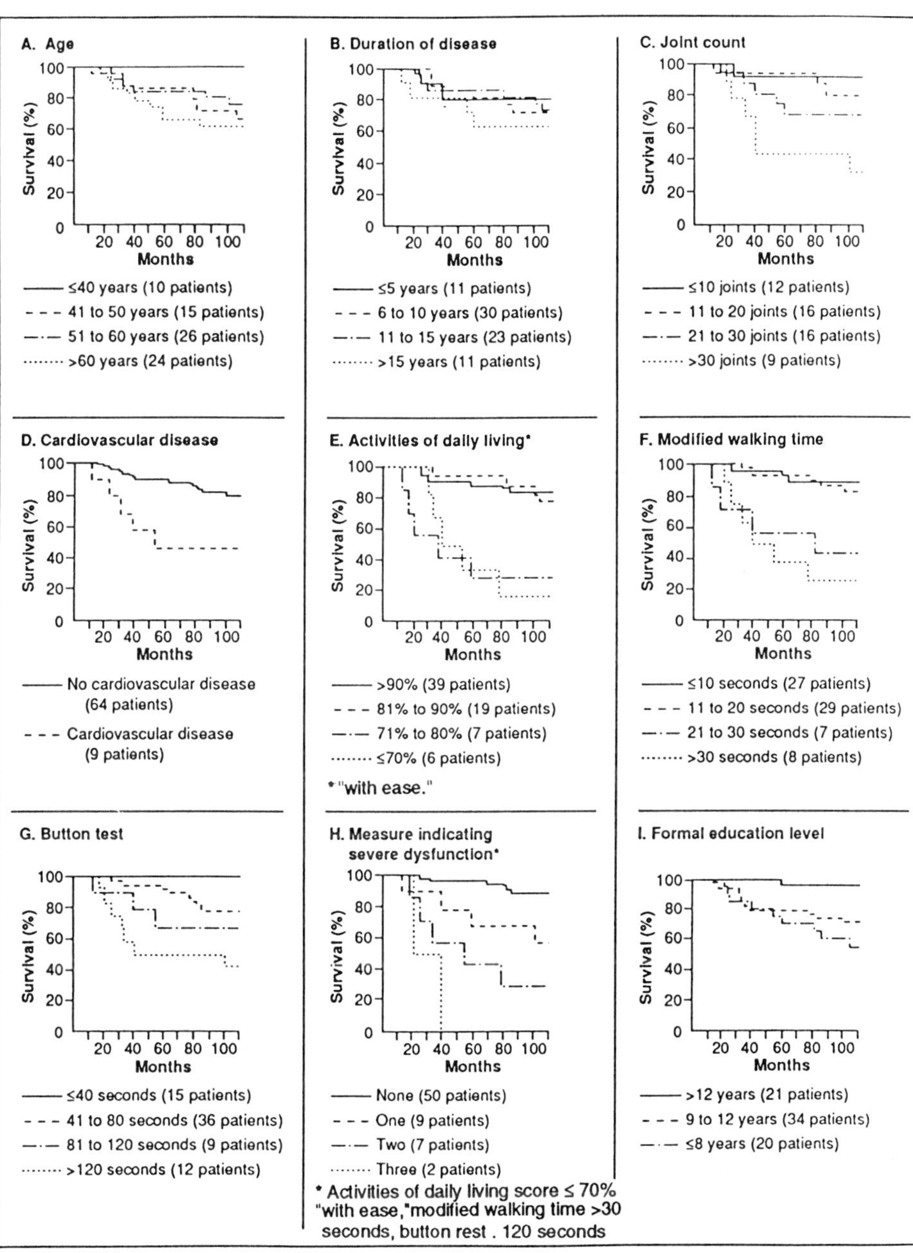
A. Age
Survival (%)
Months
≤40 years (10 patients)
41 to 50 years (15 patients)
51 to 60 years (26 patients)
>60 years (24 patients)

B. Duration of disease
Survival (%)
Months
≤5 years (11 patients)
6 to 10 years (30 patients)
11 to 15 years (23 patients)
>15 years (11 patients)

C. Joint count
Survival (%)
Months
≤10 joints (12 patients)
11 to 20 joints (16 patients)
21 to 30 joints (16 patients)
>30 joints (9 patients)

D. Cardiovascular disease
Survival (%)
Months
No cardiovascular disease
(64 patients)
Cardiovascular disease
(9 patients)

E. Activities of daily living*
Survival (%)
Months
>90% (39 patients)
81% to 90% (19 patients)
71% to 80% (7 patients)
≤70% (6 patients)
* "with ease."

F. Modified walking time
Survival (%)
Months
≤10 seconds (27 patients)
11 to 20 seconds (29 patients)
21 to 30 seconds (7 patients)
>30 seconds (8 patients)

G. Button test
Survival (%)
Months
≤40 seconds (15 patients)
41 to 80 seconds (36 patients)
81 to 120 seconds (9 patients)
>120 seconds (12 patients)

H. Measure indicating
severe dysfunction*
Survival (%)
Months
None (50 patients)
One (9 patients)
Two (7 patients)
Three (2 patients)
* Activities of daily living score ≤ 70%
"with ease,"modified walking time >30
seconds, button rest . 120 seconds

I. Formal education level
Survival (%)
Months
>12 years (21 patients)
9 to 12 years (34 patients)
≤8 years (20 patients)

cardiovascular disease (beyond hypertension) (Fig. 16D), baseline functional status in activities of daily living (Fig. 16E), physical measures of functional status, including modified walking time (Fig. 16F) and button test (Fig. 16G), were significant predictors of higher mortality rates (40,68). Five-year survivals were in the range of 85–95% in individuals with favorable values, versus 45–55% in patients with unfavorable baseline values for most of these measures.

Significant correlations were seen between baseline values for questionnaire and physical measures of functional capacity, as expected. Therefore, mortality patterns were analyzed according to whether patients showed 0, 1, 2, or 3 severely dysfunctional values at baseline for questions concerning activities of daily living, walking time, or the button test. Dysfunctional values were defined as activities of daily living scores of less than 80% "with ease," modified walking time of more than 30 s, and button test of more than 120 s (see Fig. 16H). The only two patients with 3 severely dysfunctional values at baseline were not alive 4 years later. The 7 patients with two severely dysfunctional values showed 5-year survival of about 40%. The nine patients with one severely dysfunctional value showed 5-year survival of about 70%. Patients who had no severely dysfunctional values showed five-year survival of about 95%—not significantly different from expected mortality in the general population.

These studies indicate that increased mortality rates in RA are predicted effectively by quantitative measures indicative of more severe clinical status, including functional status measures. Evidence for dose–response relations can be seen between the number of baseline measures indicating severe dysfunction and subsequent mortality. Furthermore, patients whose functional status was not compromised substantially showed mortality rates similar to those expected in the general population matched for age and gender. Overall, more severe dysfunction is associated with higher mortality rates in RA patients.

The importance of functional status is also extensively documented in data from the four ARAMIS treatment centers to predict mortality (166) (Table 16). In data from Saskatoon, functional status was highly significant in regresson analyses, while in Wichita the HAQ score, noted as disability index, was a highly significant predictor of mortality. Indeed, in all studies in which it has been examined, functional status has been a significant predictor of mortality, often generally of equal or greater importance than laboratory or imaging data.

Morality rates in patients with severe RA over long periods may be in the ranges seen in cardiovascular and neoplastic diseases. A comparison of mortality in three chronic diseases, predicted according to baseline markers, although not at disease onset, is depicted in Figure 17. Survival at 5 years in coronary artery disease (170) in 1978 before the era of coronary artery bypass surgery, in 601 nonoperative patients seen at the Cleveland Clinic (see Fig. 17A), was 45% in those with three involved vessels or left coronary artery involvement, versus 85% in individuals with one non–left-coronary involved vessel. Survival at 5

Table 16 Stepwise Cox Proportional Hazards Models to Analyze Mortality Over 30 Years in Patients with RA at 3 Treatment Centers

Step	Variable	Coefficient	Coeff./ (S.E.)	Relative Risk[a] (R.R.)	95% C.I. for R.R.	Improve p-value
Saskatoon						
1	Age	.075	15.18	1.078/Year	(1.067–1.088)	<.001
2	Nodules	.290	2.59	1.336/+	(1.073–1.664)	<.001
3	Functional Class	.216	3.31	1.241/Unit	(1.092–1.410)	<.001
4	Sex	.436	4.34	1.547/M:F	(1.270–1.884)	<.001
5	Prednisone	.352	3.52	1.422/+	(1.169–1.729)	<.001
6	Rales	.370	2.92	1.447/+	(1.130–1.854)	.002
7	Number of Joints	.012	2.13	1.012/Joint	(1.001–1.024)	.003
8	Loglatex	.032	2.05	1.032/Log	(1.002–1.064)	.022
9	Anorexia	.303	2.09	1.354/+	(1.019–1.801)	.026
10	Mean BP	.009	2.21	1.009/mmHg	(1.001–1.016)	.048
11	ESR	.004	2.06	1.004/mmHr	(1.001–1.007)	.034
12	Joint Swelling	.593	1.53	1.809/+	(0.848–3.858)	.092
Wichita						
1	Age	.076	10.57	1.079/Year	(1.064–1.094)	<.001
2	Sex	.516	3.57	1.675/M:F	(1.262–2.223)	<.001
3	Disability Index	.285	2.93	1.330/Unit	(1.099–1.610)	<.001
4	Smoking	.387	3.77	1.472/Pack	(1.204–1.800)	<.001
5	GI History	.457	2.71	1.579/+	(1.135–2.197)	.001
6	Prednisone	.474	3.36	1.606/+	(1.219–2.116)	.001
7	Loglatex	.048	2.08	1.049/Log	(1.003–1.097)	.004
8	Education	− .072	− 2.79	0.931/Year	(0.885–0.973)	.006
9	Mean BP	.017	3.05	1.017/mmHg	(1.006–1.028)	.010
10	ESR	.007	2.59	1.007/mmHr	(1.002–1.013)	.011
11	Nodules	.217	1.26	1.243/+	(0.886–1.744)	.217
Stanford						
1	Age	.064	8.74	1.006/Year	(1.051–1.082)	<.001
2	Rales	.292	2.29	1.339/+	(1.042–1.719)	.003
3	Sex	.360	2.19	1.434/M:F	(1.039–1.978)	.025
4	Number of Joints	.036	1.98	1.037/Joint	(1.001–1.074)	.037
5	Prednisone	.253	1.60	1.288/+	(0.945–1.755)	.113

[a]Relative Risk = relative multiplicative effect of the variable on the hazard function corresponding to a 1 unit change in that variable only.

Source: Ref. 166.

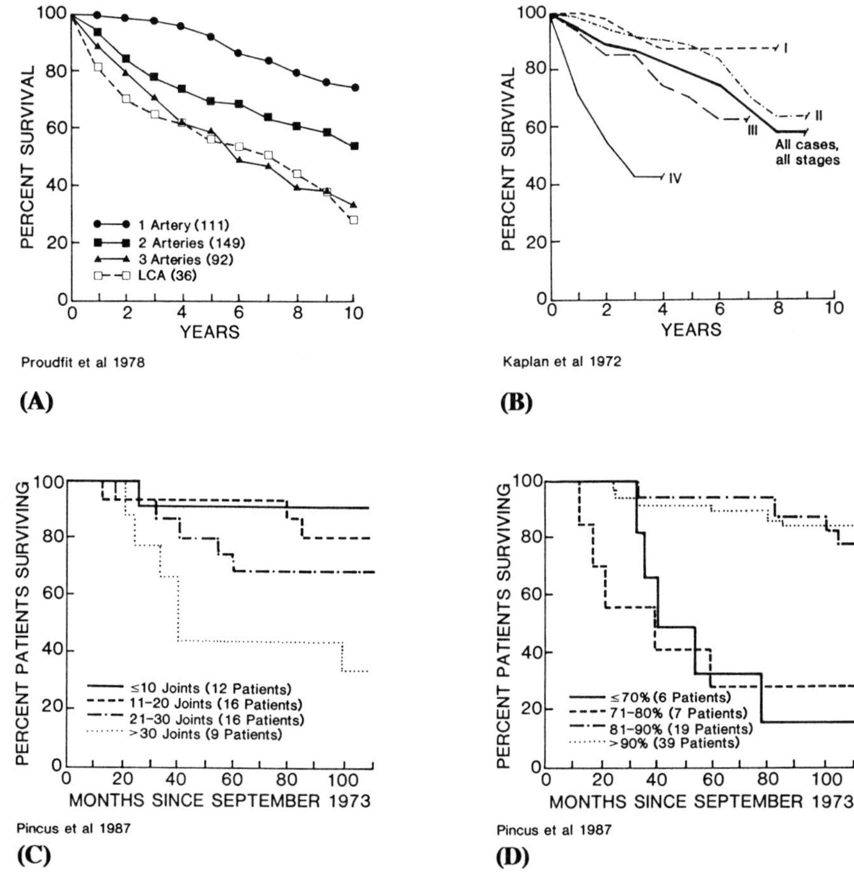

Fig. 17 Examples of survival analyses in cardiovascular, neoplastic and rheumatic disease based on specific disease markers at baseline, including (A) the number of coronary arteries involved in coronary artery disease, (B) the anatomical stage in Hodgkin's disease, (C) the number of involved joints, and (D) functional status in RA. Patients with the most severe clinical status show survivals of 40–60% over the subsequent 5 years, including patients with three involved vessels or left coronary artery disease, Stage IV Hodgkin's disease, and more than 30 involved joints or poor functional status in RA. (From Refs. 3, 8.)

years in Hodgkin's disease (171) at Stanford University in 1972, before widespread use of chemotherapy and linear accelerator therapy (see Fig. 17B) was about 85% in patients with Stage I disease versus about 45% in those with Stage IV disease. Analyses in RA indicate that the joint count (see Fig. 17C) or activities of daily living questionnaire scores (see Fig. 17D) predict that certain patients will show 5-year survival patterns in the range of patients with three-vessel coronary artery disease or Stage IV Hodgkin's disease (169,170). It must be emphasized that a smaller proportion of RA patients appear in the poorest prognostic category compared to patients with cardiovascular or neoplastic diseases, and that many patients with coronary artery disease and Hodgkin's disease patients were studied earlier in the disease course than were the patients with RA. Nonetheless, certain patients with RA have a poor prognosis for survival, comparable with those seen for certain patients with cardiovascular and neoplastic diseases.

Many patients with RA are not seen until long after disease is established, therefore, they are not treated aggressively until irreversible damage is present. Earlier recognition and treatment of RA may prevent the progression of clinical status to levels projecting 5-year survivals of less than 50%, comparable to those seen in three-vessel coronary artery disease or Stage IV Hodgkin's disease.

C4. Traditional Paradigm. Outcomes in different patients with RA are explained largely on the basis of differences in health care system variables, without consideration of possible differences in patient characteristics.

Paradigm Shift. Outcomes in different patients with RA over long periods are explained in large part on the basis of endogenous patient variables, identified by the marker of formal education level.

Comment. An underlying assumption in modern health care is that different outcomes in different patients result from differences in health care system variables e.g., differences between drugs in clinical trials. This paradigm is most effectively applied in short-term studies, but as the observation period is lengthened, patient characteristics appear to show increasing importance. For example, recent studies in RA suggest that formal education level, as a marker of differences in patient characteristics, is highly predictive of morbidity (Fig. 18) and mortality (Figs. 19 and 20) over 9 years (see Chapter 13). The associations between formal education level and outcome are not explained by treatments used, age, duration of disease, functional status measures, or any other baseline variable (68).

Further analyses of 385 RA patients seen at a University Clinic, Veterans Administration Hospital, and private practice settings, indicate poorer clinical status in individuals with low levels of formal education, according to all indicators examined (Table 17), including joint count, erythrocyte sedimentation rate, grip strength, walking time, and questionnaire self-assessment measures (69).

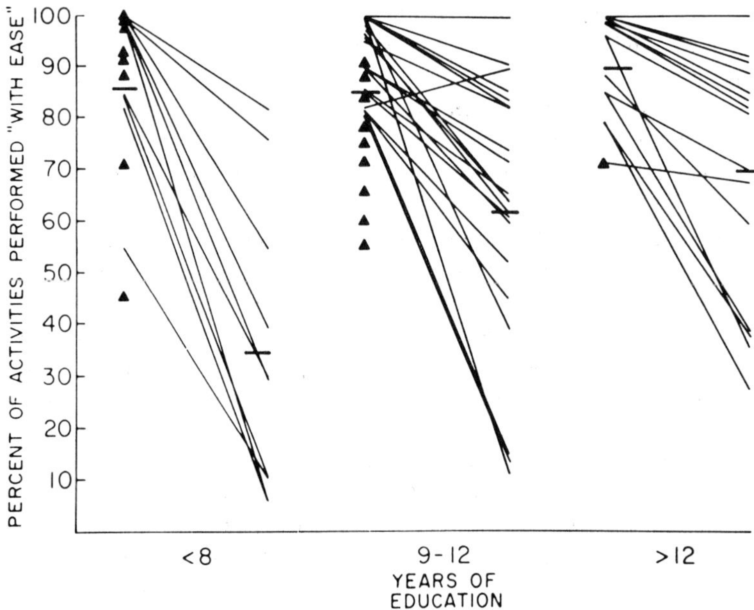

Fig. 18 Changes over 9 years in functional capacity determined by responses to questions in 50 patients with RA. The percentage of 87 questions to which patients responded that they could perform "with ease" is depicted, with patients categorized into three groups according to formal educational level. Patients who had died over the 9 years are depicted by triangles. Significant declines are seen in most patients, with significant differences between declines in grade-school education versus other patients. (From Ref. 68.)

Fig. 19 Analysis of survival in 75 patients with RA over nine years. (A) Survival of 75 patients over a period of 110 months, categorized into three groups according to formal education (numbers in parentheses indicate total number within each group). (B) Survival of a subset of 48 patients between ages 45 and 64 years, encompassing the group with accelerated mortality in RA, classified according to years of formal education (numbers in parentheses indicate total number within each group. (C) Survival of 75 patients from onset of disease (rather than from quantitative assessment) over a period of 30 years categorized into three groups according to years of formal education (numbers at the bottom indicate the numbers of patients at risk in each category at 5-year intervals). (From Ref. 68.)

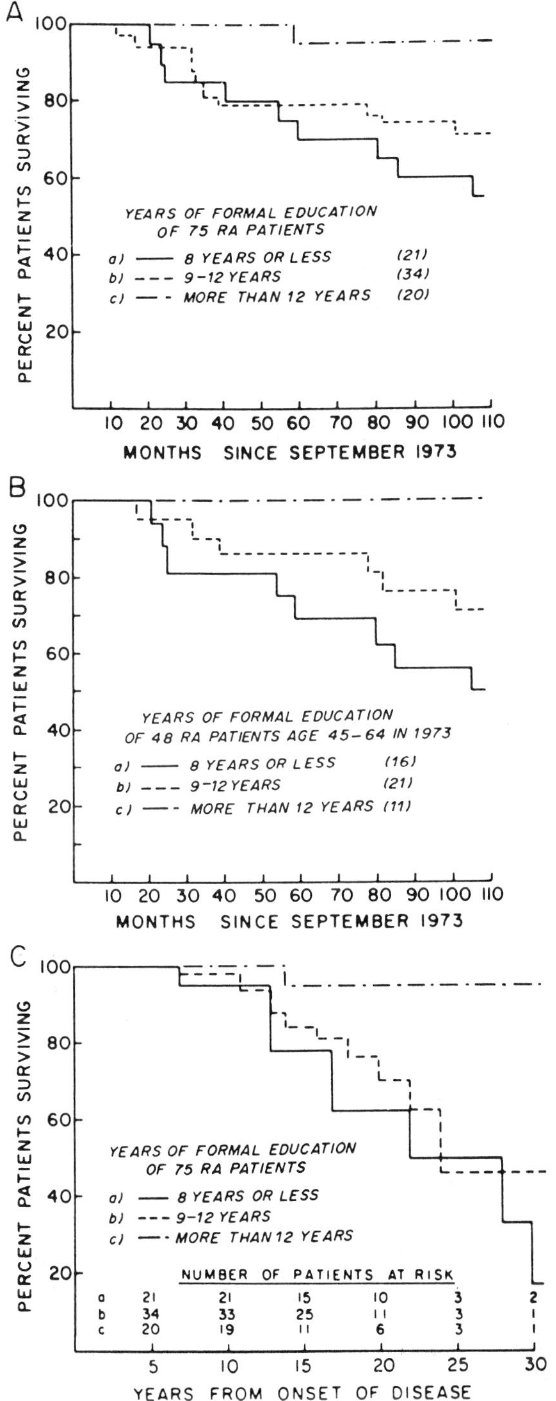

A
100
80
PERCENT PATIENTS SURVIVING
60
40
20
YEARS OF FORMAL EDUCATION
OF 75 RA PATIENTS
a)   8 YEARS OR LESS   (21)
b)   9-12 YEARS   (34)
c)   MORE THAN 12 YEARS   (20)
10 20 30 40 50 60 70 80 90 100 110
MONTHS SINCE SEPTEMBER 1973
B
100
80
PERCENT PATIENTS SURVIVING
60
40
20
YEARS OF FORMAL EDUCATION
OF 48 RA PATIENTS AGE 45-64 IN 1973
a)   8 YEARS OR LESS   (16)
b)   9-12 YEARS   (21)
c)   MORE THAN 12 YEARS   (11)
10 20 30 40 50 60 70 80 90 100 110
MONTHS SINCE SEPTEMBER 1973
C
100
80
PERCENT PATIENTS SURVIVING
60
40
20
YEARS OF FORMAL EDUCATION
OF 75 RA PATIENTS
a)   8 YEARS OR LESS
b)   9-12 YEARS
c)   MORE THAN 12 YEARS
NUMBER OF PATIENTS AT RISK
a   21   21   15   10   3   2
b   34   33   25   11   3   1
c   20   19   11   6   3   1
5   10   15   20   25   30
YEARS FROM ONSET OF DISEASE

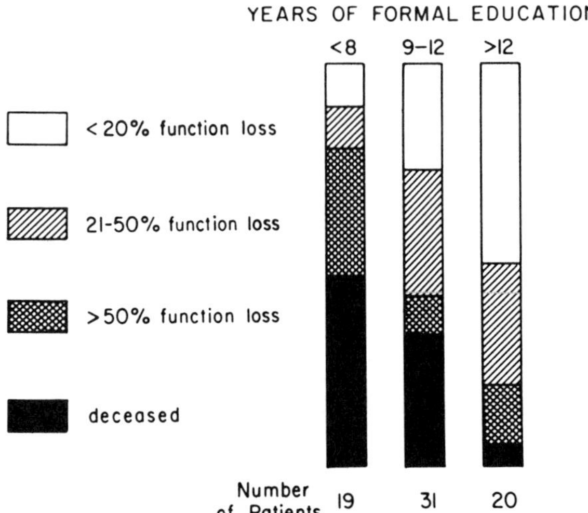

Fig. 20   Analysis of morbidity and mortality in 70 patients with rheumatoid arthritis over 9 years. Note evidence of dose–response relations in three groups according to formal education level: patients with 8 or fewer years of education included almost half who did not survive and very few good courses; patients with more than 12 years of formal education included almost half with relatively good courses. (From Ref. 68.)

These findings are also not explained by age, duration of disease, race, or clinical setting.

These studies in patients with RA may be interpreted to suggest that differences in patients according to socioeconomic status variables such as formal education level may be important, although relatively neglected, variables associated with different outcomes in patients with RA and other chronic diseases. Formal education level may identify the contribution of the *patient*, in contrast to health professionals and the medical care system, in the outcomes of disease.

D.   Treatment of Rheumatoid Arthritis

D1.   Traditional Paradigm.   ''The majority of patients can control RA satisfactorily with well-accepted, conservative regimens'' (2).

Paradigm Shift.   ''RA remains a serious threat to lifestyle, to livelihood and to life itself . . . mortality was associated not only with poor performance of tests of joint function but also with low socioeconomic status, the presence of extra-articular disease, and with rheumatoid factor positivity'' (172).

Comment.   The relatively optimistic views expressed in Figures 1 and 2, at the beginning of this chapter, that 70–80% of patients are ''controlled'' with

Table 17 Mean Values for Laboratory, Physical, and Self-Report Measures of Disease Status in 385 Rheumatoid Arthritis Patients, Classified According to Level of Formal Education

Disease status measure	Patients classified according to formal education level					
	All patients	Grade school	Some high school	High school graduate	Some college or more	P^a
Laboratory measures						
ESR (mm/h)	40.1	48.3	49.4	34.7	31.2	0.002[b]
Joint count (number of painful joints)	12.1	16.3	15.1	9.1	9.8	0.001[c]
Physical measures						
Grip strength (mmHg)	98.8	93.7	92.1	97.9	109.8	0.079
Walking time(s)	10.3	11.2	10.0	10.6	9.4	0.424[b]
Button test(s)	62.5	80.5	61.3	60.8	49.8	0.003[b]
Self-report measures						
ADL difficulty scale (1–4)	1.97	2.26	2.04	1.86	1.77	<0.001
ADL pain scale (1–4)	2.37	2.62	2.56	1.86	2.13	0.001[c]
ADL dissatisfaction scale (1–4)	2.26	2.54	2.41	2.26	2.05	0.006
Visual analog pain scale (0–10)	5.12	5.75	5.85	4.89	4.34	0.074
Global self-assessment (1–4)	2.68	3.09	2.70	2.55	2.44	<0.001

ESR, erythrocyte sedimentation rate; ADL, activities of daily living.
[a]By analysis of covariance, after controlling for age, sex, clinical setting, and disease duration.
[b]$P<0.05$ after adjustment for multiple comparisons.
[c]$P<0.01$ after adjustment for multiple comparisons.
Source: Adapted from Ref. 69.

first-line nonsteroidal anti-inflammatory drugs (NSAIDs) (see Fig. 1), and that use of second-line drugs may be deferred for several years after disease onset (see Fig. 2), may be valid if applied to all individuals who meet ARA Criteria for RA, many of whom have a self-limited process rather than a progressive disease, as discussed in the foregoing (see Paradigm A2). However, first- and second-line therapies do not "control" RA in most patients over extended periods, during which clinical progression is usually seen (29–36,38–41).

The teaching that most patients with RA can be controlled with first-line therapies may have partly contributed to poor long-term results in treatment of this disease. Many family practitioners, internists, and even rheumatologists, have been taught to defer second-line therapy for months and years, based on the "conventional wisdom" presented in Figures 1 and 2. Aggressive interventions have been pursued only after patients develop evidence of early erosions, which indicate irreversible changes, sometimes associated with clinical deformities. It should be emphasized that it has not been definitively documented that early treatment will lead to better outcomes, although, in most studies, it has been suggested that earlier therapies are certainly not likely to result in poorer outcomes. The deferral of treatment until deformities develop may partially account for poor outcomes in patients with RA (42).

D2. Traditional Paradigms. Second-line drugs for RA are "remission-inducing" (155).

Paradigm Shift. All available second-line drugs for RA are effective in certain patients over short intervals, and effective in a few patients over long periods, but long-term remission with use of currently available drugs according to traditional approaches is quite rare.

Comment. In the rheumatology literature, second-line drugs, such as gold salts, penicillamine, hydroxychloroquine, corticosteroids, methotrexate, azathioprine, and cyclophosphamide, have been described as "remission-inducing" (155). Indeed, during the year 1993, the authors have continued to note use of the term "remittive therapy" or "remission-inducing therapy" in rheumatology lectures and clinical practice, as well as reports in the rheumatology literature. Evidence that these terms are inappropriate includes:

Marginal Benefits Are Often Exaggerated

Although many reports suggest that slowing of radiographic progression may be documented in use of second-line drugs, thoughtful reviews by Ianuzzi, Kushner and colleagues (29,173) indicate that slowing of radiographic progression is relatively unusual. Indeed, among 18 published studies (Table 18), only 4 provided probable support for this concept, and 11 showed no support whatsoever (29). Radiographic progression, therefore, does not appear to be affected reproducibly in most patients with RA by available drug therapy, at least as used according to the traditional approaches outlined in Figure 2.

Table 18 Analyses of Studies in Which Slowing of Radiographic Progression in Rheumatoid Arthritis is Reported: Number of Studies Providing Different Levels of Support for This Concept

Drug used	Strong support	Probable support	Doubtful support	No support	Total
Gold salts	1	2		3	6
Penicillamine			1	1	2
Antimalarials			1	4	5
Azathioprine				1	1
Cyclophosphamide	1		1	2	4
Total	2	2	3	11	18

Source: Adapted from Refs. 29, 173.

*A Sustained Remission Longer than 3 Years Is Seen in Fewer Than 1%
of Patients Treated With Second-Line Agents*

A review of 485 patients who were treated with second-line drugs indicated evidence of remission in only about 18% (174). Equally important, fewer than 50% of these remissions were sustained for even 1 year, and fewer than 10% were sustained for longer than 3 years (Fig. 21). Therefore, fewer than 1.8% of patients treated with second-line agents in a rheumatology practice experienced a sustained remission that lasted longer than 3 years (174). These data appear applicable to most rheumatology care settings, in that no data have been reported to suggest better results from other locales.

*Fewer Than One in Five Patients Begun on Therapies With Second-Line
Agents Continue to Take These Agents 2 Years Later*

Over the last decade, several investigators have recognized that most courses of second-line drugs taken by patients with RA are discontinued within 2 years in most patients (175–177), despite continued progression of RA. An elegant study was performed by Thompson and colleagues (178) of 251 courses of therapy with four second-line drugs, gold salts, penicillamine, azathioprine, or hydroxychloroquine, in 154 patients (Fig. 22). Clinical efficacy was reported within the first 6 months in about 50% of these courses, reflecting documented benefit in clinical trials (see Fig. 22A and 22B) with little difference between the four second-line agents. However, fewer than 50% of courses were continued over longer than 1 year, fewer than 20% were continued beyond 2 years, and fewer than 10% were continued beyond 3 years (see Fig. 22C). Most courses were discontinued because of inefficacy or toxicity, rather than remission (178).

With the introduction of methotrexate into clinical care for RA (179–181), a considerably longer continuation has been seen compared to other second-line

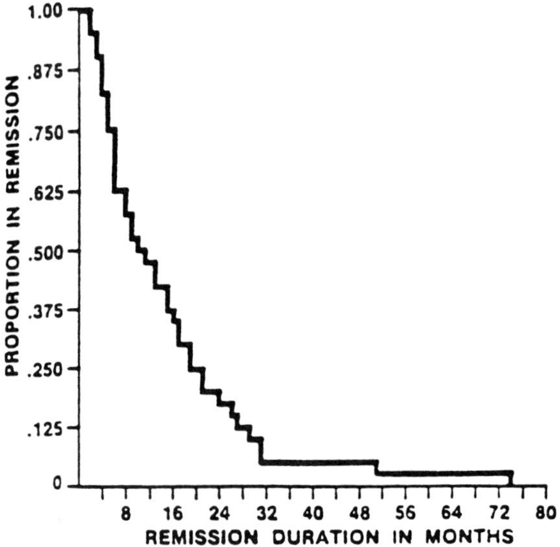

Fig. 21 Analysis of duration of remission in RA patients in a clinical practice. The initial survey involved 485 patients of whom 86 (18%) appeared to have a clinical remission. Of these remissions, 80% ended by 24 months and 90% by 36 months. Therefore, fewer than 2% of patients treated with second-line agents experienced remissions longer than 3 years. (From Ref. 174.)

agents. In a study in one large private practice (Fig. 23), 50% of the courses of methotrexate were continued 5 years after they were begun, in contrast to fewer than 25% of courses of other second-line drugs (182,183). In another study from 7 rheumatology private practices (184) (Fig. 24), no differences were seen in estimated continuation of injectable gold salts, penicillamine, azathioprine, or hydroxychloroquine. These results were very similar to the study in London by Thompson and colleagues (178), although the estimated continuation at three years was more in the range of 30% than 10% (as had been observed in London (178) 5 years earlier). Continuation of methotrexate was significantly longer—50% of courses were continued at 5 years—whereas courses of oral gold salts were significantly shorter than courses of other second-line drugs (see Fig. 24).

Although improving results with methotrexate are encouraging, long-term studies indicate that remission is unusual and that sustained remission is rare in the treatment of RA with second-line drugs. Loss of efficacy with time is frequent in use of second-line therapies, despite effective short-term results. Loss of efficacy may be based on a number of mechanisms, including tachyphylaxis, regression toward the mean (43), or multiple drug resistance (185), but this phenomenon has not been studied extensively in RA. It is also possible that

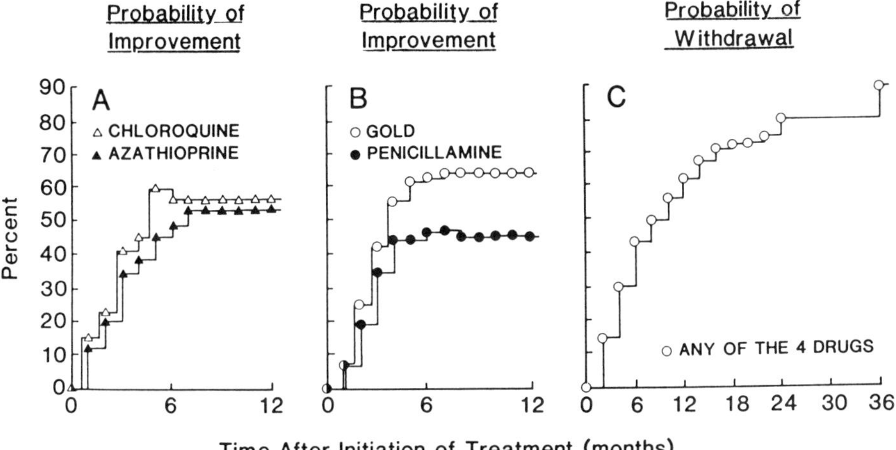

Fig. 22 Analysis of results of treatment with chloroquine, azathioprine, gold, and penicillamine. At 6 months, about 50% of patients responded to each of the agents, without significant differences among the agents (A, B). However, 50% of patients had withdrawn from treatment by 12 months, 80% by 24 months, and 90% by 36 months (C). These data indicate relatively poor clinical responses over prolonged periods using these second-line agents. (Adapted from Ref. 178.)

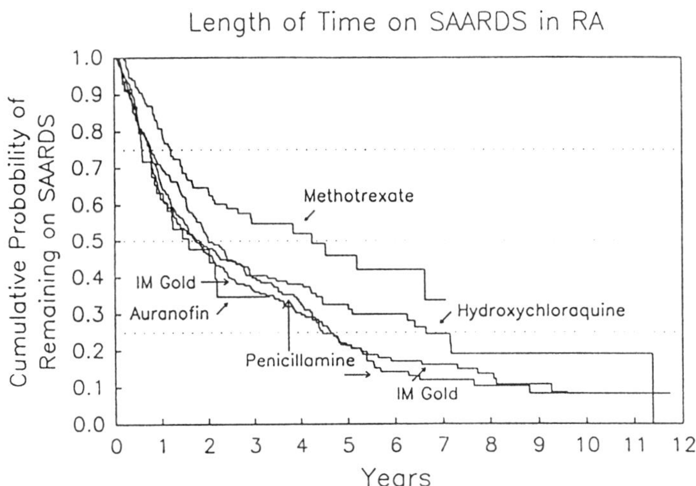

Fig. 23 Product limit (Kaplan-Meier) cumulative survival analysis for SAARD. Difference in cumulative survival is significant at the 0.001 level in Mantel-Cox and Breslow tests. (From Ref. 182.)

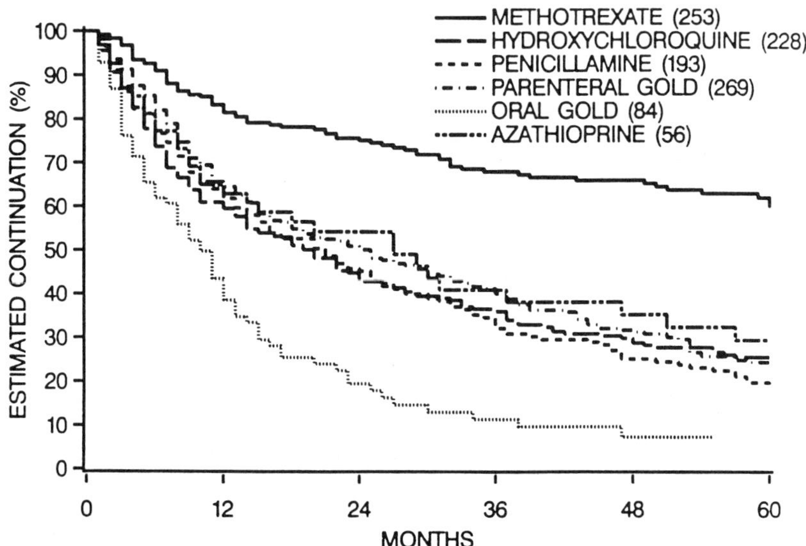

Fig. 24   Probability of continuation of courses of second-line drugs in 532 patients with RA over 60 months. Courses that were continued at the time of observation were censored. Differences between MTX and all other drugs are statistically significant. Differences between oral gold and all other drugs are statistically significant ($P < 0.001$). Differences among other drugs are not statistically significant (From Ref. 184.)

courses of drugs might be continued over longer periods if used earlier in the disease course, when they might be more effective. Further investigation of mechanisms concerning loss of efficacy of both first-line nonsteroidal anti-inflammatory drugs as well as second-line drugs may be of considerable value in efforts to improve results of treatment in patients with RA.

D3.   Traditional Paradigm.   Data from randomized controlled clinical trials may be applied effectively to describe the long-term course of RA.

Paradigm Shift.   Data from randomized controlled clinical trials provide a foundation for recognizing that a drug is more effective than placebo and has acceptable toxicity for use in clinical practice, but these data are often not applicable to describe long-term results of treatment of RA, owing to intrinsic limitations of the randomized controlled clinical trials methodology.

Comment.   The randomized controlled clinical trial is the foundation for studies of therapies in any disease, providing an approach in which patients are not selected for a given therapy on the basis of potential biases on the part of health professionals, patients, or other variables (186,187). A primary concern in the performance of clinical trials involves potential methodologic errors, including protocol violations, noncompliant patients, or transcription errors, missing data, and others. However, relatively little has been written concerning limitations to clinical trials, *intrinsic* to the methodology itself, which limits generalizability of results of clinical trials, despite rigorous attention to methodological requirements, such as random allocation, double-blind treatment protocols, appropriate patient selection, scrupulous completion of data forms, and proper statistical methodology (43,187). Some methodological limitations of clinical trials of greatest interest are summarized in the following.

Exclusion Criteria

Exclusion criteria provide a strategy in a clinical trial to circumvent variables, such as comorbidities, prior treatment with the study drug, and others that might confound a comparison of two treatment programs. However, the process of selection into a clinical trial itself introduces substantial bias, as most patients with a chronic disease such as RA may not meet inclusion criteria and are ineligible for participation (187). Most patients with RA have comorbidities (see Paradigm A4), some of which are severe and will limit participation. Furthermore, many patients have been treated with various drugs before being seen in a clinical trial study center and, therefore, may not be eligible for participation in a clinical trial. As noted previously (187), in most clinical trials conducted at Vanderbilt University since 1984, fewer than 10% of more than 1000 patients with RA were eligible for participation; in several trials, fewer than 1% of these patients were eligible, thereby limiting generalizability of results (187). It is unfortunate that exclusion criteria in clinical trials in RA are often quite rigorous. Although exclusion criteria may appear to provide a higher level of ''scientific'' uniformity, they may severely limit generalizability of the findings. The process of randomization will generally allow adjustment for possible confounding variables in various groups.

Inflexible Dosage

Most clinical trials include an inflexible dosage schedule, often fixed entirely, but, if not fixed, requiring protocol-directed adjustments that differ markedly from usual clinical practice. Furthermore, most patients with RA are taking additional drugs for the extensive comorbidities seen in this disease, as well as for RA; use and dosage of these additional drugs, such as nonsteroidal anti-inflammatory drugs, corticosteroids, and H_2-blockers, are often fixed, or a patient must drop out if an adjustment is made. Ironically, as in the case of exclusion criteria, such adjustments, which may appear to provide a higher degree of ''control'', or ''scientific'' validity, are generally unnecessary. The process of randomization itself is designed to adjust for changes in different treatment groups, and further flexibility in dosage of the test treatment as well as other treatments in clinical trials in RA might extend their generalizability.

Statistically Significant Differences Are Often Interpreted as Clinically Significant Differences

In many clinical trials in RA, differences between a placebo and a treatment are statistically significant but, on close examination, often fail to reveal substantial clinical benefit. For example, in hundreds of trials of nonsteroidal anti-inflammatory drugs, a change in joint counts generally involves an improvement of less than 30% (so that a joint count of 15 tender or swollen joints would be reduced to fewer than 11). Even though a statistically significant benefit is documented, the potential clinical significance tends to be exaggerated in reports of the trial results, and, understandably, in the promotional literature of companies which then bring the test drug to market.

An interesting example of this problem can be found in the analyses of results of treatment with various second-line drugs and placebos in randomized controlled clinical trials conducted by the Cooperative Systematic Studies of the Rheumatic Diseases (CSSRD). Differences were seen between various second-line drugs and the placebo in all of these studies (Fig. 25) (188). However, examination of these differences reveals them to be rather marginal, at best. In no trial were 50% of patients improved by more than 20% in more than four measures of clinical status, such as number of swollen joints, number of tender joints, physician or patient global impression of status, grip strength, walk time, pain, questionnaire, or laboratory measure. These data suggest that results using various drugs in these studies differ from placebo, but none provide the effectiveness that patients and physicians would like to see.

It may be worthwhile to consider more stringent criteria for advances in treatment than the traditional $p < 0.05$, which indicates a 1 in 20 chance that a result, such as a difference between a placebo and a drug, may occur by chance. For example, it might be required that a new nonsteroidal anti-inflammatory drug cannot be considered a meaningful advance in RA unless it effects a reduction in joint count in at least 50% of patients, rather than in the ''average'' patient.

The Time Frame of Observations in Clinical Trials is Relatively Short

Most clinical trials conducted in patients with RA have included periods of 2–12 months, and only one trial has been conducted over a period longer than 24 months (36 months). Therefore, apparent differences between long-term performance of drugs may not be recognized in short-term clinical trials. For example, in all trials of clinical efficacy of nonsteroidal anti-inflammatory drugs (NSAIDs), meaningful differences between any of the different types of drugs are unusual and inconsistent (189). However, in analyses of data in 532 patients from 7 rheumatology private practices (190), courses of acetylated salicylates (other than plain aspirin, i.e., coated aspirin or long-acting acetylated salicylates) were continued significantly longer in each practice compared with other NSAIDs, including nonacetylated salicylates, propionic acids, and other NSAIDs (Fig. 26).

Important differences in results of short-term clinical trials versus long-term clinical studies can also be seen in studies of second-line drugs. In clinical

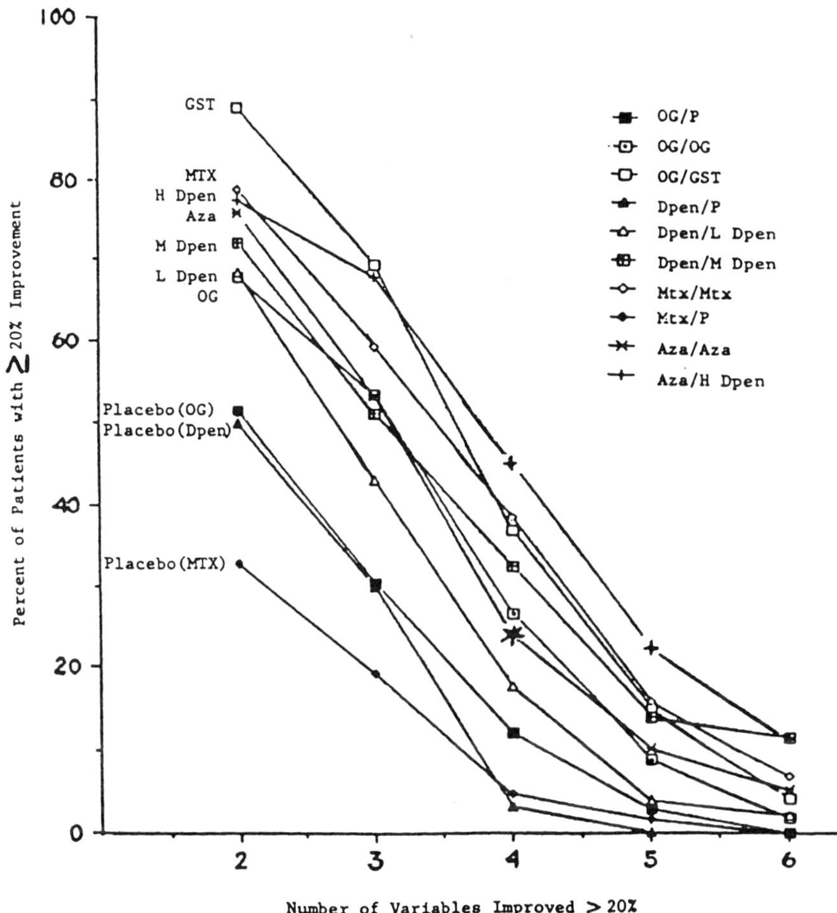

Fig. 25 Percentages of patients receiving various drugs or placebo in four studies by the Cooperative Systematic Studies Rheumatic Disease group, who demonstrated ≥20% improvement in 2, 3, 4, 5, or 6 of the measured variables. GST, gold sodium thiomalate; MTX, methotrexate; H Dpen, 750 mg/day D-penicillamine; Aza, azathiprine; M Dpen, 500 mg/day D-penicillamine; L Dpen, 125 mg/day D-penicillamine; OG, oral gold; P, placebo. (From Ref. 188.)

trials and meta-analyses (Fig. 27; See Chapter 17), methotrexate, injectable gold, and penicillamine (as well as sulfasalazine) were found to be equivalent in efficacy (191). By contrast, methotrexate was continued substantially longer than other second-line drugs over a 5-year period. To attempt to reconcile these differences, a second set of analyses was performed in the patients from 7 private practices in whom continuation of first- and second-line drugs had been studied (see Fig. 24). A subset of all courses was studied that included only the *first*

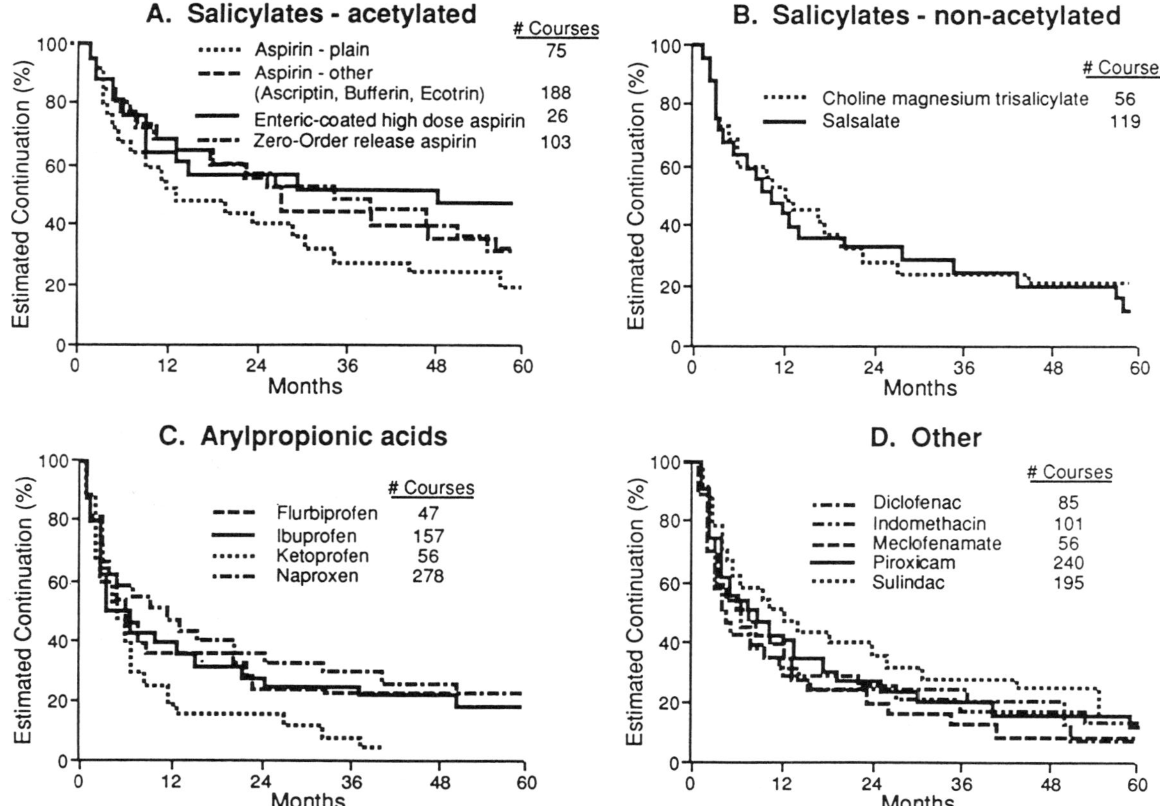

Fig. 26 Probability of continuation of 1775 courses of 15 NSAIDs taken by 532 patients with RA in seven rheumatology private practices. Differences between acetylated salicylates other than aspirin and other drugs were statistically significant. (From Ref. 190.)

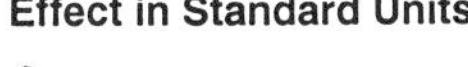

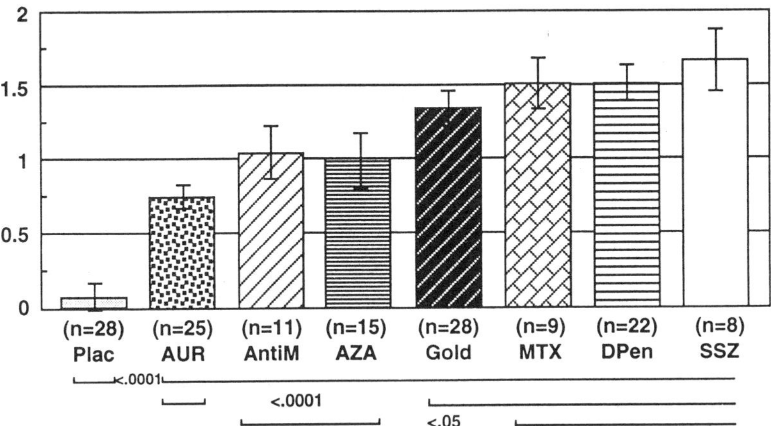

Fig. 27 Standard composite treatment effect: Composite of grip strength (adjusted for disease duration and trial length), tender joint count (adjusted for initial TJC and blinding), and ESR. (From Ref. 191.)

course of a second-line drug taken by an individual patient (rather than all courses) over a period of only 12 months (rather than over 60 months) (Fig. 28) (184). These conditions were quite similar to those in a clinical trial in which methotrexate, auranofin, and the combination of these drugs were compared (Fig. 29), and found to provide comparable clinical results (192). Over 12 months, no significant differences were seen in estimated continuation of methotrexate versus auranofin, and only minor differences were seen in continuation of other second-line drugs (Fig. 28B). These results are in marked contrast with results seen over 60 months (Fig. 28A). The data provide an explanation of apparently conflicting results in use of second-line drugs in clinical trials over relatively short periods versus clinical experience over long periods.

These findings suggest that results of clinical trials should be considered as providing an initial foundation for documenting efficacy and lack of toxicity of new therapies, but should be supplemented with data concerning long-term results of treatment. It might be reasonable to suggest to the Food and Drug Administration (FDA) a requirement that patients in any clinical trial involving a chronic disease such as RA be monitored over 5 subsequent years to characterize better results of treatment over clinically meaningful periods.

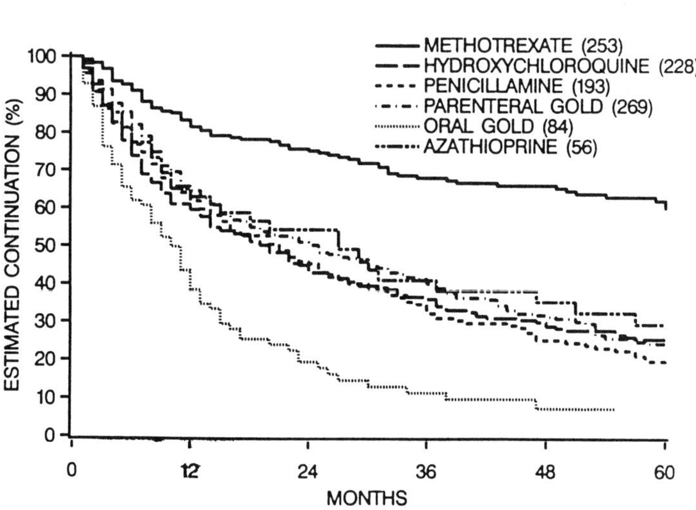

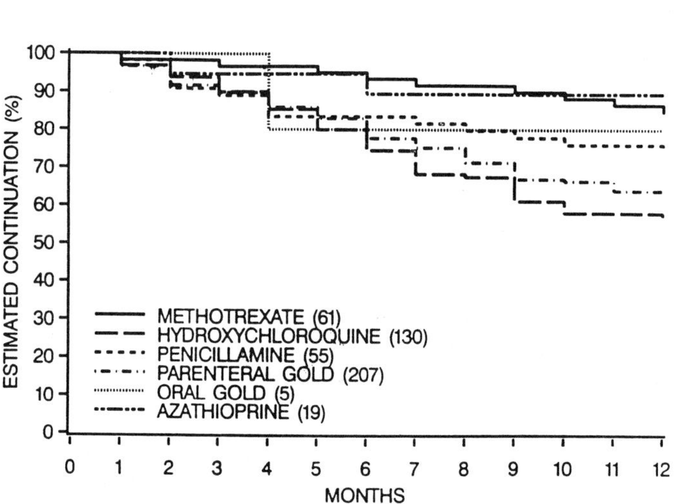

Fig. 28 (A) Estimated continuation of all 1083 courses of second-line therapy in 532 patients with RA over 60 months. Differences between methotrexate and all other drugs, as well as between oral gold (auranofin) and all other drugs, are statistically significant ($P < 0.001$); differences among other drugs are not significant. (B) Estimated continuation of 477 courses of initial second-line therapy in the same 532 patients over 12 months. Differences between methotrexate and oral gold (auranofin) are not statistically significant and are considerably less apparent than in A, in which estimated continuation was studied for all courses over 60 months. (From Ref. 184.)

Paradigm Shift. Combination therapy involving multiple second-line drugs may be appropriate to control RA in most patients, as patients generally experience progressive disease with poor outcomes, and toxicity of combination therapy does not appear significantly greater than with single second-line drug therapy.

Comment. The concept of combination therapy has provided substantial advances in the management of patients with neoplastic disease over the last 25 years. The rationale for such therapy is that a single drug may not provide optimal benefit, whereas drugs that have different mechanisms may be used effectively in combination to improve results of treatment. The dosage of a drug used in combination generally is lower than when the drug is used alone, to reduce toxicity of multiple drugs.

In RA, traditional paradigms (see Figs. 1 and 2) suggested that combination therapy would not be necessary for patients, as results of single therapies were thought to be quite good in most instances. However, with information over the last decade that these results were not as successful as had been hoped, an interest in "remodeling the pyramid" (8,193–195), with earlier use of second-line therapies, as well as combination therapy, has emerged over the last decade. Many randomized controlled clinical trials have indicated that combinations do not appear more effective than single therapies over periods of 12 months or longer (196), which has discouraged many observers from interest in the potential of combination therapy in patients with RA. For example, the study conducted by the CSSRD compared results of therapy using methotrexate, auranofin (oral gold), or a combination of these two drugs (192) (Fig. 29) and indicated similar results with use of these three regimens.

The studies of combination therapy in RA illustrate some of the problems in application of results of clinical trials over relatively brief periods to longer periods, with important implications for how these trials might be conducted in RA (115). In the trial shown in Figure 29, no differences were documented between methotrexate and auranofin, mimicking results over 1 year in clinical practice in patients who had not been treated with previous second-line antirheumatic drugs (Fig. 28), conditions very similar to this clinical trial. However, in the clinical studies of all courses of second-line drugs over 5 years, highly significant differences were seen in continuation of methotrexate or auranofin (see Fig. 28). If differences could not be documented between methotrexate and auranofin, it would be unlikely that any advantages for combination therapy of methotrexate *and* auranofin could be documented.

Some of the examples of greater effectiveness of combination than single drug therapy are seen in studies of polymyositis and systemic lupus erythematosus (SLE) nephritis, which are briefly summarized to illustrate problems in analysis of combination therapy in RA.

In studies of polymyositis at the Mayo Clinic, a comparison was made between corticosteroids only versus azathioprine plus corticosteroid therapy.

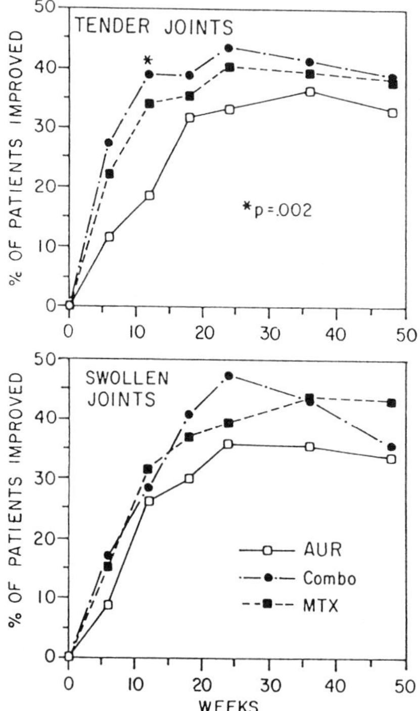

Fig. 29 Results of a randomized clinical trial in 297 patients with RA treated with auranofin (AUR), methotrexate (MTX), or auranofin plus methotrexate (Combo), illustrating percentages of patients with ≥50% meaningful improvement in tender or swollen joints. Final results showed no significant differences among the three groups. (From Ref. 192.)

Over 3 months, no differences (Table 19) were seen between the 2 regimens (197). However, over 3 years, meaningful advantages were seen for the combination of azathioprine plus corticosteroids than for corticosteroids alone, when a functional, rather than laboratory, measure was used (198). These data, which suggest that a combination of azathioprine with prednisone is of greater benefit over long periods, illustrate both the advantages of using a functional measure as well as long-term results to assess the outcomes of treatment of a rheumatic disease.

In SLE nephritis, several studies of combinations of cytotoxic drugs plus corticosteroids versus corticosteroids alone came to different conclusions. Some studies concluded that corticosteroids alone were as effective as corticosteroids plus cytotoxic drugs (199,200), and others concluded that addition of cytotoxic drugs presented a significant advantage (201). In metanalysis of all available

Table 19 Results in Treatment of Polymyositis With Prednisone Plus Azathioprine Versus Prednisone Plus Placebo Over 3 Months, 1 Year, and 3 Years

	Prednisone plus Azathioprine	Prednisone plus placebo	P value
Results at 3 mo.			
Days to normalize CPK	69.4	53.5	0.21
Change in muscle strength score	+6.5	+1.1	0.58
Change in inflammation on biopsy	+1.79	+1.65	0.80
Results at 1 yr			
Functional grade disability	3.0	3.6	<0.01
Results at 3 yr			
Functional grade disability	2.1	3.0	<0.01

CPK, creatine phosphokinase.
Sources: Modified from Refs. 197, 198.

studies (202), Felson, Anderson, and Meenan documented that the addition of cytotoxic drug therapy clearly presented meaningful advantages over corticosteroids alone for treatment of SLE nephritis.

Another approach to document potential advantages of combination versus single drug therapy involves lengthening the time frame for clinical trials, such as those conducted in SLE nephritis at the National Institutes of Health (NIH) (203–205). In these studies, maintenance of renal function in SLE was significantly greater in patients treated with cyclophosphamide and corticosteroids and somewhat better in patients treated with azathioprine and corticosteroids than in those treated with corticosteroids alone (Fig. 30). However, in Figure 20, *even after 5 years* no meaningful differences were seen in results of the various treatment programs. These data suggest that the potential advantages of an additional drug may not be documented until treatment has been continued for longer than five years.

These examples suggest that potential advantages of combination therapy may be underestimated in standard clincial trials over relatively short time periods. In RA, 99% of clinical trials have been conducted over less than 1 year, and none has been conducted for longer than 3 years. These findings present a rationale for conducting clinical trials and clinical observational studies in RA for periods as long as 5 years, or even longer, to identify potential advantages of combination second-line therapy over single second-line drug therapies.

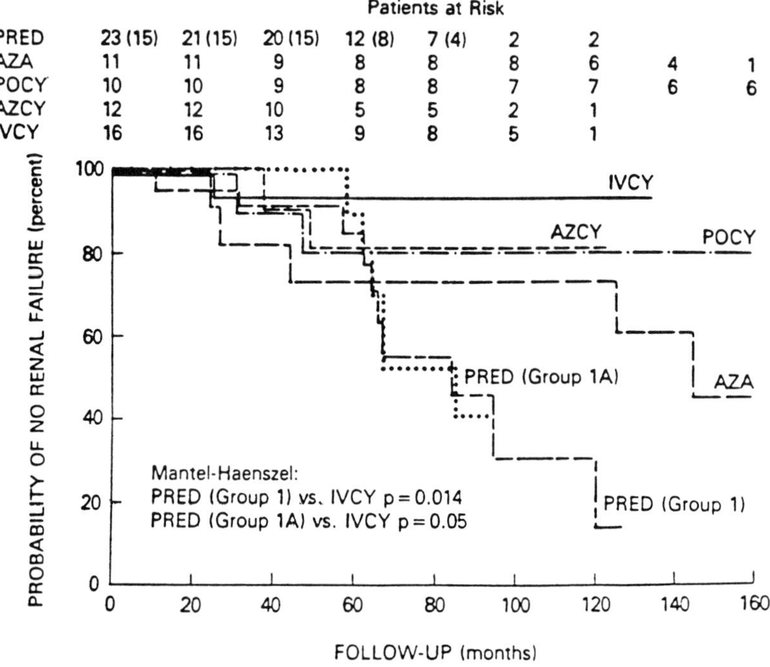

Fig. 30 Probability of maintaining life-supporting renal function in long-term randomized clinical trials of 72 high-risk patients with active SLE nephritis, according to treatment group: PRED, prednisone; AZA, azathioprine; POCY, oral cyclophosphamide; AZCY, combined oral azathioprine and cyclophosphamide; IVCY, intravenous cyclophosphamide. 95% confidence intervals at 7 years: group 1, 09.73–0.23; group 1A, 0.76–0.06, group 2, 0.98 to 0.48; group 3, 1.00–0.55; group 4, 1.00–0.57; group 5, 1.00–0.81. (From Ref. 205.)

III. CONCLUSION

This chapter is directed to documentation of the rationale for a meaningful paradigm shift in the approach to a patient with RA over the late 1980s and early 1990s. We hope the information provides a helpful Introduction to the detailed chapters by experts presented in the remaining chapters in this book. The new information presented should provide new solutions for the problems of patients with RA.

REFERENCES

1. Kelley WN, Harris ED, Jr, Ruddy KS, Sledge CB. *Textbook of rheumatology*, Philadelphia: W.B. Saunders, 1981:779.

2. McCarty DJ. *Arthritis and allied conditions: a textbook of rheumatology*, 10th Ed. Philadelphia: Lea & Febiger, 1985:675.

3. Pincus T, Callahan LF: Reassessment of twelve traditional paradigms concerning the diagnosis, prevalence, morbidity and mortality of rheumatoid arthritis. Scand J Rheumatol [Suppl] 1989; 79:67–95.

4. Kuhn TS. *The Structure of Scientific Revolutions*, 2nd Ed. Chicago: University of Chicago Press, 1970.

5. Engel GL. The need for a new medical model: a challenge for biomedicine. Science 1977; 196:129–136.

6. Holman HR. The "excellence" deception in medicine. Hosp Pract 1976; 11:11–21.

7. Wolfe F: Rheumatoid arthritis. In: Bellamy N, *Prognosis in the rheumatic diseases*. Dordrecht: Kluwer Academic Publishers, 1991:37–82.

8. Pincus T, Callahan LF: Remodeling the pyramid or remodeling the paradigms concerning rheumatoid arthritis—lessons from Hodgkin's Disease and coronary artery disease. J Rheumatol 1990; 17:1582–1585.

9. Wolfe F, Pincus T. Standard self-report questionnaires in routine clinical and research practice—an opportunity for patients and rheumatologists. J Rheumatol 1991; 18:643–646.

10. Pincus T. New concepts in prognosis of rheumatic diseases for the 1990s. In: Bellamy N, *Prognosis in the rheumatic diseases*. Dordrecht: Kluwer Academic Publishers, 1991:451–492.

11. Pincus T, Wolfe F. Treatment of rheumatoid arthritis: Challenges to traditional paradigms. Ann Intern Med 1992; 117:169–170.

12. Pincus T. The paradox of effective therapies but poor long-term outcomes in rheumatoid arthritis. Semin Arthritis Rheum 1992; 21:2–15.

13. Pincus T, Callahan LF. The 'side effects' of rheumatoid arthritis: joint destruction, disability and early mortality. Br J Rheumatol 1993; 32:(suppl 1):28–37.

14. Dawson MH, Boots RH. Recent studies in rheumatoid (chronic infectious, atrophic) arthritis. N Engl J Med 1933; 208:1030–1035.

15. Forestier J. Rheumatoid arthritis and its treatment by gold salts. J Lab Clin Med 1935; 20:827–840.

16. Cecil RL, Kammerer WH, DePrume FJ. Gold salts in the treatment of rheumatoid arthritis: a study of 245 cases. Ann Intern Med 1942; 16:811–827.

17. Keane WF, Forestier F, Kassam Y, Buchanan WW, Rooney PJ. The history of gold therapy in rheumatoid disease. Semin Arthritis Rheum 1985; 14:180–186.

18. Ropes MW, Bennett GA, Cobb S, Jacox RF, Jessar RA. 1958 revision of diagnostic criteria for rheumatoid arthritis. Bull Rheum Dis 1958; 9:175–176.

19. Arnett FC, Edworthy SM, Bloch DA, et al. The American Rheumatism Association 1987 revised criteria for the classification of rheumatoid arthritis. Arthritis Rheum 1988; 31:315–324.

20. Lichtenstein MJ, Pincus T. Rheumatoid arthritis identified in population based cross sectional studies: low prevalence of rheumatoid factor. J Rheumatol 1991; 18:989–993.

21. Mikkelsen WM, Dodge HJ, Duff IF, Kato H. Estimates of the prevalence of rheumatic diseases in the population of Tecumseh, Michigan, 1959–60. J Chronic Dis 1967; 20:351–369.

22. Adler E, Abramson JH, Elkan Z, Ben Hador S, Goldberg R. Rheumatoid arthritis in a Jerusalem population. 1. Epidemiology of the disease. Am J Epidemiol 1967; 85:365–377.

23. Valkenberg HA, Ball J, Burch TA, Bennett PH, Laurence JS. Rheumatoid factors in a rural population. Ann Rheum Dis 1966; 25:497–507.

24. Burch TA, O'Brien WM, Lawrence JS, Bennett PH, Bunim JJ. A comparison of the prevalence of rheumatoid arthritis (RA) and rheumatoid factor (RF) in Indian tribes living in Montana mountains and in Arizona desert [Abstract]. Arthritis Rheum 1963; 6:765.

25. O'Sullivan JB, Cathcart ES. The prevalence of rheumatoid arthritis: follow-up evaluation of the effect of criteria on rates in Sudbury, Massachusetts. Ann Intern Med 1972; 76:573–577.

26. Mikkelsen WM, Dodge H. A four year follow-up of suspected rheumatoid arthritis: the Tecumseh, Michigan, Community Health Study. Arthritis Rheum 1969; 12:87–91.

27. Baum J, Ziff M. Laboratory findings in rheumatoid arthritis. In: McCarty DJ. *Arthritis and Allied Conditions: A Textbook of Rheumatology.* 10th ed. Philadelphia: Lea & Febiger, 1985:643–659.

28. Carson DA. Rheumatoid factor. In: Harris ED, Jr, Ruddy S, Sledge CB eds. *Textbook of rheumatology, 2nd ed..* Philadelphia: WB Saunders, 1985:664–676.

29. Ianuzzi L, Dawson N, Zein N, Kushner I. Does drug therapy slow radiographic deterioration in rheumatoid arthritis? N Engl J Med 1983; 309:1023–1028.

30. Scott DL, Grindulis KA, Struthers GR, Coulton BL, Popert AJ, Bacon PA. Progression of radiological changes in rheumatoid arthritis. Ann Rheum Dis 1984; 43:8–17.

31. Fuchs HA, Kaye JJ, Callahan LF, Nance EP, Pincus T. Evidence of significant radiographic damage in rheumatoid arthritis within the first 2 years of disease. J Rheumatol 1989; 16:585–591.

32. Pincus T, Callahan LF, Sale WG, Brooks AL, Payne LE, Vaughn WK. Severe functional declines, work disability, and increased mortality in seventy-five rheumatoid arthritis patients studied over nine years. Arthritis Rheum 1984; 27:864–872.

33. Sherrer YS, Bloch DA, Mitchell DM, young DY, Fries JF. The development of disability in rheumatoid arthritis. Arthritis Rheum 1986; 29:494–500.

34. Scott DL, Symmons DPM, Coulton BL, Popert AJ. Long-term outcome of treating rheumatoid arthritis: results after 20 years. Lancet 1987; 1:1108–1111.

35. Yelin E, Meenan R, Nevitt M, Epstein W. Work disability in rheumatoid arthritis: effects of disease, social, and work factors. Ann Intern Med 1980; 93:551–556.

36. Meenan RF, Yelin EH, Nevitt M, Epstein WV. The impact of chronic disease: a sociomedical profile of rheumatoid arthritis. Arthritis Rheum 1981; 24:544–549.

37. Wolfe F, Cathey MA. The assessment and prediction of functional disability in rheumatoid arthritis. J Rheumatol 1991; 18:1298–1306.

38. Pincus T, Callahan LF. Taking mortality in rheumatoid arthritis seriously—predictive markers, socioeconomic status and comorbidity. J Rheumatol 1986; 13:841–845.

39. Mitchell DM, Spitz PW, Young DY, Bloch DA, McShane DJ, Fries JF. Survival, prognosis, and causes of death in rheumatoid arthritis. Arthritis Rheum 1986; 29:706–714.

40. Pincus T, Callahan LF, Vaughn WK. Questionnaire, walking time and button test measures of functional capacity as predictive markers for mortality in rheumatoid arthritis. J Rheumatol 1987; 14:240–251.

41. Pincus T. Is mortality increased in rheumatoid arthritis? J Musculoskel Med 1988; 5:27–46.

42. Ragan C, Farrington E. The clinical features of rheumatoid arthritis: prognostic indices. JAMA 1962; 181:663–667.

43. Pincus T. Rheumatoid arthritis: disappointing long-term outcomes despite successful short-term clinical trials. J Clin Epidemiol 1988; 41:1037–1041.

44. Wolfe F, Ross K, Hawley DJ, Roberts FK, Cathey MA. The prognosis of rheumatoid arthritis and undifferentiated polyarthritis in the clinic. J Rheumatol 1993 (in press).

45. Masi AT, Feigenbaum SL, Kaplan SB. Articular patterns in the early course of rheumatoid arthritis. Am J Med 1983; 75(suppl 6A):16–26.

46. Pincus T, Callahan LF, Burkhauser RV. Most chronic diseases are reported more frequently by individuals with fewer than 12 years of formal education in the age 18–64 United States population. J Chronic Dis 1987; 40:865–874.

47. Antonovsky A. Social class and the major cardiovascular diseases. J Chronic Dis 1968; 21:65–106.

48. Hinkle LE Jr, Whitney LH, Lehman EW, et al. Occupational, education, and coronary heart disease: risk is influenced more by education and background than by occupational experiences, in the Bell System. Science 1968; 161: 238–246.

49. Marmot MG, Rose G, Shipley M, Hamilton PJS. Employment grade and coronary heart disease in British civil servants. J Epidemiol Community Health 1978; 32:244–249.

50. Weinblatt E, Ruberman W, Goldberg JD, Frank CW, Shapiro S, Chaudhary BS. Relation of education to sudden death after myocardial infarction. N Engl J Med 1978; 299:60–65.

51. Rose G, Marmot MG. Social class and coronary heart disease. Br Heart J 1981; 45:13–19.

52. Weinblatt E, Goldberg JD, Ruberman W, Frank CW, Monk MA, Chaudhary BS. Mortality after first myocardial infarction: search for a secular trend. JAMA 1982; 247:1576–1581.

53. Ruberman W, Weinblatt E, Goldberg JD, Chaudhary BS. Education, psychosocial stress and sudden cardiac death. J Chronic Dis 1983; 36:151–160.

54. Ruberman W, Weinblatt E, Goldberg JD, Chaudhary BS. Psychosocial influences on mortality after myocardial infarction. N Engl J Med 1984; 311:552–559.

55. Buring JE, Evans DA, Fiore M, Rosner B, Hennekens CH. Occupation and risk of death from coronary heart disease. JAMA 1987; 258:791–792.

56. Matthews KA, Kelsey SF, Meilahn EN, Kuller LH, Wing RR. Educational attainment and behavioral and biologic risk factors for coronary heart disease in middle-aged women. Am J Epidemiol 1989; 129:1132–1144.

57. Lebowitz MD. The relationship of socio-environmental factors to the prevalence of obstructive lung diseases and other chronic conditions. J Chronic Dis 1977; 30:599–611.

58. Margolis PA, Greenberg RA, Keyes LL, et al. Lower respiratory illness in infants and low socioeconomic status. Am J Public Health 1992; 82:1119–1126.

59. Greenberg ER, Chute CG, Stukel T, et al. Social and economic factors in the choice of lung cancer treatment. N Engl J Med 1988; 318:612–617.

60. Steinhorn SC, Myers MH, Hankey BF, Pelham VF. Factors associated with survival differences between black women and white women with cancer of the uterine corpus. Am J Epidemiol 1986; 124:85–93.

61. Farley TA, Flannery JT. Late-stage diagnosis of breast cancer in women of lower socioeconomic status: public health implications. Am J Public Health 1989; 79:1508–1512.

62. Cella DF, Orav EJ, Kornblith AB, et al. Socioeconomic status and cancer survival. J Clin Oncol 1991; 9:1500–1509.

63. Kogevinas M, Marmot MG, Fox AJ, Goldblatt PO. Socioeconomic differences in cancer survival. J Epidemiol Community Health 1991; 45:216–219.

64. Zapka JG, Stoddard AM, Costanza ME, Greene HL. Breast cancer screening by mammography: utilization and associated factors. Am J Public Health 1989; 79:1499–1502.

65. White L, Katzman R, Losonczy K, et al. Associations of cognitive impairment with low education in three established populations for epidemiologic studies of the elderly. J Clin Epidemiol 1993.

66. Liu IY, LaCroiz AZ, White LR, Kittner SJ, Wolf PA. Cognitive impairment and mortality: a study of possible confounders. Am J Epidemiol 1990; 132 136–143.

67. Evans DA, Beckett LA, Albert MS, et al. Level of education and change in cognitive function in a community population of older persons. Ann Epidemiol 1993; 3:71–77.

68. Pincus T, Callahan LF. Formal education as a marker for increased mortality and morbidity in rheumatoid arthritis. J Chronic Dis 1985; 38:973–984.

69. Callahan LF, Pincus T. Formal education level as a significant marker of clinical status in rheumatoid arthritis. Arthritis Rheum 1988; 31:1346–1357.

70. Mitchell JM, Burkhauser RV, Pincus T. The importance of age, education, and comorbidity in the substantial earnings losses of individuals with symmetric polyarthritis. Arthritis Rheum 1988; 31:348–357.

71. Pincus T, Mitchell JM, Burkhauser RV. Substantial work disability and earnings losses in individuals less than age 65 with osteoarthritis: comparisons with rheumatoid arthritis. J Clin Epidemiol 1989; 42:449–457.

72. Callahan LF, Smith WJ, Pincus T. Self-report questionnaires in five rheumatic diseases: comparisons of health status constructs and associations with formal education level. Arthritis Care Res 1989; 2:122–131.

73. Engle EW, Callahan LF, Pincus T, Hochberg MC. Learned helplessness in systemic lupus erythematosus: analysis using the Rheumatology Attitudes Index. Arthritis Rheum 1990; 33:281–286.

74. Callahan LF, Bloch D, Pincus T. Identification of work disability in rheumatoid arthritis: physical, radiographic and laboratory variables do not add explanatory power to demographic and functional variables. J Clin Epidemiol 1992; 45:127–138.

75. Hannan MT, Anderson JJ, Pincus T, Felson DT. Educational attainment and osteoarthritis: differential associations with radiographic changes and symptom reporting. J Clin Epidemiol 1992; 45:139–147.

76. Kitagawa, EM, Hauser, PM. *Differential Mortality in the United States: A Study in Socioeconomic Epidemiology*, Cambridge: Harvard University Press, 1973:i–225.

77. Fuchs VR. Economics, health and post-industrial society. Milbank Mem Fund Q Health Soc 1979; 57:153–182.

78. Guralnik JM, Kaplan GA. Predictors of healthy aging: prospective evidence from the Alameda County Study. Am J Public Health 1989; 79:703–708.

79. Navarro V. Race or class versus race and class: mortality differentials in the United States. Lancet 1990; 336:1238–1240.

80. Rogot E, Sorlie PD, Johnson NJ. Life expectancy by employment status, income, and education in the National Longitudinal Mortality Study. Public Health Rep 1992; 107:457–461.

81. Black Research Working Group. *Inequalities in health (the black report)*, London: Department of Health and Social Security, 1980.

82. Pamuk ER. Social class inequality in mortality from 1921 to 1972 in England and Wales. Popul Stud 1985; 39:17–31.

83. Barker DJP, Osmond C. Infant mortality, childhood nutrition, and ischaemic heart disease in England and Wales. Lancet 1986; 1:1077–1081.

84. Blaxter M. Evidence of inequality in health from a national survey. Lancet 1987; 2:30–33.

85. Carstairs V, Morris R: Deprivation. explaining differences in mortality between Scotland and England and Wales. Br Med J 1989; 299:886–889.

86. Latour J, López V, Rodriguez M, Nolasco A, Alvarez-Dardet C. Inequalities in health in intensive care patients. J Clin Epidemiol 1991; 44:889–894.

87. LaVecchia C, Negri E, Pagano R, Decarli A. Education, prevalence of disease and frequency of health care utilisation: the 1983 Italian National Health Survey. J Epidemiol Community Health 1987; 41:161–165.

88. Kunst AE, Looman CWN, Mackenbach JP. Socio-economic mortality differences in the Netherlands in 1950–1984: a regional study of cause-specific mortality. Soc Sci Med 1990; 31:141–152.

89. Lagasse R, Humblet PC, Lenaerts A, Godin I, Moens GFG. Health and social inequities in Belgium. Soc Sci Med 1990; 31:237–248.

90. Jacobsen BK, Thelle DS. Risk factors for coronary heart disease and level of education: the Tromso Heart Study. Am J Epidemiol 1988; 127:923–932.

91. Måseide P. Health and social inequity in Norway. Soc Sci Med 1990; 31:331–342.

92. Lindgärde F, Furu M, Ljung B-O. A longitudinal study on the significance of environmental and individual factors associated with the development of essential hypertension. J Epidemiol Community Health 1987; 41:220–226.

93. Diderichsen F. Health and social inequities in Sweden. Soc Sci Med 1990; 31:359–367.

94. Koskenvuo M, Kaprio J, Kesäniemi A, Sarna S. Differences in mortality from ischemic heart disease by marital status and social class. J Chronic Dis 1980; 33:95–106.

95. Poikolainen K, Eskola J. The effect of health services on mortality: decline in death rates from amenable and non-amenable causes in Finland, 1969–81. Lancet 1986; 1:199–202.

96. Salonen JT. Socioeconomic status and risk of cancer, cerebral stroke, and death due to coronary heart disease and any disease: a longitudinal study in eastern Finland. J Epidemiol Community Health 1982; 36:294–297.

97. Lahelma E, Valkonen T. Health and social inequities in Finland and elsewhere. Soc Sci Med 1990; 31:257–265.

98. Dennis BH, Zhukovsky GS, Shestov DB, et al. The association of education with coronary heart disease mortality in the USSR Lipid Research Clinics Study. Int J Epidemiol 1993; 22:420–427.

99. Araki S, Murata K. Social life factors affecting the mortality of total Japanese population. Soc Sci Med 1986; 23:1163–1169.

100. Kagamimori S, Iibuchi Y, Fox J. A comparison of socioeconomic differences in mortality between Japan and England and Wales. World Health Stat Q 1983; 36:119–128.

101. Siskind V, Copeman R, Najman JM. Socioeconomic status and mortality: a Brisbane area analysis. Community Health Stud 1987; 11:15–23.

102. Pearce NE, Davis PB, Smith AH, Foster FH. Social class, ethnic group, and male mortality in New Zealand, 1974–8. J Epidemiol Community Health 1985; 39:9–14.

103. Kaplan GA, Seeman TE, Cohen RD, Knudsen LP, Guralnik J. Mortality among the elderly in the Alameda County Study: behavioral and demographic risk factors. Am J Public Health 1987; 77:307–312.

104. Branch LG, Ku L. Transition probabilities to dependency, institutionalization, and death among the elderly over a decade. J Aging Health 1989; 1:370–408.

105. Snowdon DA, Ostwald SK, Kane RL. Education, survival, and independence in elderly Catholic sisters, 1936–1988. Am J Epidemiol 1989; 120:999–1012.

106. Rogers RG: Living and dying in the USA: sociodemographic determinants of death among blacks and whites. Demography 1992; 29:287–303.

107. Guralnik JM, Land KC, Blazer D, Fillenbaum GG, Branch LG. Educational status and active expectancy among older blacks and whites. N Engl J Med 1993; 329:110–116.

108. Keil JE, Sutherland SE, Knapp RG, Lackland DT, Gazes PC, Tyroler HA. Mortality rates and risk factors for coronary disease in black as compared with white men and women. N Engl J Med 1993; 329:73–78.

109. Castaner A, Simmons BE, Mar M, Cooper R. Myocardial infarction among black patients: poor prognosis after hospital discharge. Ann Intern Med 1988; 109:33–35.

110. Epstein AM, Stern RS, Tognett J, et al. The association of patients' socioeconomic characteristics with the length of hospital stay and hospital charges within diagnosis-related groups. N Engl Med 1988; 318:1579–1585.

111. Marmot MG, Kogevinas M, Elston MA. Social/economic status and disease. Annu Rev Public Health 1987; 8:111–135.
112. Marmot MG, McDowall ME. Mortality decline and widening social inequalities. Lancet 1986; 2:274–276.
113. Smith GD, Bartley M, Blane D. The Black report on socioeconomic inequalities in health 10 years on. Br Med J 1990; 301:373–377.
114. Pincus T. Formal education level—a marker for the importance of behavioral variables in the pathogenesis, morbidity, and mortality of most diseases [editorial]? J Rheumatol 1988; 15:1457–1460.
115. Pincus T, Callahan LF. Associations of low formal education level and poor health status: behavioral, in addition to demographic and medical, explanations? J Clin Epidemiol 1994 (in press)
116. Nicassio PM, Wallston KA, Callahan LF, Herbert M, Pincus T. The measurement of helplessness in rheumatoid arthritis. The development of the Arthritis Helplessness Index. J Rheumatol 1985; 12:462–467.
117. Callahan LF, Brooks RH, Pincus T. Further analysis of learned helplessness in rheumatoid arthritis using a "Rheumatology Attitudes Index." J Rheumatol 1988; 15:418–426.
118. Berkson J. Limitations of the application of fourfold table analysis to hospital data. Biometric Bull 1946; 2:47–53.
119. Pincus T, Callahan LF, Mitchell JM. Increased mortality in rheumatoid arthritis is explained in part on the basis of extensive comorbidity with other diseases. Arthritis Rheum 1987; 30(suppl 4):S12 (Abstract).
120. *Balliere's clinical rheumatology, vol. 2*, London. WB Saunders, 1988.
121. Nevitt MC, Yelin EH, Henke CJ, Epstein WV. Risk factors for hospitalization and surgery in patients with rheumatoid arthritis: implications for capitated medical payment. Ann Intern Med 1986; 105:421–428.
122. Sherrer YS, Bloch DA, Mitchell DM, Roth SH, Wolfe F, Fries JF. Disability in rheumatoid arthritis: comparison of prognostic factors across three populations. J Rheumatol 1987; 14:705–709.
123. Lubeck DP, Spitz PW, Fries JF, Wolfe F, Mitchell DM, Roth SH. A multicenter study of annual health service utilization and costs in rheumatoid arthritis. Arthritis Rheum 1986; 29:488–493.
124. Pincus T, Callahan LF, Brooks RH, Fuchs HA, Olsen NJ, Kaye JJ. Self-report questionnaire scores in rheumatoid arthritis compared with traditional physical, radiographic, and laboratory measures. Ann Intern Med 1989; 110:259–266.
125. Bombardier C, Ware J, Russell IJ, et al. Auranofin therapy and quality of life in patients with rheumatoid arthritis: results of a multicenter trial. Am J Med 1986; 81:565–578.
126. Meenan RF, Pincus T. The status of patient status measures. J Rheumatol 1987; 14:411–414.
127. Brooks RH, Callahan LF, Pincus T. Use of self-report activities of daily living questionnaires in osteoarthritis. Arthritis Care Res 1988; 1:23–32.
128. Hawley DJ, Wolfe F. Sensitivity to change of the Health Assessment Questionnaire (HAQ) and other clinical and health status measures in rheumatoid arthritis: results of short term clinical trials and observational studies versus long term observational studies. Arthritis Care Res 1992; 5:130–136.

129. Fries JF, Spitz P, Kraines RG, Holman, HR. Measurement of patient outcome in arthritis. Arthritis Rheum 1980; 23:137–145.

130. Meenan RF, Gertman PM, Mason JH. Measuring health status in arthritis: the Arthritis Impact Measurement Scales. Arthritis Rheum 1980; 23:146–152.

131. Pincus T, Summey JA, Soraci SA Jr, Wallston KA, Hummon NP. Assessment of patient satisfaction in activities of daily living using a modified Stanford health assessment questionnaire. Arthritis Rheum 1983; 26:1346–1353.

132. Tugwell P, Bombardier C, Buchanan WW, Goldsmith CH, Grace E, Hanna B. The MACTAR Patient Preference Disability Questionnaire—an individualized functional priority approach for assessing improvement in physical disability in clinical trials in rheumatoid arthritis. J Rheumatol 1987; 14:446–451.

133. Liang MH, Fossel AH, Larson MG. Comparisons of five health status instruments for orthopedic evaluation. Med Care 1990; 28:632–642.

134. Kazis LE, Callahan LF, Meenan RF, Pincus T. Health status reports in the care of patients with rheumatoid arthritis. J Clin Epidemiol 1990; 43:1243–1253.

135. Pincus T, Brooks RH, Callahan LF. Reliability of grip strength, walking time and button test performed according to a standard protocol. J Rheumatol 1991; 18:997–1000.

136. Kaye JJ, Nance EP, Callahan LF, et al. Observer variation in quantitative assessment of rheumatoid arthritis: part II. A simplified scoring system. Invest Radiol 1987; 22:41–46.

137. Feigenbaum PA, Medsger TA Jr, Kraines RG, Fires JF. The variability of immunologic laboratory tests. J Rheumatol 1982; 9:408–414.

138. Pincus T, Callahan LF. Rheumatology Function Tests: grip strength, walking time, button test and questionnaires document and predict longterm morbidity and mortality in rheumatoid arthritis. J Rheumatol 1992; 19:1051–1057.

139. Olsen NJ, Callahan LF, Brooks RH, et al. Associations of HLA-DR4 with rheumatoid factor and radiographic severity in rheumatoid arthritis. Am J Med 1988; 84:257–264.

140. Fuchs HA, Callahan LF, Kaye JJ, Brooks RH, Nance EP, Pincus T. Radiographic and joint count findings of the hand in rheumatoid arthritis: related and unrelated findings. Arthritis Rheum 1988; 31:44–51.

141. Angell M. Disease as a reflection of the psyche [editorial]. N Engl J Med 1985; 312:1570–1572.

142. Spergel P, Ehrlich GE, Glass D. The rheumatoid arthritic personality: a psychodiagnostic myth. Psychosomatics 1978; 19:79–86.

143. Pincus T, Callahan LF. Depression scales in rheumatoid arthritis: criterion contamination in interpretation of patient responses. Patient Educ Couns 1993; 20:133–143.

144. Pincus T, Callahan LF, Bradley LA, Vaughn WK, Wolfe F. Elevated MMPI scores for hypochondriasis, depression, and hysteria in patients with rheumatoid arthritis reflect disease rather than psychological status. Arthritis Rheum 1986; 29:1456–1466.

145. Peck JR, Smith TW, Ward JR, Milano R. Disability and depression in rheumatoid arthritis: a multi-trait, multi-method investigation. Arthritis Rheum 1989; 32:1100–1106.

146. Blalock SJ, DeVellis RF, Brown GK, Wallston KA. Validity of the Center for Epidemiological Studies Depression Scale in arthritis populations. Arthritis Rheum 1989; 32:991–997.

147. Callahan LF, Kaplan MR, Pincus T. The Beck Depression Inventory, Center for Epidemiological Studies Depression Scale (CES-D), and General Well-being Schedule Depression Subscale in rheumatoid arthritis: criterion contamination of responses. Arthritis Care Res 1991; 4:3–11.

148. Hawley DJ, Wolfe F. Anxiety and depression in patients with rheumatoid arthritis: a prospective study of 400 patients. J Rheumatol 1988; 15:932–941.

149. Stein MJ, Walston KA, Nicassio PM. Factor structure of the Arthritis Helplessness Index. J Rheumatol 1988; 15:427–432.

150. DeVellis RF, Callahan LF. A brief measure of helplessness in rheumatic disease: the helplessness subscale of the Rheumatology Attitudes Index. J Rheumatol 1993; 20:866–869.

151. Hawley DJ, Wolfe F, Cathey MA. The sense of coherence questionnaire in patients with rheumatic disorders. J Rheumatol 1992; 19:1912–1918.

152. Callahan LF, Pincus T. The Sense of Coherence Scale in rheumatoid arthritis. 1994. (submitted)

153. Lorig K, Seleznick M, Lubeck D, Ung E, Chastain RL, Holman HR. The beneficial outcomes of the arthritis self-management course are not adequately explained by behavior change. Arthritis Rheum 1989; 32:91–95.

154. Lorig K, Chastain RL, Ung E, Shoor S, Holman HR. Development and evaluation of a scale to measure perceived self-efficacy in people with arthritis. Arthritis Rheum 1989; 32:37–44.

155. Kelley, WN, Harris, ED Jr, Ruddy S, Sledge CB, eds. *Textbook of rheumatology*, 2nd. Ed. Philadephia: W.B.Saunders, 1985.

156. Kelley, WN, Harris, ED Jr, Ruddy S, Sledge CB. *Textbook of rheumatology*, Ed. 3rd. Philadelphia: W.B.Saunders, 1989:943.

157. When are corticosteroids worth the risk for rheumatoid arthritis patients? J Musculoskel Med 1984; 1:48–53.

158. Allebeck P, Ahlbom A, Allander E. Increased mortality among persons with rheumatoid arthritis, but where RA does not appear on death certificate: eleven year follow-up of an epidemiological study. Scand J Rheumatol 1981; 10:301–306.

159. Cobb S, Anderson F, Bauer W. Length of life and cause of death in rheumatoid arthritis. N Engl J Med 1953; 249:553–556.

160. *Prognosis in the rheumatic diseases,* Dordrecht:Kluwer Academic Publishers, 1991.

161. Monson RR, Hall AP. Mortality among arthritics. J Chronic Dis 1976; 29:459–467.

162. Rasker JJ, Cosh JA. Cause and age at death in a prospective study of 100 patients with rheumatoid arthritis. Ann Rheum Dis 1981; 40:115–120.

163. Vandenbroucke JP, Hazevoet HM, Cats A. Survival and cause of death in rheumatoid arthrits: a 25-year prospective followup. J Rheumatol 1984; 11:158–161.

164. Mutru O, Laakso M, Isomäki H, Koota K. Ten year mortality and causes of death in patients with rheumatoid arthritis. Br Med J 1985; 290:1811–1813.

165. Vollertsen RS, Conn DL, Ballard DJ, Ilstrup DM, Kazmar RE, Silverfield JC. Rheumatoid vasculitis: survival and associated risk factors. Medicine (Baltimore) 1986; 65:365–375.

166. Wolfe F, Mitchell DM, Sibley JT, et al. The mortality of rheumatoid arthritis. Arthritis Rheum 1994 (in press)

167. Duthie JJR, Brown PE, Truelove LH, Baragar FD, Lawrie AJ. Course and prognosis in rheumatoid arthritis: a further report. Ann Rheum Dis 1964; 23:193–204.

168. Rasker JJ, Cosh JA. The natural history of rheumatoid arthritis: a fifteen year follow-up study. The prognostic significance of features noted in the first year. Clin Rheumatol 1984; 3:11–20.

169. Gordon DA, Stein JL, Broder I. The extra-articular features of rheumatoid arthritis: a systematic analysis of 127 cases. Am J Med 1973; 54:445–452.

170. Proudfit WL, Bruschke AVG, Sones FM Jr. Natural history of obstructive coronary artery disease: ten-year study of 601 nonsurgical cases. Prog Cardiovasc Dis 1978; 21:53–78.

171. Kaplan HS. Survival as related to treatment. In: Kaplan HS, *Hodgkin's disease*. Cambridge: Harvard University Press, 1972:360–388.

172. McCarty, D.J. *Arthritis and allied conditions: a textbook of rheumatology*, 11th Ed. Philadelphia:Lea & Febiger, 1989. pp. 735.

173. Kushner I. Does aggressive therapy of rheumatoid arthritis affect outcome [editorial]. J Rheumatol 1989; 16:1–4.

174. Wolfe F, Hawley DJ. Remission in rheumatoid arthritis. J Rheumatol 1985; 12:245–252.

175. Richter JA, Runge LA, Pinals RS, Oates RP. Analysis of treatment termination with gold and antimalarial compounds in rheumatoid arthritis. J Rheumatol 1980; 7:153–159.

176. Amor B, Herson D, Cherot A, Delbarre F. Polyarthrites rhumatoïdes évoluant depuis plus de 10 ans (1966–1978). Analyse de l'évolution et des traitements de 100 cas. Ann Med Interne (Paris) 1981; 132:168–173.

177. Situnayake RD, Grindulis KA, McConkey B. Long term treatment of rheumatoid arthritis with sulphasalazine, gold, or penicillamine: a comparison using life-table methods. Ann Rheum Dis 1987; 46:177–183.

178. Thompson PW, Kirwan JR, Barnes CG. Practical results of treatment with disease-modifying antirheumatoid drugs. Br J Rheumatol 1985; 24:167–175.

179. Hoffmeister RT. Methotrexate in rheumatoid arthritis. Arthritis Rheum 1972; 15(suppl):S114. (Abstract)

180. Hoffmeister RT. Methotrexate therapy in rheumatoid arthritis: 15 years experience. Am J Med 1983; 75(suppl 6A):69–73.

181. Hoffmeister RT. The early years, uncontrolled studies. In: Wilke WS, *Methotrexate therapy in rheumatic disease*. New York: Marcel Dekker, Inc., 1989: 37–43.

182. Wolfe F, Hawley DJ, Cathey MA. Termination of slow acting antirheumatic therapy in rheumatoid arthritis: a 14-year prospective evaluation of 1017 consecutive starts. J Rheumatol 1990; 17:994–1002.

183. Wolfe F, Cathey MA. Analysis of methotrexate treatment effect in a longitudinal observational study: utility of cluster analysis. J Rheumatol 1991; 18:672–677.

184. Pincus T, Marcum SB, Callahan LF. Long-term drug therapy for rheumatoid arthritis in seven rheumatology private practices: II. Second-line drugs and prednisone. J Rheumatol 1992; 19:1885–1894,.

185. Wilske KR. Inverting the therapeutic pyramid: observations and recommendations on new directions in rheumatoid arthritis based on the author's experience. Semin Arthritis Rheum[Suppl 1] 1993; 23:11–18.

186. Friedman, LM, Furberg, CD, DeMets, DL *Fundamentals of clinical trials,* Littleton:John Wright - PSG Inc., 1984. 1–225.

187. Feinstein AR. An additional basic science for clinical medicine: II. the limitations of randomized trials. Ann Intern Med 1983; 99:544–550.

188. Paulus HE, Egger MJ, Ward JR, Williams HJ. Cooperative Systematic Studies of Rheumatic Diseases Group: analysis of improvement in individual rheumatoid arthritis patients treated with disease-modifying antirheumatic drugs, based on the findings in patients treated with placebo. Arthritis Rheum 1990; 33:477–484.

189. Gotzche PC. Sensitivity of effect variables in rheumatoid arthritis: a meta-analysis of 130 placebo controlled NSAID trials. J Clin Epidemiol 1990; 43:1313–1318.

190. Pincus T, Marcum SB, Callahan LF, et al. Long-term drug therapy for rheumatoid arthritis in seven rheumatology private practices: I. Nonsteroidal anti-inflammatory drugs. J Rheumatol 1992; 19:1874–1884.

191. Felson DT, Anderson JJ, Meenan RF. The comparative efficacy and toxicity of second-line drugs in rheumatoid arthritis: results of two metaanalyses. Arthritis Rheum 1990; 33:1449–1461.

192. Williams HJ, Ward JR, Reading JC, et al. Comparison of auranofin, methotrexate, and the combination of both in the treatment of rheumatoid arthritis: a controlled clinical trial. Arthritis Rheum 1992; 35:259–269.

193. Wilske KR, Healey LA. Remodeling the pyramid—a concept whose time has come. J Rheumatol 1989; 16:565–567.

194. Fries JF. Reevaluating the therapeutic approach to rheumatoid arthritis: the ''sawtooth'' strategy. J Rheumatol 1990; 17[Suppl 2]:12–15.

195. McCarty DJ. Suppress rheumatoid inflammation early and leave the pyramid to the Egyptians. J Rheumatol 1990; 17:1115–1118.

196. Paulus HE. The use of combinations of disease-modifying antirheumatic agents in rheumatoid arthritis. Arthritis Rheum 1990; 33:113–120.

197. Bunch TW, Worthington JW, Combs JJ, Ilstrup DM, Engel AG. Azathioprine with prednisone for polymyositis: a controlled, clinical trial. Ann Intern Med 1980; 92:365–369.

198. Bunch TW. Prednisone and azathioprine for polymyositis: long-term followup. Arthritis Rheum 1981; 24:45–48.

199. Donadio JV Jr, Holley KE, Wagoner RD, Ferguson RH, McDuffie FC. Treatment of lupus nephritis with prednisone and combined prednisone and azathioprine. Ann Intern Med 1972; 77:829–835.

200. Hahn BH, Kantor OS, Osterland CK. Azathipprine plus prednisone compared with prednisone alone in the treatment of systemic lupus erythematosus: report of a prospective controlled trial in 24 patients. Ann Intern Med 1975; 83:597–605.

201. Cade R, Spooner G, Schlein E, et al. Comparison of azathioprine, prednisone, and heparin alone or combined in treating lupus nephritis. Nephron 1973; 10:37–56.

202. Felson DT, Anderson J. Evidence for the superiority of immunosuppressive drugs and prednisone over prednisone alone in lupus nephritis: results of a pooled analysis. N Engl J Med 1984; 311:1528–1533.

203. Steinberg AD, Decker JL. A double-blind controlled trial comparing cyclophosphamide, azathioprine and placebo in the treatment of lupus glomerulonephritis. Arthritis Rheum 1974; 17:923–937.

204. Klippel JH. Studies in the treatment of lupus nephritis, 599–602. In: Decker, J.L., moderator. Systemic lupus erythematosus: evolving concepts. Ann Intern Med 1979; 91:587–604.

205. Austin HA,III, Klippel JH, Balow JE, et al. Therapy of lupus nephritis: controlled trial of prednisone and cytotoxic drugs. N Engl J Med 1986; 314:614–619.

1

The Pathogenesis of Rheumatoid Arthritis

Gabriel S. Panayi

United Medical and Dental Schools of Guy's and St. Thomas's Hospitals
London, England

I. INTRODUCTION

In the recent past, our view of the pathogenesis of rheumatoid arthritis (RA) was that of a relatively simple process based on the formation of immune complexes and the activation of the complement cascade. Although this may still be true for some of the inflammation seen in the joint and for the pathogenesis of extra-articular features, such as vasculitis, the major contributor to the pathogenesis of the synovitis and the joint destruction is now thought to be cellular mechanisms initiated by the activation of T lymphocytes.

The normal synovial membrane (SM) consists of a loose areolar connective tissue that contains some blood vessels and is lined by the synovial-lining layer. This is not a true epithelium, as it does not possess a basement membrane. It is two- to three-cell–layers thick and consists of macrophages (type A cells) and synoviocytes (type B cells). The normal synovial membrane has only a minor infiltrate of lymphocytes and macrophages within the connective tissue. In RA the picture changes dramatically. The whole synovial membrane becomes hyperplastic and hypertrophic, which is detectable clinically as soft-tissue swelling of the joint. This swelling is partly due to edema fluid, consequent to increased vascular permeability, but mainly to the entry of leukocytes from the bloodstream and the local proliferation of synoviocytes, blood vessels, and lymphatics. The leukocytes that enter the joint are neutrophils, T and B lymphocytes, and monocytes. The neutrophils are not retained within the synovium, but accumulate within the synovial fluid where they constitute most of the cell population. The T lymphocytes accumulate as perivascular lymphocytic aggregates intimately

75

intermingled with dendritic antigen-presenting cells (1). Other T cells are found scattered within the synovial tissue but, interestingly, are not found within the lining layer. The B lymphocytes and plasma cells are found scattered either diffusely within the tissue or as well-organized and discrete lymphoid follicles. Macrophages are found within the perivascular lymphocytic aggregates, the synovial-lining layer, and scattered diffusely within the connective tissue. The increased numbers of macrophages, which have arrived there after migrating from the blood, and of synoviocytes, which have arisen by local proliferation, results in the lining layer becoming several cell layers thick. There is an expansion in the number of blood vessels and of lymphatics within the synovial membrane. The postcapillary venules have high, plump, and activated endothelial cells, and it is here that most leukocyte migration is believed to occur. Little is known about the state of the lymphatics within the rheumatoid synovial membrane.

For these changes to come about, a series of complex events have to take place and, for ease of understanding, they can be conveniently divided into different stages, although it must be clearly understood that, in the fully developed lesion, all stages are likely to be operating. This is the probable explanation of why most investigators have found a variable histological picture in different parts of the same synovial membrane. These stages may be classified as follows:

Stage 1: Initiation
Stage 2: Recruitment
Stage 3: Amplification and joint destruction
Stage 4: Repair

The merit of this classification (Fig. 1) is that it helps when thinking of possible targets for the development of new therapies. It may also help in defusing the present debate on which is the most important cell in the pathogenesis of RA, whether T cell, macrophage, or synoviocyte, by focusing on the cellular interactions that are taking place within the synovium and that have different cellular protagonists at different times. However, the merit of any scheme is whether it has any usefulness in practice, and only time will settle that question.

II. STAGE 1: INITIATION

The initiation of RA is shrouded in mystery. We do not know whether the disease has a long latent interval, or whether it arises suddenly following some unknown insult. A recent study from Finland has produced evidence that antibodies to the stratum corneum of the rat esophagus, which are thought to be highly specific for RA, may be found in the sera of individuals years before the onset of disease (2). If confirmed, this then has important implications for screening and, possibly, for active treatment during the pre- or subclinical phases of the disease to abort its full-blown development. Such preventive measures are being attempted in

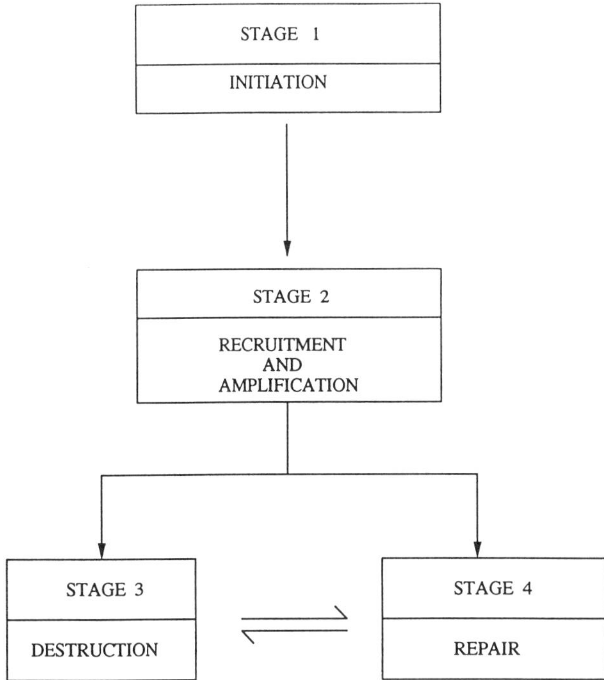

Fig. 1 The different stages in the pathogenesis of rheumatoid arthritis; they may be present at the same time, but in different parts of the same synovial membrane.

type I juvenile diabetes, in which disease markers have been better characterized, but as yet, with only limited success.

A. Epidemiological Studies

Epidemiological studies have not uncovered any obvious predisposing factor or event before the onset of RA. The impressive difference in prevalence of RA in the Xhosa of South Africa between those who live in a rural environment (3), where RA is absent, and those who live in the Soweto township (4), in which the prevalence and severity are similar to neighboring whites living in Johannesburg, does not help in unraveling this mystery, as the differences between the two environments are too many and complex. In our own study (5) comparing the clinical expression of RA in Greek and British patients with the disease, we found that the less severe disease in the former could not be entirely accounted for by differences in the prevalence of the histocompatibility antigen HLA-DR4, which was significantly lower in the Greeks, but that environmental factors may also be of importance. Of these, we singled out the immunosuppressive effects of sunshine (6) and dietary differences, such as the higher consumption of olive oil with its anti-inflammatory properties (7), as being of possible relevance.

B. Immunogenetic Studies

The best clue to the initiating event in RA is provided by immunogenetic studies. Rheumatoid arthritis is strongly associated with HLA-DR4 and HLA-DR1 in most populations yet studied (see Chapter 3). The main, if not sole, function of HLA-DR molecules is to present antigen to T cells as the first step in their activation. Antigen-presenting cells (macrophages, dendritic cells, and B lymphocytes) take up antigens by phagocytosis and processes them into antigenic fragments that are then presented on the surface of the antigen-presenting cell in the groove of the HLA molecule. A plausible hypothesis can be constructed on the premise that the articular cartilage contains autoantigens to which the individual is not tolerant; this is not unlikely, since the articular cartilage does not possess a vascular or lymphatic supply, both of which are necessary for the entry of antigens into the systemic circulation and of immune cells into the target tissue. Several possibilities can then be invoked for the initiation and maintenance of RA. First, it is possible that it could be initiated by an external agent acting in "a hit-and-run" manner such that it does not persist, but causes release of sequestered autoantigens so that RA is subsequently maintained by the induction of autoimmunity. Second, a molecular mimicry scenario would propose that transient infection with an agent that has sequences identical with a sequestered cartilage autoantigen could initiate the whole event. Third, an endogenous virus could be activated within the chondrocyte, leading to damage of the cartilage, with the release of autoantigens and the initiation of autoimmunity. Interestingly, in the transgenic TNFα mouse, it is necessary for the transgene to be expressed by the chondrocytes before destructive, inflammatory arthritis can be induced (8; Kollias G, personal communication). Several autoantigens have been proposed, but their exact role in the etiopathogenesis of RA is still unclear. These autoantigens include type II collagen (9,10), cartilage proteoglycan (11), and heat-shock proteins (12,13). We have not been able to demonstrate, by a limiting dilution analysis technique, an increased frequency of T cells responding to the mycobacterial 65-kDa heat-shock protein in the synovial fluid, as compared with the peripheral blood of patients with RA (14); a higher frequency in the fluid should have been found if the 65-kDa heat-shock protein was indeed operating as an antigen within the joint. Although T-cell clones to these antigens have been grown, their response is not restricted by HLA-DR4, which questions their relevance in view of the importance of HLA-DR4 relevance in view of the importance of HLA-DR4 in antigen presentation.

Another form of antigen that can be presented by HLA-DR molecules is superantigen. Superantigen is presented by macrophages or other antigen-presenting cells, without any processing, to the V_β chain of the T-cell receptor; superantigens can bind to different HLA-DR molecules, but bind to a single or only a limited number of T-cell receptor V_β chains. Thus, a superantigen may interact with different DR molecules and is, therefore, not restricted by any particular major histocompatibility complex (MHC) molecule, but only to a restricted set of T cells characterized by a particular V_β T-cell receptor. Following this interaction, the T cell is activated to release lymphokines and to proliferate. Superantigens may be of bacterial origin, such as the staphylococcal exotoxins, or of viral origin. Evidence for viral superantigens in human disease is still limited, although human immunodeficiency virus (HIV) may be such a candidate. The possible involvement of superantigens in RA has been raised by the observation that one-third of synovial fluids, from patients with RA, have expanded usage of the $V_\beta 14$ T-cell receptor chain (15). Usage of this T-cell receptor V_β chain is rare in the blood of normal individuals. Indeed, some of the RA patients did not use this V_β chain in their blood T cells, but did so in the joint cells. However, other investigators have not observed this restriction, whereas still others have found that $V_\beta 2$ (16) or other V_β may or may not be expanded in the joint (for more extended reviews see Refs. 17,18). These differences mean that more work needs to be done before a consensus will be reached.

The failure to find a restricted T-cell population in the joint may, however, be due to several other factors, which need to be considered. First, in lesions in which the antigen involved is known, such as the skin in tuberculoid leprosy, the frequency of antigen-specific T cells is of the order of 1:300–1:1500 (19–22). Clearly, attempts to detect this population by the approaches now being used for the rheumatoid joint are doomed to failure. The most rational approach is to clone the T cells responding to the ''rheumatoid antigen''; as this is unknown, this cannot be done. Second, bacterial superantigens bind to the DR molecules expressed on rheumatoid synoviocytes and stimulate them to produce cytokines (23). This mechanism, if operative in the RA synovial membrane, could explain the failure to find a restricted population of T cells within the joint. The weakness of this hypothesis is that it explains neither the restriction of the disease to the diarthrodial joints, nor its association with HLA-DR4/DR1. Third, the use of transgenic animals has shown that an erosive synovitis, similar to that of RA, may be produced without the initial participation of T cells. One model is the mouse transgenic for the *tax* gene of the human T-cell lymphotropic virus type 1 (HTLV-I) in which there is up-regulated production of several cytokines within the joint (24). The other is the mouse transgenic for the human tumor necrosis factor-alpha (TNF-α) gene which produces large amounts of TNF-α within the joint (8). Again, the weakness of both these models is that they do not account for the HLA-DR association of the disease. They do suggest, however, possible mechanisms by which the disease could become self-perpetuating after some unknown initiating event.

III. STAGE 2: RECRUITMENT

The hypertrophy of the synovium that takes place during rheumatoid inflammation is largely the result of two processes: the entry of leukocytes from the blood, and the expansion by cell division of synoviocytes, lymphatic cells, and endothelial cells already present within the synovium. This stage 2 of recruitment must follow the presumed initiation event, or stage 1, described in the foregoing (see Fig. 1). Some support for this staging is provided by the observations that the earliest change observed in the rheumatoid synovium is a perivascular aggregate of lymphocytes and increased thickness of the synovial lining layer. This stage is critically dependent on activation of endothelial cells (EC) by cytokines to facilitate the entry of leukocytes into the joint (Table 1).

Stage 2 comes about as a result of the interactions of antigen-presenting cells and T cells during stage 1 of initiation. The T cell releases interferon gamma (IFN-γ) and interleukin-2 (IL-2). As a consequence, the endothelial cells are activated by IFN-γ and TNF-α so that they are more adhesive for blood leukocytes, thereby facilitating their entry into the synovium; in addition, activated EC secrete a large number of cytokines, which act on other cells as well on EC in an autocrine manner (Table 2). Endothelial cells have several roles to play in the pathophysiology of rheumatoid synovitis (Fig. 2), which will be considered in this review. Interferon gamma will also activate macrophages so that they, in turn, release other monokines, such as TNF-α and IL-1. Let us consider these processes, which are illustrated in Fig. 3, in greater detail.

Table 1 Cytokines Activating Endothelial Cells and the Adhesion Molecules Up-Regulated as a Consequence

Cytokine	Adhesion molecule[a]
Tumor necrosis factor-α	VCAM-1
Interleukin-4	
Interleukin-1	
Interferon gamma	ICAM-1
Interleukin-1	
Tumor necrosis factor-α	
Interleukin-1	ELAM-1
Tumor necrosis factor-α	
Interferon gamma	

[a]VACM-1, vascular cell adhesion molecule 1; ICAM-1, intercellular adhesion molecule 1; ELAM-1, endothelial leukocyte adhesion molecule 1.

Table 2 Cytokines Produced by Endothelial Cells

Cytokine	Cell target	Function
IL-1	Lymphocytes,	Inflammation
	Monocytes	Acute-phase response
		Hematopoiesis
IL-6	Lymphocytes	Acute-phase response
		Hematopoiesis
IL-8	Neutrophils	Leukocyte recruitment
		Leukocyte activation
MCP[a]	Monocytes	Leukocyte recruitment
G-, M-, GM-CSF	Neutrophils	Hematopoiesis
	Monocytes	Leukocyte recruitment
	Eosinophils	Leukocyte activation

[a]MCP, monocyte chemotactic proteins(s).

A.   Leukocyte–Endothelial Cell Interactions

The important leukocytes from the present point of view are monocytes and T lymphocytes. The process can be divided into distinct phases (see Fig. 3): *phase I*, EC adherence; *phase II*, EC and tissue transmigration; *phase III*, retention within the tissue because of adhesion to connective tissue matrix fibrillar components; and *phase IV*, homo- and heterotypic adhesion between different cells. Phase I has been recently reviewed (25).

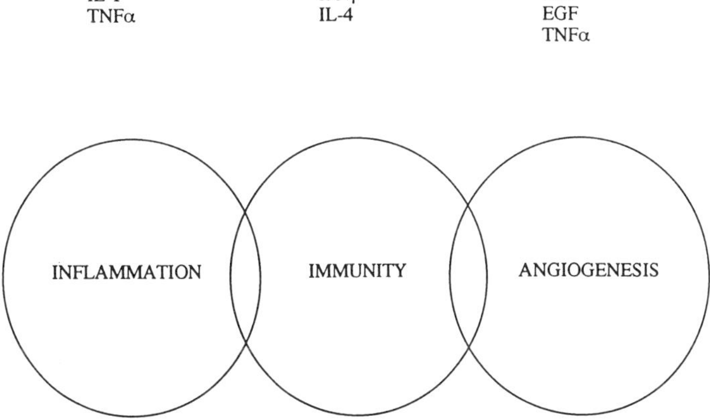

Fig. 2 Effects of different cytokines on endothelial cell functions.

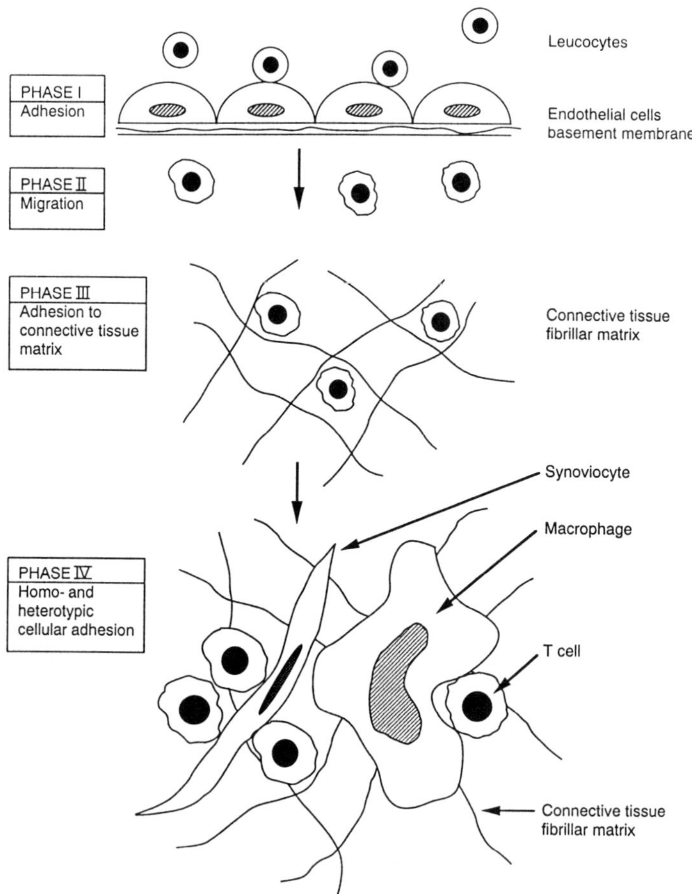

Fig. 3   The different phases in the exit from the circulation and migration through the tissue of leukocytes (neutrophils, monocytes, lymphocytes).

The Entry, Persistence, and Maturation of Monocytes in the Synovium

Phase I.   Monocytes (MO) are constantly leaving the circulation to enter tissues. The first stage of migration is by adhesion onto EC through the CD14 receptor on their surface binding to an unknown ligand on the EC (26), lymphocyte function associate antigen 1 (LFA-1) (27), and the complement receptor CR3 (28). The subsequent phases of migration have not been investigated in detail, but it is assumed that phase II is brought about by the release of enzymes, phase III by the adhesion onto extracellular matrix components, and phase IV by homo- and heterotypic intercellular adhesion, which is considered in greater detail later.

Monocytes are not a recirculating cell and have a finite life span that can be extended if they mature into tissue macrophages (MAC). Recent work has shown that monocytes will die by apoptosis, or programmed cell death, unless they are rescued by inflammatory cytokines, such as IL-1, TNF-α, and granolocyte–macrophage colony-stimulating factor (GM-CSF) (29). It is, therefore, probable that the increased numbers of monocytes found in the rheumatoid synovial membrane is the consequence of two interrelated processes: increased entry into the synovial membrane and increased survival because of the outpouring of inflammatory cytokines within the joint. Because of this increased entry and survival of monocytes, there is a large and obvious increase in the number of mature tissue macrophages seen within the synovial membrane. Of the many monokines produced by monocytes, the two of greatest importance are IL-1 and TNF-α. They have almost completely overlapping functions (Table 3), although some workers have proposed that TNF-α may be higher in a lymphokine cascade than IL-1 and, thus, able to regulate its function. Monocytes mature into macrophages, and this can be accelerated by cytokines, such as GM-CSF and 1, 25-dihydroxyvitamin D3 (30). Macrophages appear to be less capable of releasing inflammatory cytokines, such as IL-1, but more able to release anti-inflammatory substances, such as interleukin 1 receptor antagonist (IL-1ra) (30,31). Sodium aurothiomalate has been shown to accelerate monocyte to macrophage maturation (32), and we have shown that it causes reduced synovial expression of cytokines such as IL-1, TNFα, IL-8, and GM-CSF (33,34). Thus, gold salts may have two important anti-inflammatory actions during the treatment of RA: decreased cytokine production, which will bring about apoptotic monocyte death; and accelerated maturation to macrophaphes, which will increase the production of anti-inflammatory factors such as IL-1ra.

Table 3   Some of the Properties of IL-1 and TNF-α of Relevance to the Pathogenesis of Rheumatoid Arthritis

Increased endothelial cell adhesion molecule expression
Collagenase and PGE_2 production
Bone and cartilage resorption
Induction of other cytokines (IL-8, IL-6, PDGF, IL-1, GM-CSF)
HLA class II expression (TNF-α only)
Acute-phase response
Stimulation of hypothalamus (fever; release of cortisol by adrenal gland)

The Entry of T Cells Into and Their Persistence in the Synovium

Phase I.   The first phase of the entry of T cells into the synovium consists of their adhesion to EC (see Fig. 3). It should be remembered that T cells can be divided into two major populations on phenotypic, as defined by monoclonal antibodies, and functional grounds; naive T cells have not been stimulated by antigen, whereas memory T cells have been. The overwhelming number of T cells belong to the memory population, and any pathogenetic scheme needs to account for this observation (35). The CD45RO-positive memory T cells show increased adhesivencss to rcsting as well as to cytokine-stimulated EC when compared with naive CD45RA-positive T cells (36), and this is enhanced by T-cell activation (37). This increased adhesiveness is due to the action of several receptor–ligand pairs on the surface of lymphocytes and EC, respectively, including LFA-1–ICAM-1, VLA-4–VCAM-1, and an unknown receptor, probably related to asialyl Lewis X, with ELAM-1 (reviewed in 38). Activated CD45RO T cells can directly act through cell-to-cell contact on endothelial cells to up-regulate the expression of endothelial adhesion ligands, thereby enhancing lymphocyte recruitment into inflammatory foci (39) and to augment endothelial permeability to macromolecules (40). We have shown that the treatment of RA patients with intramuscular sodium aurothiomalate decreased synovial membrane expression of ELAM-1 (41).

Phase II.   The subsequent steps of migration through the EC layer and basement membrane of the postcapillary venule are not fully understood, but are thought to involve LFA-1–ICAM-1 (42). The T cells may use enzymatic activity to breach this barrier, but little is known about such a process, although activated lymphocytes are known to secrete several endo- and exopeptidases. Once having arrived in the tissue, T cells may be retained there by several mechanisms.

Phase III.   One is their adherence to connective tissue components such as fibronectin, collagen, and laminin by integrins such as VLA-4, VLA-5, and VLA-6 (43,44).

Phase IV.   Another is the adhesion to other cells found within the synovium; when the adhesion is to cells of a different phenotype (synoviocytes, macrophages, antigen-presenting cells), it is known as heterotypic adhesion, and an example of this is the adhesion of synovial T cells to synoviocytes, which is partially mediated by CD2–LFA-3 interactions (45). When it is to other lymphocytes, it is known as homotypic adhesion and is mediated by VLA-4 (46), CD44 (47), and LFA-1 (48), and their respective ligands. All these mechanisms collectively ensure that T cells are recruited into, and retained within, the RA synovial membrane.

IV. STAGE 3: AMPLIFICATION AND JOINT DESTRUCTION

Amplification and joint destruction, stage 3 of the pathogenetic scheme, is characterized by the release of cytokines, neuropeptides, enzymes, and other inflammatory mediators that are responsible for the inflammatory changes and the destruction of bone and articular cartilage so characteristic of RA. These changes are too diverse to be covered in detail here; selected areas have been covered in recent reviews [neuropetides (2), radicals (49), and prostanoids (50)] and should be consulted by those interested in them. Here we shall confine ourselves to reviewing the role of cytokines and of some important enzymes.

A. Cytokines in the Amplification of Inflammation

Immediately we come up against a difficulty. It has proved very difficult to demonstrate production, whether mRNA or protein, of the "classic" T-cell lymhokines, such as IL-2, TNF-β (lymphotoxin), and IFN-γ, within the RA synovial membrane. These lymphokines are produced by T cells involved in cell-mediated immunity (Fig. 4 depicts the properties and interactions of the proposed two major functional subsets of memory T cells.) As such, their production is demanded by the hypothesis that places the activation of "rheumatoid-specific" T cells at the apex of the immunopathogenetic scheme for RA (see Fig. 6). Indeed, the presence of abundant IL-2 mRNA (51–53), but little or no IL-2 protein, within the RA synovial membrane has been taken as evidence that T cells are being energized once they arrive within the joint (54,55); this has been adduced as evidence that other cells, in particular macrophages, are at the center of the pathogenesis of RA. Evidence from the skin lesions of tuberculoid leprosy, which are driven by type 1 T helper cells (T_H1), shows that the T-cell lymphokines, IL-2, and IFN-γ, can be demonstrated only by using very sensitive techniques, such as the polymerase chain reaction (56). This technique has shown that T cells within the lesion belonged to the T_H1 subset, as T_H2 lymphokines, such as IL-4 and IL-5, were not found. The T-cell clones, isolated from the lesions, produced T_H1 lymphokines when stimulated in vitro, confirming the direct evidence obtained from the polymerase chain reaction experiments (57). There is now accumulating evidence that the same may be true for the RA synovial membrane; thus, T cells cloned from the joint produce T_H1 lymphokines when stimulated. These findings are not surprising when one considers that the frequency of antigen-specific T cells found within a lesion that are specific for that antigen is low (see foregoing). It has proved even more difficult to demonstrate T_H2 lympokines, especially IL-4 (58), than T_H1 lymphokines within the RA synovial membrane. Thus, it may be concluded that rheumatoid-specific T cells secrete sufficient T_H1 lymphokines to maintain the cell-mediated drive. However, it is known from experiments with rodent or human lymphoid cells that T_H2 lymphokines can inhibit the activities of T_H1 T cells; the failure to

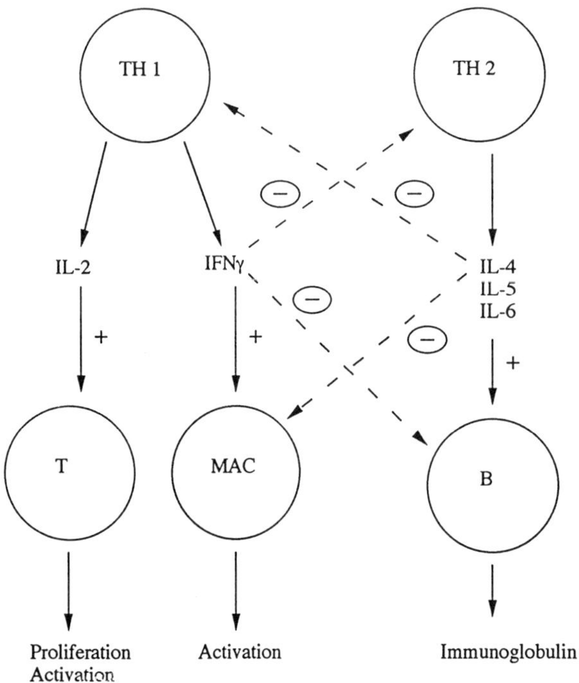

Fig. 4 A schematic representation of the lymphokines and functions of the T_H1 T cells, which are involved in cell-mediated immunity, and of T_H2 T cells, which are involved in humoral immunity. Positive (+) and negative (−) signals are shown.

demonstrate such lymphokines in the RA synovial membrane suggests that this may be one mechanism by which disease is maintained. It is not surprising, therefore, that parenteral administration of IL-4 is being considered for the treatment of RA.

Virtually all T cells entering the joint are memory T cells with some of the characteristics of activation, such as increased adherence and migration through endothelial cell monolayers, and HLA-DR positivity (Table 4), but they are not specific for the rheumatoid antigen; their exact role in the pathogenesis of RA is unclear. They may be providing unknown lymphokines necessary for the regulation, both positive and negative, of chronic inflammation. The stimulus for the production of lymphokines may be through the adhesive interactions that they undergo during the many phases of their entry into the synovium. Thus, it is known that T cells can activate endothelial cells through direct cell-to-cell contact (39,40) and that they themselves may be activated by this contact (6). We have shown, through the formation of sheep red blood cell rosettes, that T cells

Table 4 Activation Markers on Rheumatoid Synovial T Cells

Marker	Status
HLA-DR	Up-regulated
VLA-1	Up-regulated
CD2R	Up-regulated
CDW60	Up-regulated
CD3	Down-regulated
CD2	Down-regulated
LFA-1	Down-regulated
Soluble IL-2R	Found in synovial fluid and blood
Soluble CD4	during active disease
Soluble CD8	
T cells at G_1 of cell cycle	

activated by their CD2 receptor transcribe the IL-6 and HLA-DR genes (59); it should be remembered that expression of IL-6 and HLA-DR are characteristics of synovial T cells (60–62). The human ligand for CD2 is LFA-3, and this is overexpressed in the rheumatoid synovial membrane (45). Finally, adhesion of T cells to fibronectin can activate the AP-1 transcription factor, which is involved in the activation of many genes involved in inflammation (63). Since we, and others (64,65), have shown that synovial T cells have enhanced binding to fibronectin, this is another augmenting mechanism that may be available to T cells in chronic inflammatory foci, independent of specific antigenic stimulation.

B. Destruction of Cartilage and Bone

Bone and cartilage destruction is mediated by two processes: invasion by the pannus and release of cytokines. The pannus may be considered an attempt at tissue repair and will be discussed at greater length later. It is believed that IL-1 and TNF-α, released from monocytes and macrophages act on the chondrocytes to initiate destruction of articular cartilage from within. Chondrocytes subject to this attack switch off synthesis of connective tissue components and release enzymes that degrade the matrix. The role of cytokines in this process has been confirmed by the induction of joint damage through the repeated intra-articular injection of recombinant IL-1 and by the destructive arthritis that develops in mice transgenic for the human TNF-α gene and for the *tax* gene of HTLV-1 (see foregoing). Once the collagen matrix of the articular cartilage is damaged, repair is impossible, and the cartilage may enter a phase of irreversible destruction from the mechanical forces acting on it; clearly, even the most effective anti-inflammatory therapy given at this stage of the disease will have little or no effect on radiological progression of the disease.

The destruction of bone is also dependent on the erosive action of the pannus and the actions of IL-1 and TNF-α, although this is a more complex process, as it involves two cells: the osteoclast and the osteoblast. This has recently been reviewed (66). However, the same endpoint can be reached as for articular cartilage; after a certain threshold of damage to the bone has been exceeded, further destruction may be determined by mechanical forces acting independently of the presence of continued inflammation.

This sequence of events provides the strongest argument for the institution of the most effective treatment of RA as soon as possible after the diagnosis has been made, since many studies have shown that most joint damage has already occurred by 5 years of disease and has reached its maximum by 10 years. It is, therefore, not justified to carry out placebo studies in RA over several months, as joint destruction will be proceeding during this time; the relative inadequacy of present treatments is no argument against the ethical imperative of providing the best available treatment to our patients.

V. STAGE 4: REPAIR

Repair of a wound is due to the formation of new blood vessels, the entry of leukocytes, and the local proliferation of fibroblasts. Remodeling takes place through the release of enzymes, the phagocytic activity of macrophages, and the laying down of new connective tissue matrix, such as collagens, by the activated fibroblasts. All these efforts collectively attempt to restore the previous status quo. There is considerable evidence that active attempts at healing are taking place within the rheumatoid synovium: new blood vessels are formed, leukocytes are recruited from the blood, and there is proliferation of synoviocytes. Remodeling is evidenced by the increased deposition of collagen, the release of enzymes, and the phagocytic activity of macrophages. Ultrastructural analysis of the latter has shown that they contain partially digested collagen fragments. Why then is wound healing considered beneficial, but rheumatoid synovitis harmful? Part of the answer is that the the former is a ''one–off'' event, whereas the latter is chronic owing to the persistent immune stimulation thought to be taking place. One of the central mediators involved in wound healing is transforming growth factor-beta (TGF-β) and, therefore, it is not surprising to find that its injection into animal joints causes a pronounced synovitis (67), mainly because of synoviocyte proliferation, whereas systemic administration will prevent experimental arthritis (68). The realization that, concurrently with the inflammatory process, there is an attempt at repair is important, as it may provide us with new concepts in therapy. The two important features of repair are new blood vessel formation and synoviocyte proliferation and activation; these will be considered further.

A. Angiogenesis

When the rheumatoid synovium is examined by immunohistochemical techniques with antibodies specific for the clotting factor VIII, which is made by endothelial cells and lymphatics, a striking proliferation of endothelial cells and lymphatics will then be seen. This is undoubtedly necessary because the hypertrophic and hyperplastic synovium, seen clinically as joint swelling, demands new blood vessels for adequate nutrition; this is exactly analogous to the angiogenesis seen in tumors. A number of factors are involved in angiogenesis, including TGF-β, GM-CSF, epidermal growth factor (EGF), acidic fibroblast growth factor, IL-1, and TNF-α, and an as yet incompletely characterized factor from a subset of synovial macrophages (69). However, the critical event in angiogenesis is the invasion of bone and articular cartilage by the pannus, which contains blood vessels. Normally, the cartilage does not have a vascular or lymphatic supply and its differentiation from mesenchyme during embryogenesis is dependent on the death of existing vessels and the inhibition of new vessel formation. This is accomplished by the release of angiogenesis-inhibiting factor from the articular chondrocytes (70). It could be that in RA chondrocytes from the articular joint cartilage do not secrete angiogenesis-inhibiting factors; this could be an important determinant in pathogenesis, as the release of previously sequestered cartilage components into the systemic circulation could lead to autoimmunization. Recently, potent angiogenesis-inhibiting substances have been isolated. One of them is fumagillin, which is a product of the fungus *Aspergillus fumigatus* and has been shown to be an effective therapy for experimental arthritis (71). It also inhibits the growth and metastatic spread of experimental tumors (71), further reenforcing the similarities noted earlier between tumors and the RA synovial membrane. Interferon alfa-2a has recently been shown to be a potent inhibitor of life-threatening hemangiomas of infancy (72). Part of its beneficial action in the treatment of RA may, therefore, be related to its angiogenesis-inhibiting properties (73). A similar action has been proposed for sodium aurothiomalate (74).

Thus, two important new therapeutic areas that have been opened up by changes in our understanding of the pathogenesis of RA are the inhibition of leukocyte adhesion to and transmigration through the blood vessel wall, and the inhibition of angiogenesis within the synovium. Further therapeutic developments in this area will undoubtedly be forthcoming in the future.

B. Synoviocyte Proliferation and Activation

Synoviocytes may be considered the specialized fibroblasts of the synovial membrane. They have secretory potential and form the type B cell of the synovial lining layer. They are the resident cell population of the synovium and undergo expansion by cell proliferation during rheumatoid synovitis. The cytokines that are involved are mainly products of the activated macrophages and include TGF-β, acidic and basic fibroblast growth factors, IL-1, TNF-α, and IL-6. Autocrine mechanisms are switched on, as the synoviocytes themselves can secrete IL-1 (75), which can act on high-affinity IL-1 receptors expressed by them (76), IL-6 (77), TGF-β (78,79), basic fibroblast growth factor (80), and epidermal growth factor, which will stimulate synoviocyte proliferation and activation. The autocrine mechanisms may account for the persistently altered phenotype of synoviocytes that is maintained even after several passages in vitro (78,81). The effects of some of these mediators can be felt remote from the joint; IL-6 will stimulate the acute-phase response from the liver and immunoglobulin and rheumatoid factor production from B lymphocytes (77).

Synoviocytes have a vast potential to secrete factors of crucial importance to the development of tissue inflammation and destruction. Stimulation of IL-1 and TNF-α causes the secretion of metalloproteases and other enzymes, including stromelysin and collagenase. In addition, TGF-β will cause the secretion of matrix metalloproteases (MMP-1, -2, -3) (82), stromelysin (83), collagenase (84), and urokinase-type plasminogen activator (85), which contribute to tissue destruction or to remodeling, depending on the stage at which that particular lesion has reached. As a counterbalance to these degradative molecules, synoviocytes produce tissue inhibitors of metalloproteases (TIMP) (83,86) and collagen. The release of plasminogen activator may augment inflammatory processes, not only because plasmin is involved in fibrinolysis, which may enhance cell migration by the deposition of fibrin degradation products, but may be important in the processes of connective tissue turnover and remodeling, inflammation, and cell migration. It has been proposed that part of the mechanism of action of D-penicillamine and of gold salts is to inhibit synoviocyte proliferation (87,88).

The release of such a variety of factors, with often opposing actions, suggests that intricate regulatory pathways are operating within the synovium. This opens up the possibility of enhancing those that are advantageous while inhibiting those that are harmful. One example is the mutual antagonism between IFN-γ and TNF-α on HLA-DR expression, proliferation, and collagenase and GM-CSF production by synoviocytes (89). This regulatory pathway may be defective in RA, in which little IFN-γ is believed to be produced. Furthermore, the ability of TGF-β to down-regulate T-cell activation (90) may be reflected in the relatively poor responses of rheumatoid T cells to stimulants, which is normalized after successful therapy with agents such as sodium aurothiomalate (91) or lymphocytapheresis (92).

VI. A SYNTHESIS

It is appropriate to attempt a synthesis of these complex events (Fig. 5), but only the major cells and pathways will be considered. Following activation of a

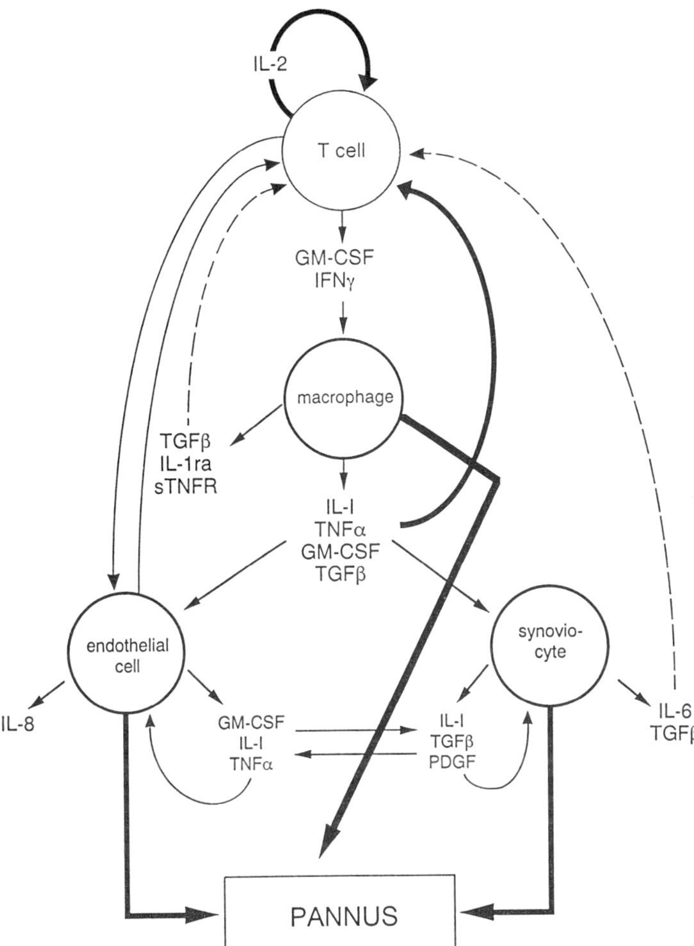

Fig. 5 A synthesis of some of the pathways involved in the pathogenesis of rheumatoid arthritis. A solid line indicates stimulatory circuits; a broken line indicates negative or suppressive circuits.

specific subset of T cells by the unknown rheumatoid antigen(s), IL-2 and IFN-γ are released; the former acts in an autocrine manner to stimulate T-cell proliferation, whereas the latter activates macrophages, endothelial cells, and synovio-cytes. Macrophages can have positive and negative influences on T-cell function by IL-1 and TGF-β, respectively. Macrophages, in a major amplification step, stimulate endothelial cell and synoviocyte proliferation and function through the release of IL-1, TNF-α, and GM-CSF. Endothelial cells then recruit into the synovial membrane and activate the inflammatory leukocytes in a mutually costimulatory process. The synoviocytes are the other major amplification step for the maintenance of synovial inflammation because of the many mediators they release that are both proinflammatory and involved in tissue repair. The crucial role of the synoviocyte is attested to by the fact that it may maintain its stimulated phenotype for several weeks or months in culture (78). The leukocytes, new blood vessels, and synoviocytes form the pannus, which is the pathological hallmark of the disease. Leukocytes, synoviocytes, and mycobacterial heat-shock protein, as a proposed rheumatoid antigen, are capable of in vitro induction of a structure resembling pannus (93). This scheme would be incomplete without including some of the negative regulatory factors: IL-1 receptor antagonist (31,94), soluble TNF receptors (95), TGF-β (96), and IL-6 (97).

VII. SUMMARY AND THERAPEUTIC IMPLICATIONS

Figure 6 shows, in summary form, the proposed etiopathogenetic mechanism for rheumatoid arthritis as a pyramid, at the apex of which is posited the initiating event, namely, the activation of the pathogenic T cell or T cells by the trimolecular complex consisting of the HLA-DR4/1 molecule, the unknown rheumatoid antigenic peptide, and the α–β T-cell receptor. Following this initiating event, several other processes are then activated, which then activate other inflammatory mechanisms, regulatory circuits, and reparative sequences. The farther down the etiopathogenetic pyramid one goes, the less likely would a single therapeutic intervention be successful. Thus, although cyclooxygenase inhibitors are very effective at the symptomatic relief of pain, they have no effect on the long-term course of the disease. It is hoped that with the definition of more specific therapeutic targets, as discussed and reviewed in this chapter, more effective and less toxic drugs will be developed. The astonishing advances in biotechnology offer the greatest hope for this, and these possibilities are discussed elsewhere in this volume (see Chapter 17).

ACKNOWLEDGMENTS

Work from the author's laboratory was funded by grants from the Arthritis and Rheumatism Council of Great Britain (U9) and an Interlaboratory Grant from the Wellcome Trust between the Rheumatology Unit, UMDS, and the Department of Medicine, University of Ioannina, Greece (Professor H. M. Moutsopoulos).

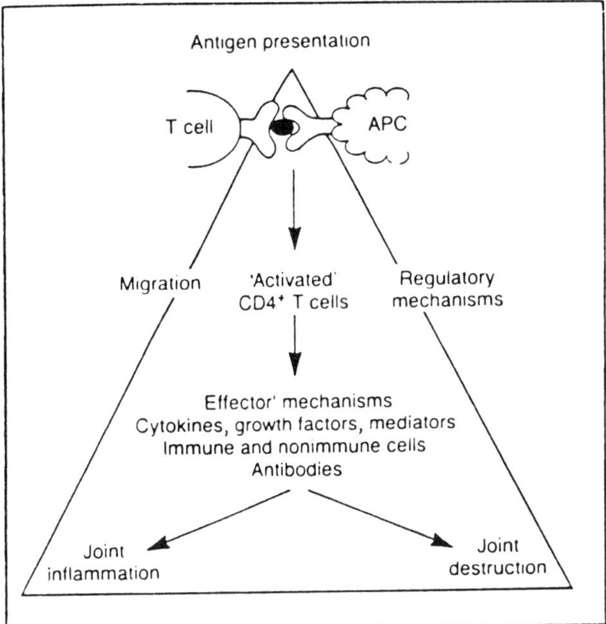

Fig. 6 The proposed pathogenesis of rheumatoid arthritis. The various "targets" that can be used for the development of new therapies are clearly seen. It should be noted that the farther down the inflammatory pyramid one goes, the greater the number of inflammatory cascades that have been activated; this would make successful therapy directed against a single mediator highly unlikely. (From Ref. 98.)

REFERENCES

1. Janossy G, Panayi GS, Duke O, Bofill M, Poulter LW, Goldstein G. Rheumatoid arthritis: a disease of T lymphocyte/macrophage immunoregulation. Lancet 1981; 2:839–842.

2. Mapp PI, Kidd BL, Gibson SJ, et al. Substance P-, calcitonin gene-related peptide- and C-flanking peptide of neuropeptide Y-immunoreactive fibres are present in normal synovium but depleted in patients with rheumatoid arthritis. Neuroscience 1990; 37:143–153.

3. Meyers OL, Daynes G, Beighton P. Rheumatoid arthritis in a tribal Xhosa population in the Transkei, Southern Africa. Ann Rheum Dis 1977; 36:62–65.

4. Solomon L, Robin G, Valkenburg HA. Rheumatoid arthritis in an urban South African negro population. Ann Rheum Dis 1975; 34:128–135.

5. Drossos AA, Lanchbury JS, Panayi GS, Moutsopoulos HM. Rheumatoid arthritis in Greek and British patients: comparative clinical, radiological, and serological study. Arthritis Rheum 1992; 35: .

6. Burkly LC, Jakubowski A, Newman BM, Rosa MD, Chi-Rosso G, Lobbo RR. Signalling by vascular adhesion molecule-1 (VCAM-1) through VLA-4 promotes CD3-dependent T cell proliferation. Eur J Immunol 1991; 21:2871–2876.

7. Kremer JM, Lawrence DA, Jubiz W, DiGiacomo R, Rynes R, Sherman M. Dietary fish oil and olive oil supplementation in patients with rheumatoid arthritis. Clinical and immunologic effects. Arthritis Rheum 1990; 33:810–820.

8. Keffer J, Probert L, Cazlaris H, et al. Transgenic mice expressing human tumour necrosis factor: a predictive genetic model of arthritis. EMBO J 1991; 10:4025–4031.

9. Londei M, Savill CM, Verhoef A, et al. Persistence of collagen type II specific T-cell clones in the synovial membrane of a patient with rheumatoid arthritis. Proc Natl Acad Sci USA 1989; 86:636–640.

10. Klimiuk PS, Clague RB, Grennan DM, Dyer PA, Smeaton I, Harris R. Autoimmunity to native type II collagen: a distinct genetic subset of rheumatoid arthritis. J Rheumatol 1985; 12:865–870.

11. Hale LP, Martin ME, McCollum DE, et al. Immunohistologic analysis of the distribution of cell adhesion molecules within the inflammatory synovial microenvironment. Arthritis Rheum 1989; 32:22–30.

12. Res PCM, Schaar CG, Breeveld FC, et al. Synovial fluid T cell reactivity against 65kD heat shock protein of mycobacteria in early chronic arthritis. Lancet 1988; 2:478–480.

13. Gaston JSH, Life PF, Bailey L, Bacon RA. Synovial fluid T cells and 65kD heat-shock protein. Lancet 1988; 2:856–858.

14. Fischer HP, Sharrock CEM, Colston MJ, Panayi GS. Limiting dilution analysis of proliferative T cell responses to mycobacterial 65-kDa heat-shock protein fails to show significant frequency differences between synovial fluid and peripheral blood of patients with rheumatoid arthritis. Eur J Immunol 1991; 21:2937–2941.

15. Paliard X, West SG, Lafferty JA, et al. Evidence for the effects of a superantigen in rheumatoid arthritis. Science 1991; 253:325–329.

16. Uematsu Y, Wege H, Straus A, et al. The T cell receptor repertoire in the synovial fluid of a patient with rheumatoid arthritis is polyclonal. Proc Natl Acad Sci USA 1991; 88:8534–38.

17. Steinmetz M, Uematsu Y. Heterogeneity of T cell repertoires in human autoimmune disease. Br J Rheumatol 1991; 30:24–27.

18. Bowness P, Bell J. T cell receptors and rheumatic disease: approaches to repertoire analysis. Br J Rheumatol 1992; 31:3–8.

19. Conceicao-Silva F, Schubach AO, Nogueria RS, Coutinho SG. Quantitation of T cells which recognize *Leishmania braziliensis braziliensis* (Lbb) antigens in lesions and peripheral blood of cutaneous or mucosal leishmaniasis patients by limiting dilution analysis. Mem Inst Oswaldo 1978; 82:118.

20. Sun J, Link H, Olsson T, et al. T and B cell responses to myelin-oligo dendrocyte glycoprotein in multiple sclerosis. J Immunol 1991; 146:1490–1495.

21. Modlin RL, Pirmez L, Hofman FM, et al. Lymphocyte bearing antigen-specific gamma delta T cells receptors accumulate in human infectious disease lesions. Nature 1989; 339:554–548.

22. Modlin RL, Melancon-Kaplan J, Young SMM, et al. Learning from lesions: patterns of tissue inflammation in leprosy. Proc Natl Acad Sci USA 1988; 85:1213–1217.

23. Mourad W, Mehindate K, Schall TJ, McColl SR. Engagement of major histocompatibility complex class II molecules by superantigen induces inflammatory cytokine gene expression in human rheumatoid fibroblast-like synoviocytes. J Exp Med 1992; 175:613–616.

24. Iwakura I, Tosu M, Yoshida E, et al. Induction of inflammatory arthropathy resembling rheumatoid arthritis in mice transgenic for HTLV-1. Science 1991; 253:1026–1027.

25. Osborn L. Leukocyte adhesion to endothelium in inflammation. Cell 1990; 62:3–6.

26. Beekhuizen H, Blokland I, Corsel-van Tilburg AJ, Koning F, van Furth R. CD14 contributes to the adherence of human monocytes to cytokine-stimulated endothelial cells. J Immunol 1991; 147:3761–3767.

27. Mentzer SJ, Crimmins MAV, Burakoff SJ, Faller DV. alpha And beta subunits of the LFA-1 membrane molecule are involved in human monocyte endothelial cell interactions. J Cell Physiol 1987; 130:410–419.

28. Beekhuizen H, Corsel-van Tilburg AJ, van Furth R. Characterisation of monocyte adherence to human macrovascular and microvascular endothelial cells. J Immunol 1990; 145:510–516.

29. Mangan DF, Wahl SM. Differential regulation of human monocyte programmed cell death (apoptosis) by chemotactic factors and pro-inflammatory cytokines. J Immunol 1991; 147:3408–3412.

30. Janson RW, Joslin FG, Arend WP. The effects of differentiating agents on IL-1 beta production in cultured human monocytes. J Immunol 1990; 145:2161–2166.

31. Dinarello CA, Thompson RC. Blocking IL-1: interleukin 1 receptor antagonist in vivo and in vitro. Immunol Today 1991; 12:404–410.

32. Harth M, McCain GA, Cousin K. The modulation of interleukin 1 production by interferon gamma, and the inhibitory effects of gold compounds. Immunopharmacology 1990; 20:125–134.

33. Farahat MNMR, Yanni G, Poston R, Panayi GS. Gold treatment in rheumatoid arthritis diminishes IL-8 expression and monocyte numbers at two weeks [abstr]. Clin Rheumatol 1992; 11:157.

34. Farahat MNMR, Yanni G, Poston R, Panayi GS. intramuscular gold diminishes macrophage numbers and monokine expression in the rheumatoid synovial membrane [abstr]. Clin Rheumatol 1992; 11:157–158.

35. Pitzalis C, Kingsley GH, Murphy J, Panayi GS. Abnormal distribution of the helper-inducer and suppressor-inducer T lymphocyte subsets in the rheumatoid joint. Clin Immunol Immunopathol 1987; 45:252–258.

36. Pitzalis C, Kingsley GH, Haskard DO, Panayi GS. The preferential accumulation of helper-inducer T lymphocytes in inflammatory lesions: evidence for regulation by selective endothelial and homotypic adhesion. Eur J Immunol 1988; 18:1397–1404.

37. Burmester GR, Strobel GF, Gohring P, Kalden JR. Adhesion of human T lymphocytes to endothelial cells isolated from the umbilical vein: II. Enhanced binding of in vitro activated T lymphocytes. Immunobiology 1987; 175:394–405.

38. Shimizu Y, Newman W, Tanaka Y, Shaw S. Lymphocyte interactions with endothelial cells. Immunol Today 1992; 13:106–112.

39. Damle NK, Eberhardt C, van der Vieren M. Direct interaction with primed CD4[+] CD45RO[+] memory T lymphocytes induces expression of endothelial leukocyte adhesion molecule-1 and vascular cell adhesion molecule-1 on the surface of vascular endothelial cells. Eur J Immunol 1991; 21:2915–2923.

40. Damle NK, Doyle LV. Ability of human T lymphocytes to adhere to vascular endothelial cells and to augment endothelial permeability to macromolecules is linked to their state of post-thymic maturation. J Immunol 1990; 144:1233–1240.

41. Corkill MM, Kirkham BW, Haskard DO, Barbatis C, Gibson T, Panayi GS. Gold treatment of rheumatoid arthritis decreases synovial expression of the endothelial leukocyte adhesion receptor ELAM-1. J Rheumatol 1991; 18:1453–1460.

42. Oppenheimer-Marks N, Davis LS, Bogue DT, Ramberg J, Lipsky PE. Differential utilization of ICAM-1 and VCAM-1 during the adhesion and transendothelial migration of human T lymphocytes. J Immunol 1991; 147:2913–1921.

43. Shimizu Y, van Seventer GA, Horgan KJ, Shaw S. Regulated expression and binding of three VLA (beta 1) integrin receptors on T cells. Nature 1990; 345:250–253.

44. Shimizu Y, Shaw S. Lymphocyte interactions with extracellular matrix. FASEB J 1991; 5:2292–2299.

45. Haynes BF, Grover BJ, Whichard LP, et al. Synovial microenvironment–T cell interactions. Human T cells bind to fibroblast-like synovial cells in vitro. Arthritis Rheum 1988; 31:947–955.

46. Bednarczyk JL, McIntyre BW. A monoclonal antibody to VLA-4 alpha chain (CDw49d) induces homotypic lymphocyte aggregation. J Immunol 1990; 144:777–784.

47. Belitsos P, Hildreth JEK, August JT. Homotypic cell aggregation induced by anti-CD44 (Pgp-1) monoclonal antibodies and related to CD44 (Pgp-1) expression. J Immunol 1990; 144:1661–1670.

48. van Kooyk Y, vande Wiel-van Kemenade P, Weder P, Kuijpers TW, Figdor CG. Enhancement of LFA-1 mediated cell adhesion by triggering through CD2 or CD3 on T lymphocytes. Nature 1989; 342:811–813.

49. Merry P, Winyard PG, Morris CJ, Grootveld M, Blake DR. Oxygen free radicals, inflammation and synovitis; the current status. Ann Rheum Dis 1989; 48:864–870.

50. Samuelsson B. Arachidonic acid metabolism: role in inflammation. Z Rheumatol 1991; 50 (suppl 1):3–6.

51. Howell WM, Warren CJ, Cook NJ, Cawley MID, Smith JL. Detection of IL-2 at mRNA and protein levels in synovial infiltrates from inflammatory arthropathies using biotinylated oligonucleotide probes in situ. Clin Exp Immunol 1991; 86:393–398.

52. Buchan G, Barrett K, Fujita T, Taniguchi T, Maini RN, Feldmann M. Detection of activated T cell products in the rheumatoid joint using cDNA probes to interleukin 2 (IL2), IL2 receptor and IFNγ. Clin Exp Immunol 1988; 71:295–301.

53. Firestein GS, Xu WD, Townsend K, et al. Cytokines in chronic inflammatory arthritis. I. Failure to detect T cell lymphokines (interleukin 2 and interleukin 3)

and presence of macrophage colony-stimulating factor (CSF-1) and a novel mast cell growth factor in rheumatoid synovitis. J Exp Med 1988; 168:1573–1586.

54. Warren CJ, Howell WM, Bhambani M, Cawley MID, Smith JL. An investigation of T cell function in the rheumatoid synovium using in situ hybridization for IL2 mRNA. Br J Rheumatol 1990; 29(suppl 2):31.

55. Howell M, Smith J, Cawley M. The rheumatoid synovium: a model for T cell anergy? [letter]. Immunol Today 1992; 13:191.

56. Yamamura M, Uyemura K, Deans RJ, et al. Defining protective responses to pathogens: cytokine profiles in leprosy lesions. Science 1991; 254:277–279.

57. Salgame P, Abrams JS, Clayberger C, et al. Differing lymphokine profiles of functional subsets of human CD4 and CD8 T cell clones. Science 1991; 254:279–282.

58. Miossec P, Naviliat M, Dupuy A, Sany J, Banchereau J. Low levels of interleukin-4 and high levels of transforming growth factor beta in rheumatoid synovitis. Arthritis Rheum 1990; 33:1180–1187.

59. Linardopoulos S, Corrigall VM, Panayi GS. Activation of HLA-DR and interleukin 6 gene transcription in resting T cells via the CD2 molecule: relevance to chronic immune-mediated inflammation. Scand J Immunol 1992;

60. Hirano T, Matsuda T, Turner M, et al. Excessive production of interleukin-6/B cell stimulatory factor-2 in rheumatoid arthritis. Eur J Immunol 1988; 18:1797–1801.

61. Wood NC, Symons JA, Dickens E, Duff GW. In situ hybridisation of IL-6 in rheumatoid arthritis. Clin Exp Immunol 1992; 87:183–189.

62. Duke O, Panayi GS, Janossy G, Poulter LW. An immunohistological analysis of lymphocyte subpopulations and their micro-environment in the synovial membranes of patients with RA using monoclonal antibodies. Clin Exp Immunol 1982; 49:23–30.

63. Yamada A, Nikaido T, Nojima Y, Schlossman SF, Morimoto C. Activation of human CD4 T lymphocytes. Interaction of fibronectin with VLA-5 receptor on CD4 cells induces the AP-1 transcription factor. J Immunol 1991; 146:53–56.

64. Garcia-Vicuna R, Humbria A, Postigo AA, et al. VLA family in rheumatoid arthritis: evidence for in vivo regulated adhesion of synovial fluid T cells to fibronectin through VLA-5 integrin. Clin Exp Immunol 1992; 88:435–441.

65. Rodriguez RM, Pitzalis C, Kingsley GH, Henderson EM, Humphries MJ, Panayi GS. T-lymphocyte adhesion to fibronectin: a possible mechanism for T cell accumulation in the rheumatoid joint. Clin Exp Immunol 1992; (in press).

66. Watrous DA, Andrews BS. The metabolism and immunology of bone. Semin Arthritis Rheum 1989; 19:45–65.

67. Allen JB, Manthey CL, Hand AR, Ohura K, Ellingsworth L, Wahl SM. Rapid onset synovial inflammation and hyperplasia induced by transforming growth factor beta. J Exp Med 1990; 171:231–247.

68. Brandes ME, Allen JB, Ogawa Y, Wahl SM. Transforming growth factor beta 1 suppresses acute and chronic arthritis in experimental animals. J Clin Invest 1991; 87:1108–1113.

69. Koch AE, Polverini PJ, Leibovich SJ. Functional heterogeneity of human rheumatoid synovial tissue macrophages. J Rheumatol 1988; 15:1058–1063.

70. Moses MA, Sudhalter J, Langer R. Identification of an inhibitor of neovascularisation from cartilage. Science 1990; 248:1408–1410.

71. Ingber D, Fujita T, Kishimoto S, et al. Synthetic analogues of fumagillin that inhibit angiogenesis and suppress tumor growth. Nature 1990; 348:555–557.

72. Ezekowitz RAB, Mulliken JB, Folkman J. Interferon alfa-2a therapy for life-threatening hemangiomas of infancy. N Engl J Med 1992; 326:1456–1463.

73. Fischer HP, Sharrock CEM, Panayi GS. High frequency of cord blood lymphocytes against mycobacterial 65 kDa heat-shock protein. Eur J Immunol 1992; 22:1667–1669.

74. Matsubara T, Ziff MA. Inhibition of human endothelial cell proliferation by gold compounds. J Clin Invest 1987; 79:1440–1446.

75. Dalton BJ, Connor JR, Johnson WJ. Interleukin-1 induces interleukin-1 alpha and interleukin-1 beta gene expression in synovial fibroblasts and peripheral blood monocytes. Arthritis Rheum 1989; 32:279–287.

76. Chin J, Rupp E, Cameron PM, et al. Identification of a high-affinity receptor for interleukin 1 alpha and interleukin 1 beta on cultured human rheumatoid synovial cells. J Clin Invest 1988; 82:420–426.

77. Guerne PA, Zuraw BL, Vaughan JH, Carson DA, Lotz M. Synovium as a source of interleukin 6 in vitro. Contribution to local and systemic manifestations of arthritis. J Clin Invest 1989; 83:585–592.

78. Bucala R, Ritchlin C, Winchester R, Cerami A. Constitutive production of inflammatory and mitogenic cytokines by rheumatoid synovial fibroblasts. J Exp Med 1991; 173:569–574.

79. Wahl SM. The role of transforming growth factor-beta in inflammatory processes. Immunol Res 1991; 10:249–254.

80. Melnyk VO, Shipley GD, Sternfeld MD, Sherman L, Rosenbaum JT. Synoviocytes synthesize, bind, and respond to basic fibroblast growth factor. Arthritis Rheum 1990; 33:493–500.

81. Ritchlin CT, Winchester RJ. Potential mechanisms for coordinate gene activation in the rheumatoid synoviocyte: implications and hypotheses. Springer Semin Immunopathol 1989; 11:219–234.

82. Okada Y, Morodomi T, Enghild JJ, et al. Matrix metalloproteinase 2 from human rheumatoid synovial fibroblasts. Purification and activation of the precursor and enzymic properties. Eur J Biochem 1990; 194:721–730.

83. MacNaul KL, Chartrain N, Lark M, Tocci MJ, Hutchinson NI. Discoordinate expression of stromelysin, collagenase, and tissue inhibitor of metalloproteinases-1 in rheumatoid human synovial fibroblasts. Synergistic effects of interleukin-1 and tumor necrosis factor-alpha on stromelysin expression. J Biol Chem 1990; 265:17238–17245.

84. Case JP, Lafyatis R, Remmers EF, Kumkumian GK, Wilder RL. Transin/stromelysin expression in rheumatoid synovium. A transformation-associated metalloproteinase secreted by phenotypically invasive synoviocytes. Am J Pathol 1989; 135:1055–1064.

85. Hamilton JA, Piccoli DS, Leizer T, Butler DM, Croatto M, Royston AK. Transforming growth factor beta stimulates urokinase-type plasminogen activator and

DNA synthesis, but not prostaglandin E2 production, in human synovial fibroblasts. Proc Natl Acad Sci USA 1991; 88:7180–7184.

86. Wright JK, Cawston TE, Hazleman BL. Transforming growth factor beta stimulates the production of the tissue inhibitor of metalloproteinases (TIMP) by human synovial and skin fibroblasts. Biochim Biophys Acta 1991; 1094:207–210.

87. Matsubara T, Hirohata K. Suppression of human fibroblast proliferation by D-penicillamine and copper sulfate in vitro. Arthritis Rheum 1988; 31:964–972.

88. Matsubara T, Saegusa Y, Hirohata K. Low-dose gold compounds inhibit fibroblast proliferation and do not affect interleukin-1 secretion by macrophages. Arthritis Rheum 1988; 31:1272–1280.

89. Alvaro Gracia JM, Zvaifler NJ, Firestein GS. Cytokines in chronic inflammatory arthritis. V. Mutual antagonism between interferon-gamma and tumor necrosis factor-alpha on HLA-DR expression, proliferation, collagenase production, and granulocyte macrophage colony-stimulating factor production by rheumatoid arthritis synoviocytes. J Clin Invest 1990; 86:1790–1798.

90. Wahl SM, Allen JB, Wong HL, Dougherty SF, Ellingsworth LR. Antagonistic and agonistic effects of transforming growth factor-beta and IL-1 in rheumatoid synovium. J Immunol 1990; 145:2514–2519.

91. Highton J, Panayi GS, Griffin J. Improvement in peripheral blood lymphocyte response to concanavalin A and pokeweed mitogen during gold treatment of rheumatoid arthritis. Agents Actions 1980; 10:507–508.

92. Emery P, Smith GN, Panayi GS. Lymphocytapheresis—a feasible treatment for rheumatoid arthritis. Br J Rheumatol 1986; 25:40–43.

93. Holoshitz J, Kosek J, Sibley R, Brown DA, Strober S. T lymphocyte–synovial fibroblast interactions induced by mycobacterial proteins in rheumatoid arthritis. Arthritis Rheum 1991; 34:679–686.

94. Schwab JH, Anderle SK, Brown RR, Dalldorf FG, Thompson RC. Pro- and anti-inflammatory roles of interleukin 1 in recurrence of bacterial cell wall-induced arthritis in rats. Infect Immun 1991; 59:4436–4442.

95. Brennan FM, Maini RN, Feldmann M. TNF alpha—a pivotal role in rheumatoid arthritis? Br J Rheumatol 1992; 31:293–298.

96. Turner M, Chantry D, Katsikis P, Berger A, Brennana FM, Feldmann M. Induction of the interleukin 1 receptor antagonist protein by transforming growth factor beta. Eur J Immunol 1991; 21:1635–1639.

97. Mihara M, Ikuta M, Koishihara Y, Ohsugi Y. Interleukin 6 inhibits delayed-type hypersensitivity and the development of adjuvant arthritis. Eur J Immunol 1991; 21:2327–2331.

98. Kingsley GH, Panayi GS, Lanchbury O. Immunol Today 1991; 12:177–179.

2

Rheumatoid Factor

Nancy J. Olsen

Vanderbilt University
Nashville, Tennessee

Pojen P. Chen

University of California, San Diego
La Jolla, California

I. INTRODUCTION

Rheumatoid factors are antibodies that recognize and bind the Fc portion of normal IgG. First described in studies by Waaler and Rose (1,2), measurement of rheumatoid factors became an important diagnostic tool useful in the identification of patients with rheumatoid arthritis. Much early interest was focused on rheumatoid factors as potential clues to the pathogenesis of this form of destructive arthritis. However, this hope was tempered by two observations. First, rheumatoid factors are commonly found in the sera of individuals with a variety of other diseases, including chronic infections and malignancies (Table 1) (3–5). Occasionally, significant titers are even found in normal individuals, and it has been estimated that 1–3 of every 1000 normal circulating human B cells are committed to produce IgM rheumatoid factor (6). Second, approximately 15% of patients who satisfy clinical criteria for rheumatoid arthritis lack detectable serum rheumatoid factors. Thus, seropositivity for rheumatoid factor is neither specific for rheumatoid arthritis nor sensitive enough to detect all individuals with this disease. Nevertheless, rheumatoid factors remain useful clinically and are of investigational interest in unraveling the pathogenesis of rheumatoid arthritis and related autoimmune diseases.

II. CLASS-SPECIFIC RHEUMATOID FACTORS

Rheumatoid factors have been identified in all of the major immunoglobulin classes (7). Routine clinical assays detect IgM rheumatoid factor and, in general, seropositivity for IgM rheumatoid factor is associated with a more severe course of rheumatoid arthritis (8). Conversely, conversion to seronegativity, as may occur with second-line therapies, is generally associated with an improved clinical status. Nevertheless, titers of rheumatoid factor in serum do not correlate with disease activity and, once seropositivity in a given patient is found, it is generally not useful to follow titers as a measure of disease status.

It has been suggested that serum levels of IgA rheumatoid factor are also associated with disease features, such as erosive radiographic changes, and may have prognostic significance (9–11). However, other studies have failed to find significant clinical associations with serum IgA rheumatoid factor (12–14), and thus the role of this autoantibody in rheumatoid arthritis remains unclear. The serum IgA rheumatoid factor may be present in either monomeric or polymeric forms. Most immunoassays detect the polymeric form, which is preponderant in both sicca syndrome and rheumatoid arthritis (15–17).

The role of IgG rheumatoid factor has been harder to elucidate owing to difficulties in establishing reliable and specific assays (18). However, it appears that elevated levels of this self-associating immunoglobulin are present in the synovial space (19), and the presence of IgG rheumatoid factor in serum may correlate with development of the extra-articular complication of vasculitis (18,20). Other studies suggest that serum levels of IgG rheumatoid factor more closely parallel changes in clinical activity than do serum levels of IgM rheumatoid factor (9,13).

The IgE rheumatoid factor has been reported to occur in serous effusions associated with rheumatoid arthritis (21), and it may be more likely elevated in patients with extra-articular manifestations (22). However, this isotype is not specific for rheumatoid arthritis, as elevated serum levels of IgE rheumatoid factor are also seen in 59% of patients with bronchial asthma (22).

Table 1 Diseases Associated with Rheumatoid Factors

Subacute bacterial endocarditis
Syphilis
Hepatitis B
Schistosomiasis
Trypanosomiasis
Nephritis associated with infected ventriculoatrial shunt
Parvovivus infection
Waldenstrom's macroglobulinemia

III. SPONTANEOUS IN VITRO RHEUMATOID FACTOR SYNTHESIS

Measurement of levels of IgM rheumatoid factor that are spontaneously synthesized by cultured peripheral blood mononuclear cells in vitro appears to be more specific for rheumatoid arthritis and more sensitive to changes in disease status than routine clinical measures of serum IgM rheumatoid factor. This difference is most likely due to the probability that in vitro levels of synthesis are more accurately reflective of what is happening at a given time point, whereas serum levels reflect cumulative activity over a previous interval. In unselected populations of patients with rheumatoid arthritis, approximately half show significant levels of spontaneous IgM rheumatoid factor synthesis, as measured by radioimmunoassay (RIA) or enzyme-linked immunosorbent assay (ELISA), and this subgroup of patients generally shows measures of more severe or active disease (23–26). In longitudinal studies, levels of in vitro IgM rheumatoid factor have been decreased during treatment with methotrexate (12,27), gold, penicillamine (28), and even with the nonsteroidal anti-inflammatory agent ibuprofen (29). However, for patients who are treated with one of these drugs, but do not derive significant clinical benefit, in vitro IgM rheumatoid factor synthesis generally does not decrease. These findings are consistent with statistical analyses of a cross-sectional population of rheumatoid arthritis patients in which IgM rheumatoid factor synthesis was correlated with disease activity, independently of second-line drug therapy (25). It is unlikely that such diverse therapeutic agents as gold and methotrexate exert these similar effects by direct actions on rheumatoid factor-producing cells. It is more likely that rheumatoid factor production reflects underlying disease activity in rheumatoid arthritis and that any significantly successful therapeutic intervention will result in decreased levels of rheumatoid factor production. Measurement of in vitro levels of IgM rheumatoid factor production may have clinical use in decisions concerning therapeutic interventions.

One recent report suggests that measurement of spontaneous in vitro IgA rheumatoid factor synthesis by blood mononuclear cells from patients with rheumatoid arthritis does not have disease correlations (30), suggesting that this isotype is not involved in disease pathogenesis in the same way as IgM rheumatoid factor.

IV. RHEUMATOID FACTORS IN THE SYNOVIAL SPACE

Rheumatoid factors of the major immunoglobulin classes have been measured in synovial fluid from patients with rheumatoid arthritis. Cultures of synovial tissue and blood from the same patient show higher levels of rheumatoid factor synthesis in the synovial cavity (31), suggesting that local synthesis within the joint space is an important in vivo source of rheumatoid factor. In addition, binding specificities of rheumatoid factors derived from the synovial space differ from those derived from peripheral blood (32), and it is possible that these locally synthesized rheumatoid factors are more pathogenic.

V. CELLULAR MECHANISMS OF RHEUMATOID FACTOR PRODUCTION

A. The Role of B Cells

As the source of autoantibodies, B cells have an important role in the immunological abnormalities of rheumatoid arthritis. However, the question of whether abnormalities are intrinsic to the B cell, or whether the B cell is dependent on signals from other cell types for expression of autoimmune features, is unresolved, and data in support of both T-dependent and T-independent rheumatoid factor production by B cells can be cited (24,33–35). The rheumatoid factor-specific B-cell precursor population may be expanded in rheumatoid arthritis patients, and normal individuals who produce high levels of in vitro IgM rheumatoid factor in response to pokeweed mitogen appear to have a larger population of B cells committed to rheumatoid factor production than do normal low producers (36).

Recent evidence suggests that a specific subset of B cells that bears the pan-T-cell antigen CD5 is responsible for production of rheumatoid factor and other autoantibodies (37,38). These CD5 B cells are analogous to Ly-1$^+$ murine B cells, which produce autoantibodies of various specificities (39). Patients with rheumatoid arthritis generally show a quantitative increase in numbers of CD5$^+$ B cells in the peripheral blood (38) and in the synovial fluid (40). The suggestion that the CD5$^+$ B-cell population is responsible for rheumatoid factor production in rheumatoid arthritis patients has been largely extrapolated from the observation that normal peripheral blood CD5$^+$ B cells produce rheumatoid factor and other autoantibodies in response to *Staphylococcus aureus* cells or Epstein–Barr virus (37,41). However, these in vitro stimuli may not activate the same B cells that respond to in vivo signals generated in the patient with rheumatoid arthritis. Furthermore, other data indicate that CD5$^-$ B cells may contribute to autoantibody production in patients with autoimmune disease (42). Therefore, the relative importance of the CD5$^+$ B-cell population in producing rheumatoid factor in rheumatoid arthritis patients remains unclear.

B. The Role of T Cells

A role of T cells in rheumatoid arthritis has been suggested by the observation that drugs or treatments that inactivate or remove T cells have therapeutic benefit. These include antithymocyte globulin (43), anti-T-cell monoclonal antibodies

(44,45), total lymphoid irradiation (46,47), thoracic duct drainage (48), cyclo-phosphamide (49), and cyclosporine (50). Anecdotal reports indicate that the profound T-cell depletion of acquired immunodeficiency syndrome (AIDS) is also associated with remission of rheumatoid arthritis (51,52). Furthermore, levels of soluble interleukin-2 (IL-2) receptors, presumably released from acti-vated T cells, correlate with disease activity in patients with rheumatoid arthritis (53,54).

Although it has been suggested that enhanced autoantibody production is a manifestation of defective T-cell control (55), the role of T cells in the synthesis of rheumatoid factor has not been established. Three observations implicate an important role for T-cell regulation of rheumatoid factor production. First, the rheumatoid factor that is produced in patients with rheumatoid arthritis is poly-clonal and probably the result of extensive mutation of a limited number of germline rheumatoid factor genes, as would occur under the influence of antigen stimulation. Second, as noted earlier, production of rheumatoid factor is not limited to IgM, but extends to other major immunoglobulin classes that are considered more T-cell-dependent. Third, B-cell malignancies are not common in patients with rheumatoid arthritis, suggesting that the activated B cells do not completely escape regulatory control (56). Furthermore, T cells are required for production of rheumatoid factor in response to immune complexes in mouse strains (57,58), and T-cell-deficient nude mice cannot mount a rheumatoid factor response to immune complexes, although the presence of rheumatoid factor precursors can be demonstrated in response to lipopolysaccharide (LPS; 59). Mice with the *xid* gene defect, which respond poorly to T-cell-independent antigens, are capable of producing rheumatoid factor in response to immune complexes (59).

T cells may control rheumatoid factor synthesis through suppressor or helper mechanisms; both may have a role. In human studies, T-cell-mediated suppression of rheumatoid factor in normal persons and in patients with rheuma-toid arthritis has been reported (23,34), and in vitro generation of suppressor T cells specific for rheumatoid factor is deficient in patients with rheumatoid arthri-tis (35), consistent with the observed selective decrease in the suppressor–inducer T-cell subpopulation (60). A role for helper T cells in promoting rheumatoid factor synthesis is suggested by the observation that isolated B cells produce lower levels of in vitro rheumatoid factor than do cultures that also contain T cells (23,33). These data suggest that T cells or T-cell cytokines may recruit additional committed B cells to produce rheumatoid factor in vivo and to sponta-neously secrete rheumatoid factor in vitro.

Nevertheless, at least some spontaneous IgM rheumatoid factor synthesis is relatively T-cell-independent, and isolated B cells can synthesize rheumatoid factor in vitro in the absence of added T cells (23). Depletion of T cells with a ricin-linked mouse antihuman–CD5 immunoconjugate results in a short-term increase in IgM rheumatoid factor synthesis, which returns to baseline as T-cell numbers are restored (61). This observation suggests that some T cells are actively involved in suppressing rheumatoid factor-committed B cells in vivo. Removal of these suppressors allows preactivated B cells to secrete antibody without T-cell help over a limited period. However, over the long-term, removal of T cells in vivo has no effect on serum rheumatoid factor titers (48), and treatment of rheumatoid factor patients with total lymphoid irradiation does not result in decreased rheumatoid factor titers, despite marked decreases in total T cells (46,47). Clearly, the issue of T-cell dependence or independence of rheumatoid factor production is complex. The two possibilities are not mutually exclusive, and some rheumatoid factor synthesis may occur independently of T cells, whereas enhancement of rheumatoid factor synthesis may rely on T-cell-mediated mechanisms.

VI. HLA-DR4 AND RHEUMATOID FACTORS

The association between rheumatoid arthritis and the *HLA-DR4* histocompatibility locus is well established (62,63). In most series, 60–65% of rheumatoid arthritis patients are positive for HLA-DR4 (64). Despite numerous studies, the relation between the presence of HLA-DR4 and seropositivity for rheumatoid factor remains somewhat controversial. Although some series indicate that HLA-DR4 is associated with seropositivity for rheumatoid factor (65–67), other series find no significant correlation (68,69). These differences may arise, at least in part, from the difficulty of defining seronegativity, as well as from geographic or ethnic differences. However, the weight of evidence seems to favor a relation between seropositivity for IgM rheumatoid factor and the presence of HLA-DR4 (64,70). In one series, including 154 white patients, 91% of the HLA-DR4-positive individuals had significant rheumatoid factor titers, whereas only 74% of seronegative patients were HLA-DR4-positive ($p < 0.01$) (64). Furthermore, there was a trend toward higher rheumatoid factor titers in the subgroup of patients positive for HLA-DR4. In addition, all 24 patients with HLA-DR4 and no other DR marker, who were classified as putative homozygotes for DR4, were seropositive for IgM rheumatoid factor. These findings are of interest in view of the independent observation that the presence of HLA-DR4 in normal individuals is associated with an increased capacity to produce IgM rheumatoid factor (36) and implicate a role for the *HLA-DR4* locus in the control of rheumatoid factor production. Precise mechanisms underlying this association remain undefined.

VII. GENETICS OF RHEUMATOID FACTORS

In addition to the histocompatibility locus, genetic loci corresponding to autoreactive antibodies are likely to have an important role in the pathogenesis of autoimmune disease. Recent advances in the characterization of genes encoding rheumatoid factors and related autoantibodies have significant implications for the relative importance of genetic and environmental factors in the pathogenesis of rheumatoid arthritis. Much of the work in this area evolved from studies of monoclonal IgM rheumatoid factors that were usually derived from patients with dysgammaglobulinemias, such as Waldenstrom's macroglobulinemia (71). A remarkable degree of cross-reactivity was demonstrated between rheumatoid factors from unrelated individuals, so that these antibodies could be separated into several major families, determined by reactivity with polyclonal anti-idiotypic reagents (71). Subsequent amino acid-sequencing data confirmed that monoclonal rheumatoid factors exhibit a high degree of homology, especially in the light chain variable regions (72). Further studies have employed monoclonal anti-idiotypic antibodies prepared against three types of immunogens: (a) synthetic peptides corresponding to the conserved sequences in critical complementarity-determining regions (CDR) of rheumatoid factor light chains, (b) isolated rheumatoid factor heavy chains, or (c) intact monoclonal rheumatoid factors (73,74). Two of three such anti-idiotypic reagents tested recognized two-thirds of a panel of 177 rheumatoid factor paraproteins (73), a further indication of the large degree of homology among these antibodies. These findings suggest that the corresponding immunoglobulin genes encoding rheumatoid factors are highly conserved in the human population.

Cloning and sequencing of germline heavy and light chain sequences for rheumatoid factors have confirmed that these autoantibodies can be encoded by a limited number of heavy and light chain variable region (v) genes (74–76). It appears that all normal individuals possess at least three rheumatoid factor-associated kappa light chain V genes, which have been designated *humkv325*, *humkv328*, and *Vg*, and these genes show only minor degrees of polymorphism, even across ethnic lines (76). At least two heavy chain V genes related to rheumatoid factors, designated *hv3005* and *hv1051*, are also present in the normal human genome, but these loci show significant polymorphisms (76).

The polymorphic nature of the heavy chain V genes suggested the possibility that differences in these loci might be related to the development of autoimmune disease. This question was examined using probes derived from the *hv3005* gene to analyze restriction fragments of genomic DNA from normal individuals and patients with rheumatoid arthritis or systemic lupus erythematosus. Of the four major hybridizing bands identified, one was deleted in approximately 20% of the autoimmune patients, but in only 5% of the normal individuals ($p < 0.01$) (77). These differences were further characterized using the polymerase chain reaction (PCR) to amplify critical DNA sequences. Individuals with the band deletion had a complete deletion of *hv3005*-like genes (78). These results suggest that the early B-cell repertoire, which has preponderantly autoreactive specificities, forms an interactive network that is critical to the development of the mature

B-cell repertoire. As the immune system develops, exogenous antigens are introduced, and the autoreactive clones are normally no longer expressed except at very low levels. If part of the neonatal autoreactive network were missing, autoreactive clones might be able to persist and expand.

Two implications can be drawn from these analyses of rheumatoid factor genes. First, the presence of genes for rheumatoid factors in normal individuals suggests that rheumatoid factors have an important role in the immune system. This could include defining the normal B-cell repertoire, as discussed earlier, as well as augmenting host defenses as part of the normal immune response (79). Second, the germline sequences for rheumatoid factors are able to encode for proteins with anti-IgG activity, suggesting that antigen-driven somatic mutation is not an absolute requirement for the generation of autoreactivity.

Rheumatoid factors in patients with rheumatoid arthritis differ in many ways from the monoclonal paraproteins used in the previously cited studies, most obviously in that they are polyclonal. Furthermore, anti-idiotypic antibodies developed against monoclonal rheumatoid factor paraproteins recognize only a few rheumatoid factors from patients with rheumatoid arthritis (80). Consequently, genetic analyses derived from the study of monoclonal paraproteins cannot be assumed to apply to patients with rheumatoid arthritis. However, several recent interesting studies have been done using monoclonal rheumatoid factors derived from patients with rheumatoid arthritis (81–88). These studies indicate that at least several germline sequences can encode proteins with rheumatoid factor activity (81). Although the number of heavy and light chain gene families that are used by these rheumatoid factors are not restricted, some of the known germline rheumatoid factor sequences appear repeatedly. Furthermore, most of the pathogenic rheumatoid factor genes that have been analyzed show similarities to those used by the naturally occurring autoantibodies and by the known fetal antibody repertoire. For example, one monoclonal rheumatoid factor derived from rheumatoid synovium had 96% homology with a known germline heavy chain V region sequence (87). Overall, the V gene usage by pathogenic rheumatoid factors at first appears to be unrestricted, since many V gene families are involved. However, on further examination, it can be shown that the V genes used are derived from the selected ''autoreactive V gene'' repertoire, which encompasses about 15% of the potentially functional repertoire of human immunoglobulin V genes. This, in turn, suggests that the pathogenic rheumatoid factors in patients with rheumatoid arthritis derive from autoantibodies that escape normal regulatory mechanisms, such as might occur during a serious infection or with transient dysfunction of normal immune mechanisms. These escaped autoreactive specificities may then be driven by antigen-specific mechanisms to become monospecific, high-affinity, pathogenic antibodies (87).

The genetic basis of pathogenic rheumatoid factor production is clearly complex. Nevertheless, recent advances in this field are allowing the development of testable hypotheses concerning the roles of genetic and environmental factors in pathogenesis. Interventions to regulate abnormal responses may not be far in the future.

REFERENCES

1. Waaler E. On the occurrence of a factor in human serum activating the specific agglutination of sheep blood corpuscles. Acta Pathol Microbiol Scand 1940; 17:172–188.
2. Rose HM, Ragan C, Pearce E, Lipman MO. Differential agglutination of normal and sensitized sheep erythrocytes by sera of patients with rheumatoid arthritis. Proc Soc Exp Biol 1948; 68:1–6.
3. Bartfield H. Distribution of rheumatoid factor activity in nonrheumatoid states. Ann NY Acad Sci 1969; 168:30–37.
4. ter Borg EJ, Van Rijswijk MH, Kallenberg CGM. Transient arthritis with positive tests for rheumatoid factor as presenting sign of shunt nephritis. Ann Rheum Dis 1991; 50:182–183.
5. Naides SJ, Field EH. Transient rheumatoid factor positivity in acute human parvovirus B19 infection. Arch Intern Med 1988; 148:2587–2589.
6. Hirohata S, Inoue T, Miyamoto T. Frequency analysis of human peripheral blood B cells producing IgM-rheumatoid factor. J Immunol 1990; 145:1681–1686.
7. Tuomi T, Aho K, Palosuo T, et al. Significance of rheumatoid factors in an eight-year longitudinal study on arthritis. Rheumatol Int 1988; 8:21–26.
8. Mongan ES, Cass RM, Jacox RF, Vaughan JH. A study of the relation of seronegative and seropositive rheumatoid arthritis to each other and necrotizing vasculitis. Am J Med 1969; 47:23–35.
9. Withrington RH, Teitsson I, Valdimarsson H, Seifert MH. Prospective study of early rheumatoid arthritis. II. Association of rheumatoid factor isotypes with fluctuations in disease activity. Ann Rheum Dis 1984; 43:679–685.
10. Teitsson I. IgA rheumatoid factor as predictor of disease activity. Scand J Rheumatol Suppl 1988; 75:233–237.
11. Winska Wiloch H, Thompson K, Young A, Corbett M, Shipley M, Hay F. IgA and IgM rheumatoid factors as markers of later erosive changes in rheumatoid arthritis. Scand J Rheumatol Suppl 1988; 75:238–243.
12. Alarcon GS, Schrohenloher RE, Bartolucci AA, Ward JR, Williams HJ, Koopman WJ. Suppression of rheumatoid factor production by methotrexate in patients with rheumatoid arthritis. Arthritis Rheum 1990; 33:1156–1161.
13. Rudge SR, Pound JD, Bossingham DH, Powell RJ. Class specific rheumatoid factors in rheumatoid arthritis: response to chrysotherapy and relationship to disease activity. J Rheumatol 1985; 12:432–436.
14. Eberhardt KB, Svensson B, Truedsson L, Wollheim FA. The occurrence of rheumatoid factor isotypes in early definite rheumatoid arthritis—no relationship with erosions or disease activity. J Rheumatol 1988; 15:1070–1074.
15. Elkon KB, Delacroix DL, Gharavi AE, Vaerman JP, Hughes GRV. Immunoglobulin A and polymeric IgA rhumatoid factors in systemic sicca syndrome: partial characterization. J Immunol 1982; 129:576–581.

16. Otten HG, Daha MR, Van Laar JM, De Rooy HH, Breedveld FC. Subclass distribution and size of human IgA rheumatoid factor at mucusal and nonmucosal sites. Arthritis Rheum 1991; 34:831–839.

17. Walker SM, McCurdy DK, Shaham B, et al. High prevalence of IgA rheumatoid factor in severe polyarticular-onset juvenile rheumatoid arthritis, but not in systemic-onset or pauciarticular-onset disease. Arthritis Rheum 1990; 33:199–204.

18. Quismorio FP, Beardmore T, Kaufman RL, Mongan ES. IgG rheumatoid factors and anti-nuclear antibodies in rheumatoid vasculitis. Clin Exp Immunol 1983; 52:333–340.

19. Johnson PM, Faulk WP. Rheumatoid factor: its nature, specificity and production in rheumatoid arthritis. Clin Immunol Immunopathol 1976; 6:414–430.

20. Theofilopoulos AN, Barutonboy G, LoSpalluto JJ, Ziff M. IgG rheumatoid factor and low molecular weight IgM. An association with vasculitis. Arthritis Rheum 1974; 17:272–284.

21. Mizushima Y, Shoji Y, Hoshi K, Kiyohawa S. Detection and clinical significance of IgE rheumatoid factor. J Rheumatol 1984; 11:22–26.

22. Gioud-Paquet M, Auvinet M, Raffin T, et al. IgM rheumatoid factor, IgA-RF, IgE-RF and IgG-RF detected by ELISA in rheumatoid arthritis. Ann Rheum Dis 1987; 46:65–71.

23. Koopman WJ, Schrohenloher RE. Enhanced in vitro synthesis of IgM-rheumatoid factor in rheumatoid arthritis. Arthritis Rheum 1980; 23:985–992.

24. Olsen N, Ziff M, Jasin HE. In vitro synthesis of immunoglobulins and IgM-rheumatoid factor by blood mononuclear cells of patients with rheumatoid arthritis. Rheumatol Int 1982; 2:59–66.

25. Olsen NJ, Callahan LF, Pincus T. In vitro rheumatoid factor synthesis in patients taking second-line drugs for rheumatoid arthritis: independent associations with disease activity. Arthritis Rheum 1988; 31:1090–1096.

26. Patel V, Panayi GS, Unger A. Spontaneous and pokeweed mitogen-induced in vitro immunoglobulin and IgM rheumatoid factor production by peripheral blood mononuclear cells in rheumatoid arthritis. J Rheumatol 1983; 10:364–372.

27. Olsen NJ, Callahan LF, Pincus T. Immunologic studies of rheumatoid arthritis patients treated with methotrexate. Arthritis Rheum 1987; 30:481–488.

28. Olsen N, Ziff M, Jasin HE. Spontaneous synthesis of IgM-rheumatoid factor by blood mononuclear cells from patients with rheumatoid arthritis. Effect of treatment with gold salts or D-penicillamine. J Rheumatol 1984; 11:17–21.

29. Cush JJ, Jasin HE, Johnson R, Lipsky PE. Relationship between clinical efficacy and laboratory correlates of inflammatory and immunologic activity in rheumatoid arthritis patients treated with nonsteroidal anti-inflammatory drugs. Arthritis Rheum 1990; 33:623–633.

30. Moore S, Ruska K, Olsen N. In vitro synthesis of total IgA but not IgA-rheumatoid factor is associated with disease activity in rheumatoid arthritis. Arthritis Rheum 1991; 34:S178.

31. Wernick RM, Lipsky PE, Marban-Arcos E, Maliakkal JJ, Edelbaum D, Ziff M. IgG and IgM rheumatoid factor synthesis in rheumatoid synovial membrane cell cultures. Arthritis Rheum 1985; 28:742–750.

32. Robbins DL, Wistar R. Comparative specificities of serum and synovial cell 19S IgM rheumatoid factors in rheumatoid arthritis. J Rheumatol 1985; 12:437–443.

33. Patel V, Panayi GS. Enhanced T helper cell function for the spontaneous production of IgM-RF in vitro in rheumatoid arthritis. Clin Exp Immunol 1984; 57:584–592.

34. Koopman WJ. Suppressor T cells prevent in vitro expression of IgM-rheumatoid factor in some healthy adults. Proc Soc Exp Biol Med 1981; 168:344–349.

35. Olsen NJ, Jasin HE. Decreased T cell-mediated suppression of IgM-rheumatoid factor synthesis in rheumatoid arthritis. Clin Immunol Immunopathol 1987; 42:38–49.

36. Olsen NJ, Stastny P, Jasin HE. High levels of in vitro IgM rheumatoid factor synthesis correlate with HLA-DR4 in normal individuals. Arthritis Rheum 1987; 30:841–848.

37. Hardy RR, Hayakawa K, Shimizu M, Hamasaki K, Kishimoto T. Rheumatoid factor secretion from human Leu-1[+] B cells. Science 1987; 236:81–83.

38. Plater-Zyberk C, Maini RN, Lam K, Kennedy TD, Janossy G. A rheumatoid arthritis B cell subset expresses a phenotype similar to that in chronic lymphocytic leukemia. Arthritis Rheum 1985; 28:971–976.

39. Hayakawa K, Hardy RR, Honda M, Herzenberg LA, Steinberg AD. Ly-1 B cells: functionally distinct lymphocytes that secrete IgM autoantibodies. Proc Natl Acad Sci USA 1984; 81:2494–2498.

40. Crow MK. Rheumatoid arthritis synovial fluid contains CD5-positive B cells. Arthritis Rheum 1989; 32:S58.

41. Casali P, Burastero SE, Nakamura M, Inghirami G, Notkins AL. Human lymphocytes making rheumatoid factor and antibody to ssDNA belong to Leu-1[+] B cell subset. Science 1987; 236:77–80.

42. Suzuki N, Sakane T, Engleman EG. Anti-DNA antibody production by CD5 + and CD5 − B cells of patients with systemic lupus erythematosus. J Clin Invest 1990; 85:238–247.

43. Shmerling RH, Trentham DE. Prolonged improvement in refractory rheumatoid arthritis after anti-thymocyte globulin therapy of brief duration [letter]. Arthritis Rheum 1989; 32:1495–1496.

44. Horneff G, Burmester GR, Emmrich F, Kalden JR. Treatment of rheumatoid arthritis with an anti-CD4 monoclonal antibody. Arthritis Rheum 1991; 34:129–140.

45. Strand V, Lipsky PE, Cannon G, Calabrese L, Weisenhutter C, Cohen S, Olsen N, Lee MJ, Lorenz TJ, Nelson B and the CD5 Plus RA Investigators Group. Effects of administration of an anti-CD5 immunoconjugate in rheumatoid arthritis: Results of two Phase II studies. Arthritis Rheum 1993; 36:620–630.

46. Kotzin BL, Strober S, Engleman EG, et al. Treatment of intractable rheumatoid arthritis with total lymphoid irradiation. N Engl J Med 1981; 305:969–976.

47. Trentham DE, Beli JA, Anderson RT, et al. Clinical and immunologic effects of fractionated total lymphoid irradiation in refractory rheumatoid arthritis. N Engl J Med 1981; 305:976–982.

48. Paulus HE, Machleder HI, Levine S, Yu DTY, MacDonald NS. Lymphocyte involvement in rheumatoid arthritis: studies during thoracic duct drainage. Arthritis Rheum 1977; 20:1249–1262.

49. Townes AS, Sowa JM, Shulman LE. Controlled trial of cyclophosphamide in rheumatoid arthritis: an 18-month double-blind crossover study. Arthritis Rheum 1972; 15:129–130.

50. Weinblatt ME, Coblyn JS, Fraser PA, et al. Cyclosporin A treatment of refractory rheumatoid arthritis. Arthritis Rheum 1987; 30:11–17.

51. Bijlsma JWJ, Derksen DWHM, Huber-Bruning O, Bordeffs JCC. Does AIDS "cure" rheumatoid arthritis? [letter]. Ann Rheum Dis 1988; 47:350–351.

52. Calabrese LH, Wilke WS, Perkins AD, Tubbs RR. Rheumatoid arthritis complicated by infection with the human immunodeficiency virus and the development of Sjogren's syndrome. Arthritis Rheum 1989; 32:1453–1357.

53. Symons JA, Wood NC, DiGiovine FS, Duff GW. Soluble IL-2 receptor in rheumatoid arthritis: correlation with disease activity, IL-1 and IL-2 inhibition. J Immunol 1988; 141:2612–2618.

54. Semenzato G, Bambara LM, Biasi D, et al. Increased serum levels of soluble interleukin-2 receptor in patients with systemic lupus erythematosus and rheumatoid arthritis. J Clin Immunol 1988; 8:447–452.

55. Golub ES. Suppressor T cells and their possible role in regulation of autoreactivity. Cell 1981; 24:595–596.

56. Carson DA, Chen PP, Fox RI, et al. Rheumatoid factor and immune networks. Annu Rev Immunol 1987; 5:109–126.

57. Coulie PG, VanSnick J. Rheumatoid factor production during anamnestic immune responses in the mouse. III. Activation of RF precursor cells induced by their interaction with immune complexes and carrier-specific helper T cells. J Exp Med 1985; 161:88–97.

58. Coulie PG, Van Snick J. Rheumatoid factor production during anamnestic immune responses in the mouse: III. Activation of RF precursor cells is induced by their interaction with immune complexes and carrier-specific helper T cells. J Exp Med 1985; 161:88–97.

59. Nemazee DA. Immune complexes can trigger specific T cell-dependent autoanti-IgG antibody production in mice. J Exp Med 1985; 161:242–256.

60. Emery P, Gentry KC, Mackay IR, Muirdern KD, Rowley M. Deficiency of the suppressor-inducer subset of T lymphocytes in rheumatoid arthritis. Arthritis Rheum 1987; 30:849–856.

61. Olsen NJ, Teal GP, Strand V. In vivo T cell depletion in rheumatoid arthritis is associated with increased IgM-rheumatoid factor synthesis. Clin. Immunol. Immunopathol. 1993; 67:124–129.

62. Stastny P. Association of the B-cell alloantigen DRw4 with rheumatoid arthritis. N Engl J Med 1978; 298:869–871.

63. Stastny P. Mixed lymphocyte cultures in rheumatoid arthritis. J Clin Invest 1978; 57:1148–1157.

64. Olsen NJ, Callahan LF, Brooks RH, et al. Associations of HLA-DR4 with rheumatoid factor and radiographic severity in rheumatoid arthritis. Am J Med 1988; 84:257–264.

65. Karr RW, Rodey GE, Lee T, Schwartz BD. Association of HLA-DRw4 with rheumatoid arthritis in black and white patients. Arthritis Rheum 1980; 23:1241–1245.

66. Dobloug JH, Forre O, Kass E, Thorsby E. HLA antigens and rheumatoid arthritis. Arthritis Rheum 1980; 23:309–313.

67. Viana Queiros M, Sancho MRH, Caetano JM. HLA-DR4 antigen and IgM rheumatoid factors. J Rheumatol 1982; 9:370–373.

68. Jaraquemada D, Ollier W, Awad J, et al. Association of HLA-DR4/Dwr and DR2,Dw2 with radiographic changes in a prospective study of patients with rheumatoid arthritis. Arthritis Rheum 1984; 27:20–25.

69. Maeda H, Juji T, Mitsui H, Sonozaki H, Okitsu K. HLA-DR4 and rheumatoid arthritis in Japanese people. Ann Rheum Dis 1981; 40:299–302.

70. Stastny P. Rheumatoid arthritis. In: Terasaki P, ed. Histocompatibility testing 1980. Los Angeles: UCLA Tissue Typing Laboratory, 1981:681–686.

71. Kunkel HG, Agnello V, Joslin FG, Winchester RJ, Capra JD. Cross-idiotypic specificity among monoclonal IgM protein with anti-gammaglobulin activity. J Exp Med 1973; 137:331–341.

72. Andrews DW, Capra JD. Complete amino acide sequence of variable domains from two monoclonal human anti-gamma globulins of the Wa cross-idiotypic group: suggestion that the J segments are involved in the structural correlate of the idiotype. Proc Natl Acad Sci USA 1981; 787:3799–3803.

73. Crowley JJ, Goldfien RD, Schrohenloher RE, et al. Incidence of three cross-reactive idiotypes on human rheumatoid factor paraproteins. J Immunol 1988; 140:3411–3418.

74. Chen PP, Olsen NJ, Yang PM, et al. From human autoantibodies to fetal antibody repertoire and B cell malignancy. Int Rev Immunol 1990; 5:239–251.

75. Jirik FR, Fong S, Heitzmann JG, et al. Cloning and sequence determination of a human rheumatoid factor light-chain gene. Proc Natl Acad Sci USA 1986; 83:2195–2199.

76. Carson DA, Chen PP, Kipps TJ. New roles for rheumatoid factor. J Clin Invest 1991; 87:379–383.

77. Yang PM, Olsen NJ, Siminovitch KA, et al. Possible deletion of a developmentally-regulated *Vh* gene in autoimmune diseases. Proc Natl Acad Sci USA 1990; 87:7907–7911.

78. Olee T, Yang PM, Siminovitch KA, et al. Molecular basis of an autoantibody-associated RFLP that confers susceptibility to autoimmune diseases. J Clin Invest 1991; 88:193–203.

79. Carson DA, Pasquali JL, Tsoukas CD, et al. Physiology and pathology of rheumatoid factors. Springer Semin Immunopathol 1981; 4:161–179.

80. Olsen NJ, Chen PP. Immunogenetics of autoantibodies and autoimmune diseases. Curr Opin Rheumatol 1991; 3:391–397.

81. Pascual V, Randen I, Thompson K, et al. The complete nucleotide sequences of the heavy chain variable regions of six monospecific rheumatoid factors derived from Epstein–Barr virus-transformed B cells isolated from the synovial tissue of patients with rheumatoid arthritis. J Clin Invest 1990; 86:1320–1328.

82. Harindranath N, Goldfarb IS, Ikematsu H, et al. Complete sequence of the genes encoding the Vh and VI regions of low- and high-affinity monoclonal IgM and IgA1

rheumatoid factors produced by CD5[+] B cells from a rheumatoid arthritis patient. Int Immunol 1991; 3:865–875.

83. Ezaki I, Kanda H, Sakai K, et al. Restricted diversity of the variable region nucleotide sequences of the heavy and light chains of a human rheumatoid factor. Arthritis Rheum 1991; 34:343–350.

84. Weisbart RH, Wong AL, Noritake D, et al. The rheumatoid factor reactivity of a human IgG monoclonal autoantibody is encoded by a variant VkII L chain gene. J Immunol 1991; 147:2795–2801.

85. Victor KD, Randen I, Thompson K, et al. Rheumatoid factors isolated from patients with autoimmune disorders are derived from germline genes distinct from those encoding the Wa, Po, and Bla cross-reactive idiotypes. J Clin Invest 1991; 87:1603–1613.

86. Soto-Gil RW, Olee T, Klink BK, et al. A systematic approach to define the germline gene counterparts of a mutated autoantibody from a rheumatoid arthritis patient. Arthritis Rheum 1992; 35:356–363.

87. Olee T, Lu EW, Huang DF, et al. Genetic analysis of self associating IgG rheumatoid factors from two rheumatoid synovia implicates an antigen driven response. J Exp Med 1992; 175:831–842.

88. Robbins DL, Kenny TP, Coloma MJ, et al. Serologic and molecular characterization of a human monoclonal rheumatoid factor derived from rheumatoid synovial cells. Arthritis Rheum 1990; 33:1188–1195.

3

HLA-DR4 and Rheumatoid Arthritis

Gerald T. Nepom

Virginia Mason Research Center
Seattle, Washington

I. INTRODUCTION

There is a strong association between rheumatoid arthritis (RA) and genes encoded by the histocompatibility locus antigen (HLA) complex on chromosome 6. This genetic association was first recognized 15 years ago by the correlation of rheumatoid disease with a serological marker associated with the HLA complex, known as DR4. In the last 15 years, remarkable progress has been made toward understanding the genes and molecules that lead to this association. Of all the autoimmune diseases, the HLA genetic association in rheumatoid arthritis is perhaps the best understood. The genes responsible for the DR4-association have been identified, cloned, and thoroughly studied, and molecular models based on an understanding of these genes form the basis for a new type of potential immunotherapeutic approach.

II. MOLECULAR BASIS FOR THE HLA-DR4-ASSOCIATION WITH RHEUMATOID ARTHRITIS

HLA-DR4 is a serologically defined marker found on HLA molecules in some individuals. Studies in the early and mid-1980s made two key observations. First, multiple different genes within the *HLA* complex on chromosome 6 encode molecules that are positive for HLA-DR4 markers. In other words, the DR4 marker is a broad and heterogeneous serological specificity that does not itself identify a unique gene. Second, the different genes that encode different DR4-positive molecules all represent alleles of each other encoded for the *HLA* locus now known as *DRB1* (1–3).

115

Detailed molecular genetic studies over the last few years have led to a comprehensive view of the gene organization of the HLA complex and its relation with DR4, summarized in Figure 1. The HLA *DRB1* locus is located in the HLA-DR region of the major histocam partibility complex (MHC) class II complex on chromosome 6. The *DRB1* locus is one of several different loci that encode DR or DR-like molecules.

The genes within the class II complex are highly polymorphic; that is, they differ in different individuals in the population. This diversity in the population is principally of two types. First, there is allelic polymorphism: over 50 alleles are known at the *DRB1* locus. Eleven of these encode polypeptides which, when expressed on the cell surface, form HLA molecules that carry the DR4 marker. Most of these 11 alleles are very rare, but four of them, termed *DRB1*0401*, *0402*, *0403*, and *0404* (also known as Dw4, 10, 13, and 14, respectively) are prevalent in white populations. These *DRB1* alleles represent different genes encoded at the same locus that differ from each other by a few amino acids. A second form of HLA genetic diversity in the population is generated by DNA recombination, in which different HLA class II haplotypes recombine with each other and, over the course of human evolution, have diversified the linkage relationships between genes at different class II loci. Thus, for example, individual *DRB1* alleles, such as *Dw4*, are found on haplotypes that carry either of two different *DQ* genes at the nearby *HLA-DQ* locus.

Both of these concepts are important for understanding the basis of the HLA-DR4 association with rheumatoid arthritis. On the one hand, polymorphism of the *DRB1* locus accounts for the presence in the population of different alleles, some of which are positive for DR4, and some of which are not. Only some of these *DR4* alleles, in turn, are associated with RA. On the other hand, ancestral recombinance, for instance, between the *DRB1* and the *DQB1* loci, forms the basis for genetic mapping studies that localize susceptibility to the *DRB1* locus itself.

All of the HLA-DR4 contribution to genetic susceptibility in whites can be accounted for by the presence of only two of the *DR4*-positive alleles, *Dw4* and *Dw14*. Thus, in separate studies in the United States, Norway, and England, patients with DR4-associated erosive RA invariably had either *Dw4* or *Dw14* as their *DR4*-positive gene (4–8,31). Several patients actually carry two such susceptibility genes, either *Dw4,Dw4* or *Dw4,Dw14*. Other linked HLA class II genes, such as *DQβ*, are less associated with disease than *Dw4* or *Dw14*, indicating the primary role of the *DRB1* locus in genetic susceptibility (5,6). Thus, individuals who are HLA *Dw4* (DRB1*0401) have a six-fold relative risk to develop RA compared to individuals in the general population (Table 1). However, only about 1 in 35 of these individuals will actually develop RA (Table 1), indicating that HLA typing would not be cost effective at this time. Even among

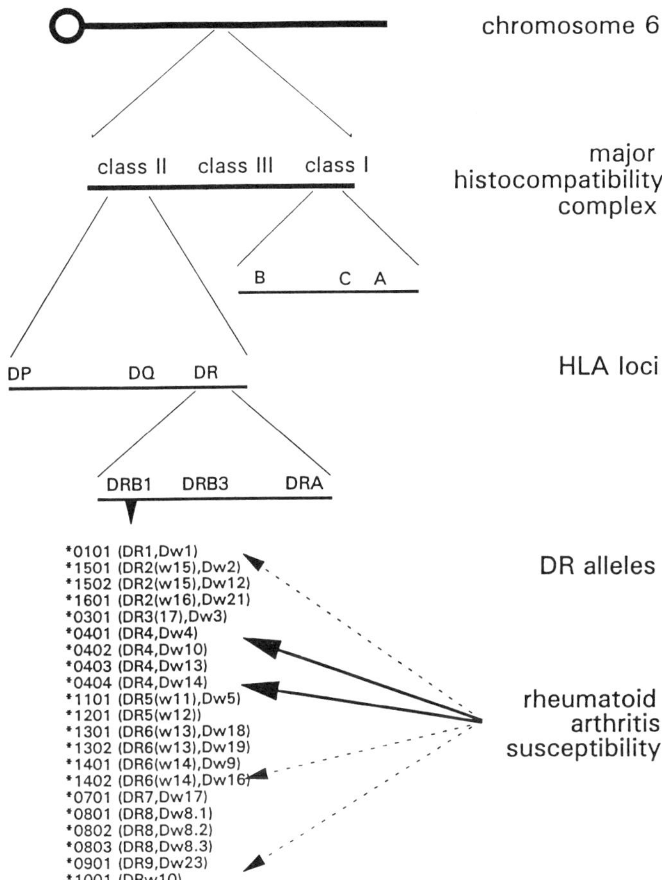

Fig. 1 Schematic gene organization of the major histocompatibility complex on chromosome 6, illustrating the localization of the major DR alleles to the *DRB1* locus within the DR region of the class II gene complex. Although only major expressed HLA loci are included in this figure, many additional genes are interspersed within this region, contributing to the potential genetic diversity of HLA-disparate individuals. The preponderant HLA genes associated with rheumatoid arthritis, *Dw4* (*DRB1*0401*) and *Dw14* (*DRB1*0404*) are *Dw4*-positive alleles of the *DRB1* locus, which encodes more than 50 different alleles in the population; among the other *DRB1* alleles shown in the figure, three [*Dw1* (*0101*), *Dw16* (*1402*), and *DR10* (*1001*)] are also associated with RA in different populations; each of these genes shares the same epitope sequence from codons 67–74.

Table 1 Estimates of Relative Risk and Prevalence for HLA Genes Associated with Rheumatoid Arthritis[a]

HLA Class II gene	Number of individuals per 10,000 population		Relative risk for individuals of this genotype compared to individuals not of this genotype	Estimated prevalence for individuals of this genotype
	with RA	without RA		
Dw4 (DRB1*0401)	50	1800	6:1	1 in 35
Dw14 (DRB1*0404)	25	500	5:1	1 in 20
Dw1 (DRB1*0101)	25	2000	1:1	1 in 80
Dw4 *or* Dw14	65	2300	6:1	1 in 35
Dw4, Dw14, *or* Dw1	90	4200	8:1	1 in 46
Dw4 *and* Dw14	15	100	116:1	1 in 7
Other	10	5800	0.12:1	1 in 580

[a]Estimates of risk of developing clinical RA among whites, based on an approximate disease prevalence of 1%. These numbers represent the upper limit of predictive value.
Adapted from: Nepom, G.T. and Nepom, B.S. Prediction of susceptibility to rheumatoid arthritis by human leukocyte antigen genotyping. In *Rheumatic Disease Clinics of North America*, G.T. Nepom, ed., **18**:785-792, 1992.

individuals who are HLA Dw4 and Dw14 in whom the relative risk to develop RA is greater than 100:1, only 1 in 7 individuals have RA (Table 1).

The *Dw4* and *Dw14* genes associated with RA differ structurally from non-*DR4* HLA genes; notably, they also differ from other *DR4*-positive alleles, such as *Dw10* and *Dw13*, which are not associated with disease. Each of these genes were cloned and sequenced in 1987 (3,9) and showed an interesting correlation: *Dw4, Dw14, Dw10*, and *Dw13* were very similar to each other. However, in one specific region of the gene, namely, the region encoding amino acids 67–74 of the HLA-DRβ polypeptide, the arthritis-associated alleles *Dw4* and *Dw14* differed from the nonassociated alleles *Dw10* and *Dw13*. This difference is illustrated in Figure 2. This region, encoding amino acids 67–74, is a highly polymorphic stretch within the *HLA-DRB1* genes. In other words, most of the *HLA-DRB1* alleles in the population carry different amino acids within this region. In fact, only three other *DRB1* genes have a similar or identical sequence from residues 67–74, namely *DRB1*0101* (*Dw1*), *DRB1*1402* (*Dw16*), *and DRB1*1001*. The presence of these other *DRB1* genes with similar sequences from residues 67–74 suggested a testable genetic hypothesis: If this sequence in the *Dw4* and *Dw14* genes is critical for RA susceptibility, then other *DRB1* alleles that carry the same sequence might also be associated with disease (10).

This hypothesis, known as the shared epitope model, adequately accounts for almost all of the known HLA contributions—both DR4 and non-DR4—to

gene	epitope sequence	prevalent population
Dw4 (DR4)	L L E Q K R A A	Caucasians
Dw14 (DR4)	L L E Q R R A A	Caucasians
Dw1 (DR1)	L L E Q R R A A	Caucasians
Dw16 (DR6)	L L E Q R R A A	Native Americans
DR10	L L E R R R A A	Asians, Spanish

Fig. 2 Rheumatoid arthritis-susceptibility genes which carry the HLA-DRB1 shared epitope sequence (codons 67–74). Each of the RA-associated genes prevalent in different ethnic groups shares a very similar amino acid sequence, either identical or with highly conservative substitutions relative to the prototype Dw4/14 sequences. The single-letter amino acid code indicates: L, leucine; E, glutamic acid; Q, glutamine; R, arginine; K, lysine; A, alanine.

rheumatoid arthritis, in all ethnic groups studied. Simply put, individuals who carry *DRB1* genes with amino acid sequences homologous to *Dw14* (i.e., LLEQ-KRAA) within the region 67–74 have a much higher than normal susceptibility to rheumatoid arthritis. Some of the study populations that support this model are indicated in Figure 2, along with the sequences of the shared epitope in non-*DR4* alleles associated with RA. In populations for which DR4 is present with a reasonable prevalence, such as most European or North American population groups, the *Dw4* and *Dw14* genes account for the preponderant susceptibility, being present in 60–80% of patients. Interestingly, in these same populations, the majority of the non-DR4 patients (from 20–40% of the total) carry the *Dw1* susceptibility gene (5,6,8). However, in population studies of groups with different ethnic backgrounds, in which Dw4 and Dw14 are not found, it is often the *Dw1* gene that is the preponderant susceptibility gene in RA (11,12). A similar story holds for both Dw16 and DR10. Native Americans in the Pacific Northwest have a high prevalence of rheumatoid arthritis. DR4, however, is only rarely found in these populations. In studies of both the Yakima nation and the Tlingit tribe, however, the *Dw16* gene was found at very high frequency and in almost all of the RA patients (13). Recent HLA studies in India and Spain in populations who also have a low prevalence of Dw4 and Dw14 have implicated the *DR10* gene in susceptibility to RA (14).

Thus, it is clear that the primary susceptibility in white populations, originally correlated with DR4, is due to the *Dw4* and *Dw14* genes at the *DRB1* locus. Analysis of non-DR4 patients remarkably demonstrates a correlation with the same shared epitope sequence present in Dw4 and Dw14. In most such studies, over 90% of patients with rheumatoid arthritis carry either one or two HLA-DRB1 molecules that carry this shared epitope (15).

III. CLINICAL HETEROGENEITY AND HLA-DR4

Rheumatoid arthritis encompasses a heterogeneous spectrum of clinical presentations. With the identification of the genetic basis for the DR4-association with RA, it was hoped that specific genetic components would correlate with subsets of the clinical spectrum and thereby provide some insight into mechanisms of pathogenesis. To some extent, this has indeed been true: The *Dw4* and *Dw14* susceptibility genes are increased in patients with the more severe erosive and progressive disease manifestations.

The concept that genetic heterogeneity parallels clinical heterogeneity is not new to rheumatology. It is well accepted that the term *juvenile rheumatoid arthritis* (JRA) represents a broad spectrum of disease categories, ranging from a pauciarticular disease presentation frequently associated with uveitis, to a rheumatoid factor-positive polyarticular symmetric arthritis, similar to the usual adult form of RA. In JRA, these clinical subsets were defined before detailed genetic analysis, but recent studies have demonstrated that each clinical subgroup has its own distinct pattern of genetic associations (Fig. 3). In fact, in JRA, only the symmetric, erosive seropositive subgroup shares the same susceptibility genes as adult RA, namely *Dw4* and *Dw14*. Other subsets of JRA are associated with other HLA genes, such as *DR5, DR6,* or *DR8* (16–19).

This same concept has been applied, a bit more tentatively, to adult rheumatoid arthritis. In general, there are three clinical variables that correlate with the MHC genetics: the spectrum of disease manifestations, the progression of disease severity, and the presence of rheumatoid factor. To some degree these coincide, since the patients with a severe progressive disease course are usually those with erosive disease of multiple joints and are usually seropositive. Although it has been universally found that these more severe patients have a very high incidence of the *Dw4* and *Dw14* susceptibility genes, it has been somewhat less clear that patients with less severe disease courses are different. To some degree, then, analysis of *DR4* susceptibility genes in RA may provide an additional predictive tool for distinguishing between patients with a likely progressive and severe disease outcome and those with a more benign clinical course.

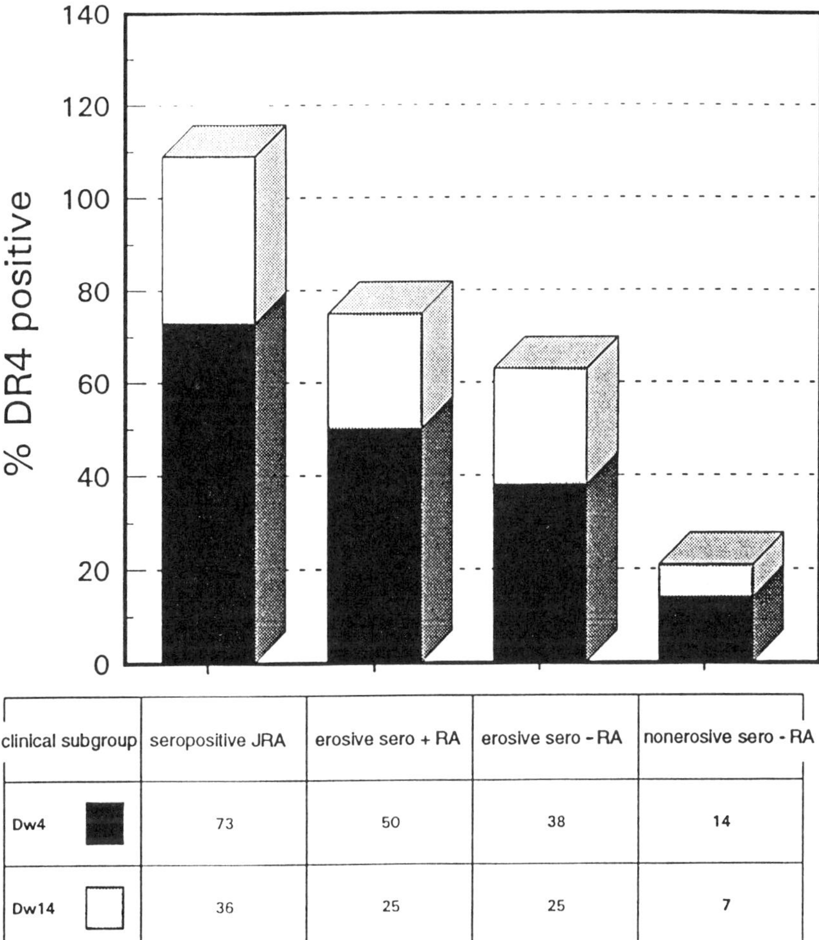

clinical subgroup	seropositive JRA	erosive sero + RA	erosive sero - RA	nonerosive sero - RA
Dw4	73	50	38	14
Dw14	36	25	25	7

Fig. 3 HLA-DR4 prevalence correlates with a spectrum of clinical heterogeneity in rheumatoid arthritis. The *Dw4* and *Dw14* susceptibility alleles are most prevalent in erosive, progressive forms of rheumatoid arthritis, both in juvenile (JRA) and adult populations, whether rheumatoid factor positive (sero + RA) or negative (sero − RA). In contrast, nonerosive, nonprogressive forms of symmetric synovitis within the RA clinical spectrum (nonerosive sero − RA) are not associated with these genes.

For example, in the Seattle studies, two groups of age-matched, elderly onset patients with RA were compared: Patients in one group had a relatively benign clinical course, responding to low doses of prednisone, and were negative for rheumatoid factor. Clinical studies had noted that disease with this phenotype often does not progress to joint destruction, a key distinction (20). The second group had more typical erosive seropositive RA. As expected, and comparable with the other population studies of seropositive erosive RA, 95% of the seropositive group carried one or more of the known susceptibility genes *Dw4, Dw14,* or *Dw1*. In contrast, the elderly onset seronegative group, without erosive changes, did not differ from the normal population in the frequencies of these alleles. In other words, there was no evidence for any contribution of HLA to the disease risk in the seronegative patient group (6).

This study of seronegative RA focused on a specific group of elderly onset patients, with a known benign clinical course, and found no HLA association. To evaluate whether this genetic correlation corresponded to the rheumatoid factor status of the patients, or whether it corresponded to the other manifestations of disease severity, we also studied a carefully selected set of seronegative adult rheumatoid arthritis patients with persistent and erosive disease who were clinically similar to the seropositive Dw4 and Dw14 patients. The seronegative patients in this study were well documented for the presence of radiographic evidence of erosive joint disease typical of RA, and were repeatedly negative for serum IgM rheumatoid factor. Eighty-one percent of these patients carried one or more of the HLA alleles previously associated with seropositive RA (i.e., the HLA alleles *Dw4, Dw14,* and *Dw1*; 21). Thus, it appears that disease severity, and particularly erosive progressive arthritis, is the primary clinical correlate of the HLA genetic predisposition, and not the presence of rheumatoid factor.

Another interesting issue relating HLA with RA is the possibility that individuals who carry more than one susceptibility allele may identify a clinically distinct phenotype. The potential exists for individuals to carry two *Dw4* genes, two *Dw14* genes, one of each, or some combination of *Dw4* or *Dw14* in association with *Dw1*. Patients with two different susceptibility genes, one inherited from each parental haplotype, tend to have the highest degree of genetic risk of RA (12,28). Interestingly, most of these patients are heterozygous for *Dw4* and *Dw14*, with one copy of each, rather than homozygous for *Dw4*, as would be expected from simple genetic models. In studies of seropositive JRA, most patients studied carried two of such susceptibility genes, usually heterozygous for *Dw4* and *Dw14* (45). Recent studies of adults with severe RA have correlated such heterozygosity with patients who manifest extra-articular disease (30,31) and have an increased need for surgical treatment (31).

These findings using DNA-based technology confirm and extend several previous reports that associated DR4 with rheumatoid factor and radiographic severity in rheumatoid arthritis (22–27). In these studies (e.g., Ref. 23), clinical criteria, such as total affected joint count, and various subjective disease status measures did not correlate with DR4-positivity, whereas radiographic indexes documenting joint space narrowing or malalignment were strongly correlated. Particularly in view of findings that significant radiographic damage occurs in RA within the first 2 years of disease (46), this association of specific HLA genes with a more progressive disease course in patients with RA raises the encouraging possibility that such specific susceptibility genes can be used as prognostic markers in early RA. Prospective studies will determine whether *Dw4* and *Dw14* genotyping will be helpful in identifying patients who, because of a likely poor clinical outcome, are good candidates for early aggressive forms of therapy.

IV. MECHANISMS TO ACCOUNT FOR THE DR4 ASSOCIATION

The structural and clinical features of the HLA susceptibility genes in RA, discussed in the foregoing, provide some direction concerning the probable mechanisms of genetic susceptibility. However, in spite of the precision with which susceptibility genes can now be identified, the precise pathogenic events mediated by these genes remain an enigma.

The genetics of RA can adequately be encapsulated in the shared epitope model, in which the sequence of amino acids from codons 67–74 of the *HLA DRB1* gene product is the principle determinant of susceptibility. Figure 4 is a schematic diagram of such an HLA molecule, highlighting the stretch of amino acids corresponding to the shared epitope. The diagram in Figure 4 represents an HLA class II molecule, composed of one α- and one β-chain, noncovalently associated to form a cell surface heterodimer. When expressed on the cell surface, this class II dimer is oriented with its key interaction domain exposed toward the extracellular environment and, more specifically, toward T cells, with their antigen-specific receptors. This interaction domain of the class II molecule is formed by both the α1- and β1-regions of the α- and β-class II polypeptides, respectively. Based on molecular-modeling comparisons with HLA class I molecules, it likely forms a deep groove, within which is the binding pocket for antigenic peptides to bind to the class II molecule (33,34). This groove is bounded on the bottom and on both sides by amino acids from the class II molecule, which create a distinct topography, consisting of pockets and bulges which, in turn, determine the precise requirements for the type of antigen that can bind. Thus, it is the specific sequence of amino acids in the class II molecule that determines the sequence and conformation of antigenic peptides that can successfully fit into the class II molecular groove. Since different HLA alleles differ in their amino acid sequences, different alleles bind different sets of antigenic peptides. It is in this sense that the HLA genes are ''permissive'' for immune

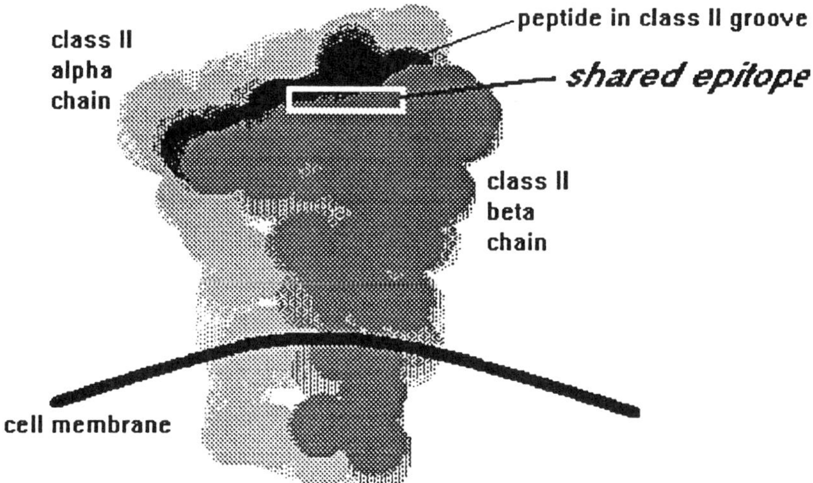

Fig. 4 A schematic—and somewhat fanciful—illustration of the class II molecule complexed with a bound peptide, illustrating the relation of the presumed shared epitope structure to contact sites on the surface of the intermolecular complex. Amino acid residues within the shared epitope are able to interact with both bound peptide and with T-cell receptor contact sites during T-cell activation.

activation, as they dictate the specificity of peptides that are permitted to bind within the class II structure.

The binding of antigenic peptide to a class II molecule is one of the first obligatory steps in specific antigen presentation. Subsequent steps that lead to T-cell activation require the recognition of the peptide–class II molecular complex by an antigen-specific T-cell receptor on an appropriate T cell, and also require the presence of various cofactors and costimulatory signals that are part of the immune recognition process. The peptide–class II interaction provides the key antigen-specific component to this interaction.

The shared epitope sequence on class II molecules associated with rheumatoid arthritis lies in an α-helical loop that forms one wall of the peptide-binding groove (see Fig. 4). As such, amino acids within the shared epitope sequence have two functional roles. On the one hand, amino acid side chains that point in toward the groove interact directly with the bound peptide. This has been directly demonstrated using site-directed mutagenesis of the amino acid at residue 71 of the Dw14 molecule (35–37). On the other hand, other residues within the shared epitope sequence, particularly 70, 74, and sometimes 67, as well as a component of amino acid 71, are oriented out of the groove, instead of into it. These amino acid residues form primary contact sites for the T-cell receptor molecule. Thus, the principal role of the shared epitope on the class II molecule is probably not just to dictate permissive peptide binding, but more likely involves direct and specific interaction with particular T-cell receptor elements.

The hypothesized disease mechanisms in which the HLA class II molecule interacts with specific T-cell receptors do not necessarily imply a primary genetic role for the T-cell receptor genes themselves. Rather, it is likely that the particular pattern of receptor usage among individual mature T cells in an individual, in concert with variation in the precursor frequency of such cells, may account for some of the seemingly low penetrance of the disease in HLA-susceptible patients.

Consideration of the molecular architecture and function of the shared epitope is leading to some interesting new therapeutic innovations. On the one hand, it is possible that blocking peptides or antagonistic peptides that bind in the class II groove can be designed such that they will displace pathogenic peptides (38,39). To make such peptide therapy relatively specific for RA, these blocking or antagonistic peptides will need to be designed such that they have stable interactions with the class II molecules that carry the shared epitope structure. Another strategy makes use of the apparent T-cell receptor interaction sites on the shared epitope, and is directed toward blocking this specific recognition with immunological reagents directed against the specific interaction sites on the T-cell receptor itself (40,41).

One presumption behind these new therapeutics is that the molecular mechanism of disease involves a straightforward antigen presentation event in which the class II molecules associated with disease trigger T-cell immunity by presentation of a pathogenic peptide. Although this is certainly a relevant and likely model for disease, it is not the only possibility. There are two variations of this model that merit serious consideration and illustrate our current state of ignorance about the underlying basis for genetic susceptibility to RA.

One of these alternative models involves the selection and maturation of potentially autoreactive T cells in individuals predisposed to disease. In this model, it is presumed that the HLA susceptibility genes such as *Dw4* or *Dw14* act during early development of the immune system to help educate maturing T cells to distinguish between self- and nonself-antigens. Indeed, this is one of the primary functions of the HLA class II genes and is a central tenet of mechanisms of immunological tolerance. With rheumatoid arthritis, it is possible that the presence of *Dw4* or *Dw14* genes during this early developmental process selects for T cells for which receptors are destined to become autoreactive and, therefore, trigger pathogenic events. Although there is as yet no direct evidence for this mechanism, in an animal model of collagen-induced arthritis, specific germline T-cell receptor genes are required along with specific HLA genes to precipitate experimentally induced autoimmune disease (42). In addition, recent studies of human T-cell receptor gene usage in peripheral blood have indicated that, indeed, there may be bias in the specificity of mature receptors based on the HLA type of the individual (43).

An additional consideration is the possibility that molecular mimicry may in some way contribute to pathogenesis associated with the shared epitope. Computer-based searches for sequence homology have demonstrated that sequences very close or identical with the shared epitope sequence are found in several microorganisms (44); however, there are no data to suggest that this potential cross-reactivity engenders a pathogenic autoimmune event. There are several interesting, but speculative, ways in which mimicry could be involved in disease onset: a pathogen could "sneak through" the immune defenses by mimicking a self-antigen; antigen presentation of a pathogen could "break tolerance" and trigger autoreactive cells directed to a self-class II molecule; or perhaps, if the shared epitope is itself a self-peptide used to maintain tolerance in the immune system, then recognition of an exogenous peptide mimic might skew the regulatory balance in favor of disease.

Efforts to verify these models and to use the structure of the shared epitope to design new immunotherapeutics represent the next step for the immunogenetic studies of RA. In this sense, the resolution of the genetic basis for the DR4 association with RA represents a beginning, not an end.

REFERENCES

1. Nepom BS, Nepom GT, Mickelson E, Antonelli P, Hansen JA. Electrophoretic analysis of human HLA-DR antigens from HLA-DR4 homozygous cell lines: correlation between beta-chain diversity and HLA-D. Proc Natl Acad Sci USA 1983; 80:6962.
2. Nepom GT, Nepom BS, Antonelli P, Mickelson E, Silver J, Goyert SM, Hansen JA. The HLA-DR4 family of haplotypes consists of a series of distinct DR and DS molecules. J Exp Med 1983; 159:394.
3. Gregersen PK, Shen M, Song Q-L, Merryman P, Degar S, Seki T, Maccari J, Goldberg D, Murphy H, Schwenzer J, Wang CY, Winchester RJ, Nepom GT, Silver J. Molecular diversity of HLA-DR4 haplotypes. Proc Natl Acad Sci USA 1986; 83:2642.
4. Nepom GT, Seyfried CE, Holbeck SL, Wilske KR, Nepom BS. Identification of HLA-Dw14 genes in DR4+ rheumatoid arthritis. Lancet 1986; 2:1002.
5. Wordsworth B, Lanchbury JSS, Sakkas LI, Welsh KI, Panayi GS, Bell JI. HLA-DR4 subtype frequencies in rheumatoid arthritis indicate that DRB1 is the major susceptibility locus within the HLA class II region. Proc Natl Acad Sci USA 1989; 86:10049.
6. Nepom GT, Byers P, Seyfried C, Healey LA, Wilske KR, Stage D, Nepom BS. HLA genes associated with rheumatoid arthritis. Arthritis Rheum 1989; 32:15.
7. Renningen KS, Spurkland A, Egeland T, Iwe T, Munthe E, Vartdal F, Thorsby E. Rheumatoid arthritis may be primarily associated with HLA-DR4 molecules sharing a particular sequence at residues 67–74. Tissue Antigens 1990; 36:235.
8. Gao X, Olsen NJ, Pincus T, Stastny P. HLA-DR alleles with naturally occurring amino acid substitutions and risk for development of rheumatoid arthritis. Arthritis Rheum 1990; 33:939.

9. Cairns J, Curtzinger J, Dahl C, Freeman S, Alter B, Bach F. Sequence polymorphism of HLA DR beta 1 alleles relating to T cell recognized determinants. Nature 1985; 317:166.

10. Gregersen PK, Silver J, Winchester RJ. The shared epitope hypothesis: an approach to understanding the molecular genetics of susceptibility to rheumatoid arthritis. Arthritis Rheum 1987; 30:1205.

11. Winchester RJ. The HLA system and susceptibility to diseases: an interpretation. In: Tan E, ed. Clinical aspects of autoimmunity. New York: Transmedica, 1986:9–26.

12. Ollier W, Thomson W. Population genetics of rheumatic diseases. In: Nepom GT, ed. Rheumatic Disease Clinics of North America. Philadelphia: WB Saunders, 1992.

13. Willkens RF, Nepom GT, Marks CR, Nettles JW, Nepom BS. The association of HLA-Dw16 with rheumatoid arthritis in Yakima Indians: further evidence for the "shared epitope" hypothesis. Arthritis Rheum 1991; 34:43.

14. Sanchez B, Moreno I, Magarino R, Garzon M, Gonzales J, Garcia A, Nunez-Roldan A. HLA-DR10 confers the highest susceptibility to rheumatoid arthritis in a Spanish population. Tissue Antigens 1990; 36:174.

15. Nepom GT, Nepom BS. Prediction of susceptibility to rheumatoid arthritis based on HLA genetics. In: Nepom GT, ed. Rheumatic Disease Clinics of North America. Philadelphia: WB Saunders, 1992.

16. Schaller JG, Hansen J. Early childhood pauciarticular juvenile rheumatoid arthritis: clinical and immunogenetic studies. Arthritis Rheum 1982; 25:S63.

17. Nepom BS. The immunogenetics of juvenile rheumatoid arthritis. In: Nepom GT, ed. Rheumatic Disease Clinics of North America. Philadelphia: WB Saunders, 1991.

18. Stastny P, Fink CW. Different HLA-D associations in adult and juvenile rheumatoid arthritis. J Clin Invest 1979; 63:124.

19. Glass D, Litvin D, Wallace K, Chylack L, Garovoy M, Carpenter CB, Schur PH. Early-onset pauciarticular juvenile rheumatoid arthritis associated with human leukocyte antigen-DRw5, iritis, and antinuclear antibody. J Clin Invest 1980; 66:426.

20. Healey LA, Sheets PK. The relation of polymyalgia rheumatica to rheumatoid arthritis. J Rheumatol 1988; 15:750.

21. Vehe R, Nepom GT, Wilske K, Healey LA, Stage D, Begovich A, Nepom BS. Rheumatoid factor positive and negative rheumatoid arthritis are immunogenetically similar. J Rheumatol 1994; 21.

22. Calin A, Elswood J, Klouda PT. Destructive arthritis, rheumatoid factor, and HLA-DR4. Arthritis Rheum 1989; 32:1221.

23. Olsen NJ, Callahan LF, Brooks RH, Nance EP, Kaye JJ, Stastny P, Pincus T. Associations of HLA-DR4 with rheumatoid factor and radiographic severity in rheumatoid arthritis. Am J Med 1988; 84:257.

24. Young A, Jaraquemada D, Awad J, Festenstein H, Corbett M, Hay FC, Roitt IM. Association of HLA-DR4/Dw4 and DR2/Dw2 with radiologic changes in a prospective study of patients with rheumatoid arthritis. Arthritis Rheum 1984; 27:20.

25. van Zeben D, Hazes JMW, Zwinderman AH, Cats A, Schreuder GMT, D'Amaro J, Breedveld FC. Association of HLA-DR4 with a more progressive disease course in patients with rheumatoid arthritis. Arthritis Rheum 1991; 34:822.

26. Alarcon GS, Koopman WJ, Acton RT, Barger BO. Seronegative rheumatoid arthritis. A distinct immunogenetic disease? Arthritis Rheum 1982; 25:502.

27. Silman A, Ollier B, McDermott M. HLA: linkage with rheumatoid arthritis or seropositivity. J Rheumatol 1988; 15:1189.

28. Rigby AS, Silman AJ, Voelm L, Gregory JC, Ollier W, Khan MA, Nepom GT, Thomson G. Investigating the HLA component in rheumatoid arthritis: an additive (dominant) mode of inheritance is rejected, a recessive mode is preferred. Genet Epidemiol 1991; 8:153.

29. Nepom B, Nepom GT, Schaller J, Mickelson E, Antonelli P, Hansen J. Characterization of specific HLA-DR4 associated histocompatibility molecules in patients with juvenile rheumatoid arthritis. J Clin Invest 1984; 74:287.

30. Hillarby M, Hopkins J, Grennan D. A re-analysis of the association between rheumatoid arthritis with and without extra-articular features, HLA-DR4 and DR4 subtypes. Tissue Antigens 1991; 37:39.

31. Weyand CM, Hicok KC, Conn DL, Goronzy JJ. The influence of HLA-DRB1 genes on disease severity in rheumatoid arthritis. Ann Intern Med 1992; 117:801.

32. Nelson J, Mickelson E, Masewicz S, Barrington R, Dugowson C, Koepsell T, Hansen J. Dw14(*DRB1*0404*) is a Dw4-dependent risk factor for rheumatoid arthritis. Tissue Antigens 1991; 38:145.

33. Bjorkman PJ, Saper MA, Samraoui B, Bennett WS, Strominger JL, Wiley DC. Structure of the human class I histocompatibility antigen, HLA-A2. Nature 1987; 329:506.

34. Brown JH, Jardetzky T, Saper MA, Samraoui B, Bjorkman PJ, Wiley DC. A hypothetical model of the foreign antigen binding site of class II histocompatibility molecules. Nature 1988; 332:845.

35. Rothbard JB, Busch R, Howland K, Bal V, Fenton C, Taylor WR, Lamb JR. Structural analysis of a peptide-HLA class II complex: identification of critical interactions for its formation and recognition by T cell receptor. Int Immunol 1989; 1:479.

36. Krieger JI, Karr RW, Grey HM, Yu W-Y, O'Sullivan D, Batovsky L, Zheng Z-L, Colon SM, Gaeta FCA, Sidney J, Albertson M, del Guercio M-F, Chesnut RW, Sette A. Single amino acid changes in DR and antigen define residues critical for peptide-MHC binding and T cell recognition. J Immunol 1991; 146:2331.

37. Hiraiwa A, Yamanaka K, Kwok WW, Mickelson EM, Masewicz S, Hansen JA, Radka SF, Nepom GT. Structural requirements for recognition of the HLA-Dw14 class II epitope—a key HLA determinant associated with rheumatoid arthritis. Proc Natl Acad Sci USA 1990; 87:8051.

38. De Magistris MT, Alexander J, Coggeshall M, Altman A, Gaeta FCA, Grey HM, Sette A. Antigen analog–major histocompatibility complexes act as antagonists of the T cell receptor. Cell 1992; 68:625.

39. Wraith DC, Smilek DE, Mitchell DJ, Steinman L, McDevitt HO. Antigen recognition in autoimmune encephalomyelitis and the potential for peptide-mediated immunotherapy. Cell 1989; 59:247.

40. Vandenbark AA, Hashim G, Offner H. Immunization with a synthetic T-cell receptor V-region peptide protects against experimental autoimmune encephalomyelitis. Nature 1989; 341:541.

41. Howell MD, Winters ST, Olee T, Powell HC, Carlo DJ, Brostoff SW. Vaccination against experimental allergic encephalomyelitis with T cell receptor peptides. Science 1989; 246:668.
42. David CS, Banerjee S. T cell receptor genes and disease susceptibility. Arthritis Rheum 1989; 32:105.
43. Gulwani-Akolkar B, Prosnett DN, Janson CH, Grunewald J, Wigzell H, Akolkar F, Gregersen PK, Silver J. T cell receptor V-segment frequencies in peripheral blood T cells correlate with human leukocyte antigen type. J Exp Med 1991; 174:1139.
44. Roudier J, Rhodes G, Petersen J, Vaughan JH, Carson DA. Hypothesis: the Epstein–Barr virus glycoprotein gp110, a molecular link between HLA DR4, HLA DR1, and rheumatoid arthritis. Scand J Immunol 1988; 27:367.
45. Vehe RK, Begovich AB, Nepom BS. HLA susceptibility genes in rheumatoid factor positive juvenile rheumatoid arthritis. J Rheumatol 1990; 17:11.
46. Fuchs H, Kaye J, Callahan L, Nance P, Pincus T. Evidence of significant radiographic damage in rheumatoid arthritis within the first 2 years of disease. J Rheumatol 1988; 16:585.

4

The Epidemiology of Rheumatoid Arthritis

Deborah P. M. Symmons and Alan J. Silman

University of Manchester
Manchester, England

I. INTRODUCTION

Epidemiology is the study of the distribution and determinants of disease in populations. Epidemiologists are interested in describing the frequency of disease and its prognosis, and in investigating risk factors for the development of the disease or its complications. In this chapter, we describe the current understanding of the incidence and prevalence of rheumatoid arthritis (RA) and discuss nongenetic risk factors for its development. The prognosis of the disease and genetic risk factors are dealt with elsewhere in this book.

II. PROBLEMS WITH DISEASE DEFINITION IN RHEUMATOID ARTHRITIS

In the field of the rheumatic diseases, before any epidemiological questions can be framed, the disease itself must be defined. It has not been easy to establish a disease definition for rheumatoid arthritis (RA) because, unfortunately, there is no single clinical, laboratory, or radiological marker that is specific for the disease. Therefore, it has been necessary to develop a set of classification criteria. Such criteria are required to distinguish mild RA from benign self-limiting synovitis at one end of the spectrum, and to distinguish severe RA from other destructive arthropathies at the other end of the spectrum. In epidemiological studies, there is also a requirement for criteria to be able to distinguish those with past, but now inactive, RA from those with normal or degenerative joints.

The first criteria set for RA was developed by a consensus of experts and accepted by the American Rheumatism Association (ARA) in 1956 (63). These criteria were subsequently revised (64) and gained widespread acceptance. They were known as the 1958 ARA criteria (Table 1). A simpler version of these criteria—called the Rome criteria—was adopted for epidemiological studies (41) (Table 2). The Rome criteria included a set for past (inactive) arthritis (Table 3). Anxieties about the specificity of the Rome criteria led to a new proposal, the New York criteria (9) (Table 4). The New York criteria never gained widespread acceptance, perhaps because no cutoff point was given for a "positive" case.

Both the Rome and New York criteria sets were developed for use in epidemiological studies. Clinical and drug studies continued to use the 1958 ARA criteria. In response to continuing criticism, a revised criteria set was proposed by the ARA in 1987 (3) (Table 5). For classification purposes patients are said to have RA if they satisfy at least four criteria. The 1987 criteria were developed to distinguish patients with established RA from those with other arthritic conditions and have not been fully evaluated in either the population setting or in patients with early RA. As well as the classic "four out of seven" list method shown in Table 5 a classification tree was developed, using the methods of recursive partitioning, which permits the substitution of one criterion for another in the case of missing values. The debate about defining RA continues, and it is likely that further refinements in classification will be necessary.

Table 1 1958 ARA Criteria for Rheumatoid Arthritis

1. Morning stiffness
2. Pain on motion or tenderness in a joint[a]
3. Swelling (soft-tissue thickening or fluid) in a joint[a]
4. Swelling (soft-tissue thickening or fluid) in another joint[a]
5. Symmetric joint swelling (simultaneous involvement of the same joint on both sides of the body)[a]
6. Subcutaneous nodules over bony prominences, on extensor surfaces, or near joints[a]
7. Radiographic changes (can include juxta-articular osteoporosis) typical of RA
8. Positive rheumatoid factor test
9. Poor mucin clot from synovial fluid
10. Synovial histopathology consistent with RA
11. Characteristic histopathology of nodules
Possible RA: two criteria for 3 weeks.
Probable RA: three or four criteria for at least 6 weeks.
Definite RA: five or six criteria for at least 6 weeks.
Classic RA: seven or more criteria for at least 6 weeks.

[a]Must be observed by a physician.
Long list of exclusions
Source: Ref. 64

Table 2 Rome Criteria for Active Rheumatoid Arthritis

1. Morning stiffness
2. Pain on movement or tenderness in a joint[a]
3. Soft-tissue swelling in a joint[a]
4. Soft-tissue swelling of another joint[a]
5. Symmetric soft-tissue joint swelling simultaneously[a,b]
6. Subcutaneous nodules[a]
7. Radiographic changes[c]
8. Positive rheumatoid factor

Three or four criteria positive: probable RA
Five or six criteria positive: definite RA
Seven or eight criteria positive: classic RA

[a]Must be observed by a physician.
[b]Does not include terminal interphalangeal joints.
[c]Can include juxta-articular osteoporosis.
Source: Ref. 41.

Table 3 Rome Criteria for Inactive Rheumatoid Arthritis

1. Past history of polyarthritis
2. Symmetric deformity of hand or foot joints
3. Radiological change
4. Positive rheumatoid factor

Two criteria positive: probable RA.
Three or four criteria positive: definite RA.

Source: Ref. 41.

Table 4 New York Criteria for Rheumatoid Arthritis

1. History of joint pain: $\geq$ three limb joints (pip/mcp, on one side counts as single joint)
2. Swelling, limitation of movement, subluxation or ankylosis of $\geq$ three limb joints *plus* symptoms of at least one joint pair. The involved joints must include at least one hand, wrist, or foot. There also must be symmetric involvement of at least one joint pair
3. Radiographic (grade 2 or more) erosive rheumatoid arthritis in hands, wrists, and feet
4. Positive serological reaction for rheumatoid arthritis

Positive: no rules or studies to indicate number and which criteria satisfied

Source: Ref. 9.

Table 5 The 1987 Revised Criteria for the Classification of Rheumatoid Arthritis (Traditional Format)

Criterion	Short title	Definition
1.[a]	Morning stiffness	Morning stiffness in and around the joints, lasting at least 1 h before maximal improvement.
2.[a]	Arthritis of three or more joint areas	At least three joint areas simultaneously have had soft-tissue swelling or fluid (not overgrowth alone) observed by a physician. The 14 possible areas are right or left PIP, MCP, wrist, elbow, knee, ankle, and MTP joints.
3.[a]	Arthritis of hand joints	At least one area swollen (as defined above) in a wrist, MCP, or PIP joint.
4.[a]	Symmetric arthritis	Simultaneous involvement of the same joint areas (as defined in 2 on both sides of the body (bilateral involvement of PIPs, MCPs, or MTPs is acceptable without absolute symmetry).
5.	Rheumatoid nodules	Subcutaneous nodules, over bony prominences, or extensor or juxtaarticular regions, observed by a physician.
6.	Serum rheumatoid factor	Demonstration of abnormal amounts of serum rheumatoid factor by any method for which the result has been positive in <5% of normal control subjects.
7.	Radiographic changes	Radiographic changes typical of rheumatoid arthritis on posteroanterior hand and wrist radiographs, which must include erosions or unequivocal bony decalcification localized in or most marked adjacent to the involved joints (osteoarthritis changes alone do not qualify).

[a]Must be present for at least 6 weeks.
Source: Ref. 3.

III. THE INCIDENCE OF RHEUMATOID ARTHRITIS

Incidence rate is the number of new cases of RA occurring in the population at risk during a given period (usually 1 year). Measuring the incidence of RA is fraught with difficulty. Two methods have been employed, both of which have flaws. The first method is to survey the same population at two time points and to estimate the number of new cases occurring between the surveys. This approach has two problems. First, a very large population survey is needed to obtain statistical precision. Second, the approach does not consider that some of the patients who develop RA after the first survey may die, and some may recover, before the second survey.

An alternative (cheaper) approach is constantly to monitor all the medical facilities to which patients from the target population who develop RA might present. The problem with this method is that some patients with RA may not seek medical help, and others may be misdiagnosed. Again it is necessary to study large populations for long periods to obtain robust estimates of incidence.

The first reliable data on the incidence of RA were based on a population survey in the North of England in 1954–1959 (46). Those classified as having RA were asked to recall their age at onset of symptoms. From these data an annual incidence of 22:1000 in adults aged over 55 was estimated. Five years later a follow-up survey found that 36 of the 620 individuals (6%) who had originally been free of RA, had now developed it. This was equivalent to an annual incidence rate of 12:1000—a figure that is much higher than those from other studies (Table 6). However, several of the studies listed in Table 6 (37,65,66) did not use standardized diagnostic criteria for RA.

All RA incidence studies to date show an increasing rate with age. The female rate is higher than the male rate at all ages. The difference between the genders is greatest in those younger than 45 and approaches equality in extreme old age.

A. Trends in Incidence

Secular trends in RA can be considered in terms of its incidence or severity. In fact, it is difficult to distinguish these concepts. Some of the criteria for defining RA (e.g., rheumatoid factor, radiological erosions) are also markers of disease severity. Thus, a reduction in the number of people satisfying these criteria might indicate an absolute decline in the incidence of the disease or a trend toward milder disease. Changes in severity might result from an improvement in the natural history of the disease or in therapy for the disease.

The Rochester Epidemiology Program at the Mayo Clinic provides an opportunity to examine changing trends in the numbers of new patients with RA who seek medical care. They reported a decline in the incidence of RA in women of about 30% between 1954 and 1974 (48). The incidence in men remained

Table 6 Incidence Studies of Rheumatoid Arthritis in Adult Populations

				Rates per 1000 persons		
Study (Ref)	Source of Cases	Year	Age range	Males	Females	Both
O'Sullivan (59)	Hospital referrals	1968			0.29	
Lawrence (46)	New cases developing between two cross-sectional surveys	1959–68	15+	8	12	10
Royal College of General Practitioners (65)	Prospective recording of new episodes in primary care	1970–72	15+	1.63	4.20	2.99
Linos et al. (48)	Retrospective review of hospital attenders	1950–74	15+	0.22	0.48	0.37
Royal College of General Practitioners (66)	Prospective recording of new episodes in primary care	1981–82	15+	1.50	3.34	2.47
Gran et al. (29)	Retrospective review of hospital attenders	1969–84		0.1	0.26	0.21
Isomaki (38)	Registration for disability	1979–84	25–64		0.70	
Hernandez-Avila et al. (37)	Biennial questionnaire survey in prospective cohort study of nurses	1976–84	30–55[a]		0.12	
Dugowson et al. (25)	Prospective notification of new referrals	1987–89	18+		0.24	
Symmons et al. (80)	Prospective monitoring of population	1990	16+	0.15	0.36	

[a]Age at baseline 10-year follow-up study.

stable during this time. A study carried out in Seattle (25) aimed to identify all female incident cases in a group health plan in 1987. The incidence rate of 0.24:1000 women was half the rate (0.48:1000 women) found in the Rochester area up to 1974. A halving of the incidence rate in women between 1976 and 1987 has also been reported from the United Kingdom (71). On the other hand, information from a population register of patients with seropositive RA in Finland showed no change in incidence between 1970 and 1980 (38).

If, as has been suggested, exposure to the environmental agent that triggers RA occurs early in life, it may be more appropriate to examine trends in the incidence of RA in patients defined by their year of birth, rather than by their year of disease onset. In a prospective study in Oberhorlen, West Germany, in the 1960s, the maximum incidence was found in those older than 65, whereas the maximum prevalence was in the decade younger than that age (7). More recently, Chan et al. (16) have reported, in a study from Worcester, Massachusetts, that the incidence of RA in those older than 50 is still high, whereas that in those younger than 50 has fallen.

There is also a widely held view that RA is declining in severity (13,45). A study from the United Kingdom has looked at three markers of disease severity (rheumatoid factor, radiological erosions, and nodules) by birth cohort (70). It found that successive generations were less likely to be positive for any of these features. Moreover, there was a severity peak in those presenting in 1960, with most birth cohorts displaying their maximum severity in that year. Population data from Finland (38) also show a fall in the proportion with RA among those who are registered as being disabled as a result of a musculoskeletal condition.

IV. PREVALENCE OF RHEUMATOID ARTHRITIS

The concept of measuring the *prevalence*—that is, all existing cases—of RA is apparently straightforward. However, in most populations the number of individuals who would satisfy the criteria for active RA (see Table 2) is small. Most people who have previously developed RA will currently have inactive disease, either because of disease remission or because of therapy. Accordingly, most point prevalence estimates will include a variable proportion of past cases. Thus, it is the cumulative life time prevalence that is being estimated, although those in whom the disease has left no stigmata will be excluded. Prevalence studies can be compared with one another only if they use the same methodology; otherwise, the proportion of the iceberg of "all RA cases ever" being detected will vary considerably.

There have been more surveys of the prevalence of RA than of any other rheumatic disease, although few studies have been sufficiently large to provide robust estimates of prevalence for all aged groups. Studies in European populations have produced remarkably consistent results, despite varying methodology. The prevalence of definite RA is about 0.8% in adults with a similar female excess to that seen in the incidence data. Tables 7–9 show the prevalence of RA in the United States, Africa, and Asia, respectively. Studies in United States white populations (15,26) have yielded results similar to those in European

Table 7 Prevalence of Rheumatoid Arthritis in North American Populations

Study (Ref.)	Population	Age	N	Males	Females	Both
				Prevalence of definite RA (%)		
Cobb et al. (17)	Pittsburgh (USA)	15+	798	0.4	1.0	0.7
Gofton et al. (27)	Haida Indians, Queen Charlotte Island	15+	209		1.0	
Mendez Bryan et al. (51)	Puerto Rico	15+	3883	0.2	0.4	
Mikkelson et al. (53)	Michigan (USA)	6+	7207	0.2	0.6	0.4
O'Brien et al. (57)	Pima Indians (USA)	30+		0.6	2.5	1.3
O'Brien et al. (57)	Blackfeet Indians (USA)	30+		1.3	1.4	1.4
Engel and Burch (26)	US adults	18–79	6672	0.46	1.7	1.0
Cathcart and O'Sullivan (15)	US whites	15+	4552			0.9
Beasley et al. (5)	Alaskan Eskimos	15+	1443	0.5	1.0	0.8
Beasley et al. (6)	Yakima Indians (USA)	18–79	501		3.4	
Harvey et al. (31)	Chippewa Indians (USA)	18+	205	4.8	8.2	6.8
Oen et al. (59)	Inuit Eskimos (Canada)	15+	2055		0.6	
Boyer et al. (10)	Yupik Eskimos	18+	4600	0.2	1.0	0.6
del Puente et al. (24)	Pima Indians (USA)	15+	1449		5.3	
Boyer et al. (11)	Southeast Alaskan Indians	19+	5169	1.3	3.5	2.4

whites. By contrast some American Indian groups (the Chippewa, Yakema, and Pima Indians) have increased prevalence rates, whereas others (Haida and Blackfeet Indians) do not. In all groups a female excess is observed.

Studies in African populations have posed a conundrum (Table 8). Studies in an urban setting, such as Soweto (74), showed a rate similar to that observed in European whites, whereas those in a rural setting (12,73) have shown a very low prevalence. In the Chinese, the prevalence is low in both a rural (4) and an urban setting (44) (Table 9). Low rates have also been reported from Indonesia (20).

Table 8 Prevalence of Rheumatoid Arthritis in African Populations

Study (Ref.)	Location	Age	N	Prevalence of definite RA (%)		
				Males	Females	Both
Lawrence et al. (47)	Kingston, Jamaica	35–64	530	1.5	2.2	1.9
Muller et al.[a] (56)	Igbo-ora, Isheri, Nigeria; and Cavalla, Liberia	5+	1027	0.8	1.2	1.0
Beighton et al. (8)	Rural, Tswana tribe Phokeng, South Africa	15+	801		0.12	
Solomon et al. (74)	Soweto, South Africa	15+	964	nil	1.4	0.9
Meyers et al. (52)	Xhosa tribe, Transkei, South Africa	15+	577		0.68	
Moolenburgh et al. (54)	Lesotho	15+	1070	nil	0.4	0.3
Brighton et al. (12)	Rural, Venda, South Africa	18+	543	nil	nil	nil[b]
Silman et al. (73)	Ibarapa, Nigeria	18+	2000	nil	nil	nil

[a]Includes "mild" disease.
[b]Prevalence of 0.03% in larger population based on cases attending local hospitals.

Table 9 Prevalence of Rheumatoid Arthritis in Asian Populations

Study (Ref.)	Population	Age	N	Prevalence of definite RA (%)		
				Males	Females	Both
Oshima (60)	Shizouka, Japan	All ages	3,000		0.8	
Shichikawa (67)	Osaka, Japan	All ages	3,000		0.2	
Wood et al. (86)	Hiroshima and Nagasaki, Japan	15+			0.4	
Shichikawa (68)	Kinki, Japan	All ages	10,272		0.3	
Kato et al. (39)	Hiroshima and Nagasaki, Japan	15+	11,393	0.4	0.7	
Schichikawa et al. (69)	Kamitonda, Japan	All ages	2,276		0.4	
Beasley et al. (4)	Kinmet, China	15+	5,629	0.2	0.4	0.3
Darmawan et al. (20)	Java, Indonesia	All ages	4,683		0.2	
Lau et al. (44)	Hong Kong	15+	2,000			0.4

Whether the variations in prevalence around the globe are due to genetic or environmental effects is still unclear. Certainly, in the Chinese, the low prevalence may be related to a low frequency of HLA-DR4 in that ethnic group.

V. GENETIC VERSUS ENVIRONMENTAL FACTORS

The debate about the relative contributions of genetic and environmental factors to the etiology of RA has been ongoing for several decades. The relation between the HLA system and RA is reviewed elsewhere in this volume (see Chapter 3). The strongest candidates for environmental triggers of RA are the sex hormones. This is suggested partly by the marked female excess in both the incidence and prevalence of RA and, partly, by the complex interrelations between pregnancy and RA.

A. Nongenetic Risk Factors

Hormones

Testosterone.   There have been several studies in both sexes exploring the relation between testosterone levels and the risk of developing RA. The case–control studies in men are summarized in Table 10. All have suggested that low testosterone levels are associated with RA. However, it is possible that the disease itself may suppress testosterone and the case–control study design cannot distinguish cause from effect. In women the picture is less clear.

Pregnancy.   It is still unclear whether pregnancy constitutes a risk factor for the development of RA. If pregnancy were a risk factor, one would expect a lower prevalence of RA among nulliparous women. In fact, the evidence suggests that nulliparity is associated with an increased risk of RA (23,65,78). It is not known whether the nulliparity is a preclinical effect of RA on reproductive

Table 10 Sex Steroid Levels in Males with Rheumatoid Arthritis

Study (Ref.)	Case *N*	Controls source	*N*	Result
Cutolo et al. (19)	7	Normal	6	Androgens ↓
Gordon et al. (28)	31	Normal	95	Serum testosterone ↓
		Ankylosing spondylitis	33	Derived free testosterone ↓
Spector et al. (77)	25	Osteoarthritis	25	Derived free testosterone ↓
Spector et al. (76)	87	Normal	141	Free testosterone ↓
		Ankylosing spondylitis	48	Serum testosterone ↓

function, or whether pregnancy itself protects against RA. It is difficult to distinguish voluntary from involuntary nulliparity. If, however, one assumed that most single women are nulliparous from choice, then this group might shed some light on the problem. In fact, marital status has little effect on the risk of RA (32,35,50,72). Evidence concerning the relation between RA and spontaneous abortion and stillbirth is also conflicting.

The Oral Contraceptive Pill.   The hypothesis that the oral contraceptive pill (OCP) protects against the development of RA originated in 1978 following an incidental finding in the Royal College of General Practitioners' (RCGP) study of the long-term risks and benefits of the OCP (85) (Table 11). This study involved a cohort of 46,000 women recruited over a 15-month period beginning in May 1968. Half the women were taking the OCP. Each woman taking the pill was matched with a woman of the same age and marital status who, up to that time, had never taken the pill. During the follow-up period, 94 new cases of RA were diagnosed. The risk of developing RA in the ''ever-takers'' was less than half (49%) that of the ''never-takers,'' with ''ex-takers'' having an intermediate risk. Subsequent follow-up of the same cohort of women has shown that this protection is not sustained (30). The initial findings of the RCGP study were supported by the Mayo Clinic's finding, noted earlier, of a decline in the incidence of RA in women, which had coincided with the introduction of the OCP in the 1960s (48).

In the 15 years since the publication of the RCGP study, there have been two further cohort studies and ten case–control studies (Table 12). Studies from the United States (24,49) and the Netherlands (33,34,82) gave conflicting results. This apparent paradox was later explained by Spector and Hochberg (75) when they divided studies up into those in which the cases were derived predominantly from a population base and those in which the cases were taken from a hospital setting. The pooled odds ratio for hospital-based cases was 0.49 (95% CI 0.39–0.63) and for population-based cases 0.95 (95% CI 0.78–1.16). Therefore, they suggested that the OCP protects against the development of severe, but not of mild, RA.

A fundamental difficulty in the interpretation of the OCP studies arises because the women have chosen whether or not to take the pill. This is not likely to be a random decision, but dictated by their lifestyle or health status. Thus, it is possible that the use of the OCP may be a surrogate for some other variable that is the true modifier of RA. This explanation is made more likely by the fact that no dose or duration effect has been convincingly demonstrated.

Postmenopausal Hormone Therapy.   There have been three studies of the effect of hormone replacement therapy (HRT) on the occurrence of RA. Their results are conflicting. The first, a case–control study (81) showed a halving of the risk of RA in those who had taken HRT. A further case–control study (14) and a retrospective cohort study (79) showed no protective effect. Again, the

Table 11 Studies of the OCP and RA

A. Cohort studies

Study (Ref.)	Yr	Place	Cohort size	Nature of cohort	Diagnostic criteria for RA
Wingrave and Kay (85)	1978	UK	46,000	Half on OCP	GP diagosis
Vessey et al. (83)	1987	Oxford	17,032	All on OCP	Hospital diagnosis
Hernandez-Avila et al. (37)	1990	USA	116,779	Nurses	ARA criteria from records

B. Case–control studies

Study (Ref.)	Year	Place	No. of cases	Source of cases	Case definitions	No. of controls	Source of controls
Vandenbroucke et al. (92)	1982	Netherlands	228	Hospital OP	Probable/definite ARA	302	Soft tissue/OA OP
Linos et al. (49)	1983	USA	229	Community	Probable/definite ARA	458	Community
Allebeck et al. (1)	1984	Sweden	76	Hospital OP	NY criteria ($>/=3$)	152	Community
del Junco et al. (22)	1985	USA	182	Community	Probable/definite ARA	182	Community
Vandenbroucke et al. (81)	1986	Netherlands	246	Hospital OP	Not stated	232	Soft tissue OA OP
Darwish and Armenian (21)	1987	Lebanon	104	Hospital OP and IP	Definite	104	Hospital OP
Spector et al. (78)	1990	England	150	Hospital OP	Definite ARA	337	OA/Community
Hazes et al. (33)	1990	Netherlands	134	Hospital OP newly diagnosed	Definite ARA	365	Soft tissue/OA
Moskowitz et al. (55)	1990	USA	71	Community	Probable/definite ARA	280	Community
Hazes et al. (34)	1990	Europe	86	Multicase families	Definite ARA	118	Sisters of cases

Table 12 Results of Studies of the OCP and RA: *Relative Risks*[a] *or Odds Ratios (95% CI) Versus Never Users*

Study (Ref.)	Ever-users	Current users	Ex-users
A. Cohort			
Wingrave and Kay (85)	0.7 (0.5–1.0)	0.5 (NS)	0.8 (NS)
Vessey et al. (83)	1.1 (0.8–1.8)	1.3 (NS)	1.0 (NS)
Hernandez-Avila et al. (37)	1.0 (0.7–1.3)	1.3 (0.3–6.5)	0.6 (0.1–2.6)
B. Case–control			
Vandenbroucke et al. (82)	0.4 (0.3–0.7)	0.5 (0.3–0.8)	0.4 (0.2–0.7)
Linos et al. (49)	1.7 (0.8–3.5)		
Allebeck et al. (1)	0.7 (0.4–1.2)	1.2 (0.6–2.5)	0.4 (0.2–0.9)
del Junco et al. (22)	1.1 (0.7–1.7)	1.3 (0.7–2.4)	1.0 (0.6–1.7)
Vandenbroucke et al. (81)	0.5 (0.3–0.9)		
Darwish and Armenian (25)	1.3 (0.6–2.6)		
Spector et al. (78)	0.6 (0.3–1.0)		
Hazes et al. (33)	0.4 (0.2–0.6)	0.6 (0.3–1.0)	
Moskowitz et al. (55)		2.0 (0.97–4.2)	1.0 (0.4–2.2)
Hazes et al. (34)	0.4 (0.1–1.2)		

[a]As estimated by Spector and Hockberg (1990).

decision to take HRT is not random; hence, the results of these studies are difficult to interpret.

Diet

There is a widespread view among patients that diet plays a part in the etiology of RA—but little epidemiological evidence to support this view. Rheumatoid arthritis may have a long latency; consequently, it is difficult to know how to focus retrospective studies. Prospective studies would require large sample sizes followed for long periods. In the absence of a specific hypothesis, it is hard to justify either approach.

Occupation

Data on the risk of RA in different occupations are scanty. There has been some suggestion of an increased risk among granite workers (42) and those in outdoor industries, such as fishing (36).

Infective Organisms

The most favored etiological model for RA is that the disease is triggered by an infection in a genetically susceptible host. A diligent search for the offending organism has, however, been unfruitful. Few infectious agents show the same geographic ubiquity as RA—although it is possible that RA might be a final common pathway following a variety of infective insults.

The strongest candidate as a viral cause for RA is the Epstein–Barr virus (EBV). Interest was first drawn following the description of an antibody to EBV in the sera of RA patients (2). It now seems that RA patients do not have an increased rate of prior EBV infection compared with normal controls, but that they have either a more severe infection, or an abnormal immune response to EBV. In countries with a low prevalence of RA (e.g., rural Africa), infection with EBV is almost universal by the age of 3. Such infection is clinically silent. In areas of high RA prevalence, infection with EBV occurs at an older age and is more likely to be clinically apparent.

Human parvovirus (HPV) is another candidate. Two papers from the United Kingdom (62,84) reported a high frequency of synovitis following HPV infection. However, neither study had an adequate control group, and none of the patients had a persistent arthritis. Some patients with early RA do have serological evidence of recent HPV infection (18), but it seems unlikely that this agent is the trigger in more than a small minority of cases of RA. It seems likely that the response to HPV is enhanced in HLA-DR4-positive persons (43). RA has some similarities to caprine arthritic encephalitis, which is a disease of goats produced by a retrovirus. However, attempts to identify a retrovirus in human RA have as yet been unsuccessful (61).

VI. SUMMARY

This chapter has summarized our current knowledge of the prevalence of RA around the globe. Rheumatoid arthritis is rare in rural Africa, among the Chinese, and in Indonesia. Genetic differences may explain some of the variation in prevalence, but environmental factors are also likely to play a part. The incidence of RA has been studied in only Western populations. There is some evidence that the incidence of RA may have fallen in young women during the 1960s and 1970s. The peak age of incidence is now in the group older than 50, whereas previously it was younger than this. It seems likely that the fall in RA incidence in young women can be attributed either directly or indirectly to the widespread use of the OCP. However, although our understanding of the genetic and nongenetic factors that make individuals susceptible to RA has grown in recent years, the initiating agent(s) of the disease remain elusive.

REFERENCES

1. Allebeck P, Ahlbom A, Ljungstrom K, Allander E. Do oral contraceptives reduce the incidence of rheumatoid arthritis? Scand J Rheumatol 1984; 13:140–146.

2. Alspaugh MA, Tan EM. Antibodies to cellular antigens in Sjogren's syndrome. J Clin Invest 1975; 55:1067–1073.

3. Arnett FC, Edworthy SM, Bloch DA, McShane DJ, Fries JF, Cooper NS, Healey LA, Kaplan SR, Liang MH, Luthra HS, Medsger TA, Mitchell DM, Neustadt DH, Pinals RS, Schauer JG, Sharp JT, Wilder RL, Hunder GG. The American Rheumatism Association 1987 revised criteria for the classification of rheumatoid arthritis. Arthritis Rheum 1988; 31:315–324.

4. Beasley RP, Bennett PH, Chun LC. Low prevalence of rheumatoid arthritis in Chinese. Prevalence survey in a rural community. J Rheumatol 1983; 10(suppl):11–15.

5. Beasley RP, Retailliau H, Healey LA. Prevalence of rheumatoid arthritis in Alaskan Eskimos. Arthritis Rheum 1973a; 16:737–742.

6. Beasley RP, Wilkens RF, Bennett PH. High prevalence of rheumatoid arthritis in Yakima Indians. Arthritis Rheum 1973b; 16:743–748.

7. Behrend T, Lawrence JS, Behrend H, Fischer K. Prevalence of rheumatoid arthritis in rural Germany. Int J Epidemiol 1972; 1:153–156.

8. Beighton P, Soloman L, Valkenburg HA. Rheumatoid arthritis in a rural South African negro population. Ann Rheum Dis 1975; 34:136–141.

9. Bennett PH, Wood PHN, eds. Population studies of the rheumatic diseases. Amsterdam: Excerpta Medica, 1968:477–478.

10. Boyer GS, Lanier AP, Templin DW. Prevalence rates of spondyloarthropathies, rheumatoid arthritis, and other rheumatic disorders in an Alaskan Inuit Eskimo population. J Rheumatol 1988; 15:678–683.

11. Boyer GS, Templin DW, Lanier AP. Rheumatic diseases in Alaskan Indians of the south east coast: high prevalence of rheumatoid arthritis and systemic lupus erythematosus. J Rheumatol 1991; 18:1477–1484.

12. Brighton SW, de la Harpe AL, van Staden DJ, Badenhorst JHM. The prevalence of rheumatoid arthritis in a rural African population. J Rheumatol 1988; 15:405–408.

13. Buchanan WW, Murdoch RM. Hypothesis: that rheumatoid arthritis will disappear. J Rheumatol 1979; 6:324–329.

14. Carette S, Carcoux S, Gingras S. Postmenopausal hormones and the incidence of rheumatoid arthritis. J Rheumatol 1989; 16:911–913.

15. Cathcart ES, O'Sullivan JB. Rheumatoid arthritis in a New England town. A prevalence study in Sudbury, Massachusetts. N Engl J Med 1970; 282:421–424.

16. Chan K-WA, Felson DT, Yood RA, Walker AM. No evidence of a secular decline in incidence of rheumatoid arthritis. Arthritis Rheum 1992; 35(suppl):5126.

17. Cobb S, Warrem JE, Merchant WR, Thompson DJ. An estimate of the prevalence of rheumatoid arthritis. J Chronic Dis 1957; 5:636–643.

18. Cohen BJ, Buckley MM, Clewley JP, Jones VE, Puttick AH, Jacoby RK. Human parvovirus infection in early rheumatoid and inflammatory arthritis. Ann Rheum Dis 1986; 45:832–838.

19. Cutolo M, Balleari E, Accardo S, et al. Preliminary results of serum androgen level testing in men with rheumatoid arthritis. Arthritis Rheum 1984; 27:958–959.

20. Darmawan J, Muirden K, Valkenburg HA, Wigley RD. The epidemiology of rheumatoid arthritis in Indonesia. Br J Rheum 1993; 32:537–540.

21. Darwish MJ, Armenian HK. A case–control study of rheumatoid arthritis in Lebanon. Int J Epidemiol 1987; 16:420–424.

22. del Junco DJ, Annegers JF, Luthra HS, Coulam CB, Kurland KT. Do oral contraceptives prevent rheumatoid arthritis? JAMA 1985; 254:1938–1941.

23. del Junco DJ, Annegers JF, Coulam CB, Luthra HS. The relationship between rheumatoid arthritis and reproductive function. Br J Rheumatol 1989; 28(suppl 1).

24. del Puente A, Knowler WC, Pettitt DJ, Bennett PH. High incidence and prevalence of rheumatoid arthritis in Pima Indians. Am J Epidemiol 1989; 129:1170–1178.

25. Dugowson CE, Koepsell TD, Voigt LF, Bley L, Nelson JL, Daling JR. Rheumatoid arthritis in women: incidence rates in group health co-operative, Seattle, Washington 1987–1989. Arthritis Rheum 1991; 34:1502–1507.

26. Engel A, Burch TA. Rheumatoid arthritis in US adults 1960–2. In: Bennett PH, Wood PHN, eds. Population studies of the rheumatic diseases. Amsterdam: Excerpta Medica, 1968.

27. Gofton JP, Robinson HS, Price GE. A study of rheumatic disease in a Canadian Indian population. II Rheumatoid arthritis in the Haida Indians. Ann Rheum Dis 1964; 23:364–371.

28. Gordon D, Beatall GH, Thomson JA, Sturrock RD. Androgenic status and sexual function in males with rheumatoid arthritis and ankylosing spondylitis. Q J Med 1986; 231:671–679.

29. Gran JT, Magnus J, Mikkelsen K, Nygaard H, Brath HK. The incidence of classical and definite rheumatoid arthritis in Lillehammer, Norway. Scand J Rheumatol 1986; 15(suppl 9):7.

30. Hannaford PC, Kay CR, Hirsch S. Oral contraceptives and RA: new data from the Royal College of General Practitioners, oral contraception study. Ann Rheum Dis 1990; 49:744–746.

31. Harvey J, Lotze M, Stevens MB, Lambert G, Jacobson D. Rheumatoid arthritis in a Chippewa band. I. Pilot screening study of disease prevalence. Arthritis Rheum 1981; 24:717–721.

32. Hawley DJ, Wolfe F, Cathey MA, Roberts FK. Marital status in rheumatoid arthritis and other rheumatic disorders: a study of 7293 patients. J Rheumatol 1991; 18:654–660.

33. Hazes JMW, Dijkmans BAC, Vandenbroucke JP, de Vries RRP, Cats A. Reduction of the risk of rheumatoid arthritis among women who take oral contraceptives. Arthritis Rheum 1990; 33:173–179.

34. Hazes JMW, Silman AJS, Brand R, Spector TD, Walker DJ, Vandenbroucke JP. Influence of oral contraception on the occurrence of rheumatoid arthritis in female sibs. Scand J Rheumatol 1990; 19:306–310.

35. Hazes JMW. Pregnancy and its effect on the risk of developing rheumatoid arthritis. Ann Rheum Dis 1991; 50:71–74.

36. Hellgren L. The prevalence of rheumatoid arthritis in different geographical areas in Sweden. Acta Rheumatol Scand 1970; 16:293–303.

37. Hernandez-Avila M, Liang MH, Willett WC, et al. Exogenous sex hormones and the risk of rheumatoid arthritis. Arthritis Rheum 1990; 33:947–953.

38. Isomaki HA. Rheumatoid arthritis as seen from official data registers. Experience in Finland. Scand J Rheumatol 1989; 79:21–24.

39. Kato H, Duff IF, Russell WJ, et al. Rheumatoid arthritis and gout in Hiroshima and Nagasaki, Japan. A prevalence and incidence study. J Chronic Dis 1971; 23:659–679.

40. Kay A, Bach F. Subfertility before and after the development of rheumatoid arthritis in women. Ann Rheum Dis 1965; 24:169–173.

41. Kellgren JH. Diagnostic criteria for population studies. Bull Rheum Dis 1962; 13:291–292.

42. Klockars M, Koskela RS, Jarvinen E, Kolari PJ, Rossi A. Silica exposure and rheumatoid arthritis: a follow-up study of granite workers. Br Med J 1987; 294:997–1000.

43. Klouda PT, Corbin SA, Bradley BA, Cohen BJ, Woolf AD. HLA and acute arthritis following human parvovirus infection. Tissue Antigens 1986; 28:318–319.

44. Lau EMC, Symmons DPM, MacGregor AJ, Bankhead CR, Donnan SPB. Low prevalence of rheumatoid arthritis in the urbanised Chinese people of Hong Kong. J Rheumatol 1993; 20:1133–1137.

45. Laurent R, Robinson RG, Beller EM, Buchanan WW. Incidence and severity of rheumatoid arthritis—the view from Australasia. Br J Rheumatol 1989; 28:360–361.

46. Lawrence JS. Rheumatism in populations. London: Heinemann, 1977.

47. Lawrence JS, Bremner JM, Ball J, Burch TA. Rheumatoid arthritis in a subtropical population. Ann Rheum Dis 1966; 25:59–66.

48. Linos A, Worthington JW, O'Fallon M, et al. The epidemiology of rheumatoid arthritis in Rochester, Minnesota: a study of incidence, prevalence and mortality. Am J Epidemiol 1980; 111:87–98.

49. Linos A, O'Fallon WM, Worthington JW, Kurland LT. Case control study of rheumatoid arthritis and prior use of oral contraceptive. Lancet 1983; 1:1299–1301.

50. Medsger AR, Robinson H. A comparative study of divorce in rheumatoid arthritis and other rheumatic diseases. J Chronic Dis 1972; 25:269–275.

51. Mendez-Bryan R, Gonzalez-Alcover R, Roger L. Rheumatoid arthritis: prevalence in a tropical area. Arthritis Rheum 1964; 7:171–176.

52. Meyers OL, Daynes G, Beighton P. Rheumatoid arthritis in a tribal Xhosa population in the Transke. Ann Rheum Dis 1977; 36:62–65.

53. Mikkelsen WM, Dodge HJ, Duff IF, Kato H. Estimates of the prevalence of rheumatic diseases in the population of Tecumseh, Michigan, 1959–60. J Chronic Dis 1967; 20:351–369.

54. Moolenburgh JD, Valkenburg HA, Fourie PB. A population study on rheumatoid arthritis in Lesotho, southern Africa. Ann Rheum Dis 1986; 45:691–695.

55. Moskowitz MA, Jick SS, Burnside S, Wallis WJ, Dickson JF. The relationship of oral contraceptive use to rheumatoid arthritis. Epidemiology 1990; 1:153–156.

56. Muller AS, Valkenburg HA, Greenwood BM. Rheumatoid arthritis in three West African populations. East Afr Med J 1972; 49:75–83.

57. O'Brien WM, Bennett PH, Burch TA, Bunim JJ. A genetic study of rheumatoid arthritis and rheumatoid factor in Blackfeet and Pima Indians. Arthritis Rheum 1967; 10:163–179.

58. Oen K, Postl B, Chalmers IM, et al. Rheumatic disease in an Inuit population. Arthritis Rheum 1986; 29:65–74.

59. O'Sullivan JB, Cathcart ES. The prevalence of rheumatoid arthritis. Follow up evaluation of the effect of criteria on rates in Sudbury, Massachusetts. Ann Intern Med 1972; 76:573–577.

60. Oshima Y. Clinical findings of collagen disease vs rheumatism. J Jpn Soc Intern Med 1960; 50:774–780.

61. Pelton BK, North M, Palmer RG, Hylton W, Smith-Burchnell CS. A search for retrovirus infection in systemic lupus erythematosus and rheumatoid arthritis. Ann Rheum Dis 1988; 47:206–209.

62. Reid DM, Reid TMS, Brown T, Rennie JAN. Human parvovirus-associated arthritis: a clinical and laboratory description. Lancet 1985; 1:422–425.

63. Ropes MW, Bennett GA, Cobb S, Jacox R, Jessar RA. Proposed diagnostic criteria for rheumatoid arthritis. Bull Rheum Dis 1956; 7:121–124.

64. Ropes MW, Bennett GA, Cobb S, Jacox R, Jessar RA. Revision of diagnostic criteria for rheumatoid arthritis. Bull Rheum Dis 1958; 9:175–176.

65. Royal College of General Practitioners. Office of Populations, Censuses and Surveys, Department of Health and Social Security. Morbidity statistics from general practice 1971–2. Second national morbidity study. London: HMSO, 1979.

66. Royal College of General Practitioners. Office of Populations, Censuses and Surveys, Department of Health and Social Security. Morbidity statistics from general practice 1981–2. Third national morbidity study. London: HMSO, 1986.

67. Shichikawa K. Epidemiology of rheumatoid arthritis. Jpn J Clin Med 1963; 21:1034–1042.

68. Shichikawa K. Prevalence of rheumatic diseases in Japan. In: Bennett PH, Wood PHN, eds. Population studies of the rheumatic diseases. Amsterdam: Excepta Medica, 1968:55–59.

69. Shichikawa K, Takenaka Y, Maeda A, Yoshino R, Tsujimoto M. A longitudinal population survey of rheumatoid arthritis in a rural district in Wakayama. Ryumachi 1981; 21(suppl):35–43.

70. Silman AJ, Davies P, Currey HLF, Evans SJW. Is rheumatoid arthritis becoming less severe? J Chronic Dis 1983; 36:891–897.

71. Silman AJ. Has the incidence of rheumatoid arthritis declined in the United Kingdom? Br J Rheumatol 1988; 27:1:77–78.

72. Silman AJ, Roman E, Beral V, Borwn A. Adverse reproductive outcomes in women who subsequently develop RA. Ann Rheum Dis 1988; 47:979–981.

73. Silman AJ, Holligan S, Birrell F, Adebajo W, Asuzu M, Thomson W. Low prevalence of rheumatoid arthritis in a rural Nigerian population [abstr]. Arthritis Rheum 1991; 34(suppl):D107.

74. Solomon L, Robin G, Valkenburg HA. Rheumatoid arthritis in an urban South African Negro population. Ann Rheum Dis 1975; 34:128–135.

75. Spector TD, Hochberg MC. The protective effect of the oral contraceptive pill on rheumatoid arthritis. Clin Epidemiol 1990; 43:1221–1230.

76. Spector TD, Ollier WER, Perry LA, Edwards A, Silman AJ, Thompson P. Testosterone levels in males: a comparative study of rheumatoid arthritis. Clin Rheumatol 1989; 8:37–41.

77. Spector TD, Perry LA, Tubb G, Silman AJ, Huskisson EC. Low testosterone levels in males with rheumatoid arthritis. Ann Rheum Dis 1988; 47:65–68.

78. Spector TD, Roman E, Silman AJ. The pill, parity and rheumatoid arthritis. Arthritis Rheum 1990; 33:782–789.

79. Spector TD, Brennan P, Harris P, Studd JW, Silman AJ. Does estrogen replacement therapy protect against rheumatoid arthritis? Ann Rheum Dis 1991; 18:1473–1476.

80. Symmons DPM, Barrett EM, Chakravarty K, Scott DGI, Silman AJ. The incidence of rheumatoid arthritis in Norfolk, England. Arthritis Rheum 1992; 35(suppl):S126.

81. Vanderbroucke JP, Witteman JCM, Valkenburg HA, Boersma JW, Cats A. Non-contraceptive hormones and rheumatoid arthritis in peri-menopausal and post-menopausal women. JAMA 1986; 255:1299–1303.

82. Vandenbroucke JP, Valkenburg HA, Boersma JW, Festen JJM, Cats A. Oral contraceptives and rheumatoid arthritis: further evidence for a preventive effect. Lancet, 1982; 2:839–842.

83. Vessey NP, Villard-Mackintosh L, Yeats D. Oral contraceptives, cigarette smoking and other factors in relation to arthritis. Contraception 1987; 35:457–465.

84. White DG, Mortimer PP, Blake DR, Woolf AD, Cohen BJ, Bacon PA. Human parvovirus arthropathy. Lancet 1985; 1:419–421.

85. Wingrave SJ, Kay CR. Reduction in the incidence of rheumatoid arthritis associated with oral contraceptives. Lancet 1978; 1:569–571.

86. Wood JW, Kato H, Johnson KG, Uda Y, Russell WJ, Duff IF. Rheumatoid arthritis in Hiroshima and Nagasaki, Japan. Prevalence, incidence and clinical characterisation. Arthritis Rheum 1967; 10:21–31.

5

Joint Assessment

Howard A. Fuchs

Vanderbilt University School of Medicine
Nashville, Tennessee

Jennifer J. Anderson

Boston University School of Medicine
Boston, Massachusetts

I. INTRODUCTION

Rheumatoid arthritis (RA) is a chronic, systemic inflammatory disease of unknown etiology that may affect any organ system. The cells lining internal body surfaces are primarily involved, with the synovial lining in the diarthrodial joints, tendon sheaths, and bursae the focus for most of this inflammation. Extra-articular manifestations are common and include inflammation of serosal surfaces elsewhere (pleurisy and pericarditis) and vasculitis. Rheumatoid nodules, scleritis, mononeuritis multiplex, and cutaneous ulceration are the most common manifestations of vasocentric inflammation in RA. Extra-articular involvement with the inflammatory process, with the exception of rheumatoid nodules, portends a much poorer prognosis for the patient with RA (1). Extensive articular involvement also portends a worse prognosis over time (2), and quantifying involvement is important for predicting morbidity and mortality.

The joint examination is the focal point of the examination of a patient with RA, both in patient care settings and in clinical trials. The articular examination enables one to establish a differential diagnosis by determining the distribution of articular inflammation, as well as the nature of the inflammation (e.g., synovial-based inflammation vs enthesitis). The assessment of disease activity and accrued damage will require quantitative measures for accurate portrayal of the disease process. This chapter deals with the formulation and use of quantitative articular assessment in RA.

II. JOINT STRUCTURE AND INFLAMMATION

Histologically, joints can be termed fibrous articulations, at which the opposing bone surfaces are connected by fibrous connective tissue; cartilaginous articulations, at which the opposing bone surfaces are connected by cartilaginous tissue; and synovial articulations, at which the opposed bone surfaces are separated by an articular cavity that is defined by the surrounding synovial tissue. The fibrous joints include the fissures in the skull or syndesmosis, which is an adjoining of bones by an interosseous ligament or membrane, as in the distal long bones of the forearm and leg. Examples of the cartilaginous articulations include symphysis pubis, manubriosternal joint, and the intervertebral disks. Involvement of these joints is not generally seen in rheumatoid arthritis due to the absence of synovial-lining cells. Hyaline cartilage covers the bony surfaces in most synovial-lined joints, with the exception of the apophyseal joints of the spine; the acromioclavicular, sternoclavicular, and temporomandibular joints, the surfaces of which are composed of primarily fibrocartilage (3). Because of these differences, inflammation in these latter joints may have different clinical signs than in the other diarthrodial joints.

The supporting structures in and around the joint include ligaments and tendons that constrain the actions of the muscles across the joint. Knowledge of the anatomy is important to ascertain the site of inflammation and to discern if the patient has RA or one of the other most common chronic inflammatory arthritidies, labeled as a group the spondyloarthropathies (psoriatic arthritis, reactive arthritis, ankylosing spondylitis, enteropathic arthritis). Rheumatoid arthritis is truly a synovial-based arthritis, whereas in the spondyloarthropathies the inflammation is often primarily at the cartilaginous insertions of ligament on bone (entheses), and synovial inflammation is then secondary; proliferative synovitis with angiogenesis and proliferation of lymphocytes and macrophages in the synovium is seen only in RA. In the small joints of the hands and feet, RA produces a typical fusiform swelling owing to the proliferation of the synovium and the presence of joint effusion; the primary finding in the small joints of the hands and feet of a patient with a spondyloarthropathy is that of a dactylitis (sausage digit) owing to inflammation at the enthesis. In addition, RA tends to be a process that involves rows of joints [e.g., metacarpophalangeal (MCP)], whereas the spondyloarthropathies often will involve rays [e.g., distal and proximal interphalangeal (DIP and PIP) and MCP joints of a finger] and often involve only weight-bearing joints. Extra-articular manifestations of RA and the spondyloarthropathies will also differ (Table 1).

A. Components of the Quantitative Articular Examination

The articular examination may separately assess tenderness, pain on motion, swelling, limitation of motion, and deformity. Tenderness, swelling, and pain

Table 1 Physical Examination Features That Distinguish Spondyloarthropathy and Rheumatoid Arthritis

Spondyloarthropathy	Rheumatoid arthritis
Asymmetric oligoarthritis	Symmetric
Preponderantly weight-bearing joints	Invariably involves hands
Dactylitis ("sausage digit")	Fusiform swelling of PIP joints
Inflammation at insertions	Synovial proliferation and inflammation
Ray distribution (e.g., entire finger)	Row distribution (e.g., all PIP joints)
± Uveitis, psoriasis, urethritis, spondylitis, gut inflammation	± Nodules, serositis, vasculitis, splenomegaly, adenopathy

on motion are primarily manifestations of acute inflammation in the joint (4), whereas limitation of motion and deformity are more a reflection of permanent structural changes. The frequency of the presence of these joint abnormalities in patients with RA seen in a cross-sectional sampling of a rheumatology clinic population, using the joint examination outlined by the American College of Rheumatology (ACR) (5), is noted in Table 2 (6). The PIP joints of the fingers, MCP, wrists, MTP, knees, and ankles had the highest frequency of swelling and tenderness. Deformities were most commonly seen in the small joints of the hands and feet. Pain on motion and limitation of motion were especially useful measures in the shoulder and hips, as these joints are difficult to assess for swelling, tenderness, and deformity. The temporomandibular, sternoclavicular, acromioclavicular, DIP of the fingers, and PIP joints of the toes uncommonly exhibited signs of inflammation.

Tenderness

Joint tenderness is generally elicited by direct palpation and is perhaps the most subjective of the components of the examination. Both patient and observer attributes, as well as the level of inflammation, will affect the level of perceived tenderness. Variation in patient pain threshold is a large confounding factor, but is less important if change over time is the outcome being evaluated. Each observer will assess tenderness differently, for both the amount of pressure and the site of application to the joint. This is especially true for inflamed joints, as patient discomfort is generally minimized during examination (for humanitarian reasons, if nothing else) and less pressure than usual may be applied. Efforts to standardize the amount of pressure applied to the joint line has included the use of a dolorimeter (7) and, more recently, a strain gauge placed between the examiner's fingers and the patient (8). The use of the dolorimeter is limited to relatively small joints and is dependent on what part of the joint it is placed. Use of the strain gauge device to determine the threshold of tenderness (scale = 0–7) may greatly reduce intraobserver variability, compared with the ACR joint

Table 2 Percentage of 189 Rheumatoid Arthritis Patients with Abnormal Findings in Specific Joints

Joint	Swelling (R/L)	Tenderness (R/L)	Pain on motion (R/L)	Limitation of motion (R/L)	Deformity (R/L)
Temporomandibular (TM)	3/4	17/17	9/11	21/21	–*
Sternoclavicular (SC)	3/3	11/12	1/1	–	0/0
Acromioclavicular (AC)	0/1	25/22	3/3	–	0/0
Shoulder	0/1	21/22	52/48	43/45	4/4
Elbow	26/29	35/31	25/23	34/31	36/32
Wrist	66/65	55/52	58/55	71/66	36/35
Metacarpophalangeal (MCP)					
Thumb	24/21	41/39	16/16	30/22	16/18
Index	82/74	51/48	24/35	31/25	39/30
Middle	67/61	45/41	24/16	32/25	36/28
Ring	50/42	41/34	23/15	31/24	34/25
Little	49/44	35/35	21/15	31/24	34/25
Proximal interphalangeal (PIP)					
Thumb	20/13	30/22	11/10	27/28	19/20
Index	36/30	40/39	23/14	35/27	24/21
Middle	40/39	46/43	27/17	37/32	32/31
Ring	31/25	40/33	21/13	27/25	27/25
Little	29/23	37/30	20/10	30/29	33/34
Distal interphalangeal (DIP)					
Index	5/3	10/4	4/2	14/13	32/33
Middle	2/1	8/6	2/2	15/11	35/27
Ring	2/1	7/4	2/2	12/10	26/22
Little	2/1	6/3	0/1	14/10	33/31
Hip	–	5/7	19/17	18/20	1/1
Knee	33/34	38/42	34/33	11/15	11/11
Ankle	40/36	38/33	34/31	29/26	5/6
Subtalar	7/6	5/5	11/10	16/14	3/3
Tarsometatarsal	11/10	11/9	19/18	23/21	3/3
Metatarsophalangeal (MTP)					
First	24/21	42/41	12/11	6/6	38/37
Second	27/22	41/39	12/7	5/4	19/19
Third	26/21	41/40	12/7	5/4	19/19
Fourth	25/20	40/40	12/8	4/4	19/18
Fifth	24/19	40/37	12/7	4/4	19/16
Proximal interphalangeal (PIP)					
First	1/2	11/8	3/3	9/9	9/8
Second	2/2	8/5	2/1	10/8	30/23
Third	3/2	7/4	2/1	8/9	20/18
Fourth	3/2	5/3	2/1	6/7	14/11
Fifth	1/2	4/3	1/1	4/3	8/5

*– = not evaluated.

Table 2 is used by the kind permission of *Arthritis and Rheumatism* and the JB Lippincott Co.

tenderness counts as used in Table 2; however, calibration of the device is crucial and may limit the practicality of this device.

The grading of the magnitude of joint tenderness varies from observer to observer (9,10). In these studies there was good agreement concerning the presence or absence of joint tenderness, but wide variation in the estimate of the magnitude. As a result, in studies requiring repeat measurements or using graded scales, all examinations need to be done by a single observer. Whether it is necessary to use graded scales versus binary (normal or abnormal) has not been determined, although for clinical trials the quantitative scale has been recommended in the past, in spite of the intraobserver variability, as the ability to show change over time may be greater.

Swelling

Swelling of a joint or periarticular structure, unlike tenderness, is always abnormal. However, the presence of swelling may be difficult to quantify owing to underlying bony proliferation from concomitant osteoarthritis of the fingers, joint deformity altering the usual joint contours, or the presence of dependent edema in the feet and ankles. Proximal interphalangeal (PIP) joint circumference may be measured by jeweler's rings, tape measure, or similar devices, but tends to be a cumbersome measure with significant interobserver error that limits its usefulness (11). As a result, quantitative assessment of swelling is usually analogous to that of tenderness, with a graded scale based on physical examination. In assessing disease activity, some investigators have felt that the joints that are both swollen and tender are more indicative of the inflammatory response, as measured by sedimentation rate and C-reactive protein (4), and would favor noting the presence of both in a particular joint in clinical trials.

Pain on Motion

Pain on motion is generally used as a surrogate for joint tenderness in joints that are difficult to palpate. In the Ritchie articular index (12) (see later), pain on motion is substituted for tenderness for the cervical spine, hips, talocalcaneal, and midtarsal joints. No current medication evaluation trial uses a separate assessment of pain on motion.

Deformity

Joint deformity in RA is very common in the small joints of the hands and feet. Swan-neck deformity describes flexion at the distal interphalangeal (DIP) joint with concomitant extension at the PIP joint of the finger. A boutonnier deformity describes flexion at the PIP joint with extension at the DIP joint of the finger. Hammertoes occur after metatarsophalangeal joint subluxation and describe the resulting flexion deformity involving both PIP and DIP joints of the toes. However, these lesions are not quantified specifically. Depending on the method of evaluation, deformity may be assessed separately from limitation of motion. In Table 2, deformity was assessed as being reducible or nonreducible.

Limitation of Motion

Arc of joint motion can be carefully measured with a goniometer, and normal values have been defined. The set of values most commonly used are those defined by the American Academy of Orthopedic Surgeons (13). A reevaluation of these norms has also been undertaken (14), but is not widely used. Tables defining the normal values can be found in these sources. Passive range of motion will exceed active range of motion in most instances; therefore, whether motion is measured actively or passively must be clearly stated.

B. Methods of Quantitative Assessment

Tenderness and Swelling

The method of examination used in Table 2 was a modification of that outlined in the *Dictionary of the Rheumatic Diseases* by the ACR Glossary Committee (5), which is as follows: for tenderness and pain on motion the same scales were used: 0 = none, 1 = minimal, 2 = wince, 3 = wince and withdraw; swelling was recorded as: 0 = none, 1 = minimal, 2 = within joint contours, and 3 = distention outside normal joint contours; limitation of motion was graded: 0 = none, 1 = <10% loss, 2 = 10–19% loss, 3 = 20–49% loss, 4 = >50% loss, and 5 = ankylosis; deformity was graded as present or absent.

In the United States, the Cooperating Clinics for the Systematic Study of the Rheumatic Diseases (CSSRD) scale for tenderness and swelling (15) is generally used in clinical trials. This scale grades tenderness and swelling, as defined by the ARA Glossary Committee for those joints included in Table 2, except the subtalar and midfoot joints are assessed as one joint.

The European League Against Rheumatism (EULAR) has designated the Ritchie articular index for joint tenderness as the preferred measure (12) in clinical trials. The grading for tenderness is also as outlined by the ACR glossary committee, but this index differs by assessing the MCP, PIP, and metatarsophalangeal (MTP) rows each as one joint instead of five separate joints. Both left and right temporomandibular, sternoclavicular, and acromioclavicular joints are graded as one, and the cervical spine is graded as a whole; the other joints are assessed separately for right and left sides. Joints that cannot be easily palpated for joint tenderness (hips, subtalar, and midfoot joints, and the cervical spine) are assessed for pain on passive motion of the joint. In the formulation of this index, the authors stressed it was designed to document changes in joint tenderness.

Adjusting for Joint Size

Lansbury proposed another approach to estimating the amount of inflammation present by factoring the size of the joint with the presence of tenderness, rather than grading the amount of tenderness for an individual joint (16). This joint count has not been widely used, however, and its relation to other outcome and process variables has not been clearly defined.

Measures of Structural Damage

Several quantitative measures of limitation of joint motion have been proposed (17,18). The joint alignment and motion scale of Speigel et al. (17) assigns a value for a range of motion for each joint, as well as an alignment score. The worse of the two determinations is the score given that joint. It has been reliable and has correlated with functional class and disease severity (19). These measures of joint motion are unlikely to be used in the short-term assessment of interventions, however, and will be of most use in longitudinal studies to determine the relative contribution of specific joint abnormalities to functional status and to predict morbidity and mortality.

C. Formulation of Reduced Joint Counts

It is time-consuming for the clinician to do a full joint count, and in daily practice it may seldom be necessary. Even in a clinical trial setting there should be little advantage to assessing joints that are seldom involved in RA. If changes in the disease are generalized (systemic) then the assessment of a limited number of more frequently involved joints may be sufficient for ascertaining changes in disease status. Also, since RA is typically symmetric in its presentation, it is possible that the assessment of one side of the body may suffice. Questions of whether such reduced joint counts are as reliable as a full joint count have been previously examined.

Prior Studies

Egger et al. (20) reduced the CSSRD joint count from 68 joints to 36 joints (Table 3), by analyzing articular examinations of patients from two medication trials, and found no major loss in sensitivity to change or in correlation with other clinical measurements. Swelling and tenderness were the characteristics included in the articular examination. Their resulting index excluded the DIP of the fingers, PIP of the toes, tarsal, shoulder, acromioclavicular, sternoclavicular, and temporomandibular joints that were included in the original CSSRD index. Thompson et al. (4) used this index, with the surface area estimates of Lansbury, as a multiplier for joints having the simultaneous presence of both swelling and tenderness of the joint; this joint count provided the best correlation with systemic inflammation as estimated by the acute-phase reactants (4). Fuchs et al. (6) compared the Thompson index with that of Egger et al. and a further reduced 28-joint index, which differs from the Egger joint count in that the shoulder joint is included, but bilateral ankle and MTP joints were excluded (see Table 3). Correlations with acute-phase reactants and walking time were higher for indices when scores were weighted for joint size, but otherwise no major differences were seen between correlations with clinical measurements and the different joint indexes.

Further Study on the Reduction in Number of Joints Assessed

Here we wish to examine the validity and sensitivity to change of three modifications of the CSSRD joint count. Each is an assessment of a subset of the 68 joints evaluated for tenderness and the 66 joints evaluated for swelling in the full CSSRD joint assessment. Table 3 indicates which joints are included in the various modifications. None include the four DIP joints of the fingers or the five PIP joints of the toes that are part of the CSSRD joint count; in Table 2, as well as in the data set used here, these joints were the ones least often swollen or tender. The Ritchie index used here was modified to separately assess each of the other joints of the CSSRD joint count, counting each MCP, PIP, and MTP joint as a separate joint, rather than counting each row of joints as a unit. The original Ritchie index also included the subtalar joint and the cervical spine, neither of which are included in the ACR joint assessment. The modified Ritchie assessment used here makes use of information on 50 joints. The other subset joint counts are the 36-joint count of Egger et al. and the 28-joint count of Fuchs et al.

The data used to address the questions of validity and sensitivity of the modified joint counts consists of a series of CSSRD joint assessments obtained on 424 patients enrolled in two comparative trials of nonsteroidal anti-inflammatory drugs (NSAIDs) in RA (21). The patients' joints were assessed first at the end of a 2-week washout period just before starting trial medications, and subsequently at several time points throughout the trial, which lasted for 12 weeks. There were 2184 joint assessments performed and 322 of the patients completed the trial with a final evaluation after either 10 or 12 weeks of treatment. The final two columns of Table 3 indicate the percentages of all of the joint assessments for these 424 subjects in which swelling and tenderness were observed in specific joints at baseline and during the trial. Comparison with Table 2 shows similar frequencies of involvement of specific sites, except for more swelling at the shoulder and midfoot joints and more tenderness at the midfoot joints.

Comparison of Reduced Joint Assessments

Table 4 summarizes the comparison of the joint count modifications. With the full CSSRD count as a standard, the various modifications are compared for

Table 3 Subsets of the CSSRD Joint Set Included in Modified Joint Counts from 2184 Articular Assessments of 424 Rheumatoid Arthritis Patients in an NSAID Clinical Trial

Joint	Ritchie	Egger	Fuchs[c]	Swelling[a] (R/L)	Tenderness[a] (R/L)
Temporomandibular	R			2/1	14/13
Sternoclavicular	R			4/3	14/13
Acromioclavicular	R			3/3	23/22
Shoulder	R[b]		F	17/14	51/48
Elbow	R	E	F	32/29	40/37
Wrist	R	E	F	65/61	62/59
Metacarpophalangeal					
First (thumb)	R		F	46/42	45/42
Second	R	E	F	68/65	55/50
Third	R	E	F	65/60	52/47
Fourth	R	E	F	37/32	36/34
Fifth	R	E	F	37/32	36/33
Proximal interphalangeal					
Thumb (interphalangeal)	R	E	F	27/23	29/26
Index	R	E	F	45/41	42/38
Middle	R	E	F	53/48	48/44
Ring	R	E	F	42/39	41/39
Little	R	E	F	33/29	35/30
Distal interphalangeal					
Index				9/7	12/9
Middle				9/6	12/9
Ring				6/5	9/8
Little				5/5	9/8
Hip	R				16/16
Knee	R	E	F	43/46	47/50
Ankle					
Mortise	R	E		46/47	48/48
Tarsus	R[b]				
Metatarsophalangeal					
First	R	E		31/29	38/37
Second	R	E		30/29	43/42
Third	R	E		29/27	42/41
Fourth	R	E		23/22	37/36
Fifth	R	E		17/16	30/29
Proximal interphalangeal (toe)					
I				7/6	13/12
II				6/7	13/13
III				6/5	12/11
IV				5/4	11/10
V				3/4	9/8

[a]Percentage of patients with tender or swollen joints (score $\geq$ 1), right and left.
[b]Subtalar (talocalcaneal) and cervical spine are also included in the full Ritchie index.
[c]R, Ritchie et al. (12); here modified to include 50 joints; E, Egger et al. (20), 36-joint count; F, Fuchs et al. (6), 28-joint count.

Table 4 Adequacy and Sensitivity of Different Joint Assessments: A Comparison of Different Scoring Methods and Joint Selections

Assessment	CSSRD	Ritchie	Egger	Fuchs
Tender joints				
Joints evaluated (N)	68	50	36	28
Joints examined (%)	100	74	53	41
Affected joints examined (%)[a]	100	90	72	58
Joint change measured (%)[b]	100	91	72	57
Sensitivity of scoring methods to detect change over time[c]				
Unweighted score	1.00	1.05	1.00	1.02
Unweighted count	1.02	1.05	0.99	0.95
Area-weighted score[d]	0.99	0.99	1.01	0.96
Area-weighted count	0.98	0.98	0.95	0.89
Swollen joints				
Joints evaluated (N)	66	48	36	28
Joints examined (%)	100	73	55	42
Affected joints examined (%)[a]	100	94	83	69
Joint change measured (%)[b]	100	91	78	62
Sensitivity of scoring methods to detect change over time				
Unweighted score	0.84	0.91	0.89	0.93
Unweighted count	0.89	0.95	0.92	0.89
Area-weighted score	0.89	0.89	0.87	0.82
Area-weighted count	0.90	0.90	0.85	0.80
Swollen and tender joints				
Sensitivity of scoring methods				
Unweighted score	0.87	0.93	0.94	0.97
Unweighted count	0.94	0.99	1.00	0.94
Area-weighted score	0.93	0.95	0.93	0.97
Area-weighted score	0.96	0.95	0.95	0.89

[a] $N = 2184$.
[b] $N = 322$.
[c] The measure of sensitivity (E), a standardized change measure, is proportional to the t-statistic. See text for description.
[d] Weighting is by joint surface area as in the Lansbury index (16).

completeness. It is clear that modified assessments, although requiring the examination of smaller proportions of the CSSRD complement, do examine affected joints preferentially. Moving from the 68-joint count to 50-, 36-, and 28-joint assessments that eliminate some less frequently affected joints, there is a steady reduction in the amount of evaluation required, but relatively higher proportions of the joints assessed are affected. This trend is even more marked for the evaluation of swelling than for those of joint tenderness. These percentages are for binary (normal or abnormal) handling of the data.

If one observes the amount of change in the binary, unweighted (for either severity of swelling or tenderness or of joint size) count occurring with each of the various modifications between the beginning and the end of the NSAID trial, it is clear that the subset modifications are identifying changes in joint tenderness in proportion to joint involvement that they detect, but that they do not detect changes in swelling to quite the same extent. This suggests that there are joints that have been excluded from these modified assessments that are more likely to have swelling change under treatment than are some of the joints that have not been excluded. There also are joints, such as the index and long finger MCP joints, that are unlikely to have swelling resolve; less change will be seen over time in indices in which these joints make up a larger proportion of the total of joints evaluated.

Sensitivity of Reduced Joint Assessments

The relative sensitivity of a variety of ways of summarizing the swelling and tenderness information available from these several reduced joint evaluations may be expressed in terms of a standardized change measure, or efficiency, E. In this context, when change is being measured within a single group of patients receiving the same treatment, E is the mean of the change in the measure between the start and the end of the trial, divided by the standard deviation (SD) of this change (Anderson JJ, and Chernoff MC. "Sensitivity to change of rheumatoid arthritis outcome measures"; manuscript in preparation), and is proportional to the t-statistic, which is used as a measure of sensitivity in a variety of formulations (22–24). The larger the value of E associated with a measure, the more sensitive it is to change (i.e., the fewer observations are needed for observed change to be statistically significant). The values of E seen in these data are quite large, ranging from 0.80 to 1.05. If $E = 0.80$ then nine observations would be needed, given the same mean change and standard deviation of change, for change to be declared statistically significant, whereas eight observations would be needed if $E = 0.85$–0.90, seven observations for $E = 0.95$–1.00, and only six if E is as high as 1.05. Thus, the joint assessment measures are all very sensitive, considerably more sensitive than some other measures often included in clinical trials, which may have values of E as low as 0.40 (25 observations needed) or 0.20 (100 observations needed) (Anderson JJ, Chernoff MC. "Sensitivity to change of rheumatoid arthritis outcome measures"; manuscript in preparation). The variability of E itself is a function of the sample size on which it is based: for $N = 322$, the SE(E) ~ 0.05; for comparing differences between highly correlated versions of the same measure with efficiencies E_1 and E_2, respectively, the SE $(E_1 - E_2) \sim 0.025$, and for the trial data of Table 4, values of E that are 0.05 apart are statistically significantly different from one another.

In Table 4, the sensitivity of a variety of scoring methods for assessments are shown. The *unweighted score* is the sum of graded levels of swelling or tenderness or both. The *unweighted count* is the number of joints that are swollen or tender or both. The *area-weighted* scores use the joint surface area estimates of Lansbury (as also used by Thompson) as a multiplier in the foregoing two methods.

Within a particular joint selection there is little difference between different joint counts. As a group, tender joint assessments in this data set have values of E that are higher (0.89–1.05) than those for the swollen joint assessments (0.80–0.93), whereas for the assessment of joints that are simultaneously tender and swollen the range is 0.87–1.00. Given the high correlations between the various joint counts, both for the type of scoring and in terms of the particular selection of joints, there are some significant differences in sensitivity between the joint selections. However, the differences are not major, nor are they entirely consistent. Among the 12 methods given in Table 4, there are at least one or two ways of scoring for which each specific joint selection is the best. The CSSRD joint selection and that of Fuchs et al. each are worst for several scoring methods, but the spread of E never exceed 0.10 for a particular scoring system. The CSSRD joint selection does least well as an unweighted score and is best as an unweighted count. The Fuchs selection of 28 joints is least sensitive when expressed as an area-weighted score or count and is most sensitive when it is used as an unweighted score.

It is generally easier to pick up change in the tender joints than in swollen joints, but the two types of changes do not always occur to the same extent. In approximately one-quarter of the patients studied here, there were discrepancies, in that the tender joint measure would improve by at least 50%, whereas the swollen joint measure would not, or vice versa. There was no particular distortion of this discrepancy between tenderness and swelling changes when the number of joints examined was reduced, or confined to the right side of the body.

Reduced Joint Assessments for the Right Side of the Body
Table 5 presents the same information for these reduced joint counts when they are restricted to the right-hand side of the body only. The patterns are similar; fewer joints to be examined, but a higher proportion of the joints assessed are affected than might be expected. The percentage of change seen is generally in keeping with the proportion of affected joints seen, and the efficiency in detecting change is relatively unimpaired.

In the most reduced version of the joint count, that of Fuchs et al. restricted to the right side of the body, only 21% of the joints are examined, which should reduce examination time considerably, and the tender joint count has 90% (0.92/ 1.02) of the efficiency of a full 68-joint CSSRD joint count for the detection of change during a clinical trial, whereas the swollen joint count has 95% (0.85/

Table 5 Adequacy and Sensitivity of Different Joint Counts Restricted to the Right Side of the Body Only

Assessment	CSSRD	Ritchie	Egger	Fuchs
Tender joint count				
Joints evaluated (N)	34	25	18	14
Joints examined (%)	50	37	26	21
Affected joints examined (%)[a]	53	46	37	31
Joint change measured (%)[b]	50	45	36	29
Sensitivity of unweighted count[c]	0.98	1.00	0.98	0.92
Swollen joint count				
Joints evaluated (N)	33	25	18	14
Joints examined (%)	50	38	27	21
Affected joints examined (%)[a]	52	48	43	36
Joint change measured (%)[b]	51	46	38	31
Sensitivity of unweighted count	0.88	0.92	0.88	0.85
Swollen and tender joint count				
Sensitivity of unweighted count	0.95	0.97	0.99	0.94

[a]$n = 2184$.
[b]$n = 322$.
[c]The measure of sensitivity (E), a standardized change measure, is proportional to the t-statistic. See text for description.

0.89) of the efficiency in detecting change of a full 66-joint CSSRD swollen joint count. Because joint assessments are generally among the most sensitive of outcomes included in a clinical trial, this relatively small drop in efficiency through the use of an abbreviated joint count should be of little importance relative to the power of clinical trials. However, without standardization of measures between trials, there would be problems in comparing the results of different trials in terms of absolute amount of improvement in the number of tender or swollen joints, owing to the different numbers of joints evaluated.

III. SUMMARY

The joint examination is the primary measure of patient status in RA patient care. Quantitative assessments are used for evaluating the effectiveness of interventions, but are not widely used clinically owing to time and economic considerations. Repeat graded assessments must be performed by the original observer, but binary (normal or abnormal) evaluations may not be as observer-dependent. Reduced quantitative joint counts for swelling and tenderness may be used with little loss of sensitivity or efficiency and are acceptable surrogates for exhaustive joint assessments. These reduced joint counts are reasonable measures to use in clinical trials and in patient care situations.

REFERENCES

1. Gordon DA, Stein JL, Broder I. The extra-articular features of rheumatoid arthritis: a systematic analysis of 127 cases. Am J Med 1973; 54:445–452.

2. Pincus T, Callahan LF. Taking mortality in rheumatoid arthritis seriously—predictive markers, socioeconomic status and comorbidity [editorial]. J Rheumatol 1987; 14:240–251.

3. Resnick D, Niwayama G. Articular anatomy and histology, In: Resnick D, ed. Bone and joint imaging. Philadelphia: WB Saunders, 1989:29.

4. Thompson PW, Silman AJ, Kirwan JR, Currey HLF. Articular indices of joint inflammation in rheumatoid arthritis: correlation with the acute-phase response. Arthritis Rheum 1987; 30:618–623.

5. Dictionary of the Rheumatic Diseases, vol I: Signs and Symptoms. New York. Contact Associates International, 1982.

6. Fuchs HA, Brooks RH, Callahan LF, Pincus T. A simplified twenty-eight-joint quantitative articular index in rheumatoid arthritis. Arthritis Rheum 1989; 32:531–537.

7. McCarty DJ, Getter RA, Phelps P. A dolorimeter for quantification of articular tenderness. Arthritis Rheum 1965; 8:551.

8. Atkins CJ, Zielinski A, Klinkhoff AV, Chalmers A, Wade J, Williams D, Schulzer M, Della Cioppa G. An electronic method for measuring joint tenderness in rheumatoid arthritis. Arthritis Rheum 1992; 35:407–410.

9. Thompson PW, Hart LE, Goldsmith CH, Spector TD, Bell MJ, Ramsden MF. Comparison of four articular indices for use in clinical trials in rheumatoid arthritis: patient, order and observer variation. J Rheumatol 1991; 18:661–665.

10. Hart LE, Tugwell P, Buchanan WW, Norman GR, Grace EM, Southwell D. Grading of tenderness as a source of interrater error in the Ritchie articular index. J Rheumatol 1985; 12:716–717.

11. Buchanan WW. Assessment of joint tenderness, grip strength, digital joint circumference and morning stiffness in rheumatoid arthritis. J Rheumatol 1982; 9:763–766.

12. Ritchie DM, Boyle JA, McInnes JM, Jasani MK, Dalakos TG, Grieveson P, Buchanan WW. Clinical studies with an articular index for the assessment of joint tenderness in patients with rheumatoid arthritis. Q J Med 1968; 37:393–406.

13. American Academy of Orthopedic Surgeons. Joint motion: method of measuring and recording. Edinburgh: Chruchill Livingstone, 1966.

14. Wright V. Measurement of joint movement. Clin Rheum Dis 1982; 8:521–725.

15. Williams HJ, Ward JR, Reading JC, Egger MJ, Grandone JT, Samuelson CO, Furst DE, Sullivan JM, Watson MA, Guttadauria M, Cathcart ES, Kaplan SB, Halla JT, Weinstein A, Plotz PH. Low-dose D-penicillamine therapy in rheumatoid arthritis: a controlled double-blind clinical trial. Arthritis Rheum 1983; 26:581–592.

16. Lansbury J, Haut DD. Quantitation of the manifestations of rheumatoid arthritis: 4. Area of joint surfaces as an index to total joint inflammation and deformity. J Am Med Sci 1956; 232:150–155.

17. Spiegel TM, Spiegel JS, Paulus HE. The joint alignment and motion scale: a simple measure of joint deformity in patients with rheumatoid arthritis. J Rheumatol 1987; 14:887–892.

18. Bosi Ferraz M, Magalhaes Oliveira L, Araujo PMP, Atra E, Walter SD. EPM-ROM scale: an evaluative instrument to be used in rheumatoid arthritis trials. Clin Exp Rheumatol 1990; 8:491–494.

19. Parker JW, Harrell PB, Alarcon GS. The value of the joint alignment and motion scale in rheumatoid arthritis. J Rheumatol 1988; 15:1212–1215.

20. Egger MJ, Huth DA, Ward JR, Reading JC, Williams HJ. Reduced joint count indices in the evaluation of rheumatoid arthritis. Arthritis Rheum 1985; 28:613–619.

21. Kolodny AL. Two double blind trials of diclofenac sodium with aspirin and naproxen in the treatment of patients with rheumatoid arthritis. J Rheumatol 1988; 15:1205–1211.

22. Anderson JJ, Felson DT, Meenan RF, Williams HJ. Which traditional measures should be used in rheumatoid arthritis clinical trials? Arthritis Rheum 1989; 32:1093–1099.

23. Gotzsche PC. Sensitivity of effect variables in rheumatoid arthritis: a meta-analysis of 130 placebo controlled NSAID trials. J Clin Epidemiol 1990; 43:1313–1318.

24. Bombardier C, Raboud J. Auranofin cooperating group. A comparison of health-related quality-of-life measures for rheumatoid arthritis research. Control Clin Trials 1991; 12:243S–256S.

6

Radiological Assessment of Joint Damage
The Premier Outcome Measure in Rheumatoid Arthritis. Current Status and Future Potential

John T. Sharp

*Emory University School of Medicine
Atlanta, and
Tifton Medical Clinic
Tifton, Georgia*

I. INTRODUCTION

Both patients and physicians are looking forward to the day when treatment of arthritis will regularly bring either cure or drug-maintained remission, at a reasonable cost and with few or no toxic side effects. Until that day comes, it behooves us to employ the resources available to achieve the most complete relief possible. But how do we measure treatment benefit? The effects of rheumatoid arthritis can be remarkably different in different patients. Some patients report extremely severe, disabling pain, but have limited objective findings and develop deformities very slowly. Others admit to only mild discomfort, but have severe inflammation and develop joint damage rapidly. Functional disability may be extreme in patients with severe pain, even in the absence of deformities or limited motion; others with less pain have minimal disability even while experiencing relentless destruction of joints. Some patients can adapt their way of living to accommodate for severe deformities and minimize the impact of the disease, but others are unable to make these adjustments. The same physical impairment in a person who does heavy labor has very different consequences than in someone who has a sedentary occupation.

Because the effects of RA are so varied, most investigators employ multiple measures simultaneously to measure disease outcome. Measures of functional and psychological impairment are particularly appropriate to evaluate the social, economic, and personal aspects of disease. The quantitation of erosions, cartilage destruction, and deformities measures the anatomical outcome of the disease. Since x-ray films, which readily detect bone and cartilage damage, represent snapshots of disease severity that are frozen in time, they are particularly useful in objectively measuring disease progression.

II. METHODS

Since 1949, when Steinbrocker proposed radiological evaluation as an aid in classifying disease severity, attempts have been made to quantify joint damage by radiological methods (1). The British recognized the need for a truly objective outcome measure and started using analysis of radiological progression in therapeutic trials in the 1950s (2,3). Early methods of radiological evaluation that assigned a single grade, usually 0–4, but 0–8 in at least one instance, to represent radiological severity, were clearly insensitive to significant changes (4–8). Subsequently, the number of newly eroded or newly narrowed joints, together with the number of joints that were judged to have significant worsening of preexisting erosions were used as the radiological outcome measurement in the Empire Rheumatism Council-sponsored study of gold therapy in the early 1960s (9).

In the early 1970s a method that scored each individual joint in the hands and wrists for erosions and joint-space narrowing was developed to describe the course of rheumatoid arthritis and to examine the question of radiological progression in a double-blind, placebo-controlled, therapeutic trial that demonstrated slowing of radiological progression by treatment with intramuscular gold (10).

Since then, several methods of radiological analysis have been proposed, and many have been employed in clinical studies (11–13). In general there are several aspects of scoring radiological abnormalities that vary among the different methods proposed. Most early methods expressed disease severity as a single score for all the joints in a given area (e.g., the hands and wrists are given a single grade of 0–4). Recent scoring methods, which have usually summed abnormalities in multiple joints of the hands and wrists, rate severity on an expanded scale from zero to several hundred points. The number and location of individual joints scored varies among investigators. Most scoring methods restrict the number of joints by scoring only those that are most likely to be involved by rheumatoid disease and are least likely to be the site of osteoarthritic or other abnormalities. For example, although the distal interphalangeal joints are often involved in RA, they are much less often attacked than the other finger joints and, because osteoarthritic changes can be a cause of confusion, these joints are not read in the scores most widely used. Some selectivity has also been practiced in choosing which metacarpocarpal and intercarpal joints are read. In addition, some studies also use foot films to assess metatarsal joints and some use knee, ankle, and elbow films to enlarge the number of joints scored to increase the sensitivity of detecting disease progression.

Scoring methods also vary relative to how many and which abnormalities are evaluated for each joint. Should a single score be given for overall severity in a given joint or separate scores for separate features (e.g., an erosion score, a joint–space-narrowing score, a subluxation score)? Some methods emphasize the number of erosions, whereas others assign an overall erosion score to represent the number and size of erosions, sometimes referred to as a *global* erosion score.

Studies using archival films to compare scoring methods have shown no significant differences between counting erosions and grading severity in individual joints. In one study, an excellent correlation was found between Larsen scores, which give an overall grade for individual joints, and a method that employed more detailed scoring of erosions and joint-space narrowing (14).

The scales used to score abnormalities also vary. Some methods use 0–5 scales, others use 0–8 and 0–16. One scale uses 0.5 increments, but most use integers to represent change. Most scales are designed to be linear in advancing from grades 1 through the maximum, the scale being conceived as a measuring device, with each grade representing a uniform quantity. However, one scale uses grade 0, skips grade 1, and then grades abnormalities 2, 3, or 4.

Equally, or more significant, is the manner in which radiological scales are used to score abnormalities. A prime objective in diagnostic radiology is to make an early diagnosis and not to miss any lesions; however, the purpose of scoring abnormalities is not to determine which reader is best at picking up early disease. Although it is important not to miss abnormalities, it is much more important to achieve consistency in scoring and to spread the scale over a wide spectrum of abnormalities, such that the score represents an accurate measurement of the extent of radiological damage over the entire span of the disease. Even a well-designed scale can be employed in such a way that all the grades are used early for slight progression of abnormalities which then leaves the measurement useless for the study of disease in the later years. Figure 1 illustrates the difference in scores assigned by two readers using the same method to score a set of 41 films. Note how much higher the scores are for less-involved films for one reader. All scales are subject to a ceiling effect, and great caution should be employed to avoid reaching the ceiling early in the evolution of abnormalities, unless a limited scale is specifically desired.

In the method that I use, individual joints are scored 0–4, according to the number of erosions when these are discrete (15). If the erosive process is confluent, erosions are scored according to the number of joint quadrants involved. A score of 5 is assigned to joints exhibiting destruction of half or more of the articular surface of at least one of the bones in the joint (e.g., the metacarpal head in an MCP joint). Joint-space narrowing is scored as 0 for none, 1 for focal or minimal narrowing, 2 for diffuse narrowing less than 50%, 3 for diffuse

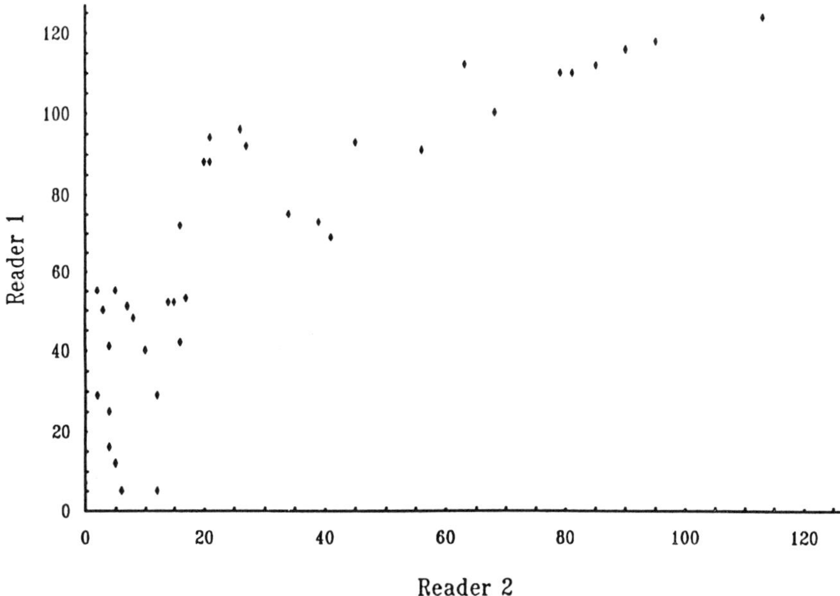

Fig. 1 Radiological scores of two readers.

narrowing greater than 50%, and 4 for ankylosis. Adding erosion scores for 34 joints and narrowing scores for 36 joints gives a maximal possible score for the hands and wrists of 314.

III. TREATMENT OF RHEUMATOID ARTHRITIS

Scoring radiological progression has been used to evaluate treatment with gold, penicillamine, azathioprine (AZA), sulfasalazine, hydroxychloroquine (Plaquenil), cyclophosphamide, and methotrexate (MTX). All double-blind, placebo-controlled, and comparison trials using radiological evaluation found by searching the National Library of Medicine files and cross-referencing techniques have been reviewed and most are included in Tables 1 and 2. The most extensive studies have been done on gold and MTX therapy, and these studies illustrate many of the problems that are encountered in radiological assessment of therapeutic effects.

Three double-blind, randomized trials examined the effect of intramuscular gold. Two compared therapeutic doses with placebo, and the third compared therapeutic with homeopathic doses. All three studies were congruent in finding benefit for gold, but in only one was treatment significantly better. In the Detroit study, patients were carefully chosen for markers of rapidly progressive disease before being randomized to treatment or placebo (16). Patients were then treated for a full 2 years: they were given gold weekly, for 20 weeks; biweekly, for 6 months; and monthly, for the remainder of the study. Most patients remained in the study for the full duration, regardless of the extent of clinical response. There was significantly less increase in erosion and joint-space–narrowing scores in the treated group, even though the number of patients in the study was small (see Table 1).

The American Rheumatism Association Cooperative Clinics sponsored a trial of gold that was conducted over 6 months (17). Numeous dropouts and the short duration of treatment compromised the study. Detailed data were not published, but the authors stated that more loss of cartilage and more erosions occurred in the placebo group ($p = 0.06$). An intention to treat analysis was not performed.

The British Empire Rheumatism Council sponsored a trial of intramuscular gold treatment, comparing weekly injections of 50 mg with 0.5 μg for 20 weeks; no maintenance gold therapy was given (9). Follow-up x-ray films were obtained at 18 and 30 months, or about 1 and 2 years after the completion of treatment. Radiographs were evaluated for the appearance of erosions or joint-space narrowing in previously uninvolved joints and for worsening of previously seen erosions. Many of the data are presented as the number of joints found to have new or worse lesions. Since the prognosis is linked for all the joints in a given patient, the appropriate data are the numbers of patients with radiographic progression, not the number of joints that progressed. For the baseline to the 18-month interval, the number of patients who had marked progression of radiological abnormalities in the wrists was substantially different between treated and control groups and was significant. Although the original report did not include an analysis, I calculate a χ^2 of 4.94 on the published figures (14 of 99 vs 28 of 100). The difference in radiological changes in the fingers was less striking and not significant (9). It is not surprising that radiographic changes were slowed in the first 18 months after initiating treatment and later resumed progression in the 18- to 30-month interval when the patients were no longer receiving gold.

Luukkainen and his colleagues compared radiological progression in patients, who stopped gold treatment because of side effects before receiving 500 mg (average 254 mg), with patients, matched for pretreatment characteristics, who received more than 500 mg (average 1858 mg) of gold; patients were started on treatment in the same time interval (18). The x-ray films were obtained between 5 and 6 years after the start of treatment. The percentage of metacarpophalangeal and metatarsophalangeal joints showing progression was significantly lower for those continuing gold, but unfortunately no data were given on the numbers of patients showing progression (see Table 2).

Table 1 Randomized, Placebo-Controlled, Double-Blind Trials That Used Radiological Assessment[a]

Author (Ref.)	Treatment	Number patients[b]	Duration	Radiological method	Result
ERC[c] (9)	A. IM gold, 1 g in 20 wk	99/100	Rx 20 wk, films at 18 and 30 mo	No. joints changed[d]	Slowing in wrist at 18 mo. No other difference between two groups
	B. IM gold, 10 μg in 20 wk	100/100			
Sigler (16)	A. IM gold, load and maintenance	13/13	24 mo	Sharp[d]	Significant slowing, erosion, and JSN scores
	B. Placebo	13/14			
ARA[c] (17)	A. IM gold, load and maintenance	20/36	27 wk	B/S/W[d]	Slowing, $p = 0.06$
	B. Placebo	19/32			
Gofton (20)	A. Oral gold, 1 yr	71/?	12 mo	B/S/W	Disagreement between 2 readers. One found difference
	B. Placebo 6 mo, then oral gold	78/?			
Borg (21)	A. Oral gold, 2 yr	67/69?	24 mo	Larsen[d]	Significantly less increase in score for gold Rx. Rates less different
	B. Placebo	65/69?			
ERC (2)	A. Cortisone	26/49	2 yr	Change	With cortisone, newly involved joints significantly less, $p < 0.05$, but % poss. new joints NS
	B. Aspirin	22/50			
MRC-Nuf[c] (3)	A. Prednisolone	41/45	2 yr	Kell[d]	Significantly fewer joints worse during prednisolone Rx
	B. Analgesics	35/39			

Study	Treatment	Patients[b]	Duration	Method	Result
Multicn[c] (26)	A. Penicillamine	?/52	12 mo	Kell	NS difference
	B. Placebo	?/53			
ARA (31)	A. Cyclophosphamide 50–150 mg/d	?20/27	32 wk	B/S/W	Analysis by number of joints, not by number patients
	B. Cyclophosphamide 5–15 mg/d	?28/37			
Shiok[c] (25)	A. Penicillamine 300–600 mg/d	?18/90	24 wk	New erosions per patient	NS difference
	B. Penicillamine 15–30 mg/d	?18/89			
Popert (30)	A. Chloroquine, 250 mg/d	24/68	1+ yr	Kell	NS difference, only patients with early disease analyzed
	B. Chloroquine, 2.5 mg/d	18/66			
Freedman (29)	A. Chloroquine	38/53	12 mo	B/S/W	Chloroquine less deterioration
	B. Placebo	39/54			
van Rit[c] (36)	A. Cyclosporine	9/17	6 mo	Kell	NS difference
	B. Placebo	13/19			

[a]Aspirin, analgesics, and homeopathic doses of medication are considered the equivalent of placebo in the studies listed here. All trials except for the ERC cortisone and MRC-Nuffield Foundation prednisolone ones were randomized and double-blind. The multicenter penicillamine, ERC cortisone, MRC-Nuffield Foundation prednisolone, and Popert chloroquine trials were stratified for selected variables.

[b]Number of patients analyzed/number of patients entered in study.

[c]ERC, Empire Rheumatism Council; ARA, American Rheumatism Association Cooperative Clinics; MRC-Nuf, Joint Committee of the Medical Research Council and Nuffield Foundation; Multicn, Multicentre Trial Group; Shiok, Shiokawa; van Ritj, van Ritjhoven.

[d]The ERC gold study counted new erosions, extension of old erosions, joints that became narrowed and assigned a progression grade. B/S/W refers to radiographic comparisons judged better, same, or worse. The ERC cortisone study evaluated narrowing, surface erosions, pocketed erosions, periosteal reaction, and subluxation. Sharp method is described in Ref. 10,15; Larsen in Refs. 7,8; and Kellgren in Ref. 4.

Table 2 Radiological Assessment in Randomized Trials Comparing Standard Treatments

Author (Ref.)	Treatment	Number	Duration	Method	Result
Luukk[a] (18)	A. IM gold >500 mg, (av 1858 mg)	32/95	5–6 yr	Larsen	Progression slowed on large dose
	B. IM gold < 500 mg (av 254 mg)	18/18			
van Riel (22)	A. IM gold	12/26	12 mo	Larsen	No statistical analysis
	B. Oral gold	14/26			
Sharp (23)	A. IM gold, initial dose, > 50 mg/wk	37/41	24 mo	Sharp	NS difference
	B. IM gold, initial dose, 25 mg/wk	38/41			
Gibson (27)	A. IM gold	20/41	24 mo	Sharp	Pen better in 2nd year
	B. Penicillamine	24/46			
vdHei[a] (32)	A. Sulfasalazinie	22/30	48 wk	Sharp	Sulfasal Rx, fewer new erosions and lower total scores, $p < 0.02$
	B. Hydroxychloroquine	28/30			
Scott (28)	A. Penicillamine	14/20	2 yr	Larsen	NS difference
	B. Hydroxychloroquine	10/23			
Berry (34)	A. Penicillamine	27/32	12 mo	B/S/W	NS difference
	B. Azathioprine	23/33			
Halberg (35)	A. Penicillamine	15/19	2 yr	Larsen	NS difference in no. patients progressing
	B. Azathioprine	10/22			
Hamdy (33)	A. Azathioprine	12/19	1 yr	Sharp	"Similar deterioration in both groups"
	B. Methotrexate	9/18			
Jeur[a] (37)	A. Azathioprine	33/33	48 wk	Sharp	MTX better than AZA for one of four methods of analysis
	B. Methotrexate	27/31			

[a]Luukk, Luukkainen; vdHei, van der Heijde; Jeur, Jeurissen.

For other abbreviations see Table 1.

The Sharp, van de Heidje, and Hamdy trials were double-blind; the Gibson, Scott, and Berry trials were single-blind; the Sharp, van der Heijde, Scott, Berry, Halberg, and Jeurissen trials were randomized; the Luukkainen patients in the high-dose gold were stratified for selected variables to match the low-dose group; the Gibson patients were stratified for selected variables.

Luukkainen et al. also reported radiological progression was slowed to a greater extent in patients started on treatment in the first 2 years after onset of arthritis than in patients treated later in their disease (19). This led them to conclude that there was little to be gained from gold treatment begun after that time. Unfortunately, the number of patients studied was small, and the radiographic data were analyzed entirely in terms of number of joints, not the number of patients. Furthermore, if the expected progression rate is greater in the first few years after onset, then slowing might be greater in this period as well, if expressed in absolute units, but might represent the same percentage slowing. The data are impressive, but additional studies need to be done to test this hypothesis.

Oral gold effectiveness was examined by Gofton et al. (20). Two readers found the mean change in radiographic score was slower in auranofin-treated than in placebo-treated patients. This difference was significant for the scores of one reader and approached significance for the second reader ($p < 0.08$). Borg et al. reported significantly less increase in absolute radiological scores among patients treated with oral gold, compared with those receiving placebo, but the difference in change of radiological deterioration rates was less impressive (21).

Oral gold was compared with intramuscular gold by van Riel et al. Radiographic progression was greater in the auranofin group, but no statistical analysis was reported; presumably, the difference was insignificant (22). Progression from baseline was significant in the auranofin group, but not in the IM gold group.

Sharp et al. compared two different dose schedules of IM gold (23). A high dose was adjusted to maintain blood levels in a predetermined range. The low dose was 25 mg/week during the loading period. No difference in radiological progression was detected after 2 years of treatment, but the power of the study was limited (power >0.70 and <0.80).

Capell et al. designed a study to compare oral gold with intramuscular gold and placebo (24). Because treatment failures, who were very common in the placebo group, were reassigned to alternative treatment, analysis was limited to the IM and oral gold groups. Radiographic progression was similar for the patients who continued in the study for 3 years, regardless of the treatment.

Cortisone and prednisolone have both been tested for their effect on radiological progression (2,3). Cortisone-treated patients had significantly fewer newly involved joints after 2 years than analgesic-treated patients, but when the data were analyzed as percentage possible joints newly involved, the difference was no longer significant. Prednisolone, given in doses that are regularly associated with potentially serious side effects, retarded the progression of radiological abnormalities more than did aspirin treatment.

Shiokawa et al. compared treatment with therapeutic doses of penicillamine, ranging from 600 to 900 mg/day, with homeopathic doses of 30–45 mg/

day (25). One observer compared x-ray films at 24 weeks with baseline ones for erosions and found the number of new erosions per assessable joint was significantly lower in the full-treatment group, but the publication does not make clear whether the number of new erosions per patient was significantly different. Another observer found no significant difference in progression of abnormalities.

A British multicenter, placebo-controlled, double-blind trial of penicillamine detected no difference in radiological progression, but it is not certain whether a detailed score of radiological changes was used in the assessment (26).

Gibson et al. compared gold with penicillamine treatment in a single-blind format (27). The x-ray films were obtained at baseline and at 1 and 2 years. There was significantly less progression of radiological scores in the penicillamine group. Unfortunately, nearly half the patients failed to finish the 2-year study. Although radiographic progression was much greater in the first year than the second, because of the large number of dropouts, this likely represents selection of patients who were doing their best to remain in the trial, rather than a lag period before drug became effective.

Scott et al. compared *d*-penicillamine with hydroxychloroquine in a 2-year single-blind trial (28). Radiological progression was less in the penicillamine group at the end of 12 months, but the difference between the two groups was not significant at 24 months.

Freedman and Steinberg conducted a double-blind study comparing chloroquine with placebo (29). At the end of 1 year, radiographic deterioration occurred in 12 of 39 control patients and in 5 of 38 treated patients. Films were scored as better, same, or worse. No statistical analysis was provided. My calculation for three grades and two groups gives a x^2 of 5.146 ($p = 0.076$ with 2 degrees of freedom).

Popert et al. compared therapeutic with homeopathic doses of chloroquine in 122 patients, but dropouts, incomplete treatment, and unavailable films reduced the number of patients who had films 12–24 months after start of treatment to 42 (30). Films of hands and feet, which were given a single grade for all abnormalities, showed no difference and no trend between groups.

The ARA Cooperative Clinics studied treatment of RA with cyclophosphamide and reported slowing of radiological progression (31). The average number of new erosions per patient per month was impressively reduced, but the data were reported as the number of joints that worsened during a 32-week trial, without reference to number of patients, and no statistical comparisons were made, so no judgment can be made concerning the significance of the difference.

van der Heijde and colleagues conducted a double-blind, randomized comparison of treatment with sulfasalazine with hydroxychloroquine (32). The median erosion scores in the hands and MTP joints and the total radiographic scores representing the sum of erosion and joint-space–narrowing scores were significantly slower in the sulfasalazine-treated group.

Hamdy et al. compared radiological progression at 24 and 52 weeks for nine patients receiving MTX and 12 receiving AZA, and found no significant difference, but the number of patients is inadequate to give the study any power for differences that were not extreme (33).

Berry et al. conducted a single-blind trial comparing penicillamine with AZA (34). Films at baseline and at 1 year were given a single grade for severity; no significant difference was found.

Halberg et al. reported that patients treated with AZA had fewer joints develop new erosions during 24 months follow-up than did patients treated with penicillamine, but the number of patients with radiological progression was not significantly different (35).

van Rijthoven et al. compared cyclosporine with placebo in 22 patients with x-ray films at baseline and at 6 months (36). Slower radiological progression in the treated patients was not significantly different, but there were many drop-outs.

Methotrexate has probably generated more interest than any other new treatment for rheumatoid arthritis in the last several decades. Controlled trials have established its effectiveness in relieving pain and improving sense of well-being and, when carefully monitored, side effects have been relatively few. Unfortunately, radiographic analysis was not included in the prerelease evaluation of MTX and, once a drug has been released, studies to adequately determine whether slowing of radiological progression is a treatment outcome are extremely difficult to organize and finance. Reports on radiological outcomes in MTX trials amply illustrate this point (see Table 3). Only one report of a double-blind, controlled study is available, and this one was not placebo-controlled. Jeurissen et al. compared MTX with AZA treatment in 64 patients (37). X-ray films were available for analysis on 57 patients at 24 weeks and on 60 patients at 48 weeks. There was significantly less progression in the MTX-treated group after 48 weeks of treatment, but there were 21 dropouts from the AZA group, and 14 of these were switched to MTX treatment. Their intention-to-treat analysis, which is otherwise a desirable method of analysis, does not deal with this problem of switching treatment during the trial. They also made the interesting observation that radiological progression was slower in both groups in the second than during the first 24 weeks of treatment.

Hanrahan et al. followed 128 patients started on MTX treatment (38). Seventy-five patients continued treatment for 2 years or longer and, of these, 47 had baseline and follow-up x-ray films. Fifteen showed marked progression of radiological abnormalities, 18 showed no progression, and the remainder had some increase in the extent of preexisting lesions, without developing new ones. No comparisons were made with other forms of treatment, but this distribution of progression is similar to that seen in general surveys of arthritis clinic patients, without consideration of treatment.

Table 3 Radiological Assessment in Observational Studies
on Methotrexate Treatment

Author (Ref.)	Number[a]	Duration	Method[b]	Result
Hanrahan (38)	47/128	2 yr	Fries	Progression in 29/47
Reykdal (39)	15/25	13–61 mo, 32.5 av	Kaye	NS difference from prior rate
Nordstrom (40)	18/27	30 mo, av	Sharp	NS difference from prior rate
Rau (41)	31/?	2–7 yr 3.9 yr, av	Larsen	Significantly slower than prior rate
Kremmer (42,43)	17/29	79–107 mo 90 mo, av	B/S/W	9/17 worse
Weinblatt (44)	10/24	70–84 mo 81 mo, av	B/S/W	6 worse, 3 same, 1 better

[a]Number of patients analyzed/number of patients entered in study.
[b]See footnote Table 1.

Reykdal et al. compared radiological progression rates before and during
MTX treatment in 15 patients given MTX for an average of 32.5 months (39).
Even though patients were not selected for the study unless they had had radiological progression during prior treatment and had exhibited "significant" clinical
response during at least 1 year of MTX treatment, the slowing of radiological
progression during MTX use was not significant. Nordstrom measured the radiological progression rate in 18 patients treated for 1–5 years (average 30 months)
with MTX and compared it with the progression rate observed in the same
patients during an average 33 months before MTX treatment; there was no
slowing (40). In contrast, Rau reported slowing of radiological progression in
31 patients during treatment with MTX for 2–7 years (average 3.9 years) as
compared with an average 2.2-year pretreatment interval when most patients had
been receiving gold therapy (41).

Among the other reports, Hamdy et al. studied a small number of patients
treated with either AZA or MTX without detecting any difference, but the power
of the study was very low (33). Kremmer et al. reported that no new lesions
were seen during the first 2 years of treatment of 22 patients, but, after 3–5 years
of treatment, radiological progression was observed in 6 of the 22 patients, and
after 79–107 months of treatment 9 of 17 patients showed progression (42,43).
No control patients were included, and no comment was made concerning progression in the 12 patients who withdrew from the study.

Weinblatt et al. reported radiographic findings on ten patients who partici-
pated in a randomized crossover trial of MTX and continued treatment for 70–84

months (average 8 months) (44). Progression of radiological abnormalities was observed in six, three patients remained stable without new lesions, and one patient exhibited articular calcification that was considered to represent healing. The radiological data in these three reports do not permit drawing any conclusions about treatment effects.

IV. CRITIQUE

Review of the studies, shown in the tables and discussed in the foregoing, prompts several generalizations. Considering what we know today about measuring radiological progression, very few of these studies were well designed and executed, and none were entirely conclusive. Only six agents have been tested in randomized, double-blind, placebo-controlled trials, and six agents in comparison trials. Many of these studies used too few patients, were too short in duration, and experienced too many dropouts. Few, if any, had a realistic strategy to salvage data of the dropouts; only one employed an intention-to-treat analysis. Power calculations were rarely presented. Many of the studies analyzed data in terms of the number of joints showing progression, without presenting data on the number of patients, and because of linkage of expected progression in joints of the same patient, this type of analysis is inappropriate.

These observations in part may reflect the period when rheumatologists were learning to setup clinical trials. They also strongly suggest that radiological assessment as a primary outcome measure was not planned in many of them, but was more of an afterthought, or a ''why not'' add-on. But in addition, these studies clearly indicate that we have been slow to appreciate several factors involved in trials. First, we are testing drugs for limited effects. If any mode of therapy were 100% successful in inducing a complete clinical remission in all patients with total cessation of radiological progression, it would not take a controlled trial to establish its worth. Second, the variability in radiological progression must be understood before a realistic estimation of the number of patients required in a study can be made (45–54). Third, radiological scores are not a uniform measure across multiple readers. An ounce of gold is the same quantity throughout the world, even though the price varies with the currency in which the price is quoted. Measuring radiological abnormalities is less precise. A score of radiographic abnormalities rendered by reader A is only approximately related to the score assigned by reader B (see Fig. 1) (7,8,13,14,55).

Physicians frequently are placed in a position of having to make judgments on the basis of incomplete data, and that is the situation here. For gold therapy, few would consider a new study comparing gold with placebo to be ethically justifiable, and differences in methods are sufficiently great to question whether a formal metanalysis of the existing studies is appropriate. Therefore, it is very unlikely there will ever be adequate data to settle the question of gold effectiveness beyond some reasonable doubt. Nevertheless, the available studies have been consistent in finding benefit from gold treatment, the difference between treatment and placebo was significant in one study of IM gold and approached significance in two others. There are reasonable explanations for these outcomes. The Detroit study, which found gold treatment to slow progression, was conducted on patients who were carefully selected for having multiple, poor prognostic indicators before randomization, treatment was continued for 2 years, and dropouts were minimal (16). The ERC study discontinued gold injections after 20 weeks (9). Interestingly, progression of radiological abnormalities in the wrists was slowed in the 0- to 18-month interval, but not in the 18- to 30-month one, a result that would be predicted if gold treatment had a limited carryover effect. The ARA study was flawed by numerous dropouts and a short interval of study (17). Even oral gold, which employs much smaller doses (about one-sixth the amount used in the IM gold studies), was better than placebo in two studies (20,21). The consistency of these observations appears to be compelling evidence to conclude that gold is effective, but before accepting this conclusion, one must ask one more question. Is it very likely that conclusively negative studies have been conducted, but not reported? Probably, if informal and retrospective (''afterthought'' hypotheses) studies that were negative or inconclusive were conducted, they have gone unreported, but I think it improbable that carefully designed, well-controlled, negative studies have been carried out and unreported. Disease progression is a central issue in the treatment of RA. The time, money, and effort required to set up a trial to adequately study the question of radiological progression is too great, and a negative finding is just as significant as a positive one, so the suspicion that reported positive studies are counterbalanced by unreported negative ones, which is often justified, would be inappropriate here. At the same time, even accepting this conclusion, the data indicate that the level of effectiveness is low.

Isolated studies that have found advantage for one drug over another in retarding radiological progression must be viewed with considerable caution. Cortisone and prednisolone may well inhibit progression when given in large doses, but it would be ill-advised to extrapolate this result to small doses. The penicillamine trials are flawed by the many dropouts and are inconclusive. Sulfasalazine deserves further study based on the van der Heijde report, but the numerous dropouts in that trial raises serious concern about the results (32).

The studies on MTX illustrate several additional important points. Most of these studies were not designed for the purpose of examining radiological progression. If radiographic analysis was even considered when the trials were designed, inadequate attention was paid to the expected rate and variance of radiological progression in the study population. Either no calculations of numbers required for the desired power were conducted, or gross errors were made in the assumptions necessary for these calculations, and few had power greater than 0.60; many had less. None of the papers failing to achieve significance commented on the power of their study. Even more important, none of these studies included a placebo control group, and only two, the small studies by Jeurissen et al. (37) and by Hamdy (33), included simultaneous, alternative treatment groups. One of these was too small to be meaningful. Three studies used historical data from previous treatment programs on the same patients to control for data collected during treatment (39–41). Under the best circumstances, comparison with the prior rate of radiological progression can give an indication of a trend, but these results are inconclusive. Most studies on radiological progression in rheumatoid arthritis have found that the rate of developing new radiological abnormalities slows with increasing duration of disease (45,51–54,56). The extent of slowing depends on the method of scoring and the reader, varying greatly between readers (see Fig. 1). Selection bias also can occur and is particularly serious when patients drop out of a study in the second treatment phase because of failure to respond. It is noteworthy that the three MTX studies that used historical data came up with opposite results. Although there is no clear reason for this difference, candidate explanations include the large number of differences in study design and an expected, "normal" decline in radiological progression rate. Pilot studies comparing progression during treatment with the prior rate to predict the value of a definitive trial should be encouraged, but small differences are likely to be misleading.

V. ARE RADIOLOGICAL SCORES RELEVANT?

If we accept the conclusion that gold is effective, how significant is slowing of radiological progression, if after 65 years of use, we can still legitimately question the value of gold treatment? Is slowing the rate of joint damage significant if it occurs in spite of continued joint pain and dysfunction? How relevant is slowing of radiological progression if patient and physician satisfaction are low because of limited or no relief of pain and no improvement in function? A loose linkage between subjective features and joint damage would account for the generally low level of satisfaction with gold therapy, in spite of its favorable effect on radiological progression, and the frequent satisfaction with MTX, in spite of its lack of demonstrated effect on joint damage. Too great a reliance on patient satisfaction could provide an inaccurate assessment of the effect of treatment on subsequent status, if slowing of radiological progression occurs "in the background."

Consider the following hypothesis. Gold therapy has multiple mechanisms of action. Attention has been focused on its effect on immune functions, but gold also is known to inhibit metalloproteases, enzymes involved in cartilage and bone breakdown (57). What if this were the main effect of gold therapy? Is a protective effect on bone and cartilage worthwhile if there are no other beneficial, pharmacological effects?

VI. JOINT DAMAGE IS ASSOCIATED WITH MANY FEATURES OF RHEUMATOID ARTHRITIS

Scores of deformities, limitation of motion and of function correlate well with radiographic scores (10,46,47,58–60). Genetic markers that predict severe disease also predict greater damage seen on radiographs (61–63). Monthly joint-swelling scores correlate with the rate of radiological progression over a 2-year follow-up (r = 0.572) (64), as do other measures of synovitis (59,65–69). Single and mean values of repeated measurements of hemoglobin and erythrocyte sedimentation rate (ESR) are related to change in radiographic scores (46,48,49,58–60,67,68,70) Patients with the highest levels of C-reactive protein show greater radiographic damage (67,70). Seropositive patients have more rapid progression of abnormalities than do seronegative patients (10,46,48,50,59, 60,71). The serum concentration of NH_2-terminal type II procollagen peptide is greater in those patients with progressive, erosive disease (72).

In general, features, such as deformities, limitation of motion when caused by joint damage, functional impairment from deformities, and pain that is due to loss of cartilage and mechanical derangement, are related to radiological abnormalities. Features that are measures of inflammatory activity when assessed at the beginning or repeatedly during a time interval predict the rate of change in radiological abnormalities. These associations establish that radiological abnormalities reflect previous disease activity and represent current disease severity. A radiological score that accurately reflects joint damage is a suitable objective measure of disease outcome.

VII. WHAT IS THE EXPECTED RATE OF PROGRESSION OF RADIOLOGICAL ABNORMALITIES?

Some investigators have published data and presented graphs depicting the progression of radiological abnormalities. These data must be interpreted with full knowledge that the units of damage vary between the different scales employed and between different readers (see Fig. 1). Given these constraints, it is clear that most observers have noted a slowing of progression with increasing duration of disease. However, there is still a legitimate concern about whether this is an artifact of the way radiographic damage is measured. How accurately do our scales reflect the real extent of joint damage? Figure 1, which illustrates how scores of joint damage vary between readers, identifies one major source of error. Scott has pointed out that a ceiling effect influences the shape of the curve of progression, an effect that most other investigators have ignored. In a recent publication cubic analysis of radiographic damage scores from multiple centers resulted in a curve of decreasing progression rate with increasing duration of disease (45). However, curve fitting by quadratic analysis and by a nonparametric method failed to confirm a decrease in progression rate over time. Observed

Table 4 Association of Radiological Findings With Clinical Variables

Clinical variable	Radiological association[a]	Ref.
Age	Predictive	59,60
HLA specificities	Rate	61–63
Nodules	Predictive	10
Rheumatoid factor	Score	10
	Rate	48
	Predictive	56,59,60,71
Deformities	Score	10,47
Limited motion	Score	10,46,47
Early radiographic score	Predictive	60
Disability index[b]	Score	58
Functional measures	Predictive	59,60
	Score	68,71
Grip strength	Predictive	59,60
Clinical activity	Predictive	65
Synovitis	Predictive	59,65,66
Joint swelling	Predictive	10,64,66
	Score	46
Ritchie index	Predictive	56,67
	Score	68
Joint scintigraphy	Predictive	69
ESR	Predictive	49,59,60,70,71
	Rate	48,61
	Score	46,68
C-reactive protein	Predictive	67,70
	Score	68
Hemoglobin (negative)	Predictive	56,58,59,67
Platelets	Predictive	59
NH_2-Terminal procollagen, type III	Predictive	72
Serum C1 esterase inhibitor	Predictive	60
Serum iron	Predictive	60
ANA	Predictive	60
Haptoglobin	Predictive	67
α_1-Antitrypsin	Score	68
Orosomucoid	Score	68
Fibrinogen	Score	68
IgM (positive)	Score	68
IgM (negative)	Predictive	67
Ceruloplasmin (negative)	Score	68
IgG (negative)	Score	68
IgA (negative)	Score	68

[a]*Rate* indicates an association between the progression of radiological abnormalities measured retrospectively and the clinical variable indicated. *Score* indicates an association of the clinical variable with the radiological score at one point in time. *Predictive* indicates the clinical variable was measured at the beginning of, or repeatedly during, an observation period and was associated with the change in radiological score at the end of that time.
[b]Fries Health Assessment Questionnaire (73).

progression rates between sequential films did not vary significantly in relation to disease duration, and calculated progression rates were almost identical for the first and last films, using patient's history to determine disease duration (45). It seems reasonable to conclude that determination of the true progression rate and the shape of the plot of radiographic scores against duration of disease awaits the development of more precise methods of measuring radiological damage and determining date of onset of disease.

VIII. FUTURE DEVELOPMENTS

Rheumatologists have become more active in conducting clinical trials and more sophisticated in carrying them out. With the present knowledge base it is possible in the immediate future to conduct definitive trials to determine the effect of treatment on radiological progression. There is sufficient information on clinical and laboratory manifestations of RA to permit selecting patients with severe disease who will have rapid radiological progression so that the number of patients studied will not need to be prohibitively large. Study protocols can be designed that will compare or combine new drugs with known effective treatment so that patients can be kept in trials long enough to get conclusive results without jeopardizing the patients' opportunity to receive disease-modifying treatment during the ''window of therapeutic opportunity.'' This is possible because data are now available on reliability of radiological scoring methods and expected progression rates to determine accurately the number of patients required in a therapeutic trial. In short, the knowledge base is now adequate for rheumatologists to fulfill their ethical and professional obligations to determine accurately the effectiveness of all currently used and proposed future treatments.

Soon this will be greatly facilitated by technical developments that will improve accuracy and facility of measuring radiological progression. Electronic storage of images—radiographic, magnetic resonance, and other—is developing rapidly and almost certainly will have a major effect on the conduct of therapeutic trials and daily rheumatological practice. Not only is software being developed that uses computed tomography (CT) or magnetic resonance images (MRI) to measure erosions in rheumatoid arthritis, but even more practical and less expensive methods may prove workable. For example, preliminary studies that use digitized data for subtraction analysis were recently presented. Improvement in resolution may be required before quantitation of small erosions will be reliable, but this method appears to be a promising approach for the measurement of change between films.

It is possible that electronically stored images can be used to measure radiological abnormalities in routine films or phosphor images. I visualize employing high-definition hand images taken in several positions and analyzing three-dimensional images with computer software to measure the volume of erosions in standard units. If such techniques improve precision of measurement of radiological progression such that error is reduced to a small fraction of the extent of change caused by disease, then radiological assessment will become a standard procedure in daily practice as well as in all therapeutic trials and the pessimism about radiographic analysis expressed by several investigators will have been proved wrong.

REFERENCES

1. Steinbrocker O, Traeger CH, Batterman RC. Therapeutic criteria in rheumatoid arthritis. JAMA 1949; 140:659–665.
2. Empire Rheumatism Council Subcommittee. Empire Rheumatism Council multi-centre controlled trial comparing cortisone acetate and acetyl salicylic acid in the long-term treatment of rheumatoid arthritis. Results of three years' treatment. Ann Rheum Dis 1957; 16:277–288.
3. Joint Committee of the Medical Research Council and Nuffield Foundation on clinical trials of cortisone, ACTH and other therapeutic measures in chronic rheumatic disease. A comparison of prednisolone with aspirin or other analgesics in the treatment of rheumatoid arthritis. Ann Rheum Dis 1959; 18:173–186.
4. Atlas of Standard Radiographs of Arthritis, vol 2. Philadelphia: FA Davis, 1963.
5. Sievers K. The rheumatoid factor in definite rheumatoid arthritis. An analysis of 1279 adult patients, with a follow-up study. Acta Rheumatol Scand Suppl 1965; 9:1–121.
6. Berens DL, Lin RK. Roentgen diagnosis of rheumatoid arthritis. Springfield, IL: Charles C Thomas, 1969.
7. Larsen A. A radiologic method for grading the severity of rheumatoid arthritis. Medical Thesis, University of Helsinki, 1974.
8. Larsen A, Dale K, Eek M. Radiographic evaluation of rheumatoid arthritis and related conditions by standard reference films. Acta Radiol Diagn 1977; 18:481–491.
9. The Research Sub-Committee of the Empire Rheumatism Council. Gold therapy in rheumatoid arthritis. Final report of a multicentre controlled trial. Ann Rheum Dis 1961; 20:315–333.
10. Sharp JT, Lidsky MD, Collins LC, Moreland J. Methods of scoring the progression of radiologic changes in rheumatoid arthritis. Arthritis Rheum 1971; 14:706–720.
11. Bluhm GB, Smith DW, Mikulaschek WM. A radiologic method of assessment of bone and joint destruction in rheumatoid arthritis. Henry Ford Hosp Med J 1983; 31:152–161.
12. Genant HK. Methods of assessing radiographic change in rheumatoid arthritis. Am J Med 1983; 75(6A):35–47.
13. Nance EP Jr, Kaye JJ, Callahan LF, Carroll FE, Winfield AC, Earthman WJ, Phillips KA, Fuchs HA, Pincus T. Observer variation in quantitative assessment of rheumatoid arthritis. Part I. Scoring erosions and joint space narrowing. Invest Radiol 1986; 21:922–927.

14. Sharp JT, Bluhm GB, Brook A, Brower AC Corbett M, Decker JL, Gennant HK, Gofton JP, Goodman N, Larsen A, Lidsky MD, Pussila P, Weinstein AS, Weissman BN, Young DY. Reproducibility of multi-observer scoring of radiologic abnormalities in the hands and wrists of patients with rheumatoid arthritis. Arthritis Rheum 1985; 28:16–24.

15. Sharp JT, Young DY, Bluhm GB, Brook A, Brower AC, Corbett M, Decker JL, Gennant HK, Gofton JP, Goodman N, Larsen A, Lidsky MD, Pussila P, Weinstein AS, Weissman BN. How many joints in the hand and wrist need to be included in a score of radiologic abnormalities? Arthritis Rheum 1985; 28:1326–1335.

16. Sigler JW, Bluhm GB, Duncan H, Sharp JT, Ensign DC, McCrum WR. Gold salts in the treatment of rheumatoid arthritis. A double-blind study. Ann Intern Med 1974; 80:21–26.

17. The Cooperating Clinics Committee of the American Rheumatism Association. A controlled trial of gold salt therapy in rheumatoid arthritis. Arthritis Rheum 1973; 16:353–358.

18. Luukkainen R, Isomaki H, Kajander A. Effect of gold treatment on the progression of erosions in RA patients. Scand J Rheumatol 1977; 6:123–127.

19. Luukkainen R, Kajander A, Isomaki H. Effect of gold on progression of erosions in rheumatoid arthritis. Better results with early treatment. Scand J Rheumatol 1977; 6:189–192.

20. Gofton JP, O'Brien WM, Hurley JN, Scheffler BJ. Radiographic evaluation of erosion in rheumatoid arthritis. Double blind study of auranofin vs placebo. J Rheumatol 1984; 11:768–771.

21. Borg G, Allander E, Lund B, Berg E, Brodin U, Pettersson H, Trang L. Auranofin improves outcome in early rheumatoid arthritis. Results from a 2-year, double blind, placebo controlled study. J Rheumatol 1988; 15:1747–54.

22. van Riel PCM, Larsen A, van de Putte LBA, Grignau FWJ. Effects of aurothioglucose and auranofin on radiographic progression in rheumatoid arthritis. Clin Rheumatol 1986; 5:359–364.

23. Sharp JT, Lidsky MD, Duffy J, Thompson HK Jr, Person BD, Masri AF, Andrianakos AA. Comparison of two dosage schedules of gold salts in the treatment of rheumatoid arthritis. Relationship of serum gold levels to therapeutic response. Arthritis Rheum 1977; 20:1179–1187.

24. Capell HA, Lewis D, Carey J. A three year follow up of patients allocated to placebo, or oral or injectable gold therapy for rheumatoid arthritis. Ann Rheum Dis 1986; 45:705–711.

25. Shiokawa Y, Horiuchi Y, Honma M, Kageyama T, Okada T, Azuma T. Clinical evaluation of D-penicillamine by multicentric double-blind comparative study in chronic rheumatoid arthritis. Arthritis Rheum 1977; 20:1464–1472.

26. Multicentre Trial Group. Controlled trial of D(−)penicillamine in severe rheumatoid arthritis. Lancet 1973; 1:275–280.

27. Gibson T, Huskisson EC, Wojtulewski JA, Scott PJ, Balme HW, Burry HC, Grahame R, Hart FD. Evidence that D-penicillamine alters the course of rheumatoid arthritis. Rheumatol Rehabil 1976; 15:211–215.

28. Scott DL, Greenwood A, Davies J, Maddison PJ, Maddison MC, Hall ND. Radiological progression in rheumatoid arthritis: do D-penicilamine and hydroxychoroquine have different effects? Br J Rheumatol 1990; 29:126–127.

29. Freedman A, Steinberg VL. Chloroquine in rheumatoid arthritis. A double blindfold trial of treatment for one year. Ann Rheum Dis 1960; 19:243–250.

30. Popert AJ, Meijers KAE, Sharp J, Bier F. Chloroquine diphosphate in rheumatoid arthritis. A controlled trial. Ann Rheum Dis 1961; 20:18–35.

31. The Cooperating Clinics Committee of the American Rheumatism Association. A controlled trial of cyclophosphamide in rheumatoid arthritis. N Engl J Med 1970; 283:883–889.

32. van der Heijde DMFM, van Reil PL, Nuvar-Zwart IH, Gribnau FW, van de Putte LB. Effects of hydroxychloroquine and sulphasalazine on progression of joint damage in rheumatoid arthritis. Lancet 1989; 1:1036–1038.

33. Hamdy H, McKendry RJR, Mierins E, Liver JA. Low-dose methotrexate compared with azathioprine in the treatment of rheumatoid arthritis. A twenty-four week controlled clinical trial. Arthritis Rheum 1987; 30:361–368.

34. Berry H, Liyanage SP, Durance RA, Barnes CG, Berger A, Evans S. Azathioprine and penicillamine in treatment of rheumatoid arthritis: a controlled trial. Br Med J 1976; 1:105–105.

35. Halberg P, Bentzon MW, Crohn O, Gad I, Halskov O, Heyn J, Ingemann M, Junker P, Lorenzen I, Moller I, Mork Hansen T, Olsen N, Pedersen G, Sorensen SF, Stage P. Double-blind trial of levamisole, penicillamine and azathioprine in rheumatoid arthritis. Dan Med Bull 1984; 31:403–409.

36. van Rijthoven AWAM, Dijkmans BA, Goei The HS, Hermans J, Montnor-Beckers ZLMB, Jacobs PCJ, Cats A. Cyclosporin treatment for rheumatoid arthritis: a placebo controlled, double-blind, multicentre study. Ann Rheum Dis 1986; 45:726–731.

37. Jeurissen MEC, Boerbooms AMT, van de Putte LBA, Doesburg WH, Lemmens AM. Influence of methotrexate and azathioprine on radiologic progression in rheumatoid arthritis. Ann Intern Med 1991; 114:999–1004.

38. Hanrahan PS, Scrivens GA, Russell AS. Prospective long-term follow-up of methotrexate therapy in rheumatoid arthritis. Br J Rheumatol 1989; 28:147–53.

39. Reykdal S, Steinsson K, Sigurjonsson K, Brekkan A. Methotrexate treatment of rheumatoid arthritis: effects on radiological progression. Scand J Rheumatol 1989; 18:221–226.

40. Nordstrom DM, West SG, Andersen PA, Sharp JT. A controlled prospective roentgenographic study of pulse methotrexate therapy in rheumatoid arthritis. Ann Intern Med 1987; 107:797–801.

41. Rau R, Herborn G, Karger T, Werdier D. Retardation of radiologic progression in rheumatoid arthritis with methotrexate therapy: a controlled study. Arthritis Rheum 1991; 34:1236–1244.

42. Kremer JM, Lee JK. The safety and efficacy of the use of methotrexate in long-term therapy for rheumatoid arthritis. Arthritis Rheum 1986; 29:822–831.

43. Kremer JM, Phelps CT. Long-term prospective study of the use of methotrexate in the treatment of rheumatoid arthritis: update after a mean of 90 months. Arthritis Rheum 1992; 35:138–145.

44. Weinblatt ME, Weissman BN, Holdsworth DE, Fraser PA, Maier AL, Falchuk KR, Coblyn JS. Long-term prospective study of methotrexate in the treatment of rheumatoid arthritis: 84-month update. Arthritis Rheum 1992; 35:129–137.

45. Sharp JT, Wolfe F, Mitchell DM, Bloch DA. The progression of erosion and joint space narrowing scores in rheumatoid arthritis during the first twenty-five years of disease. Arthritis Rheum 1991; 34:660–668.

46. de Carvalho A, Graudal H. Relationship between radiologic and clinical findings in rheumatoid arthritis. Acta Radiol Diagn 1980; 21:797–802.

47. Fuchs HA, Callahan LF, Kaye JJ, Brooks RH, Nance EP, Pincus T. Radiographic and joint count findings of the hand in rheumatoid arthritis: related and unrelated findings. Arthritis Rheum 1988; 31:44–51.

48. de Carvalho A, Graudal H. Radiographic progression of rheumatoid arthritis related to some clinical and laboratory parameters. Acta Radiol Diagn 1980; 21:551–555.

49. Scott DL, Grindulis KA, Struthers GR, Coulton BL, Popert AJ, Bacon PA. Progression of radiologic changes in rheumatoid arthritis. Ann Rheum Dis 1984; 43:8–17.

50. Scott DL, Coulton BL, Popert AJ. Long term progression of joint damage in rheumatoid arthritis. Ann Rheum Dis 1986; 45:373–378.

51. Larsen A, Thoen J. Hand radiography of 200 patients with rheumatoid arthritis repeated after an interval of one year. Scand J Rheumatoid 1987; 16:395–401.

52. Scott DL, Dawes PT, Fowler PD, Shadforth MF. Calculating radiological progression in rheumatoid arthritis. Clin Rheumatol 1986; 5:445–449.

53. DeCarvalho A, Graudal H, Jorgensen B. Radiologic evaluation of the progression of rheumatoid arthritis. Acta Radiol Diagn 1980; 21:115–121.

54. DeCarvalho A, Graudal H, Jorgensen B. Evaluation of the progression of rheumatoid arthritis. Significance of age at onset and sex. Acta Radiol Diagn 1980; 21:545–550.

55. Larsen A, Edgren J, Harju E. Laasonen L, Reitamo T. Interobserver variation in the evaluation of radiologic changes of rheumatoid arthritis. Scand J Rheumatol 1979; 8:109–112.

56. Eberhardt KB, Truedssou L, Petterson H, Svensson B, Stigsson L, Eberhardt JL, Wollheim FA. Disease activity and joint damage progression in early rheumatoid arthritis: relation to IgG, IgA, and IgM rheumatoid factor. Ann Rheum Dis 1990; 49:906–909.

57. Brinkerhoff CE. Joint destruction in arthritis: metaloproteinases in the spotlight. Arthritis Rheum 1991; 34:1073–1075.

58. Denver Data Bank. unpublished.

59. Young A, Corbett M, Winfield J, Jaqueremada D, Wiliams P, Papasavvas G, Hay F, Roitt I. A prognostic index for erosive changes in the hands, feet, and cervical spines in early rheumatoid arthritis. Br J Rheumatol 1988; 27:94–101.

60. Luukkainen R, Kaarela K, Isomaki H, Martio J, Kiviniemi P, Rasanen J, Sarna S. The prediction of radiological destruction during the early stage of rheumatoid arthritis. Clin Exp Rheumatol 1983; 1:295–298.

61. Stockman A, Emery P, Doyle T, Hopper J, Tait B, Muriden K. Relationship of progression of radiographic changes in hands and wrists, clinical features and HLA-DR antigens in rheumatoid arthritis. J Rheumatol 1991; 18:1001–1007.

62. Griffin AJ, Wooley P, Panayi GS, Batchelor JR. HLA DR antigens and disease expression in rheumatoid arthritis. Ann Rheum Dis 1984; 43:218–221.

63. Young A, Jaraquemada D, Awad J, Festenstein H, Corbett M, Hay FC, Roitt IM. Association of HLA-DR4/Dw4 and DR2/Dw2 with radiologic changes in a

prospective study of patients with rheumatoid arthritis. Arthritis Rheum 1984; 27:20–25.

64. Sharp JT, Lidsky MD, Duffy J. Clinical responses during gold therapy for rheumatoid arthritis: changes in synovitis, radiologic detectable erosive lesions, serum proteins, and serologic abnormalities. Arthritis Rheum 1982; 25:540–549.

65. Young A, Corbett M, Brook A. The clinical assessment of joint inflammatory activity in rheumatoid arthritis related to radiological progression. Rheumatol Rehabil 1980; 19:14–19.

66. Ingeman-Nielsen M, Halskov O, Hansen TM, Halberg P, Stage P, Lorenzen I. Clinical synovitis and radiological lesions in rheumatoid arthritis. A prospective study of 25 patients during treatment with remission-inducing drugs. Scand J Rheumatol 1983; 12:237–240.

67. Sjoblom KG, Saxne T, Petterson H, Wollheim FA. Factors related to the progression of joint destruction in rheumatoid arthritis. Scand J Rheumatol 1984; 13:21–27.

68. Wollheim FA, Pettersson H, Saxne T, Sjoblom KG. Radiographic assessment in relation to clinical and biochemical variables in rheumatoid arthritis. Scand J Rheumatol 1988; 17:445–453.

69. Mottonen TT, Hannonen P, Toivanen O, Rekonen A, Oka M. Value of joint scintigraphy in the prediction of erosions in early rheumatoid arthritis. Ann Rheum Dis 1988; 47:183–197.

70. Amos RS, Constable TJ, Crockson RA, Crockson AP, McConkey B. Rheumatoid arthritis: relation of serum C-reactive protein and erythrocyte sedimentation rates to radiographic changes. Br Med J 1977; 1:195–197.

71. Scott DL, Symmons DPM, Coulton BL, Popert AJ. Long-term outcome of treating rheumatoid arthritis: results after 20 years. Lancet 1987; 1:1108–1111.

72. Horslev-Petersen K, Bentsen KD, Engstrom-Laurent A, Junker P, Halberg P, Lorenzen I. Serum amino terminal type III procollagen peptide and serum hyaluronan in rheumatoid arthritis: relation to clinical and serological parameters of inflammation during 8 and 24 months' treatment with levamisole, penicillamine, or azathioprine. Ann Rheum Dis 1988; 47:116–126.

73. Fries JF, Spitz P, Kraines RG, Holman HR. Measurement of patient outcome in arthritis. Arthritis Rheum 1980; 23:137–145.

7

Health Status Assessment

Robert F. Meenan

Boston University School of Public Health
Boston, Massachusetts

I. INTRODUCTION

During the past two decades, questionnaires designed to measure health status have become an important approach to patient assessment in the rheumatic diseases in general and in rheumatoid arthritis (RA) in particular (1). Health status assessments have become a standard method of measurement in RA clinical trials (2), and they will likely become a standard method for assessing RA patients in office practice as well (3). This chapter reviews the concept of health status assessment, the content and characteristics of the general and arthritis-specific health status questionnaires that have been studied in patients with RA, and the prospects for further development and application of these interesting approaches to patient assessment.

II. THE CONCEPT OF HEALTH STATUS ASSESSMENT

In general terms, the basic model for health status assessment combines the measurement of key symptoms with the measurement of physical, mental, and social well-being (4). The nature of the symptoms assessed and the content and number of measures used to assess physical, mental, and social well-being will vary with the purposes of the particular health status measure. Greenfield and Nelson have recently depicted what they term a "health status target" that consists of five concentric circles beginning in the center with biological status and progressing outward through rings for physical health, mental health, social health, and quality of life (5).

Traditional patient assessments in RA have emphasized the biological and, to a lesser extent, the physical rings of this health status target. Measures, such as erythrocyte sedimentation rate, rheumatoid factor titer, joint count, and radiographic score are primarily measures of biological status. Other traditional measures, such as grip strength, walk time, and American College of Rheumatology (ACR) Functional Classification (6) focus exclusively on the physical aspect of health status.

It is important to recognize the basic limitation of such measures: they are not the things the patient with RA is primarily concerned about. The patient wants to feel better and function at a level as close to normal as possible; a lower joint count, a stronger grip strength, and a lower sedimentation rate may or may not be associated with such improvements. These measures are at best substitutes or proxies for the real health status goals of rheumatological care, and the proxy relationship, as the patient well knows, may be a relatively weak one.

What patients are basically interested in is good health, which may be more appropriately defined as a state of physical, mental, and social well-being, and as the absence of symptoms (7). One of the major features of the new approaches to health status assessment in RA is that they are specifically designed to address one or more of these central components of health status. The physical function measures they incorporate seek to assess the patient's ability to carry out complex musculoskeletal activities, such as walking up stairs, getting dressed, or doing household chores. Mental health is usually conceptualized in terms of psychological well-being and assessed by measuring depression, anxiety, or other mood states. The cognitive element of mental health is not included in RA-oriented instruments because it has so little relevance to the disease. Social function may be measured by assessing interactions with family, friends, and groups in either a qualitative or quantitative sense. It also may be assessed by examining the patient's ability to carry out a primary social role as a worker, homemaker, or student.

The symptom element of health status in RA is usually assessed in terms of pain. Pain, in turn, is conceptualized as a health status component that incorporates elements of physical, mental, and social health. A recent study indicates that fatigue and difficulty sleeping are also symptoms that bother many people with RA (8), but measures of these two symptoms are not incorporated into available health status questionnaires for RA.

Quality of life, the outermost ring in the health status target, incorporates biological, physical, mental, and social well-being, but it also includes such things as the person's environment, economic resources, and education. True quality of life measures are not used frequently in medical care research because the concept incorporates many variables that are not directly affected by traditional medical care. However, some investigators use the term health-related quality of life to refer to a concept that is reasonably similar to health status. Others add additional dimensions to health status by considering such features as health satisfaction and health perceptions. In this review, the focus is on health status, and the emphasis is on physical function, psychological status, social activities, and pain. Two other reviews of questionnaire-based assessments for RA and other rheumatic diseases have recently been published (9,10), as have two useful volumes on the general topics of quality of life–health status assessment for clinical research and clinical practice (11,12).

III. INSTRUMENTS FOR RHEUMATOID ARTHRITIS HEALTH STATUS ASSESSMENT

A. General Questionnaires

Health status assessments, including those that have been designed for, or used extensively to, study patients with RA, come in a variety of configurations. Guyatt et al. (13) have suggested that these measures be grouped into two major categories, generic health status assessments and arthritis-specific assessments, based on their primary purpose and content. The generic instruments, in turn, can be subcategorized into general health profiles, utility measures, and single-item self-rating health scales. This typology will be used to describe a selected set of questionnaire-based health status instruments that are now available for assessing patients with RA.

The key instruments for this purpose are listed in Table 1. For the most part, each of these instruments has been documented to have the necessary

Table 1 Measurement Characteristics of Generic and Arthritis-Specific Health Status Questionnaires

Instrument[a]	Reliability[a]	Validity[a]	Mode of administration	Administration time (mins)
Generic health profiles				
Rand HIS	+	+	Self-report	60
SIP	+	+	Interviewer/self-report	20–30
Utility measures				
QWB	?	+	Interviewer	?
PUMS	?	?	Interviewer	30
Arthritis-specific				
AIMS	+	+	Self-report	20
FSQ	+	+	Self-report	15–20
HAC	+	+	Interviewer/self-report	20/<5
MHAQ	+	+	Self-report	<5
MACTAR	+	+	Interviewer	10–20

[a] +, property tested; Rand HIS, Rand Health Insurance Study; SIP, Sickness Impact Profile; QWB, Quality of Well-Being; PUMS, Patient Utility Measurement Set; ?, property unknown; AIMS, Arthritis Impact Measurement Scaler; FSQ, Functional Status Questionnaire; HAQ, Health Assessment Questionnaire; MHAQ, Modified HAQ; MACTAR, McMaster–Toronto Arthritis Questionnaire.
Source: Ref. 9.

measurement characteristics of reliability, validity, and precision (14). Acceptable *reliability* indicates that the assessment is consistent in its measurement behavior, for example, in a test–retest format. Acceptable *validity* means that the instrument actually assesses the construct that it was designed to measure. This is demonstrated for criterion validity by showing high correlations between scores derived from the health status assessment and scores derived from other measures of a related construct. For example, the mobility scale in a health status questionnaire can be validated against walk time, or the mood scale can be validated against a depression inventory. *Precision* refers to the accuracy of the measure. This has two elements: stability and sensitivity. *Stability* means that the results of the health status assessment will not change in the absence of an intervention, whereas *sensitivity* means that the scores will change substantially in conjunction with an effective treatment.

One of the key issues in the development and widespread application of health status assessments in RA is the recognition that these measurement characteristics of reliability, validity, and precision represent the scientific, psychometric basis for any patient assessment approach (15). The old distinction between subjective and objective measures that for years induced a preference for observable measurements in the assessment of patients with RA is now known to be a relatively unimportant one. In fact, the critical measurement characteristics of many of the older, objective assessments were never documented. Recent studies suggest that the new, questionnaire-based health status assessments have measurement characteristics of reliability, validity, and sensitivity that equal or exceed those of more traditional measures (16).

Two generic health profiles that have been used to study patients with RA are the Sickness Impact Profile (SIP) and the Rand Health Insurance Study batteries (Rand HIS). These instruments were among the pioneering efforts in health status assessment. They are designed as generic measures that can be used to assess the major dimensions of health status in general populations and in patients with various types of illness, including arthritis. Their major advantage is that they permit health status comparisons to be made across different groups and different diseases, a property that is particularly important for health policy research and other approaches that involve resource allocation decisions. Their main limitation for arthritis-related uses is that they do not focus specifically on elements of functional and health status, such as hand dexterity and pain, that are particularly relevant to patients with arthritis. This may make them less sensitive as well as less relevant.

The Rand Health Insurance Study batteries were developed by Brook and colleagues, in the late 1970s, as part of a major study to examine the effect of different types of health insurance on medical care utilization (17). A key issue in this study was whether different levels of utilization would be associated with different health status outcomes, and the HIS batteries were developed to address this question. In keeping with the World Health Organization model of health status, the HIS batteries assess physical, psychological, and social function, plus general health perceptions. The physical scales include activities of daily living, role activities, household tasks, leisure, and physical activity. The psychological batteries include anxiety and depression, and the social batteries include social interaction and social participation in community and family. The main relevance of the Rand HIS batteries for RA is that this instrument is the direct ancestor of the Arthritis Impact Measurement Scales, an important arthritis-assessment questionnaire, and of the 36- and 20-item short-form instruments (SF 36 and SF 20) that have been developed by Ware and colleagues (18). These abbreviated instruments are coming into widespread use in health care and health policy research.

The Sickness Impact Profile (SIP) contains 136 true–false items and assesses 12 aspects of health status (19). Three of these (ambulation, body care, and mobility) may be combined into a physical function measure, and four (emotional behavior, social interaction, alertness behavior, and communication) may be combined into a psychosocial component. The five other assessments in the instrument are work, sleep and rest, eating, home management, and recreation and pasttimes. The scoring for each item uses predetermined weights derived from rater panels that estimated the relative severity of each level of dysfunction. A total score for the SIP may be computed by summing the two multiscale and five single-scale components of health status. The SIP may be completed in a self-assessment format or may be administered by an interviewer. It takes approximately 30 min to complete. Deyo has shown that it can be used effectively to assess health status in patients with RA (20).

The profile approach to health status assessment, as exemplified by the SIP and the Rand HIS batteries, is conceptually limited in assessing individual patients, because it does not incorporate the patient's unique preferences for different states of health. One person, for example, may place a higher value on maintaining mobility, whereas another may place a higher value on avoiding pain. Utility instruments attempt to take these preferences into account. There are two general approaches to utility measurement, the multiscale- and single–scale-rating approaches, and at least one of each has been used to study patients with RA.

The Quality of Well-Being Scale (QWB) is a utility-based assessment that is the forerunner of all the multidimensional health status questionnaires. It was originally developed in 1970 by Bush and colleagues as the Index of Well-Being (21). The QWB assesses health status within three areas, mobility, physical activity, and social activity, with each area having four or five levels of performance (22). A person can be classified as belonging to one of a number of possible combinations that represent particular levels of health status, each of which is valued for its usefulness based on preferences obtained from rater panels. The value of each health status combination is modified by the presence or absence of common symptoms that have also been rated by a panel. The overall QWB score then places each individual on a scale ranging from 0 (dead) to 1 (healthy). Scale scores can be combined with estimates of prognosis (transition) to calculate the quality-adjusted life years (QALYS) lost to the disease.

Weights for the various health states in the QWB have been developed for patients with RA (23). Another study has demonstrated the sensitivity of the QWB to treatment with auranofin in patients with RA (24). The QWB has also been used in Oregon to develop a priority ranking for the treatment of specific diseases in an attempt to ration care and thereby control costs in the state's Medicaid program. This is at once an interesting and worrisome application for health status assessment.

The second type of utility approach to health status assessment involves asking patients to incorporate all aspects of their health status into a single rating. In this approach, various techniques are used to ascertain a patient's preferences for their current health status in comparison with reference states of health. Typical approaches, which generally derive from economics and require a formal, interviewer-based assessment, include the rating scale, the standard gamble, the time trade-off, and willingness to pay. Torrance has compared these techniques and recommends the rating scale as the easiest to use (25).

Bombardier and colleagues employed an instrument called the Patient Utility Measurement Set (PUMS) in a study of auranofin therapy and quality of life in patients with RA (26). This approach seeks to measure the value to a person of his or her health status by determining the risks or sacrifices he or she would be willing to undertake to improve it. The PUMS approach requires each patient to rate their current and prestudy health status on a single visual analog scale, labeled health at one end. Time trade-off techniques are then used to ascertain how much risk each patient would accept as part of a hypothetical new treatment that would make him or her fully healthy. The formulation and scoring of these choices is a complex process that involves a detailed methodology and a trained interviewer. The PUMS approach demonstrated that patients treated with auranofin rated their current health status as significantly better than did patients receiving placebo. The magnitude of this treatment effect was similar to that detected by other health status and traditional measures in this trial.

The benefit of utility-based approaches is that they allow comparisons across disease states, permit the risks and benefits of therapy to be incorporated into a single measure, and facilitate the appropriate weighing of health status components within a single score. These weights may be rater-panel derived, as in the QWB, or may be implicitly derived patient-specific weights, as in the PUMS. The problem with utility-based approaches, particularly the patient-specific trade-off approach exemplified by PUMS, is that highly detailed protocols and trained interviewers must be used and, even then, many patients have trouble providing consistent answers to the trade-off questions involved. Thus the PUMS-approach is not well-suited to routine clinical trials or to office-based health status assessment.

B. Arthritis-Specific Questionnaires

Most of the work on health status assessment in RA has involved the development and testing of arthritis-specific questionnaires. The year 1980 was a watershed that saw the publication of major reports on the Arthritis Impact Measurement Scales (AIMS), the Health Assessment Questionnaire (HAQ), and the Functional Status Index (FSI), the forerunner of the Functional Status Questionnaire. In subsequent years, the Modified Health Assessment Questionnaire (MHAQ) and the McMaster Toronto Arthritis Patient Preference Disability Questionnaire (MACTAR) have been developed and tested. Each of these is a multidimensional health status assessment that was originally developed for use in patients with RA and other rheumatic diseases. These five arthritis-specific, multidimensional health status questionnaires differ in their component items and scales (Table 2) and in their length and mode of administration (see Table 1). The AIMS and FSQ, for example, measure psychological status (affective function), whereas the HAQ does not. The HAQ and MHAQ take considerably less time to complete than the others, and all but the MACTAR are self-administered. Each seems to possess acceptable measurement characteristics of reliability and validity, but these properties have not been equally documented for all the instruments (27). Most importantly, these assessments have roughly similar sensitivities to the effects of therapy in patients with RA (28).

Jette, a physical therapist, developed the original FSI primarily as a measure of physical function (29). This questionnaire measure assessed three distinct dimensions—dependence, pain, and difficulty—in the performance of 18 activities of daily living, using a score of 0–4 for each of the three dimensions. The FSI was used to study the function of community-based geriatric populations and was administered by an interviewer. It was also used to assess the response to inpatient arthritis unit therapy for RA (30). The Functional Status Questionnaire (FSQ), a major revision of this approach was reported in 1986 (31). The FSQ is a self-administered instrument that has been reliable and valid for assessing health status in patients with arthritis and other chronic diseases.

The Arthritis Impact Measurement Scales (AIMS) is a multidimensional, self-administered questionnaire that was developed specifically for assessing the response of arthritis patients to therapeutic interventions (32). The original AIMS instrument contains 45 health status questions, grouped into nine component scales that assess mobility, physical activity, dexterity, household activities, activities of daily living, anxiety, depression, social activity, and pain. Each scale contains four to seven items, and each item, depending on the phrasing of

Table 2 Items Covered in Arthritis Multidimensional Functional Status Questionnaires by Component

Item	AIMS[a]	FSQ[a]	HAQ[a]	MHAQ[a]
Symptoms	+	+	+	◆
Physical function				
Bed activities	−	−	−	−
Transfers	−	−	+	+
Dexterity	+	−	+	−
Ambulation	+	+	+	+
Mobility restriction/confinement	+	+	−	−
Basic ADL				
Bathing	+	+	+	+
Grooming	●	−	+	−
Dressing	+	+	+	+
Feeding	−	+	+	+
Toileting	+	−	+	−
Instrumental ADL				
Indoor home chores	+	+	−	−
Outdoor home chores/shopping	+	+	+	+
Community travel/drive car	+	+	+	−
Work/school	●	+	−	−
Affective function				
Anxiety	+	+	−	−
Depression	+	+	−	−
Emotional control	−	−	−	−
Self-esteem	−	−	−	◆
Intellectual functioning	−	−	−	−
Communication	−	−	−	−
Sleep/rest	−	−	−	−
General health perceptions	+	+	−	◆
Social function				
Interaction	+	+	−	−
Support/network	●	+	−	−
Activities/leisure	−	+	−	−

[a] −, Activity not covered; +, activity covered; ◆, covered in ALI version of MHAQ; ●, covered in AIMS2 version of AIMS.
Source: Ref. 27.

the question, contains two to six possible responses. Scale scores are adjusted to fall within a range of 0–10. These scales can be combined into three-component (physical, psychological, pain) and five-component (upper extremity, lower extremity, psychological, social, and pain) models of health status (33). The AIMS takes 15–20 min to complete, and it has been used in several RA treatment studies (34). It has been translated into a variety of languages, and modified versions have been developed for assessing health status in juvenile arthritis and in elderly patients with arthritis (35,36). Both a short version (37) and a longer version of the original questionnaire (38) have been developed for use in clinical practice and clinical research, respectively.

The Health Assessment Questionnaire (HAQ) is based on a model with four dimensions: disability, discomfort, drug side effects, and dollar costs. The HAQ is primarily used in a short, self-administered format that requires less than 5 min to complete (39). It comprises 20 questions, grouped into eight areas of daily function. Patients report their difficulty in performing each activity on a 0–3 scale that incorporates the need to use a device or help from another person. The individual item scores are summed into an overall HAQ score that ranges from 0 (excellent function) to 3 (very poor function). The HAQ short form has been validated in patients with rheumatoid arthritis and has been used in a variety of clinical trials and health care research studies in RA (40,41). It is also been incorporated into the National Health and Nutrition Examination Study as a general measure of functional ability. The longer version of the HAQ, which includes questions dealing with the discomfort, drug side effect, and dollar cost dimensions, takes approximately 20 min to complete and includes items on pain, economic status, and side effects.

The Modified Health Assessment Questionnaire (MAHQ) was developed by Pincus and colleagues as a briefer version of the parent HAQ (42). It assess physical function using eight of the HAQ questions and the same four difficulty-oriented response options. The MHAQ has been incorporated by its developers into another format, called the Activities and Lifestyle Index, that includes the MHAQ, a 10-cm pain visual analog scale, scales to assess dissatisfaction and pain in the same eight activities of daily living, a global self-report of health status, and a rheumatology attitudes index, designed to assess learned helplessness. The measurement properties of the MHAQ have been documented as being similar to those of the parent HAQ. The MHAQ/ALI approach has been used in a number of studies of patients with RA (43).

The McMaster Toronto Arthritis Patient Preference Disability Questionnaire (MCTAR) is the newest health status assessment designed specifically for use in patients with RA (44). It differs from the other arthritis-specific assessments in two major ways. First, it requires a semistructured interview to elicit patient responses. Patients are asked to designate key areas of function, based on their own preferences, in which they would like to see improvement. Patients are first asked, in general, to list areas or activities in which they have a problem owing to their arthritis. They are then prompted about difficulties they are experiencing in specific areas, including household activities, work activities, leisure time activities, and social activities. Finally, they are asked to rank these activities in terms of which they would most like to be able to do. The top five priority functions are then used as signal assessments to detect therapeutic response. The sensitivity of this approach has been shown to be comparable with that of a standard health status questionnaire in a study of methotrexate therapy for RA (45).

III. CURRENT AND FUTURE USES

The most obvious use for health status assessment is as an outcome measure in clinical trials of RA therapy. The AIMS and HAQ, in particular, are already being used widely for this purpose. In addition to clinical research applications, there are several potential uses for these questionnaires in clinical practice. Deyo and Carter have summarized these as follows: monitor disease progression, screen for functional problems, assess therapeutic response, improve doctor–patient communication, assess quality of care, and provide case-mix adjustment for comparing outcomes between patient groups and physician practices (46).

Health status questionnaires have already been used to track the progression and outcome of RA and to document the severe effects of this chronic, frequently disabling illness. By using the MAHQ, Pincus and Callahan showed that 5-year mortality in RA exceeded 50% in a group of 75 patients who had substantial disability at baseline (47). Other studies in RA have also demonstrated this link between baseline health status and later morbidity and mortality (48,49). Since it has been shown that health status in RA predicts medical care utilization over time (50), these assessments can also be used to adjust for case mix in physician profiling and other types of medical outcomes and cost research.

Health status assessments may become particularly useful as tools to identify problem areas in individual patients that merit physician attention. This type of questionnaire could be used to supplement the routine history and physical examination of an RA patient, in much the same way that many physicians currently employ general history intake questionnaires in their practices. Health status questionnaires may generate uniquely helpful information, since they focus on functional disability, an area of major concern to patients that physicians, particularly trainees, are likely to overlook (51). Even when the attempt is made to informally assess health status, as on a 4-point scale, physicians and their patients with RA frequently disagree on their ratings of the patient's physical and mental health status (52). This finding supports the need for the use of the more formal, multidimensional questionnaire approach to health status assessment in clinical practice.

Health status assessments also have the potential to provide monitoring information to physicians about individual patients. In this use, health status assessment could be performed on a routine basis, with the results presented to the physician in an organized, flow-chart format, similar to the way in which laboratory test results are currently obtained and reported. The conceptual appeal of using health status questionnaires to identify problems and monitor progress in individual patients is that the information obtained could lead to more timely and effective treatment and, ultimately, to better medical care process and outcomes. Unfortunately, studies that have examined this use of health status assessments have so far failed to show that the information has an effect on the process or outcome of care (53,54). However, additional studies are needed to examine whether this finding would change with physician education and more timely feedback. At the very least, the availability of health status information on a more or less regular basis may improve physician–patient communication by stimulating discussion on topics that are of great concern to patients.

Although there is major potential for the application of health status assessments in the clinical care of RA, there are several barriers that must be overcome before these questionnaires come into widespread use. These barriers are of two major types: educational and logistical (55). Physicians need to be educated about the strong measurement properties of these instruments. Clinical practitioners, just like clinical researchers before them, must come to recognize that these "soft" questionnaires produce "hard" measures of patient status. Physicians also need to become familiar with the meaning of health status scales and the interpretation of health status scores, just as they now understand the meaning of a sedimentation rate and know how to interpret a change in that measure. Paradoxically, familiarity may only come with more routine use, whereas more routine use may only come with more familiarity.

The logistical barriers include the length and scoring of the questionnaires. Lengthy questionnaires, such as the AIMS, that have usefulness in clinical research are not easy to use in clinical practice. Their completion time is relatively long, and there is no simple way to calculate and report the scores. Shorter questionnaires are more applicable for clinical practice. Studies have shown that well-designed short versions of arthritis health status questionnaires have sensitivity to change that is comparable with the longer versions (56,57). However, a virtual turnkey operation, similar to the way in which laboratory tests are ordered and reported, will have to be developed before one can expect busy practitioners to routinely collect health status information. Computer-based approaches to questionnaire administration and scoring may ultimately overcome many of these logistical barriers (58). The ultimate question then becomes how to pay for questionnaire administration and scoring and, in particular, whether third-party payers or administrators will cover or at least share the costs. Administrators and payers may, in fact, become the driving force behind the routine use of health status questionnaires as they seek additional information to use in managing health care (59).

Questionnaires for health status assessment have come a long way in the past two decades. From their initial appearance as relatively crude instruments that focused primarily on physical function, they have evolved into carefully designed self-assessment questionnaires that assess the full range of health status. There have proved their value in clinical research to the point at which they are now widely accepted as instruments that should be routinely used in tandem with traditional disease activity measures to assess therapeutic response. During the coming two decades, the next generation of these assessments will be automated, physicians and trainees will become better educated about the interpretation of health status scores, and health status assessment of patients with RA will become a routine part of clinical practice.

REFERENCES

1. Meenan RF, Pincus T. The status of patient status measures. J Rheumatol 1987; 14:411–413.
2. Felson DT, Anderson JJ, Boers M, Bombardier C, Chernoff M, Fried B, Furst D, Goldsmith L, Kieszak S, Lightfoot R, Paulus H, Tugwell P, Weinblatt M, Widmark R, Williams HJ, Wolfe F. American College of Rheumatology core set of disease activity measures for use in rheumatoid arthritis clinical trials. Arthritis Rheum 1993; 36:729–740.
3. Wolfe F, Pincus T. Standard self-report questionnaires in routine clinical and research practice: an opportunity for patients and rheumatologists J Rheumatol 1991; 18:643–646.
4. Patrick A, Bush JW, Chen MM. Toward an operational definition of health. J Health Soc Behav 1973; 14:6–23.
5. Greenfield S, Nelson EC. Recent developments and future issues in the use of health status assessment measures in clinical settings. Med Care 1992; 30:MS23–MS41.
6. Hochberg MC, Chang RW, Dwosh I, Lindsey S, Pincus T, Wolfe F. The American College of Rheumatology 1991 revised criteria for the classification of global funtional status in rheumatoid arthritis. Arthritis Rheum 1992; 35:498–502.
7. World Health Organization. Constitution of the World Health Organization. Geneva: WHO, 1978.
8. Mason JH, Silverman S, Weaver AL, Simms RW. Fibromyalgia impact assessment: a comparison with rheumatoid arthritis. Arthritis Care Res 1991; 4:S23.
9. Bell MJ, Bombardier C, Tugwell P. Measurement of functional status, quality of life, and utility in rheumatoid arthritis. Arthritis Rheum 1990; 33:591–601.
10. Liang MH, Katz JN, Ginsburg K. Chronic rheumatic disease. In: Spilker B, ed. Quality of life assessments in clinical trials. New York: Raven Press, 1990:441–458.
11. Spilker B, ed. Quality of life assessments in clinical trials. New York: Raven Press, 1990.

12. Lohr KN, ed. Advances in health status assessment: proceedings of a conference. Med Care 1992; 30(5 suppl):MS1–MS293.

13. Guyatt GH, van Zanten SJOV, Feeney DH, Patrick DL. Measuring quality of life in clinical trials: a taxonomy and review. Can Med Assoc J 1989; 140:1441–1448.

14. Guyatt GH, Jaescke R. How to develop and validate a new quality of life instrument. In: Spilker B, ed. Quality of life assessments in clinical trials. New York: Raven Press, 1990:47–57.

15. Feinstein AR. Clinical biostatistics XLI: hard science, soft data, and the challenge of choosing clinical variables in research. Clin Pharmacol Ther 1977; 22:485–492.

16. Pincus T, Callahan LF, Brooks RW, Fuchs HA, Olsen NJ, Kaye JJ. Self-report questionnaire scores in rheumatoid arthritis compared with traditional physical, radiographic and laboratory measures. Ann Intern Med 1989; 110:259–266.

17. Brook RH, Ware JE, Davies-Avery A, et al. Overview of adult health status measures fielded in Rand's health insurance study; general health perceptions battery. Med Care 1979; 17(suppl 7):95–97.

18. Ware JE, Sherbourne CD. The MOS 36-item short form health survey (SF-36): conceptual framework and item selection. Med Care 1992; 30:473–481.

19. Bergner M, Bobbitt RA, Carter WB, Gilson BS. The sickness impact profile: development and final revision of a health status measure. Med Care 1981; 19:787–805.

20. Deyo RA, Inui TS, Lenninger J, Overman SS. Measuring functional outcome in chronic disease: a comparison of traditional scales and self-administered health status questionnaires in patients with rheumatoid arthritis. Med Care 1983; 21:180–191.

21. Kaplan RM, Bush JW, Berry CC. Health status: types of validity for an index of well-being. Health Serv Res 1976; 11:478–507.

22. Kaplan RM, Anderson JP. The General Health Policy Model: update and applications. Health Serv Res 1988; 23:203–235.

23. Balaban DJ, Sagi PV, Goldfarb NI, Nettler S. Weights for scoring the QWB instrument among RA patients: a comparison to general population weights. Med Care 1986; 24:973–980.

24. Bombardier C, Roboud J, the Auranofin Cooperating Group. A comparison of health related quality of life measures for rheumatoid arthritis research. Control Clin Trials 1991; 12:243S–256S.

25. Torrance G. Utility approach to measuring health-related quality of life. J Chronic Dis 1987; 40:593–600.

26. Bombardier C, Ware J, Russell IJ, Larson M, Chalmers A, Read JL, the Auranofin Cooperating Group. Auranofin therapy and quality of life in patients with rheumatoid arthritis: results of a multicenter trial. Am J Med 1986; 81:565–578.

27. Guccione AA, Jette AM. Multidimensional assessment of functional limitations in patients with arthritis. Arthritis Care Res 1990; 3:44–52.

28. Liang MH, Larson MG, Cullen KE, Schwartz JA. Comparative measurement efficiency and sensitivity of five health status instruments for arthritis research. Arthritis Rheum 1985; 28:542–547.

29. Jette AM. Functional status instrument: reliability of a chronic disease evaluation instrument. Arch Phys Med Rehabil 1980; 61:395–401.

30. Shope JT, Banwell BA, Jette AM, Kulik CL, Edwards NL. Functional status outcome after treatment for rheumatoid arthritis. Clin Rheum Pract 1983; Nov:243–248.

31. Jette AM, Davies AR, Cleary PD, Calkins DR, Rubenstein LV, Fink A, Kosecoff J, Young RT, Brook RH, Delbanco TL. The Functional Status Questionnaire: reliability and validity when used in primary care. J Gen Intern Med 1986; 1:143–149.

32. Meenan RF, Gertman PM, Mason JH. Measuring health status in arthritis: the Arthritis Impact Measurement Scales. Arthritis Rheum 1980; 23:146–152.

33. Mason JH, Anderson JJ, Meenan RF. A model of health status for rheumatoid arthritis: a factor analysis of the Arthritis Impact Measurement Scales. Arthritis Rheum 1988; 31:714–720.

34. Anderson JJ, Firschein HE, Meenan RF. Sensitivity of a health status measure to short-term clinical changes in arthritis. Arthritis Rheum 1989; 32:844–850.

35. Coulton CJ, Zborowsky E, Lipton J, Newman AJ. Assessment of the reliability and validity of the Arthritis Impact Measurement Scales for children with juvenile arthritis. Arthritis Rheum 1987; 30:819–824.

36. Hughes SL, Edelman P, Chang RW, Singer RH, Schuette P. The GERI-AIMS: reliability and validity of the Arthritis Impact Measurement Scales adapted for elderly respondents. Arthritis Rheum 1991; 34:856–865.

37. Wallston KA, Brown GK, Stein MJ, Dobbins CJ. Comparing the short and long versions of the Arthritis Impact Measurement Scales. J Rheumatol 1989; 16:1105–1109.

38. Meenan RF, Mason JH, Anderson JJ, Guccione AA, Kazis LE. AIMS2: the content and properties of a revised and expanded Arthritis Impact Measurement Scales health status questionnaire. Arthritis Rheum 1992; 35:1–10.

39. Fries JF, Spitz P, Kraines G, Holman HR. Measurement of patient outcome in arthritis. Arthritis Rheum 1980; 23:137–145.

40. Nevitt MC, Yelin EH, Henke CJ, Epstein WV. Risk factors for hospitalization and surgery for rheumatoid arthritis: implications for capitated medical payments. Ann Intern Med 1986; 105:421–428.

41. Wolfe F, Kleinheksel SM, Cathey MA, Hawley DJ, Spitz PW, Fries JF. The clinical value of the Stanford Health Assessment Questionnaire functional disability index in patients with rheumatoid arthritis. J Rheumatol 1988; 15:1551–1556.

42. Pincus T, Summey JA, Soraci SA Jr, Wallston KA, Hummon NP. Assessment of patient satisfaction in activities of daily living using a modified Stanford Health Assessment Questionnaire. Arthritis Rheum 1983; 26:1346–1353.

43. Callahan LF, Brooks RH, Summey JA, Pincus T. Quantitative pain assessment for routine care of rheumatoid arthritis patients using a pain scale based on activities of daily living and a visual analogue pain scale. Arthritis Rheum 1987; 30:630–636.

44. Tugwell P, Bombardier C, Buchanan WW, Grace E, Goldsmith CH, Hanna B. The MACTAR patient preference disability questionnaire: an individualized functional priority approach for assessing improvement in physical disability in clinical trials in rheumatoid arthritis. J Rheumatol 1987; 14:446–451.

45. Tugwell P, Bombardier C, Buchanan WW, Goldsmith C, Grace E, Bennett KJ,

Williams HJ, Egger M, Alarcon GS, Guttadauria M, Yarboro C, Polisson RP, Szydlo L, Luggen ME, Billingsley LM, Ward JR, Marks C. Methotrexate in rheumatoid arthritis: impact on quality of life assessed by traditional standard item and individualized patient preference health status questionnaires. Arch Intern Med 1990; 150:59–62.

46. Deyo RA, Carter WB. Strategies for improving and expanding the application of health status measures in clinical settings: a researcher-developer viewpoint. Med Care 1992; 30:MS176–MS186.

47. Pincus T, Callahan LF, Vaughn WK. Questionnaire, walking time and button test measures of functional capacity as predictive markers for mortality in rheumatoid arthritis. J Rheumatol 1987; 14:240–251.

48. Sherrer YS, Bloch DA, Mitchell DH, Roth SH, Wolfe F, Fries JF. Disability in rheumatoid arthritis: comparison of prognostic factors across three populations. J Rheumatol 1987; 14:705–709.

49. Kazis LE, Anderson JJ, Meenan RF. Health status as a predictor of mortality in rheumatoid arthritis in a 5 year study. J Rheumatol 1990; 17:609–613.

50. Lubeck DP, Spitz PW, Fries JF, Wolfe F, Mitchell DM, Roth SH. A multicenter study of annual health service utilization and costs in rheumatoid arthritis. Arthritis Rheum 1986; 29:488–493.

51. Calkins DR, Rubenstein LV, Cleary PD, Davies AR, Jette AM, Fink A, Kosecoff J, Young RT, Brook RH, Delbanco TL. Failure of physicians to recognize functional disability in ambulatory patients. Ann Intern Med 1991; 114:451–454.

52. Kwoh CK, O'Connor GT, Regan-Smith MG, Olmstead EM, Brown LA, Burnett JB, Hochman RF, King K, Morgan GJ. Concordance between clinician and patient assessment of physical and mental health status. J Rheumatol 1992; 19:1031–1037.

53. Kazis LE, Callahan LF, Meenan RF, Pincus T. Health status reports in the care of patients with rheumatoid arthritis. J Clin Epidemiol 1990; 43:1243–1253.

54. Rubenstein LV, Calkins DR, Young TR, Cleary PD, Fink A, Kosecoff J, Jette AM, Davies AR, Delbanco TL, Brook RH. Improving patient function: a randomized trial of functional disability screening. Ann Intern Med 1989; 111:836–841.

55. Bergner M, Barry MJ, Bowman MA, Doyle MA, Guess HA, Nutting PA. Where do we go from here: opportunities for applying health status assessment measures in clinical settings. Med Care 1992; 30:MS219–MS230.

56. Lorish CD, Abraham N, Austin JS, Bradley LA, Alarcon GS. A comparison of the full and short versions of the Arthritis Impact Measurement Scales. Arthritis Care Res 1991; 4:168–173.

57. Katz JN, Larson MG, Phillips CB, Fossel AH, Liang MH. Comparative measurement sensitivity of short and longer health status measures. Med Care 1992; 30:917–925.

58. Rosen MF, Coalson D, Hayward RJ, Schmittner J, Thisted RA, Apfelbaum JL, Stocking CB, Cassel CK, Pompei P, Ford DE, Steinberg EP. Can patients use an automated questionnaire to define their current health status? Med Care 1992; 30:MS74–MS84.

59. Ellwood PM. Outcomes management: a technology of patient experience. N Engl J Med 1988; 318:1549–1556.

8

The Morbidity of Rheumatoid Arthritis

Simon Donnelly

Whipps Cross Hospital
London, England

David L. Scott

King's College Hospital
London, England

I. INTRODUCTION

Rheumatoid arthritis (RA) has a profound effect on most aspects of patients' lives in proportion to its severity. As with any potentially chronic and disabling condition, patients are justified, quite correctly, in requesting of their physicians accurate information concerning their future health status and likely prognosis following treatment. How can we accurately define, map, and influence the future course of any given patient with RA? Reliable prognostic information is of considerable benefit for patients and their employers, hospital resource planners and health administrators, insurance agencies, as well as for the accurate assessment of cases of medicolegal importance. Despite this, morbidity of RA has as yet been relatively overlooked in major textbooks of medicine and rheumatology (1,2). This is partly because morbidity of RA is not easily measurable by a single standardized and reproducible method. There are a variety of interrelated dimensions that contribute to the morbidity of the disease; for example, the inexorable failure of major joint systems, extra-articular features such as nodules and vasculitis, adverse reactions and inefficacy with antirheumatic drugs, availability and standard of medical facilities, as well as individual lifestyle inclusive of income, education level, and marital status, to name but a few. Prognosis is influenced by a relative lack of overall standardized indices of disease morbidity

207

that could be used to predict individual outcome and thus plan treatment. Despite such limiting factors, functional outcome, as measured by health status questionnaires, is directly associated with long-term outcome and morbidity and can be used to assess many aspects of the natural history of treated rheumatoid arthritis. Prevention or reduction of the long-term morbidity of RA, the alleviation of its associated disability, and the control of pain remain the principal therapeutic goals in the treatment of RA.

The first meaningful attempts to measure outcome followed the development of the Steinbrocker functional classes in 1949 (3). Before this, it had been assumed that the course of rheumatoid arthritis was toward inevitable improvement; in fact, this concept of a favorable outcome had been suggested in major American textbooks as recently as 1985 "RA is, in the majority of instances a disease with a good prognosis" (4) and a British text in 1986 "only a minority of hospitalized patients develop severe progressive destructive disease" (1). The design of studies to assess the outcome of rheumatoid arthritis is made complex by its chronic nature. Most investigations into the treatment of RA are short-term and of less than 2 years duration. Although many demonstrate a benefit in the short-term course of disease, they cannot be used to extrapolate to define overall outcome and prognosis. The studies in which patients have been observed over more than 5 years demonstrate severe morbidity. There are considerable variations within morbidity studies of arthritis. The source of patient selection is a suggested determining factor for prognosis and morbidity. In general, studies of patients identified in the community have demonstrated less marked increases in morbidity than those selected by investigations of hospital inpatients with rheumatoid arthritis. However, that patients in whom the diagnosis of RA is made in a nonclinical setting will subsequently fulfill the diagnostic criteria for definite RA in only a third or fewer of cases 3–5 years later, may explain much of this apparent difference.

II. THE COURSE OF RHEUMATOID ARTHRITIS

The course of rheumatoid arthritis has been divided arbitrarily into progressive disease, an intermittent course, and cases with long clinical remissions. The latter are really a variant of intermittent disease. This division was established by the classic studies undertaken by Short et al. (5–7). Patients with severe extraarticular disease form a fourth group and can be termed "malignant" rheumatoid, although such cases are uncommon. Most patients attending specialist rheumatology units have progressive, seropositive, erosive rheumatoid disease. Patients may show a rapid or a slow course, but the end results are similar, with disabling destructive disease predominating. This pattern of inexorable progression is among the most characteristic features of rheumatoid arthritis.

The difference between progressive and intermittent disease was illustrated in a study of 293 patients and appropriate controls from North America (6). The investigation was initiated in 1929 and was based on patients having a clinical diagnosis of RA admitted to the Massachusetts General Hospital between 1930 and 1936. The series was terminated after 300 patients were entered, and subsequent review in 1937 excluded 7 cases on diagnostic grounds, leaving 293 patients in the series. An aged- and sex-matched series of controls without arthritis was established in 1936 and 1937. The patients' disease course was divided into the period before hospital admission and the period after admission, which extended over years and decades. The disease course before hospitalization was progressive in 213 cases (73%) and intermittent in 80 cases (27%). Those patients who were said to have an intermittent course spent, on average, 65% of the duration of their disease before hospitalization in remission. Most attacks of arthritis were brief, lasting less than 1 year. The intermissions extended over variable periods; half the patients had brief attacks, with brief remissions, and 31 of the 80 patients had brief attacks and long remissions.

A problem with such an early study is disease classification. The most influential criteria for the diagnosis of rheumatoid arthritis were established in 1958 (8) and were unavailable when Short and his colleagues collected their series. Similarly, the criteria for disease remission have been established only subsequently (9). It is likely that many of their cases would not be classified as RA by present criteria, and disease remission in their patients would not fulfill the current definition.

The nature and distribution of joint involvement is important in the course of RA. There are three related questions relevant to this issue: What joints are involved in early RA; what are the changes in the type of joint involvement in the first few years of RA; and what are the long-term changes in joint involvement over 10 years or more? These questions have been examined separately in individual studies. The first question concerns the type and incidence of joint involvement early in the course of RA. This was studied in detail by Fleming et al. in 1976 (10). They looked at 102 patients seen within 1 year of the onset of symptoms. They found the joints most frequently affected were metacarpophalangeal (MCP), proximal interphalangeal (PIP), and wrists, followed by metatarsophalangeal (MTP) and shoulders. The hips were least often affected. The arthritis was preponderantly peripheral. These patients were followed prospectively for a mean of 4.5 years; eventually more severe disease was found to be associated with early wrist and MTP joint involvement.

The second question concerns the natural history of early joint changes in RA. This was described in a retrospective study of 44 patients with classic disease followed up for over 5 years (11). Three types of joint involvement were described. First, a large group of joints that are involved in the first year and remain involved throughout the disease course. Second, a smaller group of joints that are uninvolved at the beginning and remain uninvolved throughout the course, or until very late. Finally, very few joints are uninvolved at the onset and become involved over time. There was little evidence of waves of new joint involvement during the first 5–10 years of disease. Although there were flares of disease activity beyond the first year of rheumatoid arthritis, in general this did not hold true for anatomical spread of the disease.

The final question involves the longer-term course of RA joint involvement. This was assessed radiologically by Scott et al. (12) in 50 RA patients, who were followed over 10 years. The amount of joint damage in all peripheral joints was determined at the beginning of the study and after 10 years. During this time, 48 of the 50 patients showed evidence of progressive joint damage. Initially, the wrists and small joints of the feet had most damage. During the 10 years of follow-up, most progression occurred in the wrist, knee, and metacarpophalangeal joints. Radiological progression was seen in both initially normal and abnormal joints. By 10 years only a few joints showed no radiological evidence of damage. Radiographic progression was evident, in spite of the fact that the joint count did not necessarily progress. Therefore, joint deformity and radiological deterioration, the hallmarks of progressive RA, can occur in the face of an apparent benefit, as measured by improved joint tenderness and swelling.

III. ASSESSING THE MORBIDITY OF RHEUMATOID ARTHRITIS

There are many determinants of morbidity in RA, and it can be assessed in several ways. Over the last decade the approaches to assessing morbidity have been divided into five broad areas: functional measures, work disability, radiological measures, joint counts, and the interactions with patient lifestyles. These are interrelated variables, but they can be considered separately.

A. Functional Measures

The initial observation that functional measurements might be important in the progression of RA was made in early studies of Duthie and by Rasker and Cosh (13–15). Measurement of the outcome of rheumatoid arthritis has since shifted from clinical measures of outcome to functional measures, which include quality of life and psychological aspects of outcome. The simple Steinbroker functional classes (Table 1) (3) have proved useful over the last 40 years, but the class definitions are global and rather vague and, therefore, are subject to inconsistent interpretations with potential for bias. They have largely been replaced by validated questionnaires of health status, such as the Health Assessment Questionnaire (HAQ) (16) and the Arthritis Impact Measurement Scale (AIMS) (17). Does the use of a questionnaire measuring health status give a more accurate prognostic guide than patient follow-up with conventional clinical and laboratory markers, such as morning stiffness, articular index, and erythrocyte sedimentation rate (ESR)? This question is important and fundamental to the way we

Table 1 Classification of Functional Capacity in Rheumatoid Arthritis[a]

Class	Definition
Class I:	Complete functional capacity with ability to carry on all usual duties without handicaps.
Class II:	Functional capacity adequate to conduct normal activities despite handicap of discomfort or limited mobility of one or more joints.
Class III:	Functional capacity adequate to perform only a few or none of the duties of the usual occupation or of self-care.
Class IV:	Largely of wholly incapacitated with patient bedridden or confined to a wheelchair, permitting little or no self-care.

[a]Steinbroker functional classes (see text).

follow-up patients with arthritis. Questionnaires concerned with health status have been in use for more than 10 years, since the original AIMS, which has recently been revised and expanded (18). The use of health status questionnaires and simplified measures of satisfaction have a number of theoretical advantages (Table 2). There are many available functional measures, and they do not give completely identical information. Some, such as the HAQ, primarily examine functional activities. Others, such as the AIMS questionnaire, also consider psychological status in detail.

Recently, health status measures have been the subject of two long-term trials by Wolfe et al. (19,20) using the same cohort of 1274 patients with rheumatoid arthritis. The conclusions are important, and it is worth considering these investigations separately. The first study (19) followed rheumatoid patients longitudinally for up to 12 years to assess the rate of disability, and how functional deterioration is most accurately predicted. They showed functional deterioration to be present very early in the course of rheumatoid patients seen at the clinic, confirming the previous findings of Sherrer et al. (21). They suggested, by extrapolation, that the preclinical progression of rheumatoid arthritis is likely to be very slow. However, following the initial presentation to the clinic, further

Table 2 The Advantages of Functional Questionnaires in RA

Feature of questionnaire	Practical advantage
Standardized and graded	Fixed endpoints can be used to define progression or outcome
Carefully validated	Can be used in a clinical or research setting
Inexpensive and self-administered	Can be completed in the clinic, at home, or by telephone
Determine outcome variables of most concern to the patient	Measure treatment satisfaction, pain, mobility, and mood

disability develops rapidly, at more than ten times the preclinical rate, so that half the patients will reach functional disease index (FDI) scores of about 1 in 2 years, 2 in 6 years, and 2.5 in 10 years; these levels corresponding to moderate, severe, and very severe loss of functional ability.

They further demonstrated that functional outcome is accurately predicted by self-assessed measures of global severity, pain, grip strength, and the initial functional disease index (FDI) itself. Other variables that showed relatively little association with long-term disability included sex, disease duration, ethnic origin, education level, ESR, and rheumatoid factor. Age at onset, however, was strongly associated with an adverse outcome, the patient of 70 years having an independent relative risk of disability 1.5 times over that of a 40-year-old.

The second study (20) divided rheumatoid patients based on disease duration and followed them over an extended period of up to 5 years. Two hundred sixty-four patients were seen early—within 2 years of disease onset (mean 0.8 years) and followed for 2 further years. Four other patient groups (561 patients in all) of disease duration 2–7, 7–12, 12–17, 17–22 years were each followed serially for 5 years. Results confirmed that functional disability, as measured by HAQ-FDI develops very early in the course of disease and continues to worsen at approximately the same rate throughout the course of rheumatoid arthritis. They showed, for example, that grip strength deteriorated by 69.3% overall to a maximal low after 21 years, but it had already fallen by 58.2% only 0.8 years after disease onset. Similarly, a HAQ-FDI of 0.88 (corresponding to a moderate functional disability) had been reached after just 0.8 years of illness and only increased to a maximum of 1.19 after 21 years. Patients' overall assessment of severity (global severity) mirrored the foregoing findings, with significant loss occurring very early in the course of rheumatoid arthritis, followed by a more gradual decline. However, there were no longitudinal changes for depression, morning stiffness, ESR, and joint count—these latter three variables being used frequently to assess the outcome of clinical trials (22). In addition, there were significant changes in measured pain and anxiety over time, demonstrating that both of these, as well as functional measures and global severity, increase longitudinally. Both of these studies included all patients attending a clinical practice, without exclusion criteria based, for example, on comorbidities or other predefined selection criteria. As such, the conclusions are representative of all RA patients attending a clinical setting, rather than population-based studies.

Pincus et al. (23) had previously demonstrated that functional capacity— as measured by activities of daily living, grip strength, and button test—was a highly significant predictor of functional decline in rheumatoid arthritis in a small number of patients 9 years apart, and confirmed their own earlier findings (24) as well as those of Mitchell et al. (25). They also showed that, in small numbers of patients having very poor scores in measures of functional capacity, 5-year survival is less than 50%, with a mortality comparable with that of high-grade

Hodgkin's disease or triple-vessel coronary artery disease. It has previously been shown that prognosis and mortality of coronary artery disease can be accurately predicted by angiography, based on the number and sites of vessels involved (26). Similarly, prognosis in Hodgkin's disease has been graded anatomically into grades 1–4 (27), with an increasing mortality that has allowed a more aggressive standardized treatment regimen, resulting in an improved prognosis. Such quantitative grading could potentially be applied to patients with RA to allow early aggressive treatment regimens based on prognosis in a similar fashion. At present, such a grading system would give most prognostic information by widespread adoption of health status measures immediately on diagnosis. As an example, HAQ-FDI scores, as applied in the foregoing studies, could be administered based upon early referral and diagnosis. This initial HAQ-FDI score in combination with physician assessment could then be used as a standard in determining how aggressive initial treatment should be. Patient follow-up, using serial HAQ scores in addition to laboratory measures and radiological progression within fixed time intervals, or by measuring the time taken to change HAQ score by a given percentage, would allow better standardization between trials and of treatment outcome and thereby a clearer means to measure morbidity.

The foregoing studies collectively demonstrate that the measurement of an initial functional index has significant prognostic implications. They suggest that long-term assessment is most accurately measured by functional indexes, including grip strength, HAQ-FDI, and global severity, and that ESR, joint count, and morning stiffness may be less reliable long-term measures of outcome.

B. Work Disability

Early evidence suggesting an association between RA and work disability was first provided by Yelin et al. in 1980 (28). Subsequently in 1987, Yelin et al. (29) followed a random sample of 353 RA patients (mean age 51 years; 72% women) who had all worked for pay at some stage during their life; 306 were working at the time of diagnosis of RA. Ten years after diagnosis, half of the patients had become unable to work, by 15 years, 60% were work incapacitated, and after 30 years, 90% could no longer work. The majority of those unable to work reported their disablement to be because of RA (127 of 149 patients). A strong predictive factor in determining the probability of work loss was the initial HAQ-FDI score. This score demonstrated a relative risk factor for future work incapacity of 3.3. Age and the number of painful joints were also predictive of work disability, both having relative risks of approximately 1.7. However, work disability was not predicted by ESR, Rh factor, or the presence and number of joint erosions. The nature of the work itself, particularly the degree of physical demand required, showed a striking effect on disability rate, and modification of the work environment to the benefit of the RA patient resulted in almost 100%

increased likelihood of maintaining employment. A separate study (30) reached similar conclusions in 405 RA patients followed prospectively. After 10 years, 50% could no longer work and, after 15 years, this had increased to 67%. Prognosis for future work disability increased roughly in parallel with increasing age. Work disability was again dependent on the degree of physical severity, so that after 10 years, 100% of patients holding a light job were still employed, whereas only 21% of those doing heavy work continued to work. Education level was also a factor in maintaining employment, with those patients who had an education level in excess of the compulsory minimum having approximately a twofold increase in future capacity to remain in employment, and those having extensive general education retained their work capacity significantly better than those with compulsory education only.

A population-based study of work disability was performed by Pincus et al. (31) using symmetric polyarthritis as a model for RA. In men (aged 18–64), 89% of those without arthritis were working, versus only 56% of those with symmetric polyarthritis (Table 3). The results for women were similar, with fewer of the female population in employment, irrespective of disease status. Calculated loss of earnings is demonstrated. Collectively, these studies reflect work disability to be a significant problem for all patients with RA, except those having lighter duties. Significant improvements can be achieved by modification of the work environment, as for the home. Where possible, employers should be counseled concerning RA patients to allow some flexibility in working hours to account for morning stiffness, disease flares, and absences for medical attendance.

Table 3 Disability and Work Status of Persons With Symmetric Polyarthritis Aged 18–64 in 1978 US Population[a]

Category of individuals	Total number (thousands)	Percentage of population	Percentage severely disabled	Percentage working	Total earnings
Males					
No arthritis	54,033	86.2	3.7	89.4	$19,360
RA[b]	855	1.4	47.0	56.1	$ 9,198 (47.5%)
Females					
No arthritis	51,520	80.5	4.5	61.6	$ 8,006
RA[b]	1,511	2.4	51.0	31.0	$ 2,122 (26.5%)

[a]Data derived from 1978 United States Security Survey of Disability and Work, weighted to be representative of the US working-age population aged 18–64.
[b]RA, symmetric polyarthritis (see text).
Source: Ref. 31

C. Radiological Measures

Gradual progression of joint damage is a characteristic of RA. This is inevitably accompanied by increasing deformity and declining function. Radiographs provide a permanent record of the joint architecture, but they are usually interpreted descriptively, rather than numerically. It is assumed that joint radiology gives a good indication of the progression of RA joint damage and its related functional outcome. For this reason radiographs have been given a central place in assessment of the progression of RA.

Scoring of Radiographs

The first approach was devised by Steinbrocker et al. (3). They defined anatomical staging of RA including joint radiology on a 1- to 4-point scale. This defined radiological stages, but was of relatively limited use for scoring progression. A set of standard radiographs was devised by Kellgren (32) graded on a simple 0–4 scale, with 0 being normal and 4 being the most severely damaged. This system was primarily designed for epidemiological studies and is of less value in assessing the progression of RA or the effects of slow-acting antirheumatic drugs (SAARDs), because it is relatively insensitive and has no grading system for individual joints of the hand.

Two methods have become standardized scoring techniques. These were developed by Sharp et al. (33) and Larsen et al. (34). Both of these are widely used, reproducible, and give more detailed information that can be used to evaluate SAARDs. Sharpe's system was first described in 1970 and looks at two categories of change: joint space loss and erosions in the hand and wrist joints. The original scoring system was for 27 joints in each hand and wrist. Subsequently, a revision in 1985 suggested scoring 17 joints for erosions and 18 joints for joint space narrowing in each hand (35). Combining individual scores for each joint gives a large scale for the total radiological score, with an overall range of 0–314.

Larsen and his colleagues used a different approach, based on standard radiographs (36). Each joint had a set of standard radiographs graded from 0 to 5, with 5 representing the most severe grade. The radiographs usually graded are those of the hands and wrists. The scores from these joints are added, with weighting for the wrist, to give a scale of 0–150.

There are several other methods of scoring hand radiographs, including those of Gofton and O'Brien (37), Bluhm et al. (38), and Genant (39). Another simple technique, proposed by Trentham and Masi (40), is to quantify progression using a carpal/metacarpal ratio.

The scoring of radiographs is reasonably reproducible. One study examined this in detail with 13 observers (radiologists and rheumatologists) each scoring up to 41 hand and wrist films from RA patients using methods that differed in terms of the total number of joints scored (35). With one such method, which included 17 areas scored for erosions and 18 for joint-space narrowing, there was good agreement (both inter- and intraobserver), based on progression across a wide spectrum of disease activity and duration. Other studies have given similar high levels of reproducibility in scoring radiographs (37).

Progression of radiographic scores correlates significantly with disease duration (40,42–44). Up to 50% of patients have erosions and joint space narrowing indicative of permanent damage within the first 2 years of disease (45–47). A therapeutic implication of this is that treatment, to be effective, should precede this period of irreversible damage.

Effects of Antirheumatic Drugs on Radiographic Progression

Three placebo-controlled, prospective randomized studies reported in the 1970s suggest a reduced rate of radiological progression results from treatment with slow-acting drugs. Two of these, by the Co-operating Clinics (48) and by Sigler et al. (49), looked at the effects of injectable gold in active RA; the third study examined the effects of cyclophosphamide (50). Altogether there were 95 patients taking gold or placebo followed over 6 months to 2 years and 64 patients taking cyclophosphamide studied for 8 months. Two of these studies used unique methods of assessing radiographic progression, and the Sigler study incorporated the Sharp index.

Set against these positive studies are six larger placebo-controlled, randomized investigations of injectable gold, penicillamine, and cyclophosphamide (51–56), from the same time period, that showed little or no effect from treatment on radiological progression. These included 677 RA patients and lasted between 6 months and 2 years. These investigations also used methods of assessing radiological progression that were unique to the studies.

There are several ways of interpreting the data from all these placebo-controlled studies. The review by Ianuzzi et al. (57) presents one of the clearest accounts of this topic (Table 4). On balance there is only weak evidence for a modifying effect of SAARDs on radiological progression after examining the available data. Small numbers of cases in each study, the effects of dropouts, the variability of patients entered and of disease duration, and the use of different approaches to measuring radiological progression, all can be used to explain the inconsistent results. A separate study from Scott et al. (58) showed that ESR falls in approximately 75% of RA patients treated with a variety of second-line agents over 1 year, but Larsen scores demonstrated radiographic deterioration to be almost universal over the same period.

There have been several more recent randomized studies examining radiographic progression. The effect of auranofin on radiological progression was studied by Borg et al. (59) in a 24-month prospective randomized, placebo-controlled study of 138 patients with early RA (joint symptoms for less than 2

Table 4 Analyses of Studies in Which Slowing of Radiographic Progression in RA is Reported. Number of Studies Providing Different Levels of Support for This Concept

	Strong support	Probable support	Doubtful support	No support	Total
Gold salts	1	2		3	6
Penicillamine			1	1	2
Antimalarials			1	4	5
Azathioprine				1	1
Cyclophosphamide	1		1	2	4
	2	2	3	11	18

Source: Ref. 57.

years). This study was analyzed on an intention-to-treat basis. By 2 years, 52% of patients assigned to take auranofin and 37% of patients assigned to take placebo remained on their original treatment regimen. There were highly significant increases in radiological scores, assessed by Larsen's method, in both groups after 2 years; but the rate of increase in radiological damage was significantly less in those patients randomized to auranofin ($p < 0.05$). Preliminary results from a recent prospective randomized study of auranofin against placebo in 60 patients with early RA by Davis et al. (60) examined progression over 2 years; when an intention-to-treat analysis of all cases was undertaken on the radiological progression over 12 months, there was also significantly less progression with the active treatment.

The effect of sulfasalazine in early RA has been examined in a study by Van der Heijde et al. (61). They compared 60 patients who received either sulfasalazine or hydroxychloroquine (Fig. 1). X-ray films of the hands and feet were available at 24 and 48 weeks in 50 cases and were scored by a modification of Sharpe's method. The increase in the number of erosions and total radiological score was significantly greater in the group taking hydroxychloroquine than in those given sulfasalazine.

An Australian comparison of sulfasalazine with penicillamine gave a less favorable impression of sulfasalazine (62). These authors studied 54 RA patients who were randomized to receive either sulfasalazine or penicillamine. Decisive clinical improvements occurred with both drugs, but each group showed radiological deterioration, with a trend toward greater deterioration with sulfasalazine, although this did not achieve significance. Thirty-three patients were assessed after 1 year of therapy and showed a mean number of new erosions of 1.79 in patients taking penicillamine and 2.23 in those taking sulfasalazine. This further illustrates that joint counts (joint tenderness and swelling) may improve following

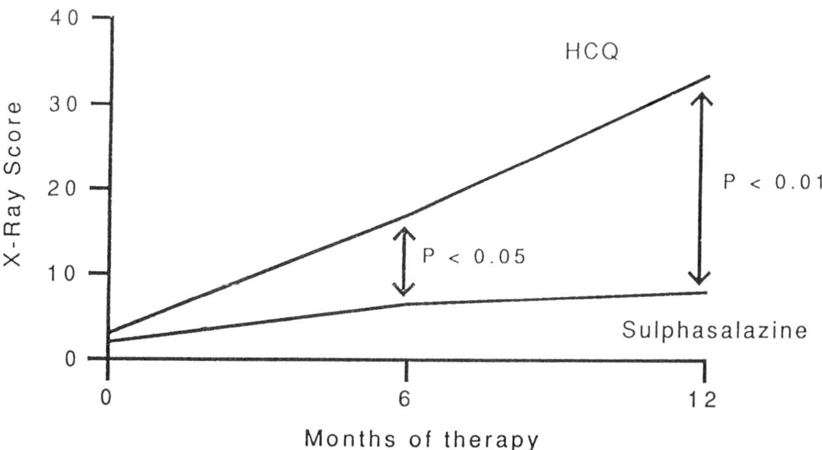

Fig. 1 Radiological progression over 12 months in patients taking sulfasalazine and hydroxychloroquine. Results from a 1-year prospective study by van der Heijde et al. (61).

SAARDs, whereas radiographs almost inevitably progress (albeit at variable rates) in spite of treatment.

One potential problem in prospective, randomized studies is the study duration. A small study of 43 RA patients randomized to receive either penicillamine or hydroxychloroquine has addressed this question (63). Radiographs were scored by Larsen's method. After 12 months of therapy, 34 patients continued receiving treatment; the patients given penicillamine had significantly less radiological progression than those given hydroxychloroquine. But after 2 years there was broadly similar amounts of progression in both groups in the 24 cases who remained on therapy (Fig. 2). This suggests that the time over which progression is studied may be relevant to the conclusions that can be drawn, and that using longer periods may alter and improve the implications and accuracy of a study. Finally, a recent study by Van der Heijde et al. (64) prospectively followed 147 patients with early arthritis (disease duration less than 1 year) for 3 years. Patients all received first- and second-line treatment as necessary, and radiographic progression was scored by a modification of the method of Sharpe. They also calculated percentage joint damage (actual score divided by maximum possible score). After 3 years, radiographic progression was evident in 70% of patients, all of whom had abnormal x-ray films at 1 year. Eighteen to twenty percent of the joints of the hands and feet were affected by 3 years, with relatively little damage per joint (only 8% of maximum possible score). The rate of progression in the first year was significantly higher than in the subsequent 2 years, and more foot joints than hand joints were affected over the entire study period. Rheumatoid factor (RF)-positive patients had more damage than RF-negative patients, with a suggestion of a small synergistic effect for HLA-DR4 positivity.

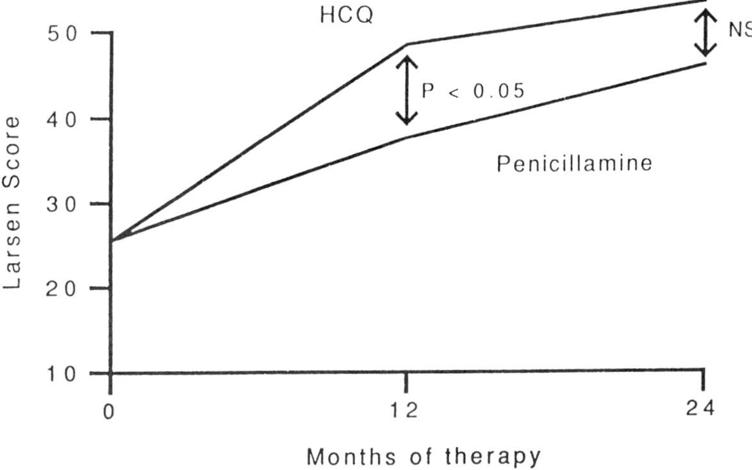

Fig. 2   Radiological progression over 24 months in patients taking penicillamine and hydroxychloroquine. Results from a prospective study by Scott *et al.*(63).

Evolving and Future Radiological Measures

Conventional radiography lacks sensitivity in early rheumatoid disease. Magnetic resonance imaging (MRI) has advantages in soft-tissue discrimination using multiplanar-imaging facilities. It has evolved to provide direct visualization of joint disease at an earlier stage and is already widely used for this purpose. The technique provides high sensitivity in early detection of joint erosions, pannus formation, cartilage destruction, subarticular cyst formation, and joint effusions (65–68). It is suggested that the early identification of erosive disease may identify a subgroup of RA with aggressive disease who would most benefit from early treatment with SAARDs (65). The use of intravenous magnetic contrast in pulse sequences allows definition of hypervascular pannus seen in acute inflammation and its differentiation from fibrous pannus, which indicates inactive disease (69,70). This is of value in detection of the response to treatment and in follow-up of RA. The expense of MRI now precludes its routine use in clinical practice, but the likely advantages in overall morbidity resulting from early appropriate use of SAARDs represent a strong argument in favor of MRI in the evaluation of early disease.

D. Joint Count

The most widely used method for assessment of joint count is the Ritchie index (71), which individually scores 52 joints for tenderness or pain on movement. Other methods used include the Lansbury index (72), which measures 86 peripheral joints accounting for the relative surface area of each joint. More simplified indexes are described by Egger et al. (73), involving 36 joints, and Fuchs et al. (74) using a 28-joint index, including 10 metacarpophalangeal (MCP), 10 proximal interphalangeal (PIP), as well as 2 shoulder, elbow, wrist, and knee joints, which gives comparable results as a measure of clinical status with traditional indexes and is more easily measured. Joint count scores have been shown to be predictive of mortality in RA in a small number of patients over 9 years of follow-up (75), but the recent long-term studies of Wolfe et al. (19,20) show that these indexes do not change significantly in the long term and, therefore, initial joint scores may not provide a reliable prognostic guide. Joint count tenderness does not correlate with radiographic score ($r = 0.01$) at any given time, and joint count swelling correlates only weakly with radiographic score ($r = 0.19$), but the correlations with joint count deformity ($r = 0.69$) and limitation of movement ($r = 0.68$) are strong, resulting in difficulty in overall standardization of joint count scores (76). There is no consensus on the optimum measurement of joint count, as prognostic assessment based upon joint tenderness and swelling may differ from that based on joint deformity and limitation of movement.

E. Patients' Lifestyle

Several underlying sociodemographic variables that are themselves interdependent might impinge on long-term outcome and morbidity. These include patient education, gender, race, income, marital status, social status, and support systems, as well as the standard and availability of medical care.

Among these, patient education has been the subject of most research. As noted already (30), the level of patient education plays an important role in potential work disability of patients with RA. Pincus and co-workers (23,75) have shown formal education level to be an independent factor influencing morbidity over 9 years. A further study of Pincus (77) in the Vanderbilt population of Tennessee shows poor clinical status occurring in patients with low formal education, as measured by joint count, ESR, grip strength, walking time, and self-assessment questionnaires, and independent of age, race, disease duration, and clinical setting. Fries et al. (78) found a negative association between years of schooling and HAQ-FDI, which was strongly apparent for men and only weakly so for women, with a suggestion that patients having the lowest number of education years probably fare worse. These results were independent of occupation and income. All of these studies measure education level by number of years spent within the educational system, and do not account for intelligence, IQ, or other individual skills; further studies are needed in this area. If it is accepted that higher education level improves general health and the outcome of RA, which has also been shown to hold true for most other chronic disease states, then additional government funding aimed toward higher education standards may be cost-effective in the long term.

Other factors, such as socioeconomic status and the availability of social support, have not been the subject of long-term studies, and a short-term study has failed to show benefit from the provision of social support (79). As already mentioned, the nature of employment in terms of physical hardship has a striking effect on overall ability to remain in employment with RA, and it is likely that the higher income results in an improved prognosis by affording access to higher standards of medical care and better education concerning diet, level of fitness, and self-discipline.

F. Comorbidities

Numerous studies have demonstrated an excess of comorbid conditions occurring in RA. A major concern in the interpretation of such data involves ''Berkson's bias'' (80): namely, the concept that comorbid conditions are more likely to be detected in a hospital setting than in the general population. This source of potential bias has been addressed in the study of Pincus (31), which used symmetric arthritis as a surrogate for RA in comparison with the general population, as representative of the United States population. The frequencies of comorbidities in those with symmetric arthritis was significantly higher than that in the general population. Therefore, it seems likely that RA patients have a predisposition to the development of most chronic disease states, resulting in an increased morbidity because of this. Mitchell et al. (25) found the median age of death in RA men and women to be 4 and 10 years earlier than in the general population. Pincus (75), in a metanalysis of causes of RA mortality, found increased mortality resulting from infection (9.4 vs 1%), renal disease (7.8 vs 1.1%), respiratory disease (7.2 vs 3.9%), and gastrointestinal disease (4.2 vs 2.4%)

A further study (81) examined RA comorbidity assessed by patient reporting and found 54% of patients reported at least one additional chronic condition, and 20% rated at least one comorbid condition as severe. Comorbidity was found to influence measures of health status as measured by AIMS and, therefore, RA studies that do not control for comorbidity are likely to overrepresent the effect of the disease.

IV. THE LONG-TERM OUTCOME OF RHEUMATOID ARTHRITIS

Several studies have examined the long-term outcome of RA and its effect on morbidity. There are nine major studies, and these are summarized in Table 5. They have examined different types of patients depending on how cases are collected. They can be divided into studies of hospital inpatients and outpatients, regional surveys, and population surveys. There are several potential weaknesses from these investigations. They may not reflect modern treatments, as their long-term nature means that therapeutic approaches have often changed by the time

Table 5 Major Morbidity Studies (Longer Than 5-Years Duration)

Study (Ref.)	Year	No. of cases		Years of observation	Patient selection source	Percentage in functional class III + IV	
		At onset	At end			At onset	At end
Short et al. (6)	1957	239	174	14	Hospital	20	63 (worse)
Ragan and Farringdon (84)	1962	500	146	13	Clinic	18	50
Duthie et al. (13)	1964	307	200	9	Hospital	65	38.5
Amor et al. (82)	1981	Not given	100	10–15	Hospital	5	35
Rasker and Cosh (14)	1984	100	65	15	Clinic (early disease)	5	51
Scott et al. (83)	1987	112	68	20	Hospital (severe disease)	77	82
Pincus et al. (24)	1984	75	55	9	Thiotepatherapy patients	12	42
Sherrer et al. (21)	1986	1043	681	12	Regional clinic and hospital	12	35
Isacson et al. (85)	1987	239	127	17	Population	9	22

results are reported. The selection of hospital patients may have included many commencing treatment late in the course of their disease, thereby invalidating potential effects of early therapy with slow-acting drugs. Diagnostic criteria or their interpretation may have been dissimilar. The centers involved in long-term studies may not see a balanced or representative group of RA patients. Despite this, much can be learned from long-term studies. The overall conclusions from all of these outcome studies suggest that up to 80% of hospital inpatients are likely to be moderately or severely incapacitated after 20 years, despite treatment, and the average outpatient with rheumatoid arthritis has a 30% chance of becoming severely disabled.

A. Studies of Hospital Inpatients

Several studies of hospital inpatients have examined between 100 and 307 patients (5,13,82,83). The patients were selected based on their requirement for hospital admission and, although they might have been expected to improve in the short-term following hospitalization, their likely long-term prognosis was poor. This concept was supported by the long-term functional outcome assessments, which were far worse than the interim results would have suggested (83). In the study of Scott et al. (83), by the end of 20 years, one-third of patients had died, and more than two-thirds were either dead or severely disabled in spite of so-called disease-modifying therapy (Table 6). However, in this study, many of the patients had advanced disease by the time of study entry, as demonstrated by a functional classification of 3 or higher in more than two-thirds of patients at baseline (see Table 6). Furthermore, joint replacement surgery in the United Kingdom is commonly associated with a prolonged waiting time of up to 2 years, and such a delay would inevitably contribute to end-stage functional impairment in these patients.

B. Studies of Hospital Outpatients

Hospital outpatient studies have been reported from several centers (14,15,24,84). The Bath series (14,15) describes the 20-year results in 100

Table 6 Changes in Functional Class over 20 Years of RA

Functional class	Initial n	5 yrs n	10 yrs n	20 yrs n
I/II	26	60	60	19
III	70	41	19	29
IV/V	16	10	11	20
Dead	0	1	17	37
Lost to follow-up	0	0	5	7

consecutive rheumatoid arthritis patients seen within 1 year of presentation. At 15 years, 65 of the patients were still alive, and 51% were in Steinbroker functional class 3 or 4. At 20 years 54 patients were still alive and 45% were in classes 3 and 4. Similar results were published by Ragan and Farringdon in 1962 (84), with 50% of their 246 patients in these classes after 13 years of observation. These outpatient studies would most closely approximate outcome and suggested morbidity for RA patients who are followed-up in hospital-based clinics.

C. Regional Survey

A regional survey, by Sherrer et al. (21) in Saskatchewan, looked at about 75% of rheumatoid arthritis patients in the province. By about 12 years, 36% of the 681 patients were in functional class III or IV. Disability developed most rapidly during the first years after disease onset and assumed a slow, nearly linear rate of increase after 10 years. A study by Mitchell (25) evaluated 805 patients in a nonhospital regional-based population and showed decreased survival for both men and women at 4 and 10 years earlier than their non-RA counterparts. The RA patients had an increased incidence of vasculitis, spinal subluxation, pulmonary disease, and infection.

D. Population Survey

There is one long-term study of RA patients in the population of Stockholm by Isacson et al. (85). This study was a 17-year follow-up of a population survey conducted during the years 1965–1967 to determine the prevalence of RA. A total of 239 RA subjects were found in a random sample of 15,268 patients (2.7%). By 1983, 112 of the patients had died, and of the 127 still living, 95 were fully evaluated. The number of patients with involvement of at least three joints (New York criteria 2: inclusive of at least one wrist, hand, or foot) had decreased from 72 to 36, and the Steinbrocker functional class remained unchanged for the group as a whole (median class 2), suggestive of a general improvement in disease outcome.

This study illustrates a number of areas of potential bias for long-term population-based studies. First, almost half of the original study subjects had died; a further 18 were inaccessible, and 14 more refused to have blood tests or radiographs, leaving only 95 patients who were evaluated. The quoted results, therefore, refer to only the milder original cases, who would have been expected to survive and to remain fit enough for further assessment including blood tests and radiographs. The patients included for assessment, therefore, would have been expected to have the best long-term outcome. Second, at follow-up, definite criteria for RA were present in only 27 patients, the diagnosis was doubtful in 44, and the remaining 24 did not appear to have RA at follow-up. These results are similar to two other population-based studies, in both of which fewer than

30% of the patients who met ARA criteria for RA at baseline also met these criteria at follow-up after 3–5 years. In the first of these, by Cathcart and O'Sullivan (86) in Sudbury, Massachusetts in 1964, 118 of 4552 patients (2.6%) met 1958 ARA criteria for definite or probable RA. At follow-up, after 3–5 years, only 27.5% still met these same criteria, leading the authors to conclude that "RA exists more frequently as a benign non-deforming condition." The present interpretation of this study is that patients previously classified as ARA probable RA include a nonspecific self-limiting form of polyarthritis that is likely to be nonprogressive in two-thirds or more of the patients. Similarly, in Tecumseh, Michigan, only 26.5% of patients who met ARA criteria for RA at baseline satisfied these criteria 4 years later (87). Thus, use of the 1958 ARA criteria has often given the impression that RA has a favorable outcome, particularly with inclusion into studies of cases of probable RA, and to a lesser extent cases of definite RA. The revised 1987 criteria (88) do not allow designation as classic, definite, or probable RA in an attempt to address this issue.

In contrast with these population studies, the studies done in a clinical setting that demonstrate progressive functional deterioration in RA patients have shown that the percentage of patients satisfying ARA criteria at follow-up remains in proportion to that at baseline. Therefore, studies of different population cohorts identifying those with RA by the 1958 ARA criteria can result in the identification of heterogeneous subsets of patients whose outcomes are not directly comparable.

E. Radiological Assessments in Long-Term Studies

The predominant conclusion is that radiological progression continues in most patients who have received even intensive therapy with SAARDs, although the lack of an untreated group prevents the ideal comparison with natural history of the disease. In the study reported by Scott et al. (77), describing the changes in 112 patients followed for 20 years at a specialist rheumatology unit, hand and wrist radiographs from the beginning and end of this period showed extensive radiological progression in most cases, despite an intensive therapy approach. The initial mean Larsen score was 32 (95% CI 8.1) and the final mean Larsen score was 77 (95% CI 12.6), although there was a small subgroup of patients who had relatively static disease without progression.

Isacson et al. (89) reported radiological changes in the knee joints of RA patients in a 17-year follow-up study. From an initial sample of 239 RA patients, identified as part of a community survey, 98 patients were available for radiological examination 17 years later. Just over half the knee joints (52%) showed radiological changes: joint-space narrowing, which was associated with active disease at follow-up. Murphy et al. (90) have outlined preliminary results of a study to determine the effects of SAARDs on the hip and knee joints over 10 years. Radiological progression (by Larsen score) occurred in knee joints; it correlated with both the initial and final ESRs and also with the area under the curve (AUC) for the ESR over the 10 years of follow-up. They concluded that control of an inflammatory index such as ESR by SAARDs may reduce radiological progression in the long term.

V. THE CAUSES OF ACCELERATED MORBIDITY IN RHEUMATOID ARTHRITIS

Numerous short-term studies over less than 2 years have demonstrated efficacy using SAARDs (91–94). The apparent paradox between the short-term improvement following second-line therapy and long-term functional disability and adverse prognosis has a number of suggested explanations.

A. Early Discontinuation of Slow-Acting Antirheumatic Drugs

For SAARDs to be effective in long-term disease suppression, they should be given continuously during the course of the disease. With the exception of methotrexate, discontinuation of second-line agents within the first 2 years of treatment probably occurs in up to 80% of cases. Wolfe and Hawley (95) have recently shown that, except for methotrexate, half of all RA patients discontinue their second-line agent within 1.5 years of commencement, either because of lack of efficacy or because of adverse reactions, and very rarely for any other cause. They studied 122 controlled, clinical trials and observational studies of SAARDs involving 16,071 patients, with a mean disease duration of 7.61 years at study entry. A recent study (96) of 191 patients taking methotrexate in severe RA showed that the probability of continuing methotrexate therapy was 65% at 2 years and almost 50% after 5 years. These patients had a long disease duration (mean 10.2 years) and 94% had received two or more second-line agents before methotrexate, of which gold was the most common (97%), followed by penicillamine (78%). This study therefore excluded a common source of bias in not excluding patients who had previously been taking SAARDs whose prognosis would be expected to be poor. Significant improvement was reported in all clinical variables of disease, including joint pain and joint swelling count, with a plateau of response achieved after 12 months and maintained until 58 months in 46% of patients. The most common reason for methotrexate discontinuation was adverse reactions (15%), of which only two (1%) were due to probable pulmonary toxicity, and both of these resolved fully following steroid therapy. In contrast, Singh et al. (97) showed that for discontinuations attributable to drug toxicity, there is little difference between methotrexate, azathioprine, and intramuscular gold at 5 years, in a large cohort of patients in the form of an observational study.

B. Early Remission With Short-Acting Antirheumatic Drugs Is Not Sustained

The recent study of Wolfe et al. (20) in the assessment of health status measures over time demonstrated that patients seen within 2 years of disease onset improved markedly and significantly in all variables inclusive of joint count, grip strength, pain score, and initial HAQ-FDI score during the initial 2-year follow-up period with treatment. However, in all time intervals studied beyond the first 2 years, functional ability worsted significantly, despite improvement in the joint count. A previous study of Wolfe et al. (98) in 485 RA patients treated with SAARDs showed evidence of early remission in approximately 18% of patients. However, fewer than 30% of these patients remained in remission 1 year later, and fewer than 10% beyond 3 years, resulting in an overall remission rate of less than 2% of patients after more than 3 years treatment with so-called disease-modifying drugs. Reasons for the nonsustained early response are unknown, but it has been suggested that there exists a therapeutic window, at the onset of disease, during which RA may be more responsive to treatment and, beyond this, irreversible changes, which include pannus formation and cartilage loss, occur, resulting in fixed deformities within the joint and a blunting of the therapeutic potential.

C. Starting Short-Acting Antirheumatoid Drugs Late in the Course of Disease

The important studies of Wolfe et al. (19,20) have shown that significant functional decline occurs at a maximum rate early in the course of RA before first clinic assessment. Radiological evidence of erosions are present in up to 50% of patients within the first 2 years of diagnosis. Most studies of long-term outcome have examined patients relatively late in the course of their disease. In the 20-year outcome study of Scott et al. (83), most cases were in the later stages and functional classes at the time of presentation to the clinic (see Table 6), with a disease duration of 1.5–10 years (median 4.5 years). In the observations of Wolfe and Hawley, already mentioned (98), the mean disease duration at entry was 7.61 years, and in almost 25% of the studies they report the mean disease duration was in excess of 10 years at onset of therapy with SAARDs. There is recent evidence that the treatment of RA with second-line agents is beginning progressively earlier in the disease (99,100). This has resulted in the establishment of early RA clinics in an attempt to initiate treatment with SAARDs as early as possible. Problems with such a concept arise because a significant proportion of early referrals, 40% in a recent study (101), will not subsequently turn out to have definite RA and, therefore, might receive potentially toxic therapy unnecessarily. Furthermore, the classic studies of Rasker and Cosh initiated treatment within 1 year in all patients, with poor long-term outcome despite this.

Long-term results showing progressive disability in most patients do not fully address the question of whether SAARDs can modify disease. Typical long-term data presently available began their observations more than 20 years ago, when many SAARDs were either unavailable or unused, the median disease duration at initial SAARD commencement was 6–8 years, and the average patient remained on disease-modifying therapy for less than 20% of the course of their disease. The most encouraging data suggesting disease modification are reported in a longitudinal study over 10 years reported by Fries (102). Three hundred seven patients were divided into two groups, one group was seen by a rheumatologist regularly and the other group who saw a rheumatologist never or only occasionally. In general, patients seen by rheumatologists had more severe disease and remained on SAARDs for 78% of their course, compared with 42% of the course for those only rarely seeing the rheumatologist. Over the 10-year follow-up period, there was essentially no disease progression in those assigned to rheumatologist care, whereas there was more typical deterioration in the patients not so managed. These results suggest that long-term disease modification can be achieved under supervision with more strict adherence to compliance.

VI. CONCLUSIONS

There is little doubt that the long-term prognosis of RA is toward inevitable functional decline, despite treatment with SAARDs. The plethora of well-conducted trials demonstrating short-term efficacy of SAARDs cannot be used to extrapolate to overall outcome and morbidity. All long-term studies have demonstrated significant morbidity of RA. At present, this is most accurately predicted by health status measures including HAQ and AIMS. There is evidence that maximum functional decline occurs early in RA and, thereafter, only relatively slowly. This suggests that treatment, to be effective, needs to be started at an early stage, perhaps in the context of an early RA referral clinic. From the outset, patients should be followed with serial functional assessments, such as HAQ-FDI, in an attempt to standardize outcome studies and rationalize treatment.

ACKNOWLEDGMENTS

Our studies have been supported by the Arthritis and Rheumatism Council and The Joint Research Board of St Bartholomew's Hospital. Dr. Scott is Muir Hambro Fellow of the Royal College of Physicians.

REFERENCES

1. Weatherall DJ, Ledingham JGG, Warrell DA, eds. Oxford textbook of medicine, 2nd ed. Oxford: Oxford University Press, 1986:16.10.

2. McCarty DJ. Arthritis and allied conditions: a textbook of rheumatology. Philadelphia: Lea & Febiger, 1985:675.

3. Steinbrocker O, Treager CH, Batterman RC. Therapeutic criteria for rheumatoid arthritis. JAMA 1949; 140:659–662.

4. Kelley WN, Harris ED Jr, Ruddy S, Sledge CB, eds. Textbook of rheumatology. Philadelphia: WB Saunders, 1985:979.

5. Short CL, Bauer W. The course of rheumatoid arthritis in patients receiving simple medical and surgical measures. N Engl J Med 1948; 238:142–148.

6. Short CL, Bauer W, Reynolds WE. Rheumatoid arthritis. Cambridge MA: Harvard University Press, 1957.

7. Short CL. Rheumatoid arthritis: types of course and prognosis. Med Clin North Am 1968; 52:549–557.

8. Ropes MW, Bennett GA, Cobb S, et al. 1958 Revision of diagnostic criteria for rheumatoid arthritis. Arthritis Rheum 1959; 2:16–20.

9. Pinals RS, Masi AT, Larsen RA. Preliminary criteria for clinical remission in rheumatoid arthritis. Arthritis Rheum 1981; 24:1308–1315.

10. Fleming A, Benn RT, Corbett M, et al. Early rheumatoid disease. II. Patterns of joint involvement. Ann Rheum Dis 1976; 35:361–364.

11. Roberts WN, Daltroy LH, Anderson RJ. Stability of normal joint findings in persistent classic rheumatoid arthritis. Arthritis Rheum 1988; 31:267–271.

12. Scott DL, Coulton BL, Popert AJ. The long term progression of joint damage in rheumatoid arthritis. Ann Rheum Dis 1986; 45:49–59.

13. Duthie JJR, Browne PE, Truelove LH, et al. Course and prognosis in rheumatoid arthritis: a further report. Ann Rheum Dis 1964; 23:193–204.

14. Rasker JJ, Cosh JA. The natural history of rheumatoid arthritis: a fifteen year follow up study. The prognostic significance of features noted in the first year. Clin Rheumatol 1984; 1:11–20.

15. Rasker JJ, Cosh JA. The natural history of rheumatoid arthritis over 20 years. Clinical symptoms, radiological signs, treatment, mortality and prognostic significance of early features. Clin Rheumatol 1987; 6(suppl 2):5–11.

16. Fries JF, Spitz PW, Kraines RG. Measurement of patient outcome in arthritis. Arthritis Rheum 1980; 23:137–145.

17. Meenan RF, Gertman PM, Mason JH. Measuring health status in arthritis: the arthritis impact measurement scales. Arthritis Rheum 1980; 23:146–152.

18. Meenan RF, Mason JH, Anderson JJ, et al. AIMS 2: the content and properties of a revised and expanded arthritis impact measurement scales health status questionnaire. Arthritis Rheum 1992; 23:1–10.

19. Wolfe F, Cathey MA. The assessment and prediction of functional disability in RA. J Rheumatol 1991; 18:1298–1306.

20. Wolfe F, Hawley DJ, Cathey MA. Clinical and health status measures over time: prognosis and outcome assessment in RA. J Rheumatol 1991; 18:1290–1297.

21. Sherrer YS, Bloch DA, Mitchell DM, et al. The development of disability in rheumatoid arthritis. Arthritis Rheum 1986; 29:494–500.

22. Paulus HE, Egger MJ, Ward JR, et al. Analysis of improvement in individual rheumatoid arthritis patients treated with disease modifying antirheumatic drugs, based on the findings in patients treated with placebo. Arthritis Rheum 1990; 33:477–484.

23. Pincus T, Callahan LF, Vaughn WK. Questionnaire, walking time and button test measure of functional capacity as predictive markers for mortality in rheumatoid arthritis. J Rheumatol 1987; 14:240–251.

24. Pincus T, Callahan LF, Sale WG, et al. Severe functional declines, worse disability and increased mortality in seventy five rheumatoid arthritis patients studied over nine years. Arthritis Rheum 1984; 27:864–872.

25. Mitchell DM, Spitz PW, Young DY, et al. Survival, prognosis and causes of death in rheumatiod arthritis. Arthritis Rheum 1986; 29:706–714.

26. Proudfit WL, Brushke AVG, Sones FM Jr. Natural history of obstructive coronary artery disease: ten-year study of 601 nonsurgical cases. Prog Cardiovasc Dis 1978; 21:5378.

27. Kaplan HS. Survival as related to treatment. In: Kaplan HS, ed. Hodgkin's disease. Cambridge MA: Harvard University Press, 1972:360–388.

28. Yelin E, Meenan R, Nevitt M, et al. Work disability among patients with rheumatoid arthritis. Ann Intern Med 1980; 93:551–556.

29. Yelin E, Henke C, Epstein W. The work dynamics of the person with rheumatoid arthritis. Arthritis Rheum 1987; 30:507–512.

30. Masikara GL, Masikara P. Prognosis of functional capacity and work capacity in rheumatoid arthritis. Clin Rheumatol 1982; 1:117–125.

31. Mitchell JM, Burkhauser RV, Pincus T. The importance of age, education, and comorbidity in the substantial earnings losses of individuals with symmetric polyarthritis. Arthritis Rheum 1988; 31:348–357.

32. Kellgren JH, Lawrence JS. Radiological assessment of rheumatoid arthritis. Ann Rheum Dis 1957; 16:485–493.

33. Sharp JT, Lidsky MD, Collins LC, et al. Methods of scoring the progression of radiologic changes in rheumatoid arthritis: correlation of radiologic, clinical and laboratory abnormalities. Arthritis Rheum 1971; 14:706–720.

34. Larsen A. A radiological method for grading the severity of rheumatoid arthritis. Academic dissertation, 1974.

35. Sharp JT, Young DM, Bluhm GB, et al. How many joints in the hands and wrists should be included in a score of radiological abnormalities used to assess rheumatoid arthritis? Arthritis Rheum 1985; 28:1326–1335.

36. Larsen A, Dale K, Eek M. Radiographic evaluation of rheumatoid arthritis and related conditions by standard reference films. Acta Radiol 1977; 18:481–491.

37. Gofton JP, O'Brien WM. Effects of auranofin on the radiological progression of joint erosion in rheumatoid arthritis. Br J Rheumatol 1982; 9(suppl 8):169–178.

38. Bluhm GB, Smith DW, Mikulaschek WM. A radiological method of assessment of bone and joint destruction in rheumatoid arthritis. Henry Ford Hosp Med J 1983; 31:152–161.

39. Genant HK. Methods of assessing radiographic change in rheumatoid arthritis. Am J Med 1983; 75(suppl 6A):37–45.

40. Trentham DE, Masi AT. Carpal:metacarpal ratio: a new quantitative measure of radiological progression of wrist involvement in rheumatoid arthritis. Arthritis Rheum 1976; 19:939–944.

41. Grindulis KA, Scott DL, Struthers GR. The assessment of radiological changes in the hands and wrists in rheumatoid arthritis. Rheumatol Int. 1983; 3:39–42.

42. Sharp JT. Radiographic evaluation in the course of rheumatoid arthritis. Clin Rheum Dis 1983; 6:541–557.

43. Weisman MH. Use of radiographs to measure outcome in rheumatoid arthritis. Am J Med 1987; 83:96–100.

44. Scott DL, Bacon PA. Joint damage in rheumatoid arthritis: radiological assessments and the effects of anti-rheumatic drugs. Rheumatol Int 1985; 5:193–199.

45. Fuchs HA, Kaye JJ, Callaghan LF, et al. Evidence of significant radiographic damage in rheumatoid arthritis within the first two years of disease. J Rheumatol 1989; 16:585–591.

46. Brook A, Corbett M. Radiographic changes in early rheumatoid disease. Ann Rheum Dis 1977; 36:71–73.

47. Mottonen TT. Prediction of erosiveness and rate of development of new erosions in early rheumatoid arthritis. Ann Rheum Dis 1988; 47:648–653.

48. Cooperating Clinics Committee of the American Rheumatism Association. A controlled trial of gold salt therapy in rheumatoid arthritis. Arthritis Rheum 1973; 16:353–358.

49. Sigler JW, Bluhm GB, Duncan H, et al. Gold salts in the treatment of rheumatoid arthritis. A double blind study. Ann Intern Med 1974; 80:21–26.

50. Cooperating Clinics Committee of the American Rheumatism Association. A controlled trial of cyclophosphamide in rheumatoid arthritis. N Engl J Med 1970; 282:883–889.

51. Shiokawa Y, Horiuchi Y, Honma M, et al. Clinical evaluation of D-penicillamine by multi-center double-blind comparative study in chronic rheumatoid arthritis. Arthritis Rheum 1977; 20:1464–1472

52. Smith SJ, Bartholomew BA, Mills DM, et al. Cyclophosphamide therapy for rheumatoid arthritis. Arch Intern Med 1975; 135:789–793.

53. Townes AS, Sowa JM, Shulman LE. Controlled trial of cyclophosphamide in rheumatoid arthritis. Arthritis Rheum 1976; 19:567–573

54. Research sub-committee of the Empire Rheumatism Council. Gold therapy in rheumatoid arthritis. Report of a multi-center controlled trial. Ann Rheum Dis 1960; 19:95–117.

55. Multi-center Trial Group. Controlled study of D-penicillamine in severe rheumatoid arthritis. Lancet 1973; 1:275–280.

56. Dixon ASJ, Davis J, Dormandy TL, et al. Synthetic D-penicillamine in rheumatoid arthritis. Double blind controlled study of a high and low dose regime. Ann Rheum Dis 1973; 34:416–421.

57. Ianuzzi L, Dawson N, Zein N, et al. Does drug therapy slow radiographic deterioration in rheumatoid arthritis? N Engl J Med 1983; 309:1023–1028.

58. Scott DL, Grindulis KA, Struthers GR, et al. Progression of radiological changes in rheumatoid arthritis. Ann Rheum Dis 1984; 43:8–17.

59. Borg G, Allander E, Lund B, et al. Auranofin improves outcome in early rheumatoid arthritis. Results from a 2 year, double-blind, placebo controlled study. J Rheumatol 1988; 15:1747–1754.

60. Davis J, Maddison P, Woolf A, et al. Auranofin effects radiographic progression in early rheumatoid arthritis. Br J Rheumatol 1990; 29(suppl 2):3.

61. van Der Heijde DM, van Riel PL, Nuver-Zwart IH, et al. Effects of hydroxychloro-quine and sulphasalazine on progression of joint damage in rheumatoid arthritis. Lancet 1989; 1:1036–1039.

62. Carroll GL, Will RK, Breidahl PD, et al. Sulphasalazine versus penicillamine in the treatment of rheumatoid arthritis. Rheumatol Int. 1989; 8:251–255.

63. Scott DL, Greenwood A, Davies J, et al. Radiological progression in rheumatoid arthritis: do D-penicillamine and hydroxychloroquine have different effects? Br J Rheumatol 1990; 29:126–127.

64. van der Heijde DMFM, van Leeuwen MA, van Riel PLCM. Biannual radiographic assessments of hands and feet in a three year prospective follow up of patients with early rheumatoid arthritis. Arthritis Rheum 1992; 35:26–34.

65. Foley-Nolan D, Stack JP, Ryan M, et al. Magnetic resonance imaging in the assessment of rheumatoid arthritis—a comparison with plain film radiographs. Br J Rheumatol 1991; 30:101–106.

66. Gilkeson G, Polisson R, Sinclair H, et al. Early detection of carpal erosions in patients with rheumatoid arthritis: a pilot study of magnetic resonance imaging. J Rheumatol 1986; 15:1361–1366.

67. Moore EA, Jacoby RK, Ellis RE, et al. Demonstation of a geode by magnetic resonance imaging: a new light on the cause of juxta-articular bone cysts in rheumatoid arthritis. Ann Rheum Dis 1990; 49:785–787.

68. Heron C. Magnetic resonance imaging in rheumatology. Ann Rheum Dis 1992; 51:1287–1291.

69. Konig H, Seiper J, Wolf K-J, Rheumatoid arthritis: evaluation of hypervascular and fibrous pannus with dynamic MR imaging enhanced with Gd-DTPA. Radiol-ogy 1990; 176:473–477.

70. Adam G, Dammer M, Bohndorf K, et al. Rheumatoid arthritis of the knee: value of gadopentetate dimeglumine-enhanced MR imaging. AJR 1991; 156:125–129.

71. Ritchie DM, Boyle JA, McInnes JM, et al. Clinical studies with an articular index for the assessment of joint tenderness in patients with rheumatoid arthritis. Q J Med 1968; 147:393–406.

72. Landsbury J, Haut DD. Quantitation of the manifestations of rheumatoid arthritis. 4. Area of joint surfaces as an index to total joint inflammation and deformity. Am J Med Sci 1956; 232:150–155.

73. Egger MJ, Huth DA, Ward JR, et al. Reduced joint count indices in the evaluation of rheumatoid arthritis. Arthritis Rheum 1985; 28:613–619.

74. Fuchs HA, Brooks RH, Callahan LF. A simplified 28 joint quantitative articular index in rheumatoid arthritis. Arthritis Rheum 1989; 32:531–537.

75. Pincus T. Is mortality increased in rheumatoid arthritis? J Musculoskel Med 1988; 5:27–46.

76. Fuchs HA, Callahan LF, Kaye JJ, et al. Radiographic and joint count findings of the hand in rheumatoid arthritis: related and unrelated findings. Arthritis Rheum 1988; 31:44–51.

77. Callahan LF, Pincus T. Formal education level as a significant marker of clinical status in rheumatoid arthritis. Arthritis Rheum 1988; 31:1346–1357.

78. Leigh JP, Fries JF. Education level and rheumatoid arthritis: evidence from five data centers. J Rheumatol 1991; 18:24–33.

79. Shearn MA, Fireman BH. Stress management and mutual support groups in rheumatoid arthritis. Am J Med 1985; 78:551–556.

80. Berkson J. Limitations of the application of fourfold table analysis to hospital data. Biomed Bull 1946; 2:47–53.

81. Berkanovic E, Margo-Lea H. Rheumatoid arthritis and co-morbidity. J Rheumatol 1990; 17:888–892.

82. Amor B, Herson D, Cherot A, et al. Follow up study of patients with rheumatoid arthritis over a period of more than ten years (1966–1978): analysis of disease progression and treatment in 100 cases. Ann Med Interne 1981; 132:168–173.

83. Scott DL, Symmons DPM, Coulton BL, et al. Long term outcome of treating rheumatoid arthritis. Results after 20 years. Lancet 1987; 1:1108–1111.

84. Ragan CH, Farringdon E. The clinical features of rheumatoid arthritis. JAMA 1962; 181:663–667.

85. Isacson J, Allander E, Brastrom LA. A seventeen year follow up of a population survey of rheumatoid arthritis. Scand J Rheumatol 1987; 16:145–152.

86. O'Sullivan JB, Cathcart ES. Follow up evaluation of the effect of criteria on rates in Sudbury, Massachusetts. Ann Intern Med 1972; 72:573–577.

87. Mikkelsen WM, Dodge HJ. A four year follow up of suspected rheumatoid arthritis: the Tecumseh, Michigan, community health study. Arthritis Rheum 1969; 12:78–91.

88. Arnett FC, Edworthy SM, Bloch DA. The American Rheumatism Association 1987 revised criteria for the classification of rheumatoid arthritis. Arthritis Rheum 1988; 31:453–457.

89. Isacson J, Brostrom LA, Allander E, et al. Radiological findings in the rheumatoid knee joint in a seventeen year follow up. Scand J Rheumatol 1987; 16: 153–159.

90. Murphy EA, Capell HA, Hunter JA. Radiological outcome 10 years after the first prescription of disease modifying therapy in rheumatoid arthritis. Br J Rheumatol 1990; 29(suppl 2):4.

91. Research Subcommittee of the Empire Rheumatism Council. Gold therapy in rheumatoid arthritis: a report of a multicenter controlled trial. Ann Rheum Dis 1960; 19:95–119.

92. Huskisson EC, Gibson TJ, Balme HW, et al. Proceedings: penicillamine or gold for rheumatoid arthritis. Multicenter trial using blind observers. The first six months. Ann Rheum Dis 1974; 33:399–406.

93. Pinals RS, Kaplan SB, Lawson JG, et al. Sulphasalazine in rheumatoid arthritis: a double blind placebo controlled trial. Arthritis Rheum 1986; 81:1427–1434.

94. Hamdy H, McKendry RJ, Mierins F, et al. Low dose methotrexate compared with azathioprine in the treatment of rheumatoid arthritis. A twenty four week controlled clinical trial. Arthritis Rheum 1987; 30:361–368.

95. Hawley DJ, Wolfe F. Are the results of controlled clinical trials and observational studies of second line therapy in rheumatoid arthritis valid and generalizable as measures of rheumatoid arthritis outcome: analysis of 122 studies. J Rheumatol 1991; 18:1008–1014.

96. Sany J, Anaya JM, Lussiez V, et al. Treatment of rheumatoid arthritis with methotrexate: a prospective open longterm study of 191 cases. J Rheumatol 1991; 18:1323–1327.

97. Singh G, Fries JF, Williams CA, et al. Toxicity profiles of disease modifying antirheumatic drugs in rheumatoid arthritis. J Rheumatol 1991; 18:188–194.

98. Wolfe F, Hawley DJ. Remission in rheumatoid arthritis. J Rheumatol 1985; 12:245–252.

99. Spector TD, Thompson PW, Evans SJW, et al. Are slow-acting anti-rheumatic drugs being given earlier in rheumatoid arthritis? Br J Rheumatol 1988; 27:498–499.

100. Young A, Cox N, Dixie J, et al. Early rheumatoid arthritis study report of first 506 patients. Arthritis Rheum 1991; 34(suppl):548.

101. Wolfe AD, Hall ND, Goulding NJ, et al. Predictors of the long term outcome of early synovitis. A five year follow up study. J Rheumatol 1991; 30:251–254.

102. Fries JF. Real disease modification; is it possible? Br J Rheumatol 1992; 31(suppl 2):266.

9

Mortality in Patients with Rheumatoid Arthritis

Heikki A. Isomäki

Rheumatism Foundation Hospital
Heinola, Finland

I. INTRODUCTION

Early studies before the era of antibiotics and glucocorticoids emphasize the importance of infections and carditis as a cause of death in patients with rheumatoid arthritis (RA). A sample of 192 autopsied patients with arthritis included 61 with rheumatoid arthritis (1). In 48 of these the cause of death was infection. Another study of 30 autopsied RA patients (some of them obviously with ankylosing spondylitis) showed that 10 deaths resulted from RA itself and 8 from its treatment (2). Carditis was the direct cause of death in 7 patients.

Later developments have greatly changed both mortality and causes of death in general and also in patients with RA. However, still today, the average life expectancy is shorter in RA patients than in the general population, and all studies of clinical patients with RA indicate an elevated mortality rate. This paper reviews studies published in the 1950s and thereafter about mortality, causes of death, and risk factors associated with premature death in RA patients. The subject has also been discussed in several earlier reviews (3–7).

II. MORTALITY RATE

The first study comparing the mortality rates of patients with RA or ankylosing spondylitis and of the general population is that of Cobb et al. from 1953 (8). In this study 583 hospitalized patients were followed for an average of 9.6 years. During that time 137 patients died, whereas the expected number of deaths based on the mortality statistics of the general population was 105.6. The standardized

235

mortality ratio (SMR; i.e., the ratio of observed to expected deaths) was 1.3, indicating a 30% increase in mortality. In the aged groups younger than 50, the SMR was 4.0 and in the older-aged groups about 1. In other words, the excess mortality was mainly due to death at a young age.

Several later studies (9–31) have not changed this general picture. Table 1 shows that the SMR has been more than unity in every published study. Variations between the different studies have been large, mainly because of differences in the patient populations and in the layout of the studies. Most studies have compared mortality with that of the general population, some with case–controls (20,27); some of the RA cohorts studied do not represent the true picture of RA, as they were selected because of sex and age (27), treatment (17), or LE cell positivity (26).

A recent, very large multicenter study from the United States and Canada includes 922 deaths among 3501 RA patients (31). The SMR was 2.4 in women, 2.1 in men, and 2.3 in all patients. The SMR ranged from 2.0 to 2.2 in three centers, reflecting community and practice data, and it was 3.1 at a tertiary referral center. In Stockholm, the SMR was 1.3 in a community-based patient sample (20) and 2.5 in hospitalized patients (21). The low mortality rate in the study of Linos et al. (18) may also be explained by the patient sample, which included all cases in the population fulfilling the diagnostic criteria for probable RA. Thus, mortality seems to be another evidence for the difference in RA between cases identified in clinical settings and all people who meet the diagnostic criteria in a population.

Table 1 Mortality in RA

Author (Ref.)	Yr	Observed deaths	Expected deaths	Obs./exp.
Cobb et al. (8)	1953	137	105.6	1.3
Duthie et al. (10)	1964	75	44.9	1.7
Uddin et al. (11)	1970	94	60	1.6
Monson et al. (14)	1976	570	307.8	1.9
Lewis et al. (17)	1980	46	40.8	1.1
Linos et al. (18)	1980	143	123.7	1.2
Allebeck et al. (20)	1981	84	62.5	1.3
Allebeck (21)	1982	473	190.9	2.5
Pincus et al. (25)	1984	20	15.2	1.3
Prior et al. (26)	1984	199	66.7	3.0
Mutru et al. (27)	1985	356	217	1.6
Mitchell et al. (28)	1986	233	154	1.5
Reilly et al. (30)	1990	63	45	1.4
Wolfe et al. (31)	1991	922	408	2.3

The other study with a very low mortality rate included mainly patients treated with azathioprine, cyclophosphamide, or chlorambucil, often in high doses, and in combination with intramuscular gold and glucocorticoids (17). Many patients in this study were initially referred with active disease requiring treatment with glucocorticoids. Despite the active disease and the unusually heavy medication, the observed mortality was almost the same as in the general population. The SMR was only 1.1, the lowest figure among all 14 published studies.

All published data indicate that mortality is increased in RA patients, especially in those younger than aged 60 (Table 2). The risk of death is about twice as high as in the general population. Estimates of loss of life expectancy vary from 3 years in women (26) to 18 years in both sexes younger than aged 50 years (9). The risk of death is higher in patients who need hospital treatment. However, the lowest SMR has been reported in hospitalized patients with cytotoxic treatment.

III. CAUSES OF DEATH

Careful analysis of causes of death has shown that RA is the underlying cause of death in almost 20% of patients (21,24,30). The most common direct causes of death in these patients are vasculitis, secondary amyloidosis, carditis, cervical myelopathy (30), or rheumatoid lung disease (28). In addition, RA is often an important contributory factor in death. Examples of this are the side effects of drugs used in the treatment of RA, or death from pneumonia in an immobilized patient.

Because only about 1% of adults suffer from RA and only one out of five of these die of RA, it is a rare cause of death in the general population. The main difference in the causes of death between RA patients and general population are deaths caused directly or indirectly by RA itself. Table 3 shows that musculoskeletal diseases (including RA) have been the cause of death in 1.3–19.7% of the

Table 2 Mortality in RA by Age

Author (Ref.)	Age (yr)	Obs./exp.	Age (yr)	Obs./exp.
Cobb et al. (8)	< 50	4.0	50 +	0.9
Duthie et al. (10)	< 60	2.1	60 +	1.4
Uddin et al. (11)	< 60	2.8	60 +	1.8
Monson et al. (14)	< 55	2.8	55 +	1.8
Lewis et al. (17)	25–64	2.3	65 +	0.7
Allebeck et al. (20)	30–59	1.0	60 +	1.4
Allebeck (21)	< 60	5.5	60 +	2.3

Table 3 Causes of Death in Patients with RA (% of All)

Author (Ref.)	ICD I infections	ICD II malignant neoplasms	ICD VII circulatory diseases	ICD VIII respiratory diseases[a]	ICD IX digestive diseases	ICD X urogenital diseases	ICD XIII Musculoskeletal diseases	ICD XVII accidents, intoxications	Others
Cobb et al. (8)	13.1	11.5	36.9	11.5	6.2	10.0	3.1[b]	0	7.7
Duthie et al. (10)	14.7	13.3	45.3	–	8.0	17.3	–	1.3	–
Uddin et al. (11)	4.3	7.4	53.2	18.1	2.1	2.1	2.1[b]	–	10.6
Monson et al. (14)	–	12.6	54.6	10.0	4.0	4.4	6.7	–	7.7
Lewis et al. (17)	–	28.3	41.3	19.6	4.3	0	2.2	0	4.3
Allebeck et al. (20)	2.4	23.8	54.8	1.2	6.0	0	4.8	–	7.1
Allebeck (21)	1.1	11.8	44.2	5.1	8.2	4.2	19.7	2.1	3.6
Prior et al. (24)	2.0	15.1	39.2	14.6	5.5	3.0	17.1	–	3.5
Pincus et al. (25)	20	25	40	5	5	0	5	0	0
Vandenbroucke et al. (26)	2.4	19.4	43.0	12.1	5.5	5.5	10.3	0.6	1.2
Mutru et al. (27)	2.0	11.8	46.6	8.1	–	11.8	8.7[b]	3.1	7.9
Mitchell et al. (28)	4.8	13.1	42.6	13.5	6.0	3.2	10.0	4.0	2.8
Scott et al. (29)	10.8	16.2	35.1	16.2	–	8.1	–	–	13.5
Reilly et al. (30)	4.8	12.7	46.0	11.1	1.6	3.2	19.0	0	1.6
Wolfe et al. (31)	7.0	11.3	47.1	18.1	5.7	1.2	1.3	2.6	5.7

[a]Includes pneumonia.
[b]RA-induced amyloidosis only.
–, not listed.

cases. The variation between different studies is greater in this disease group than in any other. There certainly are differences in the patient samples, but it is very likely that much of the variation can be explained by inaccurate classification of death.

Death certificate data, in which RA is rarely mentioned, are another source of error (32–34). This may introduce a serious bias in results, especially if the study sample is not a cohort of patients with established RA, but includes only cases in which RA is mentioned in the death certificates. Studies based on death certificate data alone (35) cannot be compared with cohort analysis. Errors in classifying the causes of death in RA patients have been treated earlier (36,37).

Secondary amyloidosis is a common finding in autopsied RA patients (38–42). Death of amyloidosis is usually caused by renal failure, but heart, intestine, and other organs may also be severely affected. The frequency of secondary amyloidosis as a cause of death has been reported in seven studies (8,11,24,27,28,30,31). It has varied from 0.2 (31) to 8.7% (27) of all causes of death. The lowest figure is from the United States, the highest from the highly selected patient population of the national Finnish rheumatism hospital. In the main, the variation probably reflects the differences in the patient populations, but the magnitude of the variation is so large that it may be a sign of true differences in the frequency of secondary amyloidosis. Amyloidosis is also a more common cause of death in European countries than in the United States in patients with juvenile RA (43).

Cardiovascular diseases are the leading cause of death in RA patients. Vasculitis (30,44) and noncoronary heart disease in men (45) are more common in RA patients than in the general population; therefore, it may be the SMR of cardiovascular diseases has been elevated in some of the studies (14,21,24). The variation between different studies is small.

Malignant neoplasms constitute about 20% of all the causes of death in general Western populations. In patients with RA the average percentage is lower, although the variation between different studies is from 7.4 (11) to 28.3% (17). The incidence of all malignant neoplasms together is not elevated in RA patients (46), and the survival of RA patients with cancer is the same as that of other cancer patients (47). The death rate is low in cancer because RA patients die of other causes before contracting cancer.

Malignant diseases of the lymphatic and myeloid system are an interesting exception to the general picture. The incidence of lymphoma, leukemia, and myeloma is higher in RA patients than in the general population (46). The highest seems to be the risk of the large-cell non-Hodgkin's lymphoma (48). This elevated risk can be explained mainly by predisposition to lymphoproliferative malignancies inherent in RA (49). In some studies, the mortality rate in lymphoproliferative malignancies has been elevated (14,24,31,50), but not in all (51).

Renal disease is well known in RA and is also a common cause of death (52). Clinical findings before death included uremia in 23% of the 132 autopsied RA patients, and in addition to amyloidosis, both vasculitis and proliferative glomerulonephritis were observed in the uremic patients (41). Many antirheumatic drugs, such as gold, penicillamine, and nonsteroidal anti-inflammatory drugs (NSAIDs) have renal side effects, but renal disease can hardly be attributed to these alone.

A common finding has been the high frequency of infections as a cause of death. The importance of infections is emphasized if infections of the respiratory and genitourinary system are classified together with those in Chapter 1 of the International Code of Diseases (ICD) (7). In a recent Japanese study (53), 20.5% of the deaths were caused by infectious diseases and, in a German autopsy study, 48% were (39). The mortality statistics indicate a serious lack of resistance to infections in RA patients (54). Consumption of NSAIDs is the main explanation for deaths of upper gastrointestinal bleeding.

IV. FACTORS PREDICTING DEATH

Mortality seems to be predicted by the clinical picture of RA, as well as by age- and sex-dependent hormonal status (55). Mortality is higher among patients with more severe disease, as assessed by the number of diagnostic criteria (19,20,56) or functional disability (19,20,57–60). Simple functional tests are able to discriminate severely disabled cohorts from RA patients with extremely high mortality (57). Extra-articular features are associated with high mortality (61). Patients with cutaneous ulcers, vasculitic rash, neuropathy, and scleritis had higher mortality than those whose disease was confined to the joints (44).

Immunoglobulin M rheumatoid factor in serum is associated with a severe clinical picture of RA and also with high mortality (20,62). Cryoglobulinemia and precipitating antibodies to soluble cellular antigens also indicate aberration of the immune system in RA, and they predicted a poor life prognosis (44). In general, however, clinical findings and health status scores seem to predict mortality better than immunological laboratory tests (63).

Mortality has been used as a measure of the efficacy of treatment in RA patients in only a few studies. Foster et al. (64) treated 16 RA patients, with necrotizing scleritis or peripheral ulcerative keratitis, with cytotoxic drugs and 18 patients with other drugs. In 10 years, only 1 patient treated with cytotoxic drugs died, and this death occurred after cytotoxic therapy was withdrawn. Nine of the patients treated with conventional drugs died. Although not randomized, this study indicates that cytotoxic drugs are able to reduce mortality in patients with necrotizing scleritis, which is often associated with generalized vasculitis (65). The lowest SMR in RA patients has been reported in hospitalized patients with an active disease and with exceptionally heavy drug treatment, including cytotoxic drugs (17). Only one of the 46 deaths in this study could be attributed directly to RA (cervical subluxation).

In a retrospective analysis of RA patients hospitalized for the first time in the 1960s, cumulative mortality in 1989 was 75% in patients never treated with intramuscular gold, 50% in patients treated with gold for less than 2 years, and only 25% in patients treated with gold for more than 10 years. The difference in mortality could not be explained by age, sex, or rheumatoid factor (66).

Alkylating cytostatic treatment (67–69) and methotrexate (70) seem to prevent progression of renal amyloidosis. The occurrence of secondary amyloidosis and the number of deaths from amyloidosis in patients with juvenile rheumatoid arthritis have declined in Finland since systematic cytostatic drug treatment was introduced for severe polyarthritis in the early 1980s (71).

Despite the scarcity of data, the mortality statistics provide evidence in favor of therapy. As stated by Vollertsen et al. (56), studies showing decreased survival associated with glucocorticoid or cytotoxic therapy may indicate selection bias. Only the most severely ill patients have been treated with these drugs.

The mortality risk of the patient is influenced not only by RA and its treatment, but also by the patient's socioeconomic status. Pincus and Callahan (72) reported increased mortality in patients with a low level of formal education: 9 out of 20 grade school-educated, 10 out of 34 high school-educated, and 1 out of 21 college-educated patients died during 9 years. This difference in mortality could not be explained by demographic or clinical variables.

The number of years of schooling completed is perhaps the best single variable describing socioeconomic status (73). It has been proposed that a low level of formal education is a composite variable that identifies behavioral risk factors predisposing to an etiology and a poor outcome in most chronic diseases (74,75). These unfavorable behaviors may include smoking, diet, an inability to cope with stress, or learned helplessness (76). It is not clear, however, whether a low educational level is an independent mortality risk or whether it reflects rather the socioeconomic status, including occupation and income (73).

V. CONCLUSIONS

The earlier concept of RA as a disease causing pain and disability, but not shortening life expectancy, is incorrect. On the contrary, in hospitalized RA patients, nearly 20% of the deaths are directly caused by RA, and it is a contributory cause of death in other patients. Consequently, the average life expectancy is shorter for RA patients than for the general population. This is illustrated in Figure 1, which shows the prevalence of Finnish individuals entitled to free medication because of RA or allied diseases. The prevalence increases almost

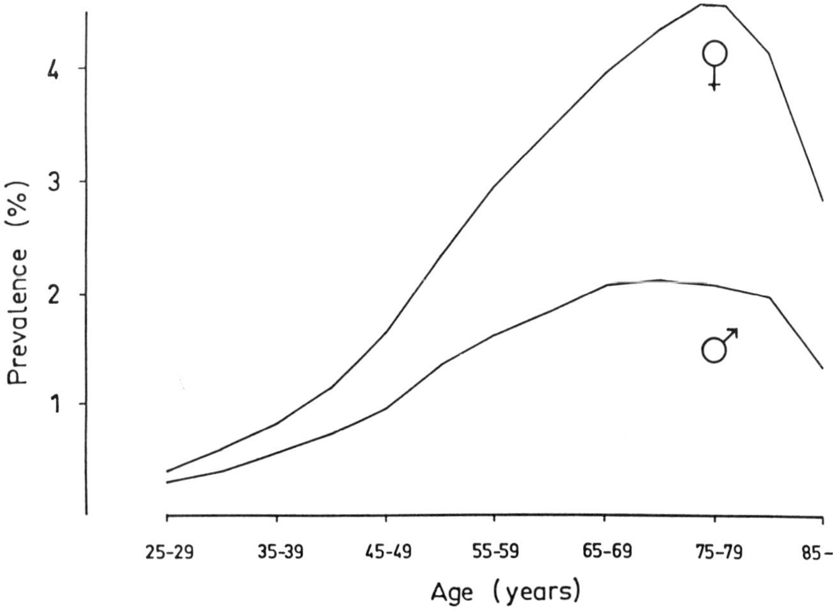

Fig. 1 Prevalence by age of individuals with free medication because of RA or other chronic arthritis (excluding SLE and other systemic connective tissue diseases and gout) in Finland in 1991.

linearly with age to 75 years, but thereafter, declines abruptly in both sexes. The loss of rheumatoid individuals through death is greater than the incidence of new cases and, therefore, the prevalence of RA declines in very old persons.

It is obvious that the risk of death in patients with RA is higher in undeveloped than in highly developed societies. Several studies have shown very low prevalences of RA in undeveloped countries. Although our current understanding of mortality in RA is drawn from a very small part of the globe (7), there are reasons to suggest that one explanation for the low prevalence is the premature death of RA patients. As society develops, patients live longer, but with severe disabilities. This was the situation in Finland in 1939, when chronic polyarthritis was the third most frequent cause of disability after mental disorders and tuberculosis. Only the new achievements in therapy have been able to reduce, first, disability and, later, mortality as well.

There is no need to overemphasize the importance of mortality in RA. Even if all deaths from RA could be prevented, the mean life expectancy of patients would increase by only a few years. Premature death is, however, the result and the ultimate end of severe disability. Improvements in the quality of life for decades by prevention of disability is important, and mortality studies may serve as a tool for investigation of the long-term efficacy of therapies. A future subject of mortality studies should be whether life expectancy can be increased by, for example, early aggressive immunosuppressive treatment.

REFERENCES

1. Fingerman DL, Andrus FC. Visceral lesions associated with rheumatoid arthritis. Ann Rheum Dis 1943; 3:168–181.
2. Rosenberg EF, Baggenstoss AH, Hench PS. The causes of death in thirty cases of rheumatoid arthritis. Ann Intern Med 1944; 20:903–919.
3. Abruzzo JL. Rheumatoid arthritis and mortality. Arthritis Rheum 1982; 25:1020–1023.
4. Cosh JA. Survival and death in rheumatoid arthritis. J Rheumatol 1984; 11:117–119.
5. Pincus T, Callahan LF. Taking mortality in rheumatoid arthritis seriously—predictive markers, socioeconomic status and comorbidity. J Rheumatol 1986; 13:841–845.
6. Pinals RS. Survival in rheumatoid arthritis. Arthritis Rheum 1987; 30:473–475.
7. Symmons DPM. Mortality in rheumatoid arthritis. Br J Rheumatol 1988; 27(suppl 1):44–54.
8. Cobb S, Anderson F, Bauer W. Length of life and cause of death in rheumatoid arthritis. N Engl J Med 1953; 249:553–556.
9. Reah TG. The prognosis of rheumatoid arthritis. Proc R Soc Med 1963; 56:813–817.
10. Duthie JJR, Brown PE, Truelove LH, Baragar FD, Lawrie AJ. Course and prognosis in rheumatoid arthritis. A further report. Ann Rheum Dis 1964; 23:193–204.
11. Uddin J, Kraus AS, Kelly HG. Survivorship and death in rheumatoid arthritis. Arthritis Rheum 1970; 13:125–130.
12. Jacoby RK, Jayson MIV, Cosh JA. Onset, early stages and prognosis of rheumatoid arthritis. A clinical study of 100 patients with 11 year follow-up. Br Med J 1973; 1:96–100.
13. Isomäki H, Mutru O, Koota K. Death rate and causes of death in patients with rheumatoid arthritis. Scand J Rheumatol 1975; 4:205–208.
14. Monson RR, Hall AP. Mortality among arthritics. J Chronic Dis 1976; 29:459–467.
15. Koota K, Isomäki H, Mutru O. Death rate and causes of death in RA patients during a period of five years. Scand J Rheumatol 1977; 6:241–244.
16. Constable TJ, McConkey B, Paton A. The cause of death in rheumatoid arthritis. Ann Rheum Dis 1978; 37:569.
17. Lewis P, Hazleman BL, Hanka R, Roberts S. Cause of death in patients with rheumatoid arthritis with particular reference to azathioprine. Ann Rheum Dis 1980; 39:457–461.
18. Linos A, Worthington JW, O'Fallon WM, Kurland LT. The epidemiology of rheumatoid arthritis in Rochester, Minnesota: a study of incidence, prevalence, and mortality. Am J Epidemiol 1980; 111:87–98.
19. Rasker JJ, Cosh JA. Cause and age at death in a prospective study of 100 patients with rheumatoid arthritis. Ann Rheum Dis 1981; 40:115–120.

20. Allebeck P, Ahlbom A, Allander E. Increased mortality among persons with rheumatoid arthritis, but where RA does not appear on death certificate. Scand J Rheumatol 1981; 10:301–306.

21. Allebeck P. Increased mortality in rheumatoid arthritis. Scand J Rheumatol 1982; 11:81–86.

22. Cosh JA, Rasker JJ. A 20 year follow-up study of 100 patients with rheumatoid arthritis. Ann Rheum Dis 1982; 41:317.

23. Rasker JJ, Cosh JA. The natural history of rheumatoid arthritis: a 15 year follow-up study. The prognostic significance of features noted in the first year. Clin Rheumatol 1984; 3:11–20.

24. Prior P, Symmons DPM, Scott DL, Brown R, Hawkins CF. Cause of death in rheumatoid arthritis. Br J Rheumatol 1984; 23:92–99.

25. Pincus T, Callahan LF, Sale WG, Brooks AL, Payne LE, Vaughn WK. Severe functional declines, work disability, and increased mortality in seventy-five rheumatoid arthritis patients studied over nine years. Arthritis Rheum 1984; 27:864–872.

26. Vandenbroucke JP, Hazevoet HM, Cats A. Survival and cause of death in rheumatoid arthritis: a 25-year prospective follow-up. J Rheumatol 1984; 11:158–161.

27. Mutru O, Laakso M, Isomäki H, Koota K. Ten year mortality and causes of death in patients with rheumatoid arthritis. Br J Med 1985; 290:1811–1813.

28. Mitchell DM, Spitz PW, Young DY, Bloch DA, McShane DJ, Fries JF. Survival, prognosis, and causes of death in rheumatoid arthritis. Arthritis Rheum 1986; 29:706–714.

29. Scott DL, Symmons DPM, Coulton BL, Popert AJ. Long-term outcome of treating rheumatoid arthritis: results after 20 years. Lancet 1987; 1:1108–1111.

30. Reilly PA, Cosh JA, Maddison PJ, Rasker JJ, Silman AJ. Mortality and survival in rheumatoid arthritis: a 25 year prospective study of 100 patients. Ann Rheum Dis 1990; 49:363–369.

31. Wolfe F, Mitchell DM, Sibleg J, Fries JF, Bloch DA, Williams CA, Spitz P, Hager M, Kleinheksal SM, Cathey MA. The mortality of 3501 persons with rheumatoid arthritis in the ARAMIS data banks. Arthritis Rheum 1991; 34(suppl):D109.

32. Atwater EC, Jacox RF. The death certificate in rheumatoid arthritis. Arthritis Rheum 1967; 10:259.

33. Lindahl BIB. The reliability of Swedish mortality statistics for rheumatoid arthritis. Scand J Rheumatol 1984; 13:289–296.

34. Laakso M, Isomäki H, Mutru O, Koota K. Death certificate and mortality in rheumatoid arthritis. Scand J Rheumatol 1986; 15:129–133.

35. Wicks IP, Moore J, Fleming A. Australian mortality statistics for rheumatoid arthritis 1950–81: analysis of death certificate data. Ann Rheum Dis 1988; 47:563–569.

36. Lindahl BIB. The causal sequence on death certificates: errors affecting the reliability of mortality statistics for rheumatoid arthritis. J Chronic Dis 1985; 38:47–57.

37. Lindahl BIB. In what sense is rheumatoid arthritis the principal cause of death? J Chronic Dis 1985; 38:963–972.

38. Mutru O, Koota K, Isomäki H. Cause of death in autopsied RA patients. Scand J Rheumatol 1976; 5:239–240.

39. Rainer F, Klein G, Schmid P, Härringer M. Untersuchungen über Art und Häufigkeit der Todesursachen bei chronischer Polyarthritis. Z Rheumatol 1978; 37:335–341.

40. Vapra AN, Pokk LR. Visceral lesions as cause of death in rheumatoid arthritis patients. Proc 10th European Rheumatology Congress, Moscow, 1983:1069.

41. Boers M, Croonen AM, Dijkmans BAC, Breedveld FC, Eulderink F, Cats A, Weening JJ. Renal findings in rheumatoid arthritis: clinical aspects of 132 necropsies. Ann Rheum Dis 1987; 46:658–663.

42. Dhillon V, Woo P, Isenberg D. Amyloidosis in the rheumatic diseases. Ann Rheum Dis 1989; 48:696–701.

43. Baum J, Gutowska G. Death in juvenile rheumatoid arthritis. Arthritis Rheum 1977; 20(suppl):253–255.

44. Erhardt CC, Mumford PA, Venables PJW, Maini RN. Factors predicting a poor life prognosis in rheumatoid arthritis: an eight year prospective study. Ann Rheum Dis 1989; 48:7–13.

45. Mutru O, Laakso M, Isomäki H, Koota K. Cardiovascular mortality in patients with rheumatoid arthritis. Cardiology 1989; 76:71–77.

46. Isomäki H, Hakulinen T, Joutsenlahti U. Excess risk of lymphomas, leukemia and myeloma in patients with rheumatoid arthritis. J Chronic Dis 1978; 31:691–696.

47. Hakulinen T, Knekt P, Uotila O, Isomäki H. Similar survival rates for rheumatoid and non-rheumatoid cancer patients. Scand J Rheumatol 1986; 15:285–289.

48. Isomäki H, Hakulinen T, Franssila K, Teppo L, Knekt P. Leukaemia and lymphoma in patients with rheumatoid arthritis. Scand J Rheumatol 1988; 17:236.

49. Silman AJ, Petrie J, Hazleman B, Evans SJW. Lymphoproliferative cancer and other malignancy in patients with rheumatoid arthritis treated with azathioprine: a 20 year follow up study. Ann Rheum Dis 1988; 47:988–992.

50. Laakso M, Mutru O, Isomäki H, Koota K. Cancer mortality in patients with rheumatoid arthritis. J Rheumatol 1986; 13:522–526.

51. Fries JF, Bloch D, Spitz P, Mitchell DM. Cancer in rheumatoid arthritis: a prospective long-term study of mortality. Am J Med 1985; 78(suppl 1A):56–59.

52. Laakso M, Mutru O, Isomäki H, Koota K. Mortality from amyloidosis and renal diseases in patients with rheumatoid arthritis. Ann Rheum Dis 1986; 45:663–667.

53. Yoshizawa H, Kudo H, Iwano K, Yamada A, Aikawa T, Miyamoto Y, Takahashi K, Saito K, Ogita T, Okudaira K. Causes of death in patients with rheumatoid arthritis. Analysis of 117 cases for 13 years. Ryumachi 1990; 30:255–263.

54. Baum J. Infection in rheumatoid arthritis. Arthritis Rheum 1971; 14:135–137.

55. Symmons DPM, Prior P, Scott DL, Brown R, Hawkins CF. Factors influencing mortality in rheumatoid arthritis. J Chronic Dis 1986; 39:137–145.

56. Vollertsen RS, Conn DL, Ballard DJ, Ilstrup DM, Kazmar RE, Silverfield JC. Rheumatoid vasculitis: survival and associated risk factors. Medicine 1986; 65:365–375.

57. Pincus T, Callahan LF, Vaughn WK. Questionnaire, walking time and button test measures of functional capacity as predictive markers for mortality in rheumatoid arthritis. J Rheumatol 1987; 14:240–251.

58. Wolfe F, Kleinheksel SM, Cathay MA, Hawley DJ, Spitz PW, Fries JF. The clinical value of the Stanford Health Assessment Questionnaire functional disability index in patients with rheumatoid arthritis. J Rheumatol 1988; 15:1480–1488.

59. Kazis LE, Anderson JJ, Meenan RF. Health status as a predictor of mortality in rheumatoid arthritis: a five-year study. J Rheumatol 1990; 17:609–613.

60. Leigh JP, Fries JF. Mortality predictors among 263 patients with rheumatoid arthritis. J Rheumatol 1991; 18:1307–1312.

61. Gordon DA, Stein JL, Broder I. The extra-articular features of rheumatoid arthritis. A systematic analysis of 127 cases. Am J Med 1975; 54:445–452.

62. Kellgren JH, O'Brien WM. On the natural history of rheumatoid arthritis in relation to the sheep cell agglutination test (SCAT). Arthritis Rheum 1971; 14:115.

63. Pincus T, Callahan LF. Reassessment of twelve traditional paradigms concerning the diagnosis, prevalence, morbidity and mortality of rheumatoid arthritis. Scand J Rheumatol Suppl 1989; 79:67–95.

64. Foster CS, Forstot SL, Wilson LA. Mortality rate in rheumatoid arthritis patients developing necrotizing scleritis or peripheral ulcerative keratitis. Effects of systemic immunosuppression. Ophthalmology 1984; 91:1253–1263.

65. Jayson MI, Jones DE. Scleritis and rheumatoid arthritis. Ann Rheum Dis 1971; 30:343–347.

66. Lehtinen K, Isomäki H. Intramuscular gold therapy is associated with long survival in patients with rheumatoid arthritis. J Rheumatol 1991; 18:524–529.

67. Berglund K, Keller C, Thysell H. Alkylating cytostatic treatment in renal amyloidosis secondary to rheumatic disease. Ann Rheum Dis 1987; 46:757–762.

68. Vouyiouka O, David J, Ansell BM, Hall A, Woo P. Mortality and morbidity of a cohort of juvenile arthritis patients with amyloidosis. Arthritis Rheum 1990; 33(suppl):S144.

69. Ahlmen M, Ahlmen J, Svalander C, Bucht H. Cytotoxic drug treatment of reactive amyloidosis in rheumatoid arthritis with special reference to renal insufficiency. Clin Rheumatol 1987; 6:27–38.

70. Tiitinen S, Kaarela K, Filipowicz-Sosnowska A, Jesien-Dudzinska E. Treatment of amyloidosis with azathioprine or colchicine or methotrexate in patients with rheumatoid arthritis in Finland and Poland. Rheumatologia 1991; 24:138–144.

71. Savolainen A, Isomäki H. Decrease in number of deaths from secondary amyloidosis in patients with juvenile rheumatoid arthritis. J Rheumatol 1993; 20:1201–1203.

72. Pincus T, Callahan LF. Formal education as a marker for increased mortality and morbidity in rheumatoid arthritis. J Chronic Dis 1985; 38:973–984.

73. Leigh JP, Fries JF. Occupation, income, and education as independent covariates of arthritis in four national probability samples. Arthritis Rheum 1991; 34:984–995.

74. Pincus T, Callahan LF, Burkhauser RV. Most chronic diseases are reported more frequently by individuals with fewer than 12 years of formal education in the age 18–64 United States population. J Chronic Dis 1987; 40:865–874.

75. Pincus T. Formal educational level—a marker for the importance of behavioral variables in the pathogenesis, morbidity, and mortality of most diseases. J Rheumatol 1988; 15:1457–1460.

76. Callahan LF, Brooks RH, Pincus T. Further analysis of learned helplessness in rheumatoid arthritis using a "rheumatology attitudes index." J Rheumatol 1988; 15:418–426.

77. Pincus T. Rheumatoid arthritis: disappointing long-term outcomes despite successful short-term clinical trials. J Clin Epidemiol 1988; 41:1037–1041.

10

The Economic Impact of Rheumatoid Arthritis

Deborah P. Lubeck

Stanford University
Stanford, California

I. INTRODUCTION

Measurement of patient outcome now encompasses many components: physical health, mental health, perceptions of well-being, treatment side effects, and cost of therapy versus benefit. Accordingly, a major research effort has been focused on developing methods for the measurement of health status and patient outcome in arthritis and other rheumatological diseases. The intent of this effort is to produce standard measures for evaluating the effects of disease, the effects of treatment, and costs of care. Although there are more and more frequent reports on the use of these measures in observational studies and clinical trials, the results are often difficult to interpret because they are couched in unfamiliar jargon and use terms, such as indirect or direct costs, quality of life, or lost productivity. As these articles appear in the literature and clinical investigators include such measures in their own work, a review of the terms and the instruments is timely.

II. ECONOMIC EFFECT OF THE RHEUMATIC DISEASES

In the United States, the rheumatic diseases are responsible for significant expenditures for medical services (1). The rheumatic diseases are also associated with lost functional capacity, resulting in severe limitations in the ability to perform work and carry out other activities of daily living, including social and leisure activities (2). These costs are certain to rise dramatically in the next decade as the proportion of persons with chronic arthritis and musculoskeletal conditions increases in parallel with the aging population (3). It is no surprise that the increasing concern with cost containment (4) will have important implications for those involved in research or treatment of the rheumatic diseases. In today's competitive health care environment, there are many policies directed at eliminating or constraining inpatient care for treatment of arthritis and policies limiting the use of expensive therapies, diagnostic tests, or restricting access to pharmaceuticals in an effort to reduce overall health expenditures.

Rheumatoid arthritis (RA), one of the most severe rheumatic conditions, afflicts approximately 6.5 million Americans, resulting in medical expenditures and work loss estimated at up to 14 billion dollars per year (5–7). Most persons with RA experience a lifetime of remission and flare-ups requiring ongoing medical supervision. Medical management of RA involves frequent monitoring, including radiographs and blood chemistries. Fortunately, many drug and therapeutic regimens produce measurable benefits and may modify the course of RA. Aspirin and over-the-counter analgesics are generally used initially to relieve symptoms of inflammation at a relatively low cost. However, many patients cannot tolerate aspirin or do not receive substantial relief, and these patients progress to nonsteroidal anti-inflammatory drugs (NSAIDs), steroids, or disease-remittive agents, such as methotrexate or gold injections. Over the past decade, orthopedic surgeons have made dramatic advances in replacing disease-damaged joints. All these therapies have had a significant effect on the individual patient's well-being and quality of life, yet they have also increased the cost of medical care for RA. To fully understand the implications of the disease and its treatment, clinicians must understand and address the economic costs and benefits of therapy, so they can make the best-informed decisions on how to care for patients to improve their functioning.

Costs of care are generally divided into three categories: (1) *direct costs* are expenditures for medical care and related items; (2) *indirect costs* are those due to lost function in one's usual activities; and (3) *intangible costs* are those associated with loss in functioning, increased pain, and reduced life quality (8). Direct costs include expenditures for physician visits, diagnostic tests, medications, hospital stays, and surgical procedures, among a long list of items. Direct costs also include expenditures on other items such as transportation to and from the doctor, higher food bills associated with a special diet, care provided in the home, or expenditures to adapt the home environment to make functioning easier. Indirect costs are measured as lost income resulting from a reduction or cessation in work (2), and losses in social and physical functioning are measured by specific instruments developed for that purpose. Numerous studies have documented these costs, which have increased over time (9–13).

The most recent driving force behind the increasing costs of medical care is the growth of high-cost medical therapies in parallel with the growing prevalence of the disease in an aging population. These include dramatic and costly

Table 1 Annual Resource Expenditures for RA, by Study (in 1990 Dollars[a])

Category of service	Lubeck et al. (13)		Meenan et al. (9)		Jacobs et al. (16)[b]		Thompson et al. (15)	
Inpatient care	$1,826	(36%)	$3,840	(66%)	$1,162	(60%)	$,614	(46%)
Outpatient care	2,184	(43%)	1,619	(28%)	796	(40%)	2,464	(44%)
Physician visits	412	(8%)	470	(8%)	166	(8%)	897	(16%)
Medications	872	(17%)	420	(7%)	114	(6%)	796	(14%)
Diagnostic tests	666	(13%)	485	(8%)	67	(3%)	363	(6%)
Miscellaneous expenditures	1,054	(21%)	321	(6%)	—	—	555	(10%)
Total costs	$5,064		$5,780		$1,958		$5,633	

[a]The estimates of the costs of the studies were updated to 1990 dollars by using the Consumer Price Index (Social Security Administration, 1991).

[b]The study by Jacobs et al. was based on costs for treatment of RA in a Medicaid population. All others were based on fee-for-service care.

surgical procedures, such as hip replacements; medications that are effective, but costly; costs of care for side effects of therapy; and increasing costs associated with less costly laboratory testing for many persons (14). The data in Table 1 are based on studies of private and Medicaid patients completed from 1975 through 1983 (9,12,15,16). The data are adjusted to 1990 dollars for comparative purposes. As can be seen in Table 1, persons with RA have significant expenditures for outpatient care. They average more than double the number of visits to a physician each year, with an average of eight visits to various specialists and general practitioners (7,13). The costs for medical care for these RA patients, some at over 5500 dollars per year, are estimated at two to three times as high as average costs for persons of similar age and sex in the general United States population (14). Additionally, the indirect costs from lost wages are often two to three times as great as direct medical expenditures (9,17). In the following sections we will look at some recent studies on the other components of medical costs associated with RA.

III. THERAPEUTIC STRATEGIES WITH ECONOMIC EFFECT

A. Hospitalization

Hospitalization is usually the largest component of the costs of care for RA (see Table 1). Hospital admissions may account for as much as two-thirds of medical expenditures for persons with late-stage disease (9,13). A study by Wolfe et al. (18) reported detail on hospitalizations for RA. In a 1-year period, 15% of 816 RA patients whose medical records were reviewed were hospitalized a total of 160 times (1.3 admissions per hospitalized patient or 0.2 hospitalizations per patient in the study group). The mean length of hospitalization was 13.1 days at an average cost of 7845 dollars (1173 dollars per patient in study group). The average cost for total joint surgery in this group was 12,287 dollars. The most commonly performed surgical procedures included reconstructive surgery of the hand or wrist and foot, followed by total knee replacement. Medical hospitalizations were mostly for the diagnosis or treatment of articular disease. In a study of Medicaid patients, surgical hospitalizations were 7900 dollars, or more than 2.5 times the cost of medical hospitalizations (16).

The Diagnosis-Related Group (DRG) classification system is the current model for payment of patients requiring hospital care in the United States. Although DRG payment originated with Medicare, approximately one-third of the states are now using systems whereby all payers (including commercial insurers) are using DRG-based prospective hospital payment. All-payer systems are a means to deter shifting costs from one payer to another. New York is one of these states, and a study by Munoz and colleagues evaluated resources for hospitalizations for rheumatology patients (19). Mean hospital costs were 5524 dollars for all patients, with the highest cost and longest stay for Medicare and Medicaid patients. These patients tend to be older and have more procedures performed on admission. Based on an all-payer system, hospitals averaged a 1000 dollar per admission loss for RA patients. These data indicate that hospitals are not recovering all costs associated with the care of RA patients, many of whom tend to be older and more severely ill than other hospitalized patients. The consequences may be that patients are discharged sooner to home or intermediate care facilities, so that hospitals do not lose funds for treating these patients during extended stays for which the hospitals will not be fully reimbursed. As a result, physicians are faced with the need to improve cost efficiency in providing care to RA patients, while still maintaining high-quality care.

One option is to provide certain therapies on an outpatient basis, rather than in the hospital. A study by Helewa and colleagues (20), based in Canada, evaluated the cost effectiveness of inpatient care compared with intensive outpatient treatment for RA patients. Patients were randomized in this study to treatment alternatives. At baseline, the two groups were similar in 19 of 20 disease characteristics (they differed only in the number of active joints involved). Evaluation not only focused on costs associated with treatment, but also the posthospital course. Inpatient therapy resulted in improved outcomes, but at approximately 2.5 times the cost of outpatient care (an additional 3000 dollars per patient). The outcomes, reflected in improvement in five clinical measures, showed improvement as early as at 7 weeks follow-up. The researchers were not able to specify, however, what factors led to the improved benefit associated with hospitalization. In comparison with the foregoing articles, the average hospital stay for these Canadian patients was longer—16 days—than the current DRG guidelines, a trend that cannot be maintained in the United States given current reimbursement policy.

In the United States, health maintenance organizations (HMOs) are associated with lower costs of care, primarily as a result of less frequent hospitalizations and shorter hospital stays in HMOs (21). When Wolfe and colleagues compared hospitalization rates across RA patients, they found admissions were reduced by 34% in HMOs (22). These studies found no qualitative differences in the type of care provided to patients in HMOs compared with those receiving care from fee-for-service (FFS) physicians. A study by Yelin and colleagues (23) found that RA patients had the same frequency and type of hospitalizations as FFS patients and similar lengths of stay. The authors did observe a difference in the frequency of ambulatory care, with fewer outpatient visits in HMOs (23). However, patients in the study by Yelin and colleagues were cared for only by rheumatologists, no matter what the setting of care, which may explain the similarity in hospitalizations. A comparison involving HMOs that do not include rheumatologists might yield different results. Although it appears that the quality of care and the types of services provided to RA patients are similar in different delivery settings, the emphasis to continue to constrain hospital costs and reduce length of stay remains very strong, and will, no doubt, increase throughout this decade.

B. Pharmaceutical Therapy

We have seen that hospitalization costs for RA are higher than average, and that patients have more frequent visits to physicians and other health care providers, especially in certain delivery settings. Drug therapy is also quite costly. In the studies reported in Table 1, medications constituted as much as 17% of total direct expenditures. The cost of drug treatment is often misinterpreted as the cost of the drug alone. This is not so. There are significant costs associated with monitoring (laboratory tests and professional visits) and treatment of side effects, both rare side effects and frequent ones. The long duration of therapy and associated monitoring can raise even relatively low drug costs to significant expenditure levels. A study by Borg and colleagues (24) reviewed all costs for treatment associated with disease-modifying antirheumatic disease drugs (DMARDs). Patients who were prescribed parenteral gold, penicillamine, or chloroquine were followed for 12 weeks. Visits for monitoring and treatment accounted for the major expense for these patients (approximately two-thirds)— costs over and above the cost of the drug and routine physician visits.

In the study of hospitalization by Wolfe and colleagues described earlier, 42.5% of medical hospitalizations were for the treatment of side effects of therapy (18). Gastrointestinal (GI) side effects (acid peptic symptoms or GI bleeding) were the most common reasons for admission, followed by fracture related to corticosteroid therapy. Another study by Bloom and colleagues focused on the costs of treatment for side effects of NSAIDs, and found that treatment costs increased by almost 50% for arthritis patients prescribed these drugs (25). Side effects again included gastritis, abdominal pain, and GI bleeding. And in the study by Jacobs and colleagues (16), 20 out of 158 patients (13%) were hospitalized for GI side effects. These patients incurred hospital charges eight times more than persons without this problem.

Rheumatologists are well aware of the adverse effects of NSAID therapy on the GI tract, and recognize that appreciable savings in medical expenditures can result from selective therapeutic use. Patients who have a history of gastric involvement may benefit from therapy approved for use in prevention of NSAID-induced gastropathy, including the use of misoprostol, antacids, or antiulcer medications (26). These drugs allow patients who previously had to discontiue NSAIDs because of side effects to continue to obtain analgesic relief. Studies of the cost-effectiveness of these drugs have found a reduction in treatment costs, at least for the initial months of prophylaxis, when compared with no therapy (27). Cost savings are attributed to reduced hospitalizations and therapy for GI treatment of side effects, such as silent ulcers. Cost savings over a longer period are more difficult to estimate. Additional work by Edelson and colleagues (28) specifies costs associated with misoprostol for different types of users. Clearly patients who have a history of gastric involvement reap the greatest benefit from these drugs because they are expected to realize cost savings associated with reduced physician visits, laboratory tests, and hospitalizations, while still obtaining the benefits of NSAIDs. Thus, the cost of prophylaxis is offset by the medical care costs that are saved. For patients who are not likely to have serious gastric side effects, or who are not likely to experience non–life-threatening side effects, the costs of the prophylaxis are not offset by cost savings for treatment not incurred. Most reviews of drug effectiveness or benefit do not address the issue of costs or the influence of clinical diversity on cost–benefit. However, there is considerable advantage in finding the best and least expensive therapeutic match for the patient.

IV. MEASURING BENEFIT OR OUTCOME

Costs of treatment should always be viewed in relation to the health outcomes associated with care because economic methods cannot adequately measure the significance of such effects as increases or decreases in pain, psychological functioning, or the effects on family or social life. Health outcomes may be reflected in single measures, such as lives saved or reduced morbidity, or in multidimensional measures incorporating physical, social, and mental functioning, and well-being. Assessment of the quality of a health outcome is an increasingly important health care goal, especially in a disease such as RA, for which the benefit is improved functioning, rather than increased life-expectancy. If economics is to have relevance for clinical decision-making, it must also consider the effects of disease and therapy on the patient's health and well-being.

Patrick and Bergner (29) and Bell and colleagues (30) review, in two very thorough articles, the major concepts and domains associated with measurement of health outcome. Health status and quality of life are often used interchangeably to encompass the broad categories of life expectancy, health impairment, functional status, health perceptions, and opportunity. The authors detail the various definitions and measurement of positive health. A wide variety of measures are available: some cover global assessment and general populations, others are intended for specific conditions or disease groups. Some measures emphasize functioning and observable behavior, whereas others emphasize the patient's subjective evaluation of well-being, symptoms, and life quality. It is important for clinicians to gain an understanding of these instruments and of their usefulness in clinical practice.

There are numerous health assessment instruments developed specifically for rheumatology that measure various dimensions of quality of life, such as symptoms, social interactions, or physical functioning. Among these are the arthritis impact measurement scales (AIMS; 31) and the Stanford Health Assessment Questionnaire (HAQ; 32). The content of these instruments, like others, focuses on physical functioning, disease symptoms, and social well-being reported in adult populations (30). Arthritis measurement instruments have been shown to be reliable and valid and have been used empirically to measure disability and to predict mortality in RA patients, and to evaluate the benefit from therapy (30–33). These instruments have also been translated and tested in other languages and for diverse ethnic groups.

A well-known method to measure overall health quality is the quality of well-being scale (QWB). The QWB is a general (in contrast to disease-specific) measure of health status, which incorporates patient preferences concerning symptoms and activities over the previous days. The QWB combines weights of the different dimensions of health states (symptom or problem complexes, mobility, physical activity, and social activity) into a single value that ranges from death to optimal functioning. The QWB has been employed in RA and compared with the AIMS, and significant association was found for the overall QWB scores with the component measures of the AIMS (34).

As indicated in Table 2, the QWB does not include other important dimensions of health status, including pain and mental health. Another important component of health status that is not covered in any of the questionnaires is fatigue. An index tapping energy–fatigue was developed for the Rand Medical Outcomes Study (MOS), an observational study of patient outcomes in different practice settings (35). This scale, along with others tapping mental health and physical functioning, has been incorporated in analyses of general populations,

Table 2 Health-Related Quality-of-Life Measure

Instrument characteristics	Instrument			
	AIMS (31)	HAQ (32)	QWB (34)	JRA (28)
Physical functioning				
Mobility	X	X	X	X
Self-care	X	X	X	X
Pain	X	X		
Role functioning				
Role limitations	X	X	X	
Social functioning	X	X		
Leisure activities	X	X		
Mental health	X	X		
Symptomatology	X	X	X	
Patient utility measures			X	

and chronic disease populations (36,37). These studies indicate that fatigue is prominent in chronic illness, and is associated with increased morbidity, often leading to work loss.

Few economists would dispute the benefit of measuring health status, because important aspects of the burden of disease are tapped. The information obtained from studies that include health assessment as a component, whether the instruments are disease-specific or generic, may be useful in evaluating the clinical effect of drug therapy or toxicity, observing specific aspects of functioning or well-being associated with the progression of RA, or in predicting utilization of health care resources for these patients. Additionally, concerns of patient populations who are not normally studied may be studied, and important effects of the disease on that population may become apparent.

One of the more recent health outcomes scales was developed by Lovell et al. (38) for juvenile rheumatoid arthritis (JRA). As mentioned by Patrick et al. (29), assessment of health outcome in pediatric and adolescent patients has been lacking, and is extremely important. Measurement scales developed for adult populations have poor reliability when applied to younger patients. Or, adult scales must be altered or administered in more expensive or time-consuming formats when applied to juveniles. Lovell's JRA scale takes approximately 10 mins to complete and can be administered in a clinic setting. The scale consists of ten items covering normal daily function including: dressing, eating, getting in and out of bed, standing, walking, and climbing. Individual items are scored on a 0–2 scale and then summed for an overall scale, ranging from 0–20. This research is important for our ability to incorporate outcome assessment in clinical practice and research in JRA.

A selected listing of health outcome measures is provided in Table 2, indicating the dimensions measured. The instruments described are short multi-item measures that have demonstrated reliability and validity in the rheumatic diseases and are short enough that they can be completed at the time of a clinic visit. Clinicians interested in conducting similar research will find the discussion of the instruments in the articles referenced here a very useful starting point.

V. MEASURING THE EFFECT OF ALTERNATIVE PATIENT CARE

Outcome assessment allows us to measure the effect of drug therapy and surgical intervention on costs of care and patient quality of life. Outcome studies and cost studies are growing in number in rheumatology, but there has been less attention toward investigating the effect of nonpharmacological and nonsurgical approaches to the management of arthritis. However, successful intervention of behaviors that decrease pain or functional limitations associated with arthritis could convey multiple health benefits and significant economic savings. The value of research investigating the effect of health education is clear.

Research evaluating health education programs developed at Stanford University (the arthritis self-management course) by Holman and Lorig (39) indicates that patients who have completed the program respond by improving their health behaviors, such as initiating regular exercise, resulting in improved health status, such as decreases in pain and functional disability, as measured by some of the standard outcome scales described in the foregoing. Furthermore, Holman and colleagues showed that the arthritis self-management course resulted in reduced health care use for participants, and that these reductions were maintained for as long as 4 years after the patient's training. Physician visits were reduced by two per year for RA patients and approximately one per year for osteoarthritis patients. These reduced visits result in savings over the 4-year period (for 1% of the estimated number of patients nationally) of 2.9 million dollars for RA and 14.5 million dollars for osteoarthritis patients. Clearly this is a substantial health benefit. Health education has a potentially significant role as a component of cost-effective and quality health services delivered by rheumatologists.

The benefit of patient education was publicly acknowledged at a conference organized by the National Arthritis Advisory Board. This meeting focused on the need for adequate financial support for arthritis patient-education programs. As described by Winfield (40), there is a forceful case for the health benefits and cost-effectiveness of education programs. However, growth of these programs is limited by the lack of capacity to obtain reimbursement. Third-party insurers generally exclude reimbursement for patient education and other preventive services. However, currently, when public policy is directed at multiple efforts toward controlling health care costs, a strong case can be made that health education is cost-effective and should be included as part of a health benefits package. Such programs will also help clinicians improve the quality of care they provide to patients, while helping control their own expenditures.

Similarly, the data reported in the foregoing for cost studies and health outcomes studies are obtained from patient self-report. Questionnaires of this type provide valuable information to assess, monitor, and predict morbidity, work disability, health services use, and mortality. Pincus and colleagues found that self-reported patient information was similar to laboratory and radiographic information in terms of providing information on management of the disease (41). However, no mechanism exists for reimbursing patients for completing these often time-consuming questionnaires. Again, this is another area for which patient care might be improved at significant cost savings.

VI. SUMMARY

Medical care in the United States is faced with a continuing and growing expenditure crisis, which has, in turn, had an influence on shaping policy and research in medicine. Current public policy attempts to contain costs by limiting patient access to certain services, and by requiring that patients and physicians bear a greater portion of costs. Although the rheumatological diseases may be treated primarily in ambulatory care settings, the high prevalence of this disease, the aging of patients, and the long duration of costly management make costs of treatment an important consideration for clinicians. Rheumatologists must become more cognizant of the cost implications of therapy and potential alternatives, while still ensuring the quality of care provided through measurement of patient outcome. This is best done by taking a proactive approach to research on the costs and outcomes of health care.

REFERENCES

1. Felts W, Yelin E. The economic impact of the rheumatic diseases in the United States. J Rheumatol 1989; 16:867–884.
2. Lubeck DP, Yelin EH. A question of value: measuring the impact of chronic disease. Milbank Q 1988; 66:444–464.
3. Waldo D, Lazenky H. Demographic characteristics and health care use and expenditures by the aged in the U.S. 1977–1984. Health Care Financing Rev. 1984; 6:1–29.
4. Ginzberg E. Sounding board: a hard look at cost-containment. N Engl J Med 1987; 316:1151–1154.
5. US Dept. of Health and Human Services. How to cope with arthritis. NIH Publication No. 82–1092). Washington DC: US Gov't Printing Office, 1981.
6. US Dept. of Health and Human Services. Medicine for laymen: arthritis. NIH Publication No. 83-1945. Washington, DC: US Gov't Printing Office, 1982.
7. Yelin EH, Felts WR. A summary of the impact of musculoskeletal conditions in the United States. Arthritis Rheum 1990; 33:750–755.
8. Hall J, Mooney G. What every doctor should know about economics. Part 1. The benefits of costing. Med J Aust 1990; 152:29–31.
9. Meenan RF, Yelin EH, Henke CJ, Curtis DL, Epstein WV. The costs of rheumatoid arthritis: a patient-oriented study of chronic disease costs. Arthritis Rheum 1978; 21:827–833.
10. Liang MH, Larson M, Thompson M, et al. Costs and outcomes in rheumatoid arthritis and osteoarthritis. Arthritis Rheum 1984; 27:522–529.
11. Meenan RF, Yelin EH, Nevitt M, et al. The impact of chronic disease. Arthritis Rheum 1981; 24:544–549.
12. Kramer JS, Yelin EH, Epstein WV. Social and economic impacts of four musculoskeletal conditions. Arthritis Rheum 1983; 26:901–907.
13. Lubeck DP, Spitz PW, Fries JF, Wolfe F, Mitchell DM, Roth SH. A multicenter study of annual health service utilization and costs in rheumatoid arthritis. Arthritis Rheum 1986; 29:488–493.
14. Epstein WV. Economics and arthritis [editorial]. Arthritis Rheum 1990; 33:746–749.
15. Thompson MS, Read JL, Hutchings HC, Paterson M, Harris ED. The cost effectiveness of auranofin: results of a randomized clinical trial. J Rheumatol 1988; 15:35–42.
16. Jacobs J, Keyserling JA, Britton M, Morgan GJ Jr, Wilkenfeld J, Hutchings HC. The total cost of care and the use of pharmaceuticals in the management of rheumatoid arthritis: the Medi-Cal program. J Clin Epidemiol 1988; 41:215–223.

17. Lubeck DP, Spitz P, Fries J. Measurement of personal costs in rheumatoid arthritis. Arthritis Rheum 25 (suppl) 1982; E64.

18. Wolfe F, Kleinheksel SM, Spitz PW, Lubeck DP, Fries JF, Young DY, Mitchell D, Roth S. A multicenter study of hospitalization in rheumatoid arthritis. Frequency, medical–surgical admissions, and charges. Arthritis Rheum 1986; 29:614–619.

19. Munoz E, Goldstein J, Benacquista T, Mulloy K, Wise L. Health care financing policy for hospitalized rheumatology patients. J Rheumatol 1989; 16:885–889.

20. Helewa A, Bombardier C, Goldsmith CH, Menchions B, Smythe HA. Cost-effectiveness of inpatient and intensive outpatient treatment of rheumatoid arthritis. A randomized, controlled trial. Arthritis Rhcum 1989; 32:1505–1514.

21. Manning WG, Leibowitz A, Goldberg GA, Rogers WH, Newhouse JP. A controlled trial of the effect of a prepaid group practice on use of services. N Engl J Med 1984; 310:1505–1510.

22. Wolfe F, Kleinheksel SM, Spitz PW, Lubeck DP, Fries JF, Young DY, Mitchell DM, Roth SH. A multicenter study of hospitalization in rheumatoid arthritis: effect of health care system, severity, and regional difference. J Rheumatol 1986; 13:277–284.

23. Yelin EH, Henke CJ, Kramer JS, Nevitt MC, Shearn M, Epstein WV. A comparison of the treatment of rheumatoid arthritis in health maintenance organizations and fee-for-service practices. N Engl J Med 1985; 312:962–967.

24. Borg G, Allander E, Goobar JE. Disease-modifying anti-rheumatic drug therapy. An expensive therapy despite inexpensive drugs. Scand J Rheumatol 1990; 19:115–121.

25. Bloom BS. Risk and cost of gastrointestinal side effects associated with nonsteroidal anti-inflammatory drugs. Arch Intern Med 1989; 149:1019–1022.

26. Garris RE, Kirkwood CF. Misoprostol: a prostaglandin E_1 analogue. Clin Pharm 1989; 8:627–644.

27. Hillman AL, Bloom BS. Economic effects of prophylactic use of misoprostol to prevent gastric ulcer in patients taking nonsteroidal anti-inflammatory drugs. Arch Intern Med 1989; 149:2061–2065.

28. Edelson JT, Tosteson ANA, Sax P. Cost-effectiveness of misoprostol for prophylaxis against nonsteroidal anti-inflammatory drug-induced gastrointestinal tract bleeding. JAMA 1990; 264:41–47.

29. Patrick DL, Bergner M. Measurement of health status in the 1990s. Annu Rev Public Health 1990; 11:165–183.

30. Bell MJ, Bombardier C, Tugwell P. Measurement of functional status, quality of life, and utility in rheumatoid arthritis. Arthritis Rheum 1990; 33:591–601.

31. Meenan RF, Yelin EH, Nevitt M. The impact of chronic disease. Arthritis Rheum 1984; 24:544–549.

32. Fries JF, Spitz P, Kraines RG, Holman HR. Measurement of patient outcome in arthritis. Arthritis Rheum 1980; 23:137–145.

33. Anderson JJ, Firschein HE, Meenan RF. Sensitivity of a health status measure to short-term clinical changes in arthritis. Arthritis Rheum 1989; 32:844–850.

34. Kaplan RM, Anderson JP, Wu AW, Mathews WC, Kozin F, Orenstein D. The quality of well-being scale: application in AIDS, cystic fibrosis, and arthritis. Med Care 1989; 27:S27–S43.

35. Stewart AL, Hays RD, Ware JE Jr. The MOS short-form general health survey. Reliability and validity in a patient population. Med Care 1988; 26:724–735.

36. Stewart AL, Greenfield S, Hays RD, et al. Functional status and well-being of patients with chronic conditions. Results from the medical outcomes study. JAMA 1989; 262:907–913.

37. Wu AW, Rubin HR, Mathews WC, et al. A health status questionnaire using 30 items from the medical outcomes study: preliminary validation in persons with early HIV infection. Med Care 1991; 29:786–798.

38. Lovell DJ, Howe S, Shear E, Hartner S, McGirr G, Schulte M, Levinson J. Development of a disability measurement tool for juvenile rheumatoid arthritis. The juvenile arthritis functional assessment scale. Arthritis Rheum 1989; 32:1390–1395.

39. Holman H, Mazonson P, Lorig K. Health education for self-management has significant early and sustained benefits in chronic arthritis. Trans Assoc Am Physicians 1989; CII:204–208.

40. Winfield JB, the ACR/AHPA/AF/NAAB task force on arthritis patient education. Arthritis patient education. Efficacy, implementation, and financing. Arthritis Rheum 1989; 32:1330–1333.

41. Pincus T, Callahan LF, Brooks RH, et al. Self-report questionnaire scores in rheumatoid arthritis compared with traditional physical, radiographic, and laboratory measures. Ann Intern Med 1989; 110:259–266.

11

Work Disability and Rheumatoid Arthritis

Edward H. Yelin

The Rosalind Russell Arthritis Center and Institute for Health Policy Studies
University of California
San Francisco, California

I. INTRODUCTION

Any clinician treating substantial numbers of persons with rheumatoid arthritis knows that the prevalence of work disability among such persons may be high, if only because he or she has completed so many forms verifying the extent of the condition as part of the process by which persons with this condition apply for benefits. However, the official work disability rate for persons with RA, represented by claims on the Social Security Disability Insurance Program and private disability policies, is dramatically lower than the actual work disability rate, represented by all those who meet the medical criteria for these programs, but who do not have the requisite work history to qualify. Some of these persons claim other entitlements, such as Supplemental Security Income benefits, but many others are not aware of them or do not qualify for them because their spouses make too much money.

In this article, I will review the definitions of disability, present data on the prevalence of this problem, describe models of its causation, and present some of the options for public policy. The data on the prevalence of work disability indicate the proportion of all persons with the condition who have stopped working and the length of time between onset of disease and work disability. The studies of the causes of work disability allow the clinician and persons with RA to predict the probability of work loss, given a matrix of medical and social characteristics of these persons and the characteristics of their jobs, and can help in devising a strategy to reduce the chance that work loss will occur.

Because of the relatively low overall prevalence of RA, there are few large, community-based studies of work disability among persons with this condition, and none that tie their work prognosis to changes in the economy at large. Thus, in the final section of this paper, I review the evidence from studies of work disability among persons with all forms of chronic disease, in general, and all forms of musculoskeletal disease, in particular, that show how changes in the economy affect persons with RA.

II. DEFINITIONS OF WORK DISABILITY

In the research literature, *work disability* is variously defined as a limitation in the capacity to work (1), by the receipt of disability benefits, or as being out of the labor force after onset of the condition (2). No definition of work disability provides an objective measure of the effect of RA on work. Rheumatoid arthritis affects self-reported work capacity in as many as 90% of the persons with this condition (1), but most persons with RA persevere, at least for several years, before they actually stop working. In turn, only a small fraction of all those who leave work before the normal age of retirement collect disability benefits (3). Accordingly, most work disability researchers concur that the best way to measure this phenomenon is to count those who have the condition, are of working ages, and are out of the labor force. In so enumerating persons with RA experiencing work disability, the researcher does not have to trust their judgment about whether the RA is a justifiable cause for being out of the labor force. However, to rely on the work capacity definition, one would have to use such an assessment, and one would probably provide too liberal an estimate of work disability. To rely on the disability benefit criterion, one would eliminate all those out of the labor force after onset of RA, but who do not qualify for the benefits for reasons having nothing to do with the RA itself.

III. IMPORTANCE OF WORK DISABILITY BECAUSE OF RHEUMATOID ARTHRITIS

Three clinical studies of the costs of rheumatoid arthritis have been conducted, all concurring that the great majority of the costs of the condition are due to wage losses owing to morbidity, rather than to direct medical care expenditures (4–6). Table 1 reviews the three studies, updating their results by stating costs in 1990 terms. The similarity of the results are remarkable, given the dramatically different populations studied and the method of analysis. Meenan et al. (4) included only those with severe RA in their study, and found that three-quarters of the annual cost of RA was due to wage losses, labeled ''indirect costs'' in the table. Liang et al. (5) included persons with RA of a wider range of severities in their study, and found that among such persons, although overall costs were

Table 1 Economic Costs of RA, by Study (in 1990 Dollars)

Study[a] (Ref.)	Direct costs	Indirect costs	Total
Meenan et al. (4)	5,767 (25%)	16,936 (75%)	22,703 (100%)
Liang et al. (5)	1,776 (15%)	10,230 (85%)	12,006 (100%)
Stone (6)	10,938 (18%)	50,764 (82%)	61,702 (100%)

[a]The estimates of the costs of the three studies were updated to 1990 dollars by using the Consumer Price Index (Social Security Administration, 1991). The Meenan et al. and Liang et al., studies used the prevalence method of estimating costs; the Stone study used the incidence method.
Source: Adapted from Ref. 28.

lower, the wage loss portion of the costs was higher. These two studies enumerated all the costs accruing to all cases of RA prevalent in a year. Stone (6) estimated the lifetime costs accruing only to those cases of RA incident in a year, but found that a similarly high proportion (82%) of all the costs of RA were due to wage losses.

IV. INCIDENCE AND PREVALENCE OF WORK DISABILITY BECAUSE OF RHEUMATOID ARTHRITIS

As is often found in studies of the effect of illness, studies conducted in clinical samples are much more specific to the illness in question, including discrete measures designed to assure the reliability of the diagnosis and the degree of severity, but these studies may not be representative of the population of persons with the condition in the surrounding area, let alone in the nation as a whole. In contrast, studies conducted in random samples of the population at large generally rely on self-report of the diagnosis and extent of symptoms, although they are more representative. Both kinds of data have been used to estimate the prevalence of work disability owing to RA (Table 2). In the three studies that used clinical samples (7–9), the authors estimate that between 51 and 59% of the persons with a work history before the onset of RA had stopped working altogether by the time the study was conducted, an average of about a decade later. The most recent of these studies (9) also reported the proportion who made changes in their work situation before leaving work. Of the 51% who stopped working altogether, roughly a tenth changed jobs, hours of work, occupation, or work rules; the remainder made no changes before stopping work. Of the 49% who continued to work, about a quarter made significant changes in work characteristics as a way of preventing work disability.

This same study used life table methods to trace the work history of the cohort of persons with RA from the date of onset until either employment ended or the study was completed. From these data, it was determined that approximately 10% of persons with RA who were employed before onset stopped working within a year after diagnosis. The proportion leaving work increased to

Table 2 Work Disability Rate Among Persons with RA,
by Study Type

Study (Ref.)	Type of sample	Work disability rate (%)
Yelin et al. (7)	Clinical	59
Reisine et al. (8)	Clinical	57
Yelin et al. (9)	Clinical	51
Pincus et al. (10)	Community	72

Source: Ref. 28.

almost 20% within 2 years of onset, to more than 30% within 5 years, to half within 10 years, and to 90% within 30. The incidence of work loss was relatively constant in each of the first 10 years after onset, never rising above 10% per year or falling below 5% per year.

Thus, the cross-sectional studies indicate that about half of working-aged persons with RA who had worked before onset are out of the labor force at any one time. The one longitudinal study indicates that the prevalence of work disability continues to increase until retirement age, sparing only about 10% of persons with RA from job loss.

As high as these rates would appear to be, the one systematic study using a national, probability sample of adults living in the community found even higher rates of work disability (10). Since this study did not verify the respondents' reports of a diagnosis of RA, the authors enumerated only persons who both reported that a physician had specifically told them they had RA and whose symptom reports of symmetric joint involvement were unambiguously consistent with a diagnosis of RA. In this study, 60% of the persons so designated as meeting these clinical criteria for RA were not working at the time of the survey. However, the authors did not stratify the sample according to the respondents' work histories. Presumably, some of these individuals had never been employed. Thus, the prevalence estimates from this study may not be too different from those made from the clinically based samples. However, whether the prevalence of work disability among persons with RA is about half or about three-quarters, it is high relative to almost all other chronic conditions (11).

V. CAUSES OF WORK DISABILITY

The high prevalence of work disability among persons with RA has made this condition a laboratory for studies of the causes of work loss after onset of illness. It was once considered a waste of time to conduct such studies. After all, whether someone with a chronic disease stops working after onset will necessarily depend on the severity of the underlying pathological disorder and symptoms, as well

as the resulting impairment. Indeed, in every study of the causes of work disability, such medical factors are associated with work outcome. However, the correlations between measures of disease and work status are relatively weak,
suggesting that much more than severity of disease and impairment determines
whether someone with RA will stop working.

Social scientists studying work disability among persons with a wide range
of conditions hypothesized that, medical severity held constant, the individual's
human capital, his or her will to work, and the demand for labor would combine
to determine whether work loss resulted after onset of illness (12). Human
capital includes the individual's education (more education presumably gives the
individual entree to less physically demanding work), income (persons with
higher incomes generally have more generous disability benefits), and particular
skills (employers might accommodate those with uncommon skills). Commitment to work would matter in the individual's decision on whether to persevere
through the pain of arthritis or would choose to apply for disability benefits (13).
A slack demand for labor would affect the work disability rate because employers
generally would prefer those without disabilities when given a choice among
workers.

These social science models of work disability derived from two principal
schools of economic thought: the first holding that an individual's ability to stave
off bad things generally (disability among them) was a function of their resources
(12), the other that rising social welfare payments (disability benefit programs
among them) were "enticing" individuals who could work to drop out of the
labor force (15).

Neither school developed a discrete set of models based on the experience
of persons trying to cope with chronic disease at the work place, but instead,
applied general models of economic behavior to the disability context. Discussion
with persons with rheumatoid arthritis indicates that their decisions about work
turn on very concrete interactions between the manifestations of their illness and
the nature of their jobs. In particular, many report having trouble interweaving
the periods of exacerbation and remission into a highly structured work schedule.
Interestingly, few reported that the brute force requirements of their jobs were
the major impediment to continued employment, primarily because most did not
have very physically demanding jobs and, in fact, had not had them in the past.

As a result of these discussions, I hypothesized that the time requirements
of jobs would have the strongest force on whether work loss developed after
onset of RA (16). In a cross-sectional study, workers who reported flexible jobs
before onset of the RA had dramatically lower work disability rates as of the
study year (7). In particular, workers who could control the time of arrival,
breaks, and departure, and those controlling the pace of work activities were less
likely to report having stopped work altogether. These social characteristics of
jobs had far stronger associations with work outcomes than measures of the

severity and impairment of the RA or overall health status, measures of the individual's human capital and commitment to work, the physical demands of jobs, or the overall demand for labor.

The findings from this cross-sectional study have since been corroborated in another cross-sectional one (8), and by a longitudinal study in which the work characteristics were measured before the change in employment status, reducing the chance that those reporting work disability were merely attributing it after the fact to the characteristics of jobs (9).

Interestingly, one does not have to rise very high in a work organization to obtain the kind of autonomy that reduces the probability of work disability, persons with supervisorial responsibilities having only slightly greater flexibility in work activities than those at the bottom of work hierarchies (16). Moreover, only the most tangible aspects of maintaining control over work activities matters. Although being able to decide when to visit one's physician, without first asking permission of a supervisor, or how to set the pace of work does matter, determining others' schedules or setting investment priorities for the firm, both of which are measures of having supreme autonomy on the job according to organizational theory (17), do not matter in determining the work disability rate (16).

Since this initial research on the causes of work disability among persons with RA was conducted, the models developed for RA have been validated for other discrete chronic conditions, including cancer (18), asthma (19), human immunodeficiency virus (HIV)-related illnesses (20), and cardiovascular disease (21), and for chronic conditions as a whole (22). That flexibility in work should affect the work disability rate in other conditions should not be surprising, since all chronic conditions involve periods of exacerbation and remission, and all have symptoms that vary within a day and among the seasons of the year.

The findings of this research concerning the social characteristics of jobs should not be misconstrued. Persons with severe RA do have a poorer work prognosis. Likewise, those with little education and scant job skills are much more likely to stop working. Finally, persons with physically demanding jobs are less likely to keep working, especially when discrete impairments that result from the RA interact with discrete physical requirements of jobs. For example, persons with impairments in their fingers whose jobs require manual dexterity are quite likely to stop working. However, all these characteristics of the persons with RA are less important as determinants of work disability status than the ability to control the time requirements of jobs. Moreover, a matrix of "good" job characteristics can make a profound difference on the probability of work disability. All else equal, the probability of work loss after onset of RA decreases by about 5% for each item of an eight-item scale measuring the flexibility of the work environment (data not published).

VI. IMPLICATIONS FOR CLINICAL AND PUBLIC POLICY

The finding that the flexibility of the work environment affects the work disability rate among persons with RA has wide-ranging implications for the clinician and for public policy. First, it enables the clinician to provide the person with RA a much more precise estimate of the risk of work loss than could be made on the basis of pathophysiological, functional, and social characteristics alone. Second, it suggests a counseling strategy relative to work. Initially, persons with RA should be encouraged to have open discussions with their employers about the kinds of changes in work rules that would reduce their risk of work loss. Such changes are consistent with the expectations placed on employers to accommodate the employment needs of all persons with disabilities under the recently enacted Americans with Disabilities Act of 1990 (23). The clinician can assist in these negotiations, providing wary employers with information about the expected productivity of the person with RA when given flexible conditions and by providing the person with RA with some concrete suggestions on what might improve their ability to maintain employment. Studies of the costs of accommodating the physical needs of persons with disabilities indicate that the median such accommodation costs less than 400 dollars, and the 90th percentile less than 1000 dollars (24). Accommodating the need for flexible work costs much less than changing the physical environment, a point that should be emphasized in discussions among the clinician, person with RA, and employer.

Clinicians must not blindly suggest that the person with RA initiate such discussions with employers, however, without first ascertaining that a particular workplace is likely to try to accommodate his or her special needs. Should it be determined that such an accommodation is unlikely to be forthcoming and that the requirements of the job do not mesh well with the nature of the RA, the clinician might refer the person with RA for occupational therapy and, perhaps, rehabilitation and training, while suggesting that the person with RA try to initiate a change in job early in the course of illness. Early changes reduce the probability of work loss later, both because employers are less likely to lay off long-term workers and because experience on the job enables the person with RA to develop strategies to compensate for the loss of physical function.

Public policy can also facilitate the development of work rules conducive to the maintenance of employment. The Americans with Disabilities Act does this at the national level by requiring job accommodation. Local governments can do their part, however, by adopting model work rules of their own, thereby demonstrating the benefits of such rules to other employers, and by staffing rehabilitation agencies with professionals who understand the job requirements of persons with RA and similar chronic conditions.

VII.   TRENDS IN WORK DISABILITY

Because RA is a *fairly* uncommon condition, affecting about 1% of adults, and because it is hard to identify in studies using self-report methods, no trend data on work disability owing to this condition are available. Instead, we are forced to rely on information about the prevalence of work disability among persons with all kinds of musculoskeletal conditions and assume (perhaps incorrectly) that the trends apply to those with RA.

Table 3 summarizes trends in labor force participation among persons with all forms of musculoskeletal conditions and among all working-aged adults in the United States for the period 1970 through 1987; reference 25 includes more detailed information for women and men, and for young and old workers. Among all persons with musculoskeletal conditions, labor force participation rates fell by 12% from 1970 to 1987. Labor force participation rates fell slightly among such persons without activity limitations, but fell even more steeply—by 16.4%—among those with activity limitations. Thus, persons with musculoskeletal conditions experienced much less access to work as the years unfolded, which is another way of stating that their work disability rates were on the rise.

In contrast, the labor force participation rate among all working-aged persons was expanding rapidly between 1970 and 1987, by 7.2% in relative terms, in the process accommodating the baby boom generation and a much larger proportion of women. This 7.2% expansion is net of an 8.3% gain among all working-aged adults without activity limitations and a slight decline—3.9%—among such persons with limitations. The latter decline was less than a quarter as large as that experienced by persons with musculoskeletal conditions and activity limitation. Thus, persons with musculoskeletal conditions fared much more poorly in the labor market than other working-aged adults, and this is true regardless of whether or not such persons had activity limitation. In addition, persons with musculoskeletal conditions fared much more poorly than they did at the beginning of the period, despite the overall growth occurring in the proportion of working-aged adults in the labor force.

Table 3   Labor Force Participation Rate Among Persons with Musculoskeletal Conditions and Among All Working-Aged Persons, US, 1970–1987

Group	Total (%)	Activity limitations (%)	Without activity limitations (%)
All working-aged persons with musculoskeletal conditions	− 12.0	− 16.4	− 1.3
All working-aged persons	−7.2	− 3.9	8.3

Source: Author's analysis of 1970–1987 National Health Interview Survey.

These data, although not specific to rheumatoid arthritis, suggest that if the work disability rate was increasing among those with musculoskeletal conditions of lower average severity, the rate among those with RA was probably increasing as well. At the very least, these findings indicate that the studies of work disability among persons with RA conducted a decade ago may not apply to those with RA of more recent onset.

VIII. CAUSE OF GROWTH IN WORK DISABILITY

Although no studies prove that the work disability rate among persons with RA is increasing, one study was recently completed to explain the overall rise in work disability rates, regardless of condition (26). That study derived from the finding that the overall rise in work disability rates was the sum of two quite distinct processes: a dramatic increase among older men and a slight decrease among younger women. This, in turn, suggested the hypothesis that the older men with disabilities were exiting from one set of industries and the younger women with disabilities were entering another. Since the major industry shedding workers was manufacturing, and the major industry hiring them was services, I analyzed the change in the proportion of these two industries's workers with disabilities over the years of the study.

Indeed, service industry, which needed workers, hired increasing proportions of workers with disabilities, whereas manufacturing, which was retrenching, hired decreasing proportions of them. In a separate analysis, I found that 96% of the variance in the work disability rate over time could be explained by the change in an industry's share of all employment. This means that persons with disabilities were one of the principal ways that the shift from a manufacturing to a services economy was accommodated. Since more discrete data on how this overall dynamic affected persons with discrete diseases was unavailable in the database analyzed, one can only speculate based on the worsening employment picture among persons with musculoskeletal conditions generally that such persons were disproportionately displaced from manufacturing industry in decline.

IX. SUMMARY

Much is known about the prevalence and causes of work disability among persons with rheumatoid arthritis. Specifically, we know that

1. Among persons with RA working before onset of the RA, between 50 and 60% stop working within a decade of onset.
2. Among such persons, 10% leave work within the first year of disease, and all but 10% leave work before the normal age of retirement.
3. Among such persons who leave work, all but a tenth do so without having made changes in the specific job, tasks, work rules, or occupation.

4. Among such persons who continue working, however, roughly a quarter made changes in their work situation.

5. Among all working-aged persons with RA, regardless of prior work history, about 60% are not in the labor force at any one time.

6. Medical severity and degree of impairment affect whether disability results after onset of RA (27).

7. The social characteristics of jobs—flexibility in the pacing and scheduling of work activities—are the strongest and most consistent set of risk factors for work disability among persons with RA.

We have also some evidence from musculoskeletal conditions generally that work disability rates are rising, although none of this evidence is specific for RA.

The clinician treating persons with RA can help them understand the work prognosis of this condition in much the same way that he or she may help them understand the probability that they will run a benign or severe course of the disease or experience a favorable or poor outcome of surgery. In turn, the astute clinician will assist such persons in determining whether their specific jobs are conducive to the maintenance of employment, and then help them negotiate the kinds of work rules that will improve the chances of a good work outcome.

ACKNOWLEDGMENT

This work was supported by the Milbank Memorial Fund, New York, New York, Multipurpose Arthritis Center Grant AM-20684, and The Rosalind Russell Arthritis Center.

REFERENCES

1. La Plante M. Data on disability from the National Health Interview Survey, 1983–1985. Report to: National Institute on Disability and Rehabilitation Research, Washington, DC, 1988.

2. Yelin E. Displaced concern: the social context of the work disability problem. Milbank Q 1989; 67 (suppl 2):114–165.

3. Chirikos T. Accounting for the historical rise in work-disability prevalence. Milbank Q 1986; 64:271–301.

4. Meenan R, Yelin E, Henke C, Curtis D, Epstein W. The costs of rheumatoid arthritis: a patient-oriented study of chronic disease costs. Arthritis Rheum 1978; 21:827–833.

5. Liang M, Larson M, Thompson M, et al. Cost and outcomes in rheumatoid and osteoarthritis. Arthritis Rheum 1984; 27:522–529.

6. Stone C. The lifetime costs of rheumatoid arthritis. J Rheumatol 1984; 11:819–827.

7. Yelin E, Meenan R, Nevitt M, Epstein W. Work disability in rheumatoid arthritis: effects of disease, social, and work factors. Ann Intern Med 1980; 93:551–556.

8. Reisine S, Grady K, Goodenow C, Fifield J. Work disability among women with rheumatoid arthritis: the relative importance of disease, social, work and family factors. Arthritis Rheum 1989; 32:539–543.

9. Yelin E, Henke C, Epstein W. The work dynamics of the person with rheumatoid arthritis. Arthritis Rheum 1987; 30:507–512.

10. Pincus T, Mitchell J, Burkhauser R. Substantial work disability and earnings losses in individuals less than 65 with osteoarthritis: comparisons with rheumatoid arthritis. J Clin Epidemiol 1989; 42:449–457.

11. Yelin E. Arthritis: the cumulative impact of a common chronic condition. Arthritis Rheum (in press).

12. Berkowitz M, Johnson W, Murphy E. Public policy toward disability. New York: Praeger, 1976.

13. Parsons D. The decline of male labor-force participation. J Polit Econ 1980; 88:117–134.

14. Levitan S, Taggart R. Jobs for the disabled. Baltimore: Johns Hopkins Press, 1977.

15. Feldstein M. Social Security and private capital accumulation: international evidence in an extended life-cycle model. Harvard Institute of Economic Research Paper (unpublished).

16. Yelin E, Nevitt M, Epstein W. Toward an epidemiology of work disability. Milbank Memorial Fund Q Health Soc 1980; 58:386–415.

17. Wright E, Martin B. The transformation of the American class structure, 1960–1980. Am J Sociol 1987; 93:1–29.

18. Greenwald H, Dirks S, Borgatta E, et al. Work disability among cancer patients. Soc Sci Med 1989; 29:0.

19. Blanc P, Yelin E. Asthma severity as a predictor of work disability among persons with asthma. Am Rev Respir Dis 1991; 143:A269.

20. Yelin E, Greenblatt R, Hollander H, et al. The impact of HIV-related illness on employment. Am J Public Health 1991; 81:79–84.

21. Murphy L. Job dimensions associated with severe disability due to cardiovascular disease. J Clin Epidemiol 1991; 44:155–166.

22. Yelin E, Henke C, Epstein W. Work disability among persons with musculoskeletal conditions. Arthritis Rheum 1986; 29:1322–1333.

23. West J. The social and policy context of the act. In: West J, ed. The Americans with Disabilities Act: from policy to practice. New York: Milbank Fund, 1991.

24. Berkeley Planning Associates. A study of accommodations provided to handicapped employees by federal contractors. Oakland, CA: Berkeley Planning Associates, 1982.

25. Yelin E, Katz P. Laborforce participation among persons with musculoskeletal conditions, 1970–1987: national estimates derived from a series of cross-sections. Arthritis Rheum 1991; 34:1361–1370.

26. Yelin E. Disability and the displaced worker. New Brunswick, NJ: Rutgers University Press, 1992.

27. Callahan L, Bloch D, Pincus T. Identification of work disability in rheumatoid arthritis: physical, radiographic, and laboratory variables do not add explanatory power to demographic and functional variables. J Clin Epidemiol 1992; 45:127–138.

28. Felts, Yelin E. 1989.

12

Psychological Dimensions of Rheumatoid Arthritis

Laurence A. Bradley

University of Alabama at Birmingham
Birmingham, Alabama

I. INTRODUCTION

The past 20 years have been distinguished by increasing recognition of the importance of the psychological dimensions of rheumatoid arthritis (RA) (1), as it now is generally accepted that psychosocial factors are associated with disease outcomes, such as pain, functional ability, and mortality (2). There also is evidence of relations among environmental and psychological factors and immune system responses (3,4).

Progress in understanding the psychological dimensions of RA has been enhanced by resolution of important conceptual and methodological problems in early research efforts, such as the use of retrospective research methods and excessive attention to negative personality characteristics among patients (5). Nevertheless, we are merely beginning to identify the complex interactions that exist among the environment, psychological status, biological processes, and clinical outcomes.

This chapter will document our current progress in this area and describe important issues for future research. The first section of the chapter examines several psychological factors that reflect primarily the effect of RA on patients' well-being and health status. These factors include depression and anxiety, pain perceptions and behavior, stress, and social relations. The next section describes cognitive and behavioral factors that influence patients' adjustment to RA, including perceptions of helplessness, control, and self-efficacy, as well as patients' adherence with their medical regimens and strategies for coping with their illnesses. Finally, the chapter concludes with a discussion of some psychological interventions used to help patients improve their health status, with emphasis on patients' abilities to maintain improvement after psychological treatment is terminated.

II. PSYCHOLOGICAL EFFECTS OF RHEUMATOID ARTHRITIS

A. Depression and Anxiety

Early studies of the emotional reactions associated with RA typically have evaluated patients with objective, standardized measures, such as the Minnesota Multiphasic Personality Inventory (MMPI; 6), Beck Depression Inventory (BDI; 7), Center for Epidemiologic Studies-Depression scale (CES-D; 8), the anxiety and depression subscales of the Arthritis Impact Measurement Scales (AIMS; 9,10), and structured psychiatric interviews (11,12). These investigations have consistently found that patients with RA show elevated levels of depression and anxiety relative to healthy controls or other patient groups. For example, the frequency with which depression and anxiety disorders are diagnosed among RA patients has ranged from 14 to 42% (e.g., 13–15).

Psychological distress appears to be associated with high levels of medical service use among patients with RA. Katz and Yelin recently found that, over a 5-year period, patients with elevated scores on a geriatric depression scale reported significantly greater numbers of physician visits and hospitalizations related to their RA than patients whose depression scores were within normal limits (16). This suggests that early identification and effective treatment of psychological distress might reduce patients' health care costs as well as improve their well-being.

However, some of the measures that are used to evaluate psychological distress, such as the MMPI and BDI, contain items that are biased because they refer to physical symptoms associated with arthritis or other chronic diseases (17,18). As a consequence, a patient might produce an elevated score on the MMPI depression scale by responding ''false'' to items such as, ''I am about as able to walk as I ever was.'' Nevertheless, elevated levels of depression and anxiety have been found among patients with RA even when relatively uncontaminated measures, such as the CES-D and structured psychiatric interviews, have been employed (13,14).

Several recent longitudinal investigations have examined changes in anxiety and depression among RA patients. It has been reported consistently that anxiety and depression levels are characterized by modest changes over periods ranging from 6 months to 5 years (19–22). For example, Hawley and Wolfe (19) found that there was a significant, albeit modest, improvement of 0.43 units in AIMS anxiety scores in 400 patients over a mean period of 3.1 years, but there was no significant change in the AIMS depression scale during the study period.

The small change in the AIMS anxiety scale was significant, in part, because of the large number of subjects examined. In a subsequent study (20) of 561 patients over periods ranging from 2 to 5 years, there was no significant change in depression; however, in contrast with the earlier investigation there was a small and significant increase in anxiety.

Some effort has been devoted to identifying the predictors of changes that do occur in depression and anxiety. Two studies (21,22) have indicated that increases in the number of tender or painful joints tend to be accompanied by increases in anxiety and depression. However, pain severity, age, lack of satisfaction with current lifestyle, and degree of functional impairment are better predictors of depression and anxiety than are joint counts and other measures of disease activity (14,19).

One might question whether disease activity would be a more powerful predictor of psychological distress if patients were studied intensively over short periods. Affleck et al. recently studied 54 patients with RA on a daily basis for 75 consecutive days (23), to examine intensively individuals and quantify their subjective experiences with a minimum of retrospective reporting bias. Disease activity did not predict daily mood, as assessed by standardized measures of depression, anxiety, and hostility, consistent with the results of previous investigations. Instead, the most significant determinants of daily mood states were age, neuroticism, and chronic pain.

B. Pain

Patients with RA suffer pain from a number of sources, including chronic inflammation and degenerative processes, which affect joint and connective tissues; systemic complications, which may damage multiple organs; and psychological factors (e.g., depression, environmental rewards) which may augment pain perception (24). The growing recognition among health care professionals of the importance of pain in patient health status is seen in recognition that pain intensity ratings represent a stronger predictor of medication usage in patients with RA than physical or psychological disabilities (25). The pain ratings also are significant determinants of patients' general health status as well as of subsequent physical disability (25).

Similar to the results of longitudinal studies of psychological distress, patients with RA report moderate increases in pain intensity levels over a 5-year period (26), and consistently patients' pain intensity ratings are significantly associated with depression (27–29). Cross-sectional studies have suggested that disease activity does not have a strong direct influence on pain ratings (e.g., 27). However, a prospective daily study (28) indicated that both disease activity and depression show positive and independent associations with pain intensity ratings over a 75-day period.

The association between psychological distress and reports of pain poses substantial difficulties for investigators. For example, patients who receive placebo capsules during a controlled trial of an analgesic medication may reduce their pain ratings substantially owing to high expectations of pain relief and improved mood induced by attention from the professional staff. Although patients receiving the analgesic also may have high expectations for relief, the placebo effect on mood and pain may reduce the power of the experiment to detect meaningful differences between the two interventions. As a consequence, a behavioral observation method that is relatively independent of mood states has been developed for assessing pain among patients with RA (29–33). This method requires trained observers to record the frequencies with which patients display specific, operationally defined pain behaviors as they perform a timed sequence of standard physical maneuvers (e.g., walking, standing, sitting, reclining). These behaviors were chosen because they reliably suggest to naive observers and physicians that individuals are experiencing pain (Table 1). A series of investigations demonstrated that the frequency counts of the seven "pain behaviors" are correlated with patients' pain and disability ratings, as well as with disease activity measures, but are independent of psychological distress (29–32). The frequency counts also are sensitive to the effects of a psychosocial intervention designed to reduce pain among patients with RA (34).

Table 1 Operational Definitions of Pain Behaviors Displayed By Patients with Rheumatoid Arthritis

Behavior	Definition
Guarding	Abnormally stiff, interrupted, or rigid movement during shifting or pacing
Bracing	Position in which an almost fully extended limb supports and maintains an abnormal distribution of weight
Grimacing	An obvious facial expression of pain, which may include a furrowed brow, narrowed eyes, tightened lips, corners of mouth pulled back, and clenched teeth
Sighing	An obvious exaggerated exhalation of air usually accompanied by a rise and fall of the shoulders
Rigidity	*Excessive* stiffness of an affected joint or body part (with the exception of fingers and toes) that is not directly involved in locomotion
Passive rubbing	Touching, resting, or holding an affected joint or body part on another body part for at least 3 consecutive seconds
Active rubbing	Massaging an affected joint or body part for at least 3 consecutive seconds

Despite the advantages associated with a measure of pain that is independent of psychological distress, the behavioral observation method is used infrequently in clinical settings owing to the professional time and expense it entails. Therefore, Anderson et al. (33) recently demonstrated that trained observers can reliably record the pain behaviors displayed by patients during physical examinations and performance of a 50-ft (15-m) walk. It remains to be determined, however, whether the behavioral observation method will be adopted for use in a large number of clinical and laboratory settings.

C. Stress

Rheumatoid arthritis produces numerous stressors in addition to psychological distress and pain. These include activity limitations and functional impairments in the home and workplace, as well as financial hardships associated with loss of income and health care costs (35–39; also see Chaps. 10, 11, and 13). Patients with RA frequently report that stress tends to precede flare-ups in disease activity (40). There is also some evidence that neural structures (e.g., hypothalamus) that are associated with stress responses may additionally be involved in the inflammatory process in RA (41,42). Therefore, investigators have begun to examine relations between stress and immune system function as well as other biological variables.

It has been reported that frequent daily stresses are associated with high proportions of B cells relative to T cells (4) and high erythrocyte sedimentation rates (ESR) (43). More complex relations also have been found in which daily stresses are associated with mood disturbances that, in turn, are related to decreases in soluble interleukin-2 receptor (sIL-2R) levels and increases in joint pain (3), a somewhat surprising finding, as sIL-2R levels are positively associated with joint inflammation in RA (44). Thus, patients' pain ratings may have varied directly as a function of the stress-induced mood disturbances, rather than changes in joint inflammation. Nevertheless, these initial studies of stress and immune system function are quite exciting, although it has yet to be determined whether stress may be causally linked with changes in biological variables (e.g., sIL-2R, substance P) that are involved in the inflammatory processes underlying RA.

D. Social Relationships

In addition to producing stressors that adversely affect patients, RA also generates negative consequences for those in the patients' families and other social networks. For example, Deyo et al. (45) found that between 43 and 52% of patients with RA report dysfunction in the areas of social interaction, communication with others, and emotional behavior, as assessed by the Sickness Impact Profile (46). Moreover, two independent studies have reported that about 60% of patients with RA experience at least one major psychosocial change related to family functioning, such as increased arguments with marital partners, changes in the health of other family members, and sexual problems (47,48). The finding of the high frequency of sexual dysfunction has been confirmed in two recent investigations (49,50).

Results similar to those just noted have been found in interviews with spouses of patients with RA. Revenson and Majerovitz (51) demonstrated that between 28 and 36% of spouses report frustration with patients' physical limitations, reductions in shared pleasurable activities with the patients, and negative changes in patients' moods. Indeed 21% of the spouses expressed fear and uncertainty concerning the implications of the patients' future health for their marriages. Although little data are available concerning associations between divorce and RA (5), Hawley et al. (52) found no higher frequency of divorce among 1267 patients with RA than among patients with noninflammatory rheumatic diseases or with national population-based divorce rates.

Several recent investigations have demonstrated that marital and family relationships have important implications for patients' health status. Reisine et al. (53) reported that relatively high levels of homemaker responsibilities (e.g., cooking, shopping, giving nurturance) at disease onset are associated with lower risk of work disability among women with RA. Two longitudinal studies also have shown that patients who are married report lower levels of functional disability (54,55). Similarly, Reisine and Fifield (55) found that marriage is associated with lower levels of pain and depression as well as disability. However, the positive effects of marriage were eliminated when patients' perceptions of social support were statistically controlled. This suggests that marital status may be merely a marker for the benefits of a supportive social network, although the married patients also perceived that they were needed more by others than did patients who were not married (56). Thus, the desire to meet the needs of spouses and other family members may provide an independent contribution to the relationship between marriage and better function among patients with RA.

E. Discussion: Psychological Effects of Rheumatoid Arthritis

Rheumatoid arthritis produces negative effects on patients' mood states, pain, and social relationships, which may be significant determinants of negative changes in patients' health status. For example, it has consistently been found that psychological distress and perceptions of pain are strongly associated. These factors, as well as marital status and social support, predict several dimensions of health status, such as functional and work disability (54,55,57,58) and use of medical services for RA (16).

One surprising finding has emerged from the literature published to date. That is, disease activity does not consistently show strong relations with pain or psychological distress. It has been suggested, however, that the potential effects of disease activity on patients' psychological reactions and pain may be modified by several cognitive and behavioral factors (19). These factors, which include patients' perceptions of helplessness, control, and self-efficacy, as well as their coping strategies and adherence with treatment regimens, are discussed in the following section.

III. COGNITIVE AND BEHAVIORAL FACTORS THAT INFLUENCE ADJUSTMENT TO RHEUMATOID ARTHRITIS

A. Learned Helplessness and Perceptions of Control

Learned helplessness refers to a phenomenon characterized by emotional, motivational, and cognitive deficits in adaptive coping with stressful situations. The deficits are produced by an individual's perception that no viable solutions are available to eliminate or reduce the source of stress (59). It has been hypothesized that learned helplessness might underlie a portion of the psychological distress and behavioral disabilities shown by patients with RA (5). That is, many patients may develop the belief that their diseases are beyond their effective control because RA is characterized by an unknown cause or cure, as well as by a chronic and unpredictable course. These patients tend to perceive that, regardless of their actions, they will not be able to substantially reduce the pain, disabilities, or other symptoms associated with their illnesses. This perception of uncontrollability may cause the patients to experience anxiety and depression (i.e., emotional deficits) that, in turn, may lead to increased pain and reduced attempts to engage in activities of daily living (i.e., motivational deficits), or to develop new means of adapting to their disabilities and distress (i.e., cognitive deficits). These deficits may be particularly profound and resistant to change among patients who view the consequences of their diseases as relatively stable over time and global in nature (i.e., adversely affecting numerous vocational, recreational, social, and marital or sexual activities).

The importance of perceptions of helplessness in adaptation to RA has been confirmed in many studies. All of these investigations have used various forms of a self-report measure, the Arthritis Helplessness Index (AHI; 60), to assess the extent to which individuals believe they can control their symptoms. For example, high levels of helplessness among patients with RA are associated with low self-esteem (60), use of maladaptive coping strategies (60–62), high levels of pain and depression (60–63), and high levels of functional impairment (64,65). Also, helplessness and the expectation that one's arthritis will become more severe in the future (i.e., hopelessness) have predicted depression and anxiety over a 4-month period, even after controlling for initial levels of depression, anxiety, and physical functioning (66). Moreover, a 3-year longitudinal study has shown that disease severity and helplessness are the best predictors of future disability in physical functioning (67,68).

The investigations on helplessness suggest that perceptions of control over symptoms (i.e., low helplessness) is desirable for patients with RA. Nevertheless, a recent study has demonstrated that patients who believe they can control their symptoms suffer psychological distress in response to increased pain unless they cognitively restructure their pain experiences (e.g., adopt the belief that pain has made life more precious) (69). In addition, Affleck et al. (70) reported that patients who perceive they have good control over the long-term course of RA tend to experience high levels of psychological distress. These studies indicate, then, that perceptions of control over RA symptoms lead to better adaptation than perceived control of the course of a disease that typically is characterized by progressive declines in health status. However, perceived symptom control also may be relatively maladaptive during a flare in disease activity and pain unless one can cognitively restructure the loss of control in a positive manner.

B. Self-Efficacy

Another cognitive factor that is closely related to perceptions of helplessness or control is self-efficacy (71; also see Chap. 21). However, in contrast with perceptions of control of numerous symptoms, self-efficacy (SE) represents a belief that one can perform *specific* behaviors or tasks to achieve specific health-related goals. There may be great variation for any individual in SE for different behaviors. For example, individuals with RA may have high SE for pacing their daily activities to reduce pain and fatigue, but they also may have low SE for performing exercises to improve their physical function.

The importance of SE is that it tends to predict health status if individuals believe that the relevant behaviors will lead to improved health status (72). Lorig et al. reported that high baseline levels of SE for pain and functional ability among patients with RA were strongly associated with low levels of pain, disability, and depression at the baseline and at a 4-month follow-up assessment (71). An independent investigation found that high SE for pain was significantly correlated with low frequencies of observable displays of pain behavior among persons with RA even after controlling for demographic factors and disease severity (73). Nevertheless, similar to the literature on perceived symptom control, high SE among patients with relatively high pain intensity levels is associated with increased depression (74).

C. Coping Strategies

Coping is defined as behaviors that are performed to manage environmental and internal demands (i.e., stressors and conflicts among them) that tax or exceed a person's resources (75). It is generally agreed that the coping process comprises several stages (76). These are (a) appraisal of the threat associated with a particular stressor; (b) performing behaviors (coping strategies) that may control the effect of the stressor; and (c) evaluating the outcomes produced by the behaviors and, if necessary, performing alternative-coping responses.

Numerous studies have been performed since 1980 on coping among patients with RA. These investigations have assessed coping primarily with three instruments: the Ways of Coping Scale (77), the Coping Strategies Questionnaire (78), and the Pain Management Inventory or PMI (79). The former instrument assesses a wide array of coping responses, but many of the scale's items may not be relevant to patients' attempts to cope with their RA symptoms (80). The latter two instruments are designed specifically for patients with chronic painful conditions. The Coping Strategies Questionnaire (78) measures seven strategies: diverting attention, reinterpreting pain sensations, use of coping self-statements, ignoring pain sensations, praying or hoping, catastrophizing, and increasing activity levels. It also asks patients to rate the effectiveness of these strategies in controlling and decreasing their pain. The PMI (79), however, assesses only active (i.e., adaptive) and passive (i.e., maladaptive) pain-coping strategies.

Despite the use of the foregoing different coping measures, passive coping strategies, such as escapist fantasies (e.g., hoping that pain will get better someday) and catastrophizing (e.g., believing that no coping strategy will effectively control symptoms) are consistently associated with high levels of psychological distress (81–85) and pain (79) among patients with RA. Conversely, psychological adjustment and relatively low levels of pain and functional impairment are associated with strategies such as attempts to derive personal meaning from the illness experience, seeking information about arthritis, focusing on positive thoughts during pain episodes, and infrequent usage of catastrophizing (e.g., 85–87).

Little effort has been devoted to identifying the determinants of patients' choices of coping strategies. However, there is evidence that the choice of coping strategies made by women with RA is influenced both by functional disability and spouse support. Manne and Zautra (88) employed causal modeling procedures to demonstrate that the use of escapist fantasies by women with RA is influenced by high functional disability, both directly and indirectly, through critical spouse responses. Psychological adjustment is negatively associated with these escapist fantasies and is positively associated with information-seeking strategies and attempts to derive meaning from the illness. The choice of these latter strategies is directly influenced by sympathetic spouse responses.

Nearly all the studies reviewed in the foregoing have consisted of cross-sectional examinations of the relations between coping strategies and patient well-being. A recent longitudinal investigation, however, used causal modeling to examine predictors of psychosocial adaptation to RA (89). It was found that low baseline levels of perceived competence (a construct similar to self-efficacy) and high helplessness contributed directly to high future levels of depression. In addition, initial levels of helplessness interacted with passive pain-coping strategies so that the presence of one of these factors led to an increase in the other. Passive-coping strategies, in turn, contributed directly to high future levels of impairment in psychosocial functions (e.g., family and social relationships, work). These data, then, represent the first evidence of causal links between perceptions of control, self-efficacy, coping strategy usage, and psychosocial adaptation to RA.

D. Adherence With Treatment Regimens

It is widely accepted that the efficacy of medical and behavioral treatment interventions is, in part, dependent on the degree to which patients perform the actions required by these interventions (90). Thus, adherence with treatment regimens may be considered to be an adaptive coping strategy for most patients with RA (Table 2).

Unfortunately, the literature indicates that adherence with medication regimens ranges from 30 to 78% among these patients (90). Correlates of low adherence include low education (91), prescription of nonsteroidal anti-inflammatory drugs (e.g., indomethacin) relative to disease-modifying agents (e.g., prednisone, D-penicillamine) (92), use of complex pharmacological regimens (93), negative interactions with physicians (94), and low levels of patient belief in the efficacy of prescribed regimens (94,95).

Similar findings have been reported for adherence with home exercise performance and splint usage. Adherence rates among RA patients for home exercise range between 39 and 65%; rates of adherence with splint usage vary from 25 to 65% (90). The only factor that consistently correlates with low adherence with these interventions is low patient belief in treatment efficacy (95,96).

Table 2 Rates and Predictors of Adherence with Treatments for Rheumatoid Arthritis

Treatment	Adherence rates (%)	Predictors of adherence
Medication	30–78	Education
		Type of medication
		Complexity of regimen
		Patient–physician interactions
		Patient belief in treatment efficacy
Home exercise	39–65	Patient belief in treatment efficacy
Splint usage	25–65	Patient belief in treatment efficacy

Relatively little attention has been devoted to the development of interventions that might enhance adherence among patients with RA. DeVellis et al. (97) has proposed a model for improving adherence that is based on patients' cognitive representations of their adherence problems, their problem-solving strategies, and appraisals of the outcomes of these strategies. The investigators tested a multicomponent intervention based on the model with 51 patients with RA, who displayed a variety of adherence problems involving exercise, rest, splint usage, and medication regimens. Patients who received the intervention were significantly more likely to report resolution of their adherence problems at a 2-week follow-up than control patients.

Feinberg (98) recently tested a similar intervention with 40 patients for whom resting hand splints were prescribed. This intervention and a standard care control procedure were administered to patients on a random basis at the initial splinting session with an occupational therapist. During the first 28 days after the initial session, patients who received the experimental intervention showed greater adherence with splint usage and reported shorter periods of morning stiffness than did control patients. These results suggest that it is possible to improve adherence to treatment regimens among patients with RA and that high adherence may be positively associated with some dimensions of health status.

E.　Discussion: Cognitive and Behavioral Variables

It has consistently been shown that patients' cognitive and behavioral responses to their illnesses are associated with their psychological adjustment and other dimensions of health status. With cognitive responses, both cross-sectional and longitudinal studies have shown that perceptions of control over RA symptoms and SE for pain and disability tend to be correlated with relatively low levels of pain, depression, and disability among patients with RA. There is also evidence that disease activity may moderate relations between patient cognition and health status. Perceptions of control and SE are associated with psychological distress when patients experience reduced control over their pain.

For behavioral responses, patients' use of coping strategies interacts with perceptions of symptom control to influence pain and functional ability (89). Use of passive strategies, such as escapist fantasy and catastrophizing, leads to increased helplessness and is consistently associated with psychological distress, pain, and functional impairment.

No data have been reported on the possible relations among perceptions of symptom control, coping strategy usage, and adherence with medical regimens. Nevertheless, patients' cognitions concerning the efficacy of their treatments and perceptions of their interactions with physicians are reliably associated with adherence.

Given the strong relations between health status and patients' cognitions and behaviors, several psychosocial interventions have been developed that may alter patients' perceptions of control or SE as well as their coping strategies and, thereby, improve pain, emotional states, or function. The major psychosocial interventions are reviewed in the following section.

IV. PSYCHOSOCIAL INTERVENTIONS

The psychosocial interventions that have been developed for patients with RA tend to share similar treatment components. These components include education, training in relaxation and other coping skills, and rehearsal of newly learned skills to help increase patients' perceptions of symptom control or SE (Table 3). The effects of nearly all of the interventions have been assessed relative to those produced by waiting list or attention–placebo control conditions. The following discussion focuses on interventions that have been subjected to the most stringent testing procedures.

Bradley et al. (34) evaluated a biofeedback-assisted, group therapy intervention that trained patients with RA and their family members in relaxation and behavioral problem-solving skills. Treatment was intended to increase patients' perceptions of control over their symptoms. The results indicated that the intervention, relative to attention–placebo and no adjunct treatment conditions, produced significant reductions in pain behavior and disease activity (i.e., joint counts) at posttreatment. A 1-year follow-up showed that patients who received the intervention reported lower levels of pain and depression than those who received no adjunctive treatment (99). Contrary to expectations, however, neither perceptions of control nor functional ability were influenced by the intervention.

Several other investigators have reported that similar interventions designed to increase perceived symptom control reduce pain among patients with RA (100–103). Only one of these interventions, however, increased functional ability and reduced joint counts among the patients (100). Moreover, all of the studies that have assessed maintenance of patient improvement have shown that the effects of treatment tend to diminish over time (34,101,102). Lack of adherence with the skills learned in treatment may be responsible for this phenomenon. Parker et al. (103) showed that patients who continued to practice their newly learned relaxation skills during a 1-year follow-up maintained improvements on pain ratings, perceptions of symptom control, and coping skill usage.

In contrast with the interventions just described, treatments based on principles of self-efficacy have tended to produce better maintenance of treatment gains. Lorig et al. (104) recently reported that the Arthritis Self-Management Program (ASMP) produced significant increases in SE for pain and other symptoms and significant reductions in pain ratings and arthritis-related physician visits among patients with RA and osteoarthritis. Moreover, these improvements were maintained for 4 years after initiation of treatment. Estimated net 4-year savings in health care costs were 648 dollars for each patient with RA. However,

Table 3 Summary of Psychosocial Interventions for Patients With Rheumatoid Arthritis

Investigation (Ref.)	Sample	Intervention	Control condition	Outcomes
Bradley et al. (34)	53 (43 women, 10 men)	Temperature biofeedback-assisted group therapy for patients and family members Monthly telephone calls from project staff during 6-mo follow-up	Group social support (attention–placebo) and no adjunct treatment	Intervention produced significant reductions in pain behavior and disease activity at posttreatment. Intervention produced significant reduction in anxiety at 6-mo follow-up.
Bradley et al. (99)	53	None; 12-mo follow-up of biofeedback-assisted group therapy	None; 12-mo follow-up of group social support and no adjunct treatment	Intervention produced significant reductions in pain ratings and depression at 12-mo follow-up.
Achterberg et al. (100)	23 women	Relaxation training and temperature biofeedback training	Physical therapy	Intervention produced significant improvements in pain ratings, joint counts, and functional ability.
Applebaum et al (101)	18 (16 men, 2 women)	Temperature biofeedback-assisted group therapy	Symptom monitoring, waiting-list control condition	Intervention produced significant improvements in pain ratings, social communication, and range of motion. Improvements were not maintained at 18-mo follow-up.

Table 3 Summary of Psychosocial Interventions for Patients With Rheumatoid Arthritis (*cont.*)

Investigation (Ref.)	Sample	Intervention	Control condition	Outcomes
Radojevic et al. (102)	59 (45 women, 14 men)	Cognitive–behavioral group therapy with family member participation or Cognitive–behavioral group therapy without family member participation	Education and family support and no adjunct treatment	Both interventions produced significant improvements in number of swollen joints and swelling severity at posttreatment and 2-mo follow-up and in joint pain at follow-up. Intervention with family participation was superior to intervention without family participation at posttreatment only.
Parker et al. (103)	83 (80 men, 3 women)	Cognitive–behavioral group therapy	Arthritis education group program and no adjunct treatment	Intervention produced significantly greater use of adaptive-coping strategies and perceived control of symptoms at 12-mo follow-up. Patients who reported high adherence with treatment during follow-up reported significant improvements in pain, perceived control of symptoms, and coping skill usage.

| Lorig et al. (104)[a] | 968 (762 women, 206 men) | Arthritis Self-Management Program (ASMP) | Standard care and participation in observational studies unrelated to prior ASMP investigations | The ASMP produced significant increases in perceived self-efficacy for pain and other symptoms and significant reductions in pain ratings and arthritis-related physician visits at 4-yr follow-up assessment. Estimated net savings in health care costs for each patient with RA was $648. |
| O'Leary et al. (105) | 30 women | Cognitive–behavioral group therapy | Provision of self-help book on arthritis | Intervention produced significant improvements in perceived self-efficacy for pain and functional ability, pain ratings, and joint counts. Changes in self-efficacy were associated with decreases in pain intensity and increases in suppressor T cells. Differences between intervention and control conditions were not maintained at 4-mo follow-up. |

[a]603 patients in this study were diagnosed with rheumatoid arthritis.

the ASMP did not alter functional ability among the patients. Lorig provides a full description of the ASMP in Chapter 21.

Similar to the results reported by Lorig et al., O'Leary and her colleagues (105) found that a psychological treatment program, relative to provision of a self-help book on arthritis, improved SE for pain and functional ability and reduced pain and joint counts among patients with RA. Indeed, increases in SE for pain were significantly associated with decreases in pain ratings and increases in suppressor T cells during treatment. These treatment effects, however, were reduced at a 4-month follow-up assessment primarily because of improvements in health status among the control patients during the follow-up period.

A. Discussion: Psychosocial Interventions

Psychosocial interventions produce reliable improvements in patients' perceptions of pain and pain behavior. However, these interventions rarely produce increases in functional ability. Moreover, with the exception of the ASMP developed by Lorig et al., the interventions studied to date have demonstrated that patients usually do not maintain their improvements following treatment.

Keefe and Van Horn (106) recently provided a model of relapse of treatment gains among patients with RA. This model suggests that relapse tends to occur when patients' symptoms increase in intensity and their perceptions of symptom control or self-efficacy are compromised. As noted by Tennen et al. (69) and Schiaffino et al. (74), these events are associated with high levels of psychological distress. Moreover, Keefe and Van Horn suggest that if patients stop their coping efforts in response to these events, they are likely to experience a major relapse in pain, function, or mood states (106).

The model just described has an important implication for psychosocial interventions. That is, these interventions might produce better maintenance of treatment gains if they include treatment components designed specifically to help patients cope with potential relapse. Keefe and Van Horn suggest that all phases of treatment should include (a) practice in identifying high-risk situations that are likely to tax patients' coping resources; (b) practice in identifying the early signs of relapse, such as increases in pain or depression; (c) rehearsal of cognitive and behavioral skills for responding to these early relapse signs; and (d) training in self-reinforcement for effective displays of coping with possible relapse.

V. SUMMARY

This chapter has documented the effect of RA on patients' well-being and health status as measured by pain, emotional states, stress, and social relationships. It also has shown that complex relations exist between patients' cognitive and behavioral responses to their illnesses and their well-being. Finally, the review has indicated that psychosocial interventions designed to influence these responses produce reliable improvements at posttreatment in patients' pain perceptions and behavior. The effects of these interventions on functional abilities, however, are quite variable, and effects on pain often diminish after treatment is terminated.

It is anticipated that several issues will receive greater attention from future investigators. First, there will be increased emphasis on longitudinal studies of the relations among patients' responses to their illnesses and their well-being and health status. The intensive daily study methodology (e.g., 23) will become an especially useful method for understanding these complex relations. Second, there will be greater use of large databases and multivariate methods of analysis to better identify causal associations among disease activity, demographic and psychological factors, and health status. Third, more effort will be devoted to understanding the relations among patients' environments (e.g., daily stress), cognitions, behaviors, and immune system responses. There also will be attempts to determine the influence of these associations on clinical status and long-term outcome (107). Finally, two important concerns will be addressed in studies of psychosocial interventions. That is, there will be modifications of current interventions so that they may have greater influence on patients' functional abilities. Efforts also will be made to help patients better maintain their improvements following treatment. Indeed, it is anticipated that the relapse prevention model (106) will have great influence on future investigators' attempts to improve long-term effects of psychosocial interventions on patients' health status.

REFERENCES

1. Burish TG, Bradley LA. Coping with chronic disease: definitions and issues. In: Burish TG, Bradley LA, eds. Coping with chronic disease: research and applications. New York: Academic Press, 1983:3–12.
2. Bradley LA. Psychosocial factors and disease outcomes in rheumatoid arthritis: old problems, new solutions, and a future agenda [editorial]. Arthritis Rheum 1989; 32:1611–1614.
3. Harrington L, Affleck G, Urrows S, et al. Temporal covariation of soluble interleukin-2 receptor levels, daily stress, and disease activity in rheumatoid arthritis. Arthritis Rheum 1993; 36:199–203.
4. Zautra AJ, Okun M, Robinson SE, et al. Life stress and lymphocyte alterations among patients with rheumatoid arthritis. Health Psychol 1989; 8:1–14.
5. Bradley LA, Anderson KO, Young LD, et al. Psychosocial aspects of arthritis. Bull Rheum Dis 1985; 35:1–12.
6. McKinley JC, Hathaway SR. The identification and measurement of the psychoneuroses in medical practice: the Minnesota multiphasic personality inventory. JAMA 1943; 122:161–167.

7. Beck AT. Depression: clinical, experimental, and theoretical aspects. New York: Harper & Row, 1967.

8. Radloff L. The CES-D scale: a self-report depression scale for research in the general population. Appl Psychol Meas 1977; 1:385–401.

9. Meenan RF, Gertman PM, Mason, JH. Measuring health status in arthritis: the arthritis impact measurement scales. Arthritis Rheum 1980; 23:146–152.

10. Meenan RF, Mason JH, Anderson JJ, et al. AIMS-2: the content and properties of a revised and expanded arthritis impact measurement scales health status questionnaire. Arthritis Rheum 1992; 35:1–10.

11. Helzer JE, Robins LN. The diagnostic interview schedule: its development, evaluation, and use. Soc Psychiat Epidem 1988; 23:6–16.

12. Spitzer RL, Williams JBW, Gibbon M, et al. Structured clinical interview for DSM-IIIR. Washington DC: American Psychiatric Association, 1990.

13. Blalock SJ, DeVellis RF, Brown GK, et al. Validity of the Center for Epidemiological Studies depression scale in arthritis populations. Arthritis Rheum 1989; 32:991–997.

14. Frank RG, Beck NC, Parker JC, et al. Depression in rheumatoid arthritis. J Rheumatol 1988; 15:920–925.

15. Ahles TA, Khan S, Yunus MB, et al. Psychiatric status of patients with primary fibromyalgia, patients with rheumatoid arthritis, and subjects without pain: a blind comparison of DSM-III diagnoses. Am J Psychiatry 1991; 148:1721–1726.

16. Katz PP, Yelin EH. Prevalence and correlates of depressive symptoms among persons with rheumatoid arthritis. J Rheumatol 1993; 20:790–796.

17. Pincus T, Callahan LF, Bradley LA, et al. Elevated MMPI scores for hypochondriasis, depression, and hysteria in patients with rheumatoid arthritis reflect disease rather than psychological status. Arthritis Rheum 1986; 29:1456–1466.

18. Peck JR, Smith TW, Ward JR, et al. Disability and depression in rheumatoid arthritis: a multi-trait, multi-method investigation. Arthritis Rheum 1989; 32:1100–1106.

19. Hawley DJ, Wolfe F. Anxiety and depression in patients with rheumatoid arthritis: a prospective study of 400 patients. J Rheumatol 1988; 15:932–941.

20. Wolfe F, Hawley DJ, Cathey MA. Clinical and health status measures over time: prognosis and outcome assessment in rheumatoid arthritis. J Rheumatol 1991; 18:1290–1297.

21. Parker J, Smarr K, Anderson S, et al. Relationship of changes in helplessness and depression to disease activity in rheumatoid arthritis. J Rheumatol 1992; 19:1901–1905.

22. Parker JC, Smarr KL, Walker SE, et al. Biopsychosocial parameters of disease activity in rheumatoid arthritis. Arthritis Care Res 1991; 4:73–80.

23. Affleck G, Tennen H, Urrows S, et al. Neuroticism and the pain–mood relation in rheumatoid arthritis: insights from a prospective daily study. J Consult Clin Psychol 1992; 60:119–126.

24. Anderson KO, Bradley LA, Young LD, et al. Rheumatoid arthritis: review of psychological factors related to etiology, effects, and treatment. Psychol Bull 1985; 98:358–387.

25. Kazis LE, Meenan RF, Anderson JJ. Pain in the rheumatic diseases. Arthritis Rheum 1983; 26:1017–1022.

26. Callahan LF, McCoy A, Smith W. Comparison and sensitivity to change of self-report scales to assess difficulty, dissatisfaction, and pain in performing activities of daily living over one and five years in rheumatoid arthritis. Arthritis Care Res 1992; 5:137–145.

27. Parker JC, Smarr KL, Angelone EO, et al. Psychological factors, immunologic activation, and disease activity in rheumatoid arthritis. Arthritis Care Res 1992; 5:196–201.

28. Affleck G, Tennen H, Urrows S, et al. Individual differences in the day-to-day experience of chronic pain: a prospective daily study of rheumatoid arthritis patients. Health Psychol 1991; 10:419–426.

29. McDaniel LK, Anderson KO, Bradley LA, et al. Development of an observation method for assessing pain behavior in rheumatoid arthritis patients. Pain 1986; 24:165–184.

30. Anderson KO, Bradley LA, McDaniel LK, et al. The assessment of pain in rheumatoid arthritis: validity of a behavioral observation method. Arthritis Rheum 1987; 30:34–43.

31. Anderson KO, Bradley LA, McDaniel LK, et al. The assessment of pain in rheumatoid arthritis: disease differentiation and temporal stability of a behavioral observation method. J Rheumatol 1987; 14:700–704.

32. Anderson KO, Keefe FJ, Bradley LA, et al. Prediction of pain behavior and functional status of rheumatoid arthritis patients using medical status and psychological variables. Pain 1988; 33:25–32.

33. Anderson KO, Bradley LA, Turner RA, et al. Observation of pain behavior in rheumatoid arthritis patients during physical examination: relationship to disease activity and psychological variables. Arthritis Care Res 1992; 5:49–56.

34. Bradley LA, Young LD, Anderson KO, et al. Effects of psychological therapy on pain behavior of rheumatoid arthritis patients: treatment outcome and six-month follow-up. Arthritis Rheum 1987; 30:1105–1114.

35. Felts W, Yelin E. The economic impact of the rheumatic diseases in the United States. J Rheumatol 1989; 16:867–884.

36. Yelin E. Arthritis: the cumulative impact of a common chronic condition. Arthritis Rheum 1992; 35:489–497.

37. Mitchell JM, Burkhauser RV, Pincus T. The importance of age, education, and comorbidity in the substantial earnings losses of individuals with symmetric polyarthritis. Arthritis Rheum 1988; 31:348–357.

38. Liang MH, Larson M, Thompson M, et al. Costs and outcomes in rheumatoid arthritis and osteoarthritis. Arthritis Rheum 1984; 27:522–529.

39. Stone CE. The lifetime economic costs of rheumatoid arthritis. J Rheumatol 1984; 11:819–827.

40. Affleck GA, Pfeiffer C, Tennen H, et al. Attributional processes in rheumatoid arthritis patients. Arthritis Rheum 1987; 30:927–931.

41. Levine JD, Collier DH, Basbaum AI, et al. Hypothesis: the nervous system may contribute to the pathophysiology of rheumatoid arthritis. J Rheumatol 1985; 12:406–411.

42. Chikanza IC, Petrou P, Kingsley G, et al. Defective hypothalamic response to immune and inflammatory stimuli in patients with rheumatoid arthritis. Arthritis Rheum 1992; 35:1281–1288.

43. Thomason BT, Brantley PJ, Jones GN, et al. The relation between stress and disease activity in rheumatoid arthritis. J Behav Med 1992; 15:215–220.

44. McFarlane AC, Brooks PM. Pschoimmunology and rheumatoid arthritis: concepts and methodologies. Int J Psychiatry Med 1990; 20:307–322.

45. Deyo RA, Inui TS, Leininger J, et al. Physical and psychosocial function in rheumatoid arthritis: clinical use of a self-administered health status instrument. Arch Intern Med 1982; 142:879–882.

46. Bergner M, Bobbitt RA, Carter WB, et al. The Sickness Impact Profile: development and final revision of a health status measure. Med Care 1981; 19:787–805.

47. Liang MII, Rogers M, Larson M, ct al. Thc psychosocial impact of systcmic lupus erythematosus and rheumatoid arthritis. Arthritis Rheum 1984; 27:13–19.

48. Yelin E, Feshbach DM, Meenan RF, et al. Social problems, services, and policy for persons with chronic disease: the case of rheumatoid arthritis. Soc Sci Med 1979; 13:13–20.

49. Blake DJ, Maisiak R, Alarcón G, et al. Sexual quality of life of patients with arthritis compared to arthritis-free controls. J Rheumatol 1987; 14:570–576.

50. Blake DJ, Maisiak R, Kaplan A, et al. Sexual dysfunction among patients with arthritis. Clin Rheumatol 1988; 7:50–60.

51. Revenson TA, Majerovitz SD. The effects of chronic illness on the spouse: social resources as stress buffers. Arthritis Care Res 1991; 4:63–72.

52. Hawley DJ, Wolfe F, Cathey MA, et al. Marital status in rheumatoid arthritis and other rheumatic disorders: a study of 7293 patients. J Rheumatol 1991; 18:654–660.

53. Reisine ST, Grady KE, Goodenow C, et al. Work disability among women with rheumatoid arthritis: the relative importance of disease, social, work, and family factors. Arthritis Rheum 1989; 32:538–543.

54. Ward MM, Leigh JP. Marital status and the progression of functional disability in patients with rheumatoid arthritis. Arthritis Rheum 1993; 36:581–588.

55. Reisine S, Fifield J. Expanding the definition of disability: implications for planning, policy, and research. Millbank Q 1992; 70:491–508.

56. Reisine S. Marital status and social support in rheumatoid arthritis [editorial]. Arthritis Rheum 1993; 36:589–592.

57. Leigh JP, Fries JF. Predictors of disability in a longitudinal sample of patients with rheumatoid arthritis. Ann Rheum Dis 1992; 51:581–587.

58. Wolfe F, Cathey MA. The assessment and prediction of functional disability in rheumatoid arthritis. J Rheumatol 1991; 18:1298–1306.

59. Garber J, Seligman MEP (eds). Human helplessness: theory and applications. New York: Academic Press, 1980.

60. Nicassio PM, Wallston KA, Callahan LF. et al. The measurement of helplessness in rheumatoid arthritis: the Arthritis Helplessness Index. J Rheumatol 1985; 12:462–467.

61. Stein MJ, Wallston KA, Nicassio PM. Factor structure of the arthritis helplessness index. J Rheumatol 1988; 15:427–432.

62. Stein MJ, Wallston KA, Nicassio PM, et al. Correlates of a clinical classification schema for the arthritis helplessness subscale. Arthritis Rheum 1988; 31:876–881.

63. Smith TW, Peck JR, Ward JR. Helplessness and depression in rheumatoid arthritis. Health Psychol 1990; 9:377–389.

64. Callahan LF, Brooks RH, Pincus T. Further analysis of learned helplessness in rheumatoid arthritis using a "rheumatology attitudes index." J Rheumatol 1988; 15:418–426.

65. DeVellis RF, Callahan LF. A brief measure of helplessness in rheumatic disease: the helplessness subscale of the rheumatology attitudes index. J Rheumatol 1993; 20:866–869.

66. DeVellis BM, Blalock SJ. Illness attributions and hopelessness depression: the role of hopelessness expectancy. J Abnorm Psychol 1992; 101:257–264.

67. Lorish CD, Abraham N, Austin J, et al. Disease and psychosocial factors related to physical functioning in rheumatoid arthritis. J Rheumatol 1991; 18:1150–1157.

68. Alarcón GS, Jackson J, Lorish CD, et al. Prediction of physical functioning (Ph F) in rheumatoid arthritis (RA): a three years analysis of a large cohort [abstract]. Arthritis Rheum 1992; 35:S100.

69. Tennen H, Affleck G, Urrows S, et al. Perceiving control, construing benefits, and daily processes in rheumatoid arthritis. Can J Behav Sci 1992; 24:186–203.

70. Affleck G, Tennen H, Pfeiffer C, et al. Appraisals of control and predictability in adapting to a chronic disease. J Pers Soc Psychol 1987; 53:273–279.

71. Lorig K, Chastain RL, Ung E, et al. Development and evaluation of a scale to measure perceived self-efficacy in people with arthritis. Arthritis Rheum 1989; 32:37–44.

72. O'Leary A. Self-efficacy and health: behavioral and stress-physiological mediation. Cogn Ther Res 1992; 16:229–245.

73. Buescher KL, Johnston JA, Parker JC, et al. Relationships of self-efficacy to pain behavior. J Rheumatol 1991; 18:968–972.

74. Schiaffino KM, Revenson TA, Gibofsky A. Assessing the impact of self-efficacy beliefs on adaptation to rheumatoid arthritis. Arthritis Care Res 1991; 4:150–157.

75. Lazarus RS, Folkman S. Stress, appraisal, and coping. New York: Springer-Verlag, 1984.

76. Manne SL, Zautra AJ. Coping with arthritis: current status and critique. Arthritis Rheum 1992; 35:1273–1280.

77. Folkman S, Lazarus R. An analysis of coping in a middle-age community sample. J Health Soc Behav 1980; 22:457–459.

78. Rosenstiel AK, Keefe FJ. The use of coping strategies in chronic low back pain patients: relationship to patient characteristics and current adjustment. Pain 1983; 17:33–44.

79. Brown GK, Nicassio PM. Development of a questionnaire for the assessment of active and passive coping strategies in chronic pain patients. Pain 1987; 31:53–64.

80. Stone AA, Greenberg MA, Kennedy-Moore E, et al. Self-report, situation-specific coping questionnaires: what are they measuring? J Pers Soc Psychol 1991; 61:648–658.

81. Revenson TA, Felton BJ. Disability and coping as predictors of psychological adjustment to rheumatoid arthritis. J Consult Clin Psychol 1989; 57:344–348.

82. Keefe FJ, Brown GK, Wallston KA, et al. Coping with rheumatoid arthritis pain: catastrophizing as a maladaptive strategy. Pain 1989; 37:51–56.

83. Parker J, McCrae C, Smarr K, et al. Coping strategies in rheumatoid arthritis. J Rheumatol 1988; 15:1376–1383.

84. Regan CA, Lorig K, Thoresen CE. Arthritis appraisal and ways of coping: scale development. Arthritis Care Res 1988; 1:139–150.

85. Brown GK, Nicassio PM, Wallston KA. Pain coping strategies and depression in rheumatoid arthritis. J Consult Clin Psychol 1989; 57:652–657.

86. Hagglund KJ, Haley WE, Reveille JD, et al. Predicting individual differences in pain and functional impairment among patients with rheumatoid arthritis. Arthritis Rheum 1989; 32:851–858.

87. Affleck G, Urrows S, Tennen H, et al. Daily coping with pain from rheumatoid arthritis: patterns and correlates. Pain 1992; 51:221–230.

88. Manne S, Zautra AJ. Spouse criticism and support: their association with coping and psychological adjustment among women with rheumatoid arthritis. J Pers Soc Psychol 1989; 56:608–617.

89. Smith CA, Wallston KA. Adaptation in patients with chronic rheumatoid arthritis: application of a general model. Health Psychol 1992; 11:151–162.

90. Bradley LA. Adherence with treatment regimens among adult rheumatoid arthritis patients: current status and future directions. Arthritis Care Res 1989; 2:S33–S39.

91. Beck NC, Parker JC, Frank RG, et al. Patients with rheumatoid arthritis at high risk for noncompliance with salicylate treatment regimens. J Rheumatol 1988; 15:1081–1084.

92. Deyo RA, Inuie TS, Sullivan B. Compliance with arthritis drugs: magnitude, correlates, and clinical implications. J Rheumatol 1981; 8:931–936.

93. Feinberg J. The effect of patient–practitioner interaction on compliance: a review of the literature and application in rheumatoid arthritis. Patient Educ Couns 1988; 11:171–187.

94. Geersten HR, Gray RM, Ward JR. Patient noncompliance within the context of seeking medical care for arthritis. J Chron Dis 1973; 26:689–698.

95. Ferguson K, Bole GG. Family support, health beliefs, and therapeutic compliance in patients with rheumatoid arthritis. Patient Couns Health Educ 1979; 1:101–105.

96. Nicholas JJ, Gruen H, Weiner G, et al. Splinting in rheumatoid arthritis. I. Factors affecting patient compliance. Arch Phys Med Rehabil 1982; 63:92–94.

97. DeVellis BM, Blalock SJ, Hahn PM, et al. Evaluation of a problem-solving intervention for patients with arthritis. Patient Educ Couns 1988; 11:29–42.

98. Feinberg J. Effect of the arthritis health professional on compliance with use of resting hand splints by patients with rheumatoid arthritis. Arthritis Care Res 1992; 5:17–23.

99. Bradley LA, Young LD, Anderson KO, et al. Effects of cognitive-behavioral therapy on rheumatoid arthritis pain behavior: one-year follow-up. In: Dubner R, Gebhart G, Bond M, eds. Pain research and clinical management, vol 3. Amsterdam: Elsevier, 1988:310–314.

100. Achterberg J, McGraw P, Lawlis GF. Rheumatoid arthritis: a study of relaxation and temperature biofeedback training as an adjunctive therapy. Biofeed Self Regul 1981; 6:207–223.

101. Applebaum KA, Blanchard EB, Hickling EJ, et al. Cognitive–behavioral treatment of a veteran population with moderate to severe rheumatoid arthritis. Behav Ther 1988; 19:489–502.

102. Radojevic V, Nicassio PM, Weisman MH. Behavioral intervention with and without family support for rheumatoid arthritis. Behav Ther 1992; 23:13–30.

103. Parker J, Frank RG, Beck NC, et al. Pain management in rheumatoid arthritis: a cognitive–behavioral approach. Arthritis Rheum 1988; 31:593–601.

104. Lorig KR, Mazonson PD, Holman HR. Evidence suggesting that health education for self-management in patients with chronic arthritis has sustained health benefits while reducing health care costs. Arthritis Rheum 1993; 36:439–446.

105. O'Leary A, Shoor S, Lorig K, et al. A cognitive–behavioral treatment for rheumatoid arthritis. Health Psychol 1988; 7:527–544.

106. Keefe FJ, Van Horn Y. Cognitive behavioral treatment of rheumatoid arthritis pain: maintaining treatment gains. Arthritis Care Res 1993; 6:213–222.

107. Rubin LA, Hawker GA. Stress and the immune system: preliminary observations in rheumatoid arthritis using an in vivo marker of immune activity [editorial]. Arthritis Rheum 1993; 36:204–207.

13

Socioeconomic Status and Rheumatoid Arthritis

Leigh F. Callahan

National Center for Chronic Disease Prevention and Health Promotion
Centers for Disease Control and Prevention
Atlanta, Georgia

I. INTRODUCTION

Socioeconomic status has been observed to be associated with the prevalence, morbidity, and mortality of most common chronic diseases (1–17). An association of socioeconomic status with mortality was recognized initially in 1851 in Britain; then in Europe and North America, and in most developing countries since World War II (2,18,19). As life expectancy increases in a society with modernization, greater differences in mortality are seen among the strata in that society (20).

Reports indicate that low socioeconomic status is associated with high disease prevalence, disability, and mortality in patients with cardiovascular disease (10,21–39), cancer (40–43), pulmonary disease (44), rheumatoid arthritis (RA; 12,45–52), systemic lupus erythematosus (SLE; 51,53–55), back pain (56,57), osteoarthritis (OA; 58), migraine headaches (59), and in the general population (1,3,4,48,60–63). This finding persists throughout the entire life span (14), and extends across many risk factors for disease (39,64–66).

Associations between socioeconomic status and health status have been noted in many different countries with different health care systems (2,3,6,17,29,30,34,41,60,66–79). In analyses of cardiovascular disease mortality over 7 years in 17,530 London civil servants, job classification explained variation in mortality considerably more than all recognized risk factors, including blood pressure, smoking, and cholesterol level (30). In eastern and southern Finland, among 1711 men born between 1900–1919, increased age, low levels of formal education, high systolic and diastolic blood pressure, and low forced vital capacity were the most significant independent predictors of disability over 25 years (71).

Several studies from Norway have noted an association between increased levels of coronary heart disease and lower levels of social class (67,68). In a rural French population, formal education level and home comfort were associated significantly with mortality (69); when education was accounted for, income was not significantly associated with mortality (69). In Australia, low socioeconomic status was associated with higher levels of mortality, and this association became more marked with increasing age (60); a negative correlation between socioeconomic index and mortality was seen for both sexes and all age groups, irrespective of the country of birth (60).

Despite an overall decline in mortality in the United States since 1960, individuals of low socioeconomic status still die at higher rates than those with high levels of socioeconomic status (17). This disparity in mortality between socioeconomic groups increased between 1960 and 1986 (17).

II. MEASURES OF SOCIOECONOMIC STATUS

Socioeconomic status has been examined according to a number of variables, including income, formal education level, occupation, home ownership, race, marital status, and so on (80–83). Although occupational, financial, and educational status are correlated, it has been proposed that each reflects different societal and individual forces associated with health and disease (84). For example, occupation reflects control over pace of work, and responsibility; income reflects medical care accessibility, home ownership, diet; and formal education indicates intelligence, time preference or willingness to delay gratification, skills for acquiring positive psychological, economic, and social resources (84).

Initially, economic development was seen as a leading explanation of declines in life expectancy in modern society. However, high levels of health in some relatively poor areas, and low life expectancy in some wealthier areas, indicate that a relation between high income and good health is not invariant (18).

The United States presents an example in which wealth and health are not well correlated. Expenditures for health care in the United States have increased at a rapid and sustained rate over the past several decades (85). The United States has the second highest per capita medical expenditures (following Sweden), and the world's finest medical system, yet a mortality rate that is higher than 18 other countries, including Spain, Italy, and Greece (20). Increased expenditures and utilization in medical care, from 6.1% of the gross national product (GNP) in 1965 to more than 14% in 1992, have not been associated with major improvements in health status. On the contrary, some observers suggest that, in some ways, the health of Americans is now worsening (86).

The number of years of formal education an individual has attained has been demonstrated in several studies to be a most important socioeconomic variable associated with good health status outcomes (1,3,8,16,25,63,84,87–94). The number of years of formal education has become a most commonly used measure of socioeconomic status in epidemiological studies (95). It is more easily and accurately measured than occupation or income, and much less likely to be influenced by disease than those variables.

The positive influence of increased formal education on health status outcomes has been hypothesized to result from several different mechanisms. The simplest is that health knowledge acquisition accompanies higher education, which can lead to improved health. However, provision of information alone appears to be a weak stimulus toward improvement in health behavior (20,96). A second hypothesis is that formal education is simply a marker for intelligence, and that good health and intelligence are correlated significantly. However, although intelligence and education are correlated significantly, studies indicating that environmental factors are the most predictive variables of failure to complete school weaken the suggestion that education is simply a proxy for intelligence (97). A third hypothesis is that both education and health are markers for an individual's willingness to delay gratification to ''invest in human capital'' (98), which may be reflected in greater compliance and health behaviors.

A fourth hypothesis on associations between education and health status is that formal education level is a marker for behavioral variables, which may favorably affect health (84,95,99). Education may enhance problem-solving abilities, efficiency in using medical services, capacity to cope with stress, social skills, psychological status, and economic skills, enabling individuals to insulate themselves from adversity or cope with adverse situations more effectively.

Formal education itself cannot account entirely for differences in health status outcomes. Therefore, the association between education levels and health status may reflect correlations between education and mediational process variables, which favorably affect health. A model illustrating a conceptual framework for such a relationship is illustrated in Fig. 1. Several exogenous elements, such as host, family, and policy factors, may influence formal education level, mediational processes, and health status outcomes. Mediational processes, such as personal health behaviors, psychological variables, and cognitive variables, are associated with health status outcomes, and these processes may be influenced by formal education, as well as exogenous factors.

III. FORMAL EDUCATION AND HEALTH STATUS OUTCOMES IN RHEUMATOID ARTHRITIS

Psychological and social characteristics of patients hospitalized for RA, hypertension, and duodenal ulcer were initially described in 1965 (45). When the patients with RA were compared with controls, the patients with RA were found to have

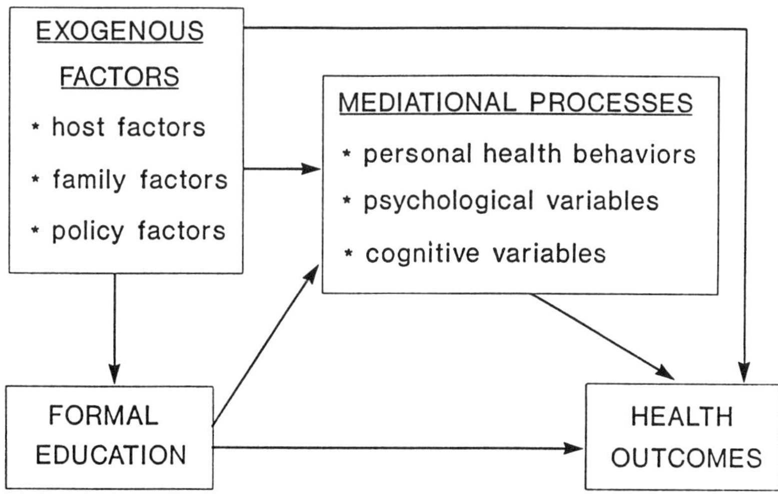

Fig. 1   A conceptual framework of health status and formal education.

lower levels of formal education, 9.0 years versus 10.4 years in the control group. The patients with RA were also unwilling to see changes in themselves.

Increased mortality and morbidity were seen in association with lower formal education levels in 75 RA patients studied 9 years apart in 1973 and 1982 (12). Nine of the 20 patients with eight or fewer years of education had died, compared with 10 of 34 with 9–12 years of education, and only 1 of 21 with more than 12 years of education ($p < 0.05$) (Fig. 2A). The mean formal education level differed significantly ($p = 0.002$) in patients who survived the 9-year period, compared with patients who died, 11.5 years versus 9.0 years. The associations between formal education level and mortality remain significant in adjusted analyses to test whether other baseline measures that differed significantly in survivors and nonsurvivors, including age, number of involved hand joints, and three measures of functional capacity (i.e., responses to questions

Fig. 2   Life tables depicting mortality in rheumatoid arthritis patients. (A) Mortality of 75 patients over a period of 110 months, categorized into three groups according to formal education level (numbers in parentheses indicate total number within each group). (B) Mortality of a subset of 48 patients between ages 45 and 64, encompassing the group with accelerated mortality in rheumatoid arthritis, categorized into three groups according to formal education level (numbers in parentheses indicate total number within each group). (C) Mortality of 75 patients over a period of 30 years categorized into three groups according to formal education level (numbers at bottom indicate numbers of patients at risk in each category at 5-year intervals). (From Ref. 12.)

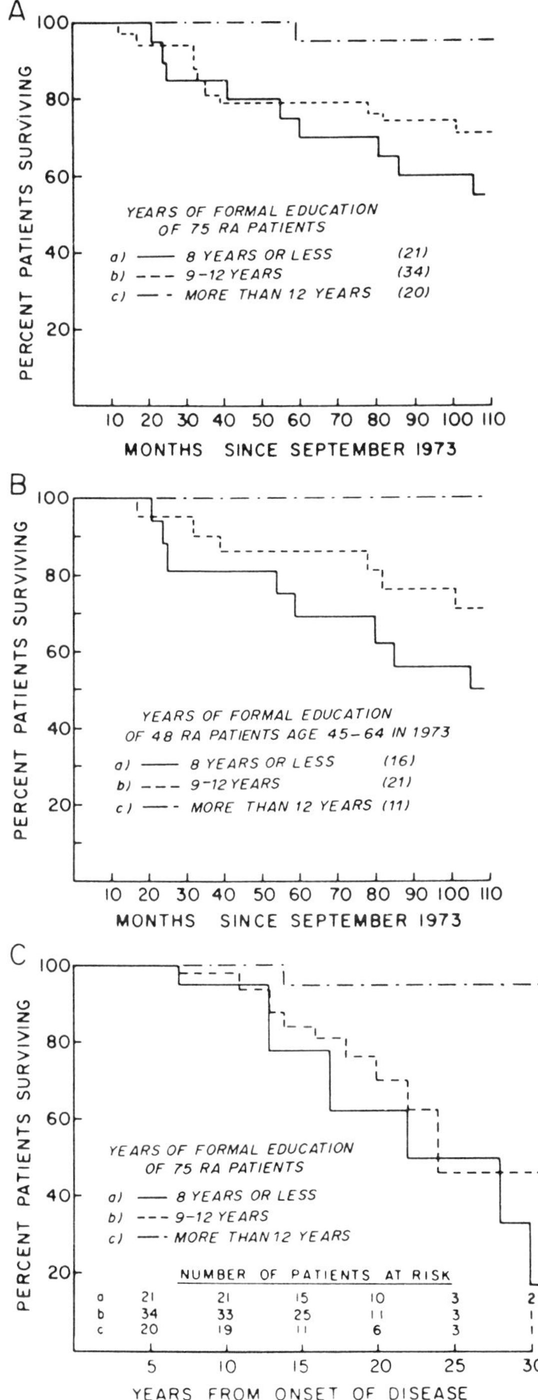

A
100
80
60
40
20
PERCENT PATIENTS SURVIVING
YEARS OF FORMAL EDUCATION
OF 75 RA PATIENTS
a) 8 YEARS OR LESS (21)
b) 9-12 YEARS (34)
c) MORE THAN 12 YEARS (20)
10 20 30 40 50 60 70 80 90 100 110
MONTHS SINCE SEPTEMBER 1973

B
100
80
60
40
20
PERCENT PATIENTS SURVIVING
YEARS OF FORMAL EDUCATION
OF 48 RA PATIENTS AGE 45-64 IN 1973
a) 8 YEARS OR LESS (16)
b) 9-12 YEARS (21)
c) MORE THAN 12 YEARS (11)
10 20 30 40 50 60 70 80 90 100 110
MONTHS SINCE SEPTEMBER 1973

C
100
80
60
40
20
PERCENT PATIENTS SURVIVING
YEARS OF FORMAL EDUCATION
OF 75 RA PATIENTS
a) 8 YEARS OR LESS
b) 9-12 YEARS
c) MORE THAN 12 YEARS
NUMBER OF PATIENTS AT RISK
a 21 21 15 10 3 2
b 34 33 25 11 3 1
c 20 19 11 6 3 1
5 10 15 20 25 30
YEARS FROM ONSET OF DISEASE

concerning activities of daily living, modified walking time, and the button test) might confound these associations.

The relative risk of mortality for patients with fewer than 11 years of formal education was 2.53. This relative risk remained above 2.20 when patients were stratified according to median levels of age, duration of disease, overall functional capacity, modified walking time, morning stiffness, number of intra-articular injections, as well as according to sex, smoking, and use of gold or oral corticosteroids. A Cox proportional hazards model, which included formal education level, overall functional capacity, age, and duration of disease, indicated that both functional capacity and formal education level were statistically significant in stepwise maximum partial likelihood ratio analyses.

The independent association between formal education level and mortality, not explained by age or duration of disease, was also documented in actuarial life table analyses, with patients stratified according to these variables. Life tables for a subset of 48 patients aged 45–64 in 1973, in whom the mean age of surviving and deceased patients was 55.1 and 55.2 respectively, indicated a pattern similar to that seen for the entire population over the 9-year period (see Fig. 2B). Patterns were also similar when mortality was depicted from onset of disease, rather than from a baseline review (see Fig. 2C). Taken together, the stratification and modeling analyses indicate that the association of formal education level and mortality is not explained by other available variables, including age, duration of disease, measures of functional capacity, and all other variables studied.

Morbidity was studied, in surviving patients, as functional capacity in activities of daily living. Almost all patients showed severe functional declines, but the magnitude of these declines differed substantially according to levels of formal education (Fig. 3). Mean functional capacity in survivors was decreased from 91.5 to 33.3% for the grade school-educated; 92.9 to 65.3% for high school-educated; and 92.4 to 69.9% for college-educated patients. Mean declines were 58.1, 28.8, and 22.3% in the three groups ($p < 0.01$). The relative risk for declines in functional capacity of 30% or more was 2.07 in individuals with fewer than 11 years of formal education, compared with more than 12 years of education. This relative risk was 2.01, adjusted for age, and 1.92, adjusted for duration of disease, as well as 1.80, adjusted for both variables, indicating that associations between morbidity and education are explained only minimally by age or duration of disease.

Overall, 79% of grade school-educated, 43% of high school-educated, and 20% of college-educated patients had either died or declined more than 50% in functional capacity over a 9-year period (Fig. 4). These associations were explained only in small part by other variables, as patients of different formal education levels were similar at baseline in age, duration of disease, measures of functional capacity, number of involved hand joints, number of severe radiographic changes, use of gold, oral corticosteroids, or other therapies.

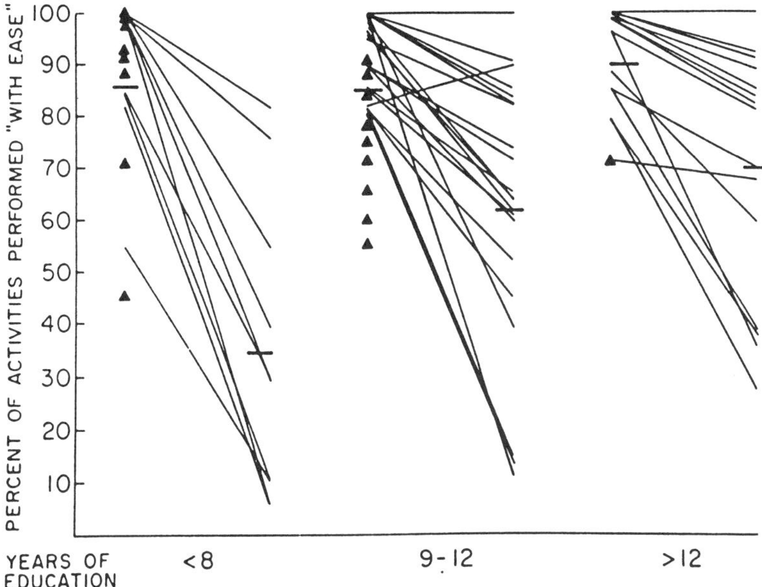

Fig. 3 Changes over 9 years in functional capacity determined by responses to questions in 50 patients with rheumatoid arthritis. The percentage of 87 questions to which patients responded that they could perform ''with ease'' is depicted, with patients categorized into three groups according to formal education level. Patients who had died over the 9 years are depicted by inverted triangles. Significant declines are seen in most patients, with significant differences between declines in grade school educated versus other patients. (From Ref. 12.)

To extend these findings, a cross-sectional study of clinical status was conducted in 385 additional patients with RA seen in a university rheumatology clinic, a Veterans' Administration medical center, or in the private practices of four rheumatologists. Patients were classified into four groups: fewer than 8, 9–11, 12, and more than 12 years of formal education. The clinical measures studied included erythrocyte sedimentation rate, joint count, grip strength, walking time, button time test, and five self-report questionnaire measures of pain, difficulty, dissatisfaction, and global status (50).

All laboratory, physical, and questionnaire measures indicated substantially poorer clinical status in patients who did not complete high school, compared with those who had completed high school (50) (Table 1). In general, the poorest results were seen in patients with only a grade school education. Progressively better results were seen in patients with some high school education, high school graduates, and patients with some college education. No differences were seen in clinical status in patients who had attended college, graduated from college, or had postgraduate education (see Table 1). Trends in clinical status according

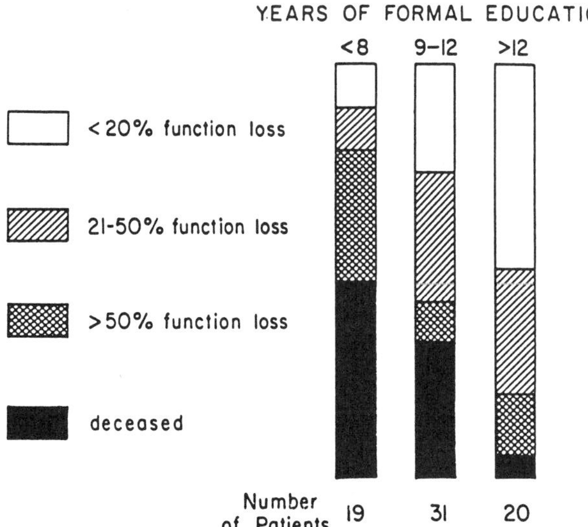

Fig. 4   Mortality and morbidity, defined as loss of functional capacity, in 75 rheumatoid arthritis patients over 9 years, with patients categorized according to number of years of formal education. (From Ref. 12.)

to formal education level were similar in all three clinical settings, although patients seen at the Veterans Administration medical center had lower levels of formal education than those seen at the university clinic and private practices. Differences in clinical status according to formal education level were not explained by age, sex, race, duration of disease, or clinical setting.

Possible associations of formal education with clinical status were analyzed in 2006 patients with RA from five clinical centers: Santa Clara, California; Saskatoon, Canada; Wichita, Kansas; Phoenix, Arizona; and Stanford, California (52). The range of formal education level among the men was greater than among the women, as seen in all studies. Patients were classified into three categories of functional status according to the Health Assessment Questionnaire (HAQ) (101) disability index and into three groups on the basis of years of education. A statistically significant inverse relation was seen between education and the HAQ scores. The relation was strong for men, with a smooth dose–response pattern, and weaker for women (Table 2). When the analyses were performed separately for the two largest centers, Wichita and Saskatoon, similar results were seen.

Longitudinal analyses were performed in this sample to study possible predictive power over 2 years for the HAQ disability index (52). As in the cross-sectional analyses, lower levels of formal education were predictive with

Table 1 Mean Values for Laboratory, Physical, and Self-Report Measures of Disease Status in 385 Rheumatoid Arthritis Patients, Classified According to Level of Formal Education

		Patients classified according to formal education level						
Disease status measure[a]	All patients	Grade school	Some high school	High school graduate	Some college	College graduate	Post-graduate	p[b]
Laboratory measures								
ESR (mm/hr)	40.1	48.3	49.4	34.7	29.3	41.8	26.6	0.002[c]
Painful joint count	12.1	16.3	15.1	9.1	10.2	9.3	8.5	0.001[d]
Physical measures								
Grip strength (mmHg)	98.8	93.7	92.1	97.9	111.6	101.6	110.9	0.079
Walk time (s)	10.3	11.2	10.0	10.6	9.6	10.2	6.5	0.424
Button test (s)	62.5	80.5	61.3	60.8	46.9	58.1	54.8	0.003[c]
Self-report measures								
ADL difficulty scale (1–4)	1.97	2.26	2.04	1.86	1.73	1.99	1.70	0.000[d]
ADL pain scale (1–4)	2.37	2.62	2.56	2.26	2.06	2.46	2.06	0.001[d]
ADL dissatisfaction scale (1–4)	2.26	2.54	2.41	2.12	2.03	2.29	1.81	0.006
Visual analog pain scale (0–10)	5.12	5.75	5.85	4.89	4.26	4.94	3.86	0.074
Global self-assessment (1–4)	2.68	3.09	2.70	2.55	2.43	2.61	2.25	0.000[d]

[a]ESR, erythrocyte sedimentation rate; ADL, activities of daily living.
[b]By analysis of covariance, after controlling for age, sex, clinical setting, and disease duration.
[c]$p < 0.05$ after adjustment for multiple comparisons.
[d]$p < 0.01$ after adjustment for multiple comparisons.
Source: Ref. 50.

Table 2 Correlation Coefficients, Cross Tabulation, and χ^2 Analyses According to Formal Education Level for Rheumatoid Arthritis Patients From Five Data Centers

Correlation coefficients of disability index with years of schooling

	Women	Men
Entire sample	−0.096	−0.361

Cross tabulations, entire sample

Disability Score	Women schooling categories			Total	Disability Score	Men schooling categories			Total
	< 12 yr	12 yr	> 12 yr			< 12 yr	12 yr	> 12 yr	
0 ≤ score < 1	112	164	222	498	0 ≤ score < 1	34	38	89	161
1 ≤ score < 2	141	203	259	603	1 ≤ score < 2	78	47	43	118
2 ≤ score ≤ 3	93	129	122	344	2 ≤ score ≤ 3	50	38	11	99
Total	346	491	603		Total	162	123	143	

χ^2 with 4 degrees of freedom: 7.68.
Probability of type I error:
0.104 in a 2-tailed test.

χ^2 with 4 degrees of freedom: 64.93.
Probability of type I error:
0.0001 in a 2-tailed test.

Source: Ref. 52.

poorer HAQ disability scores in men, and weakly associated in women, even with adjustment for age, sex, labor force status, occupation, marital status, race, income, erythrocyte sedimentation rate, rheumatoid factor titer, number of tender joints, and duration of disease.

Several studies have indicated higher levels of depression and learned helplessness in individuals with RA who had fewer years of formal education (102–105). Higher scores on the Beck Depression Inventory, the Center for Epidemiologic Studies Depression Scale (CES-D), and the Anxiety and Depression Subscales of the General Well Being Schedule were noted in individuals with fewer years of formal education (105). Increased levels of learned helplessness, assessed according to a rheumatology attitudes index, have also been shown to be associated with fewer years of formal education in patients with SLE (51,106), OA, fibromyalgia, and scleroderma (51,104).

IV. POSSIBLE MECHANISMS OF ACTION AND IMPLICATIONS FOR HEALTH POLICY

The mechanism whereby formal education is associated with health status is poorly understood. Social stratification results in an unequal distribution of desirable resources in society (96). This view would suggest that the recognized associations between low education and high mortality would be explained by unequal distribution of medical and health-promoting resources. However, disparities in mortality among socioeconomic strata are seen in many countries with adequate nutrition, housing, water, and waste disposal (2,18,20). Furthermore, universal access to health care has not diminished associations between socioeconomic status and health; indeed, evidence for widening social inequalities in health has been presented in the United Kingdom, where the National Health Service is available (13). The advances in public health and the access to private individual health care explain only a small component of associations between socioeconomic status and health, and other mechanisms must be sought.

The associations between education and mortality affirm the need to recognize the importance of this variable in policy and clinical situations. Since it has been noted that medical care can explain no more than 10% of the variation in health status (107), some medical economists argue that greater reductions in morbidity and mortality are possible through expenditures on education, rather than on medical care (87,98). However, the percentage of our gross national product that is spent on health care is much greater than the percentage spent on education.

Although education appears a powerful predictor of health status, data concerning formal education level are not collected in usual clinical practice. Therefore, extensive medical databases may include diagnoses, date of birth, religion, dates of admission, dates of surgery, and such, on all patients admitted to hospitals, but these databases rarely include information concerning education level. Because the education level is a powerful predictor of morbidity and mortality in many diseases, often as powerful a predictor of clinical status as age or duration of disease (51), it would appear desirable that this variable should be collected in routine care.

Since formal education itself cannot account entirely for differences in health status outcomes, variables, such as personal health behaviors, psychological variables, and cognitive variables, appear likely mediators of the associations. It might be preferable to collect data concerning potential mediational variables in routine clinical care, in addition to education, but if resources are not available to collect further data, the simple variable formal education level should be collected.

The consideration of reimbursement for interventions designed to modify directly a potential mediational variable, such as perceived learned helplessness, in patients with arthritis might also be considered. Patient education interventions have been demonstrated to result in improved knowledge, self-care behavior, pain behavior, psychological status, and health status (104,108–110). In a meta-analysis of 15 studies concerning potential effects of psychoeducational interventions on disability, pain, and depression in individuals with chronic rheumatoid arthritis or osteoarthritis, patient education was found to contribute to health status above and beyond standard clinical care (108). In present health care practice, patient education is generally not reimbursable, whereas reimbursement for expensive and extensive high technology tests is provided without question. A change in policy might facilitate improvement in outcomes for patients with arthritis.

Health education programs may lead to improved outcomes in a chronic disease through changes in a mediational variable, rather than through changes in knowledge. This finding emerged initially from studies of the Arthritis Self-Management Course (111) developed at Stanford University. This course consists of six weekly 2-hour sessions taught by two trained lay-leaders who, follow a standardized protocol (111). The course content includes the pathophysiology of osteoarthritis and rheumatoid arthritis, design of individual exercise and relaxation programs, an overview of medication effects and treatment of arthritis, joint protection methods, nutrition practices, decision-making about nontraditional remedies, physician–patient communications, and techniques for solving arthritis-related problems. It is taught using experiential and interactive methods. The course has been documented to result in improved functional outcomes (112).

Examination of mechanisms whereby the Arthritis Self-Management Course led to positive effects on health outcome led to unexpected observations. It was initially thought that improved outcomes would result from provision of knowledge concerning arthritis. Although there was an overall increase in knowledge concerning arthritis, no association was found between increased knowledge and improved outcomes. A second hypothesis was that improved outcomes resulted from changes in patient behavior, such as increased exercise, better drug compliance, and so on; however, only weak associations were found between changes in behavior and changes in health status (112).

A third hypothesis studied was that the improved health outcomes resulted from a patient's improvement in perceived self-efficacy (113). Perceived self-efficacy, a concept initially described by Bandura, involves a belief that one can perform a specific behavior or task in the future (114). It refers to personal judgments concerning one's abilities to perform in a given domain of activity. Perceived self-efficacy was the most significant correlate of improved health outcomes in results from the Arthritis Self-Management Course.

Improvements in scores for perceived learned helplessness have also been documented after completion of two self-care intervention models (104), and these decreases were sustained at 8 and 12 months. Although higher perceived learned helplessness scores were found in individuals with lower levels of education, formal education level was not associated with the degree of change in perceived learned helplessness. This finding suggests that interventions targeted toward decreasing learned helplessness in individuals with fewer years of formal education might be worthy of further study.

REFERENCES

1. Stockwell EG. A critical examination of the relationship between socioeconomic status and mortality. Am J Public Health 1963; 53:956–964.
2. Antonovsky A. Social class, life expectancy and overall mortality. Milbank Mem Fund Q 1967; 45(pt 1):31–73.
3. Kitagawa EM, Hauser PM. Differential mortality in the United States: a study in socioeconomic epidemiology. Cambridge: Harvard University Press, 1973:i–255
4. Nagi MH, Stockwell EG. Socioeconomic differentials in mortality by cause of death. Health Serv Rep 1973; 88:449–456.
5. Yeracaris CA, Kim JH. Socioeconomic differentials in selected causes of death. Am J Public Health 1978; 68:342–351.
6. Holme I, Helgeland A, Hjermann I, Leren P, Lund-Larson PG. Four-year mortality by some socioeconomic indicators: the Oslo study. J Epidemiol Community Health 1980; 34:48–52.
7. Laughton KB, Buck CW, Hobbs GE. Socio-economic status and illness. Milbank Mem Fund Q 1958; 36:46–57.
8. Leigh JP. Education, occupational status, and illness. WAC 1982; 9:441–456.
9. Wan T. Social differentials in selected work-limiting chronic conditions. J Chronic Dis 1972; 25:365–374.
10. Lehman EW. Social class and coronary heart disease: a sociological assessment of the medical literature. J Chronic Dis 1967; 20:381–391.

11. Leigh JP. Direct and indirect effects of education on health. Soc Sci Med 1983; 17:227–234.

12. Pincus T, Callahan LF. Formal education as a marker for increased mortality and morbidity in rheumatoid arthritis. J Chronic Dis 1985; 38:973–984.

13. Marmot MG, McDowall ME. Mortality decline and widening social inequalities. Lancet 1986; 2:274–276.

14. Marmot MG, Kogevinas M, Elston MA. Social/economic status and disease. Annu Rev Public Health 1987; 8:111–135.

15. Syme SL, Berkman LF. Social class, susceptibility and sickness. Am J Epidemiol 1976; 104:1–8.

16. Guralnik JM, Land KC, Blazer D, Fillenbaum GG, Branch LG. Educational status and active life expectancy among older blacks and whites. N Engl J Med 1993; 329:110–116.

17. Pappas G, Queen S, Hadden W, Fisher G. The increasing disparity in mortality between socioeconomic groups in the United States, 1960 and 1986. N Engl J Med 1993; 329:103–109.

18. Grosse RN, Auffrey C. Literacy and health status in developing countries. Annu Rev Public Health 1989; 10:281–297.

19. Fuchs VR. Some economic aspects of mortality in developed countries. In: Perlman M, ed. The economics of health and medical care. London, Macmillan, 1974:174–193.

20. Sagan LA. True causes of sickness and well-being: the health of nations. New York, Basic Books, 1987.

21. Weinblatt E, Ruberman W, Goldberg JD, Frank CW, Shapiro S, Chaudhary BS. Relation of education to sudden death after myocardial infarction. N Engl J Med 1978; 299:60–65.

22. Ruberman W, Weinblatt E, Goldberg JD, Chaudhary BS. Education, psychosocial stress and sudden cardiac death. J Chronic Dis 1983; 36:151–160.

23. Ruberman W, Weinblatt E, Goldberg JD, Chaudhary BS. Psychosocial influences on mortality after myocardial infarction. N Engl J Med 1984; 311:552–559.

24. Syme SL, Hyman MM, Enterline PE. Some social and cultural factors associated with the occurrence of coronary heart disease. J Chronic Dis 1964; 17:277–289.

25. Hinkle LE Jr, Whitney LH, Lehman EW, Dunn J, Benjamin B, King R, Plakun A, Flehinger B. Occupation, education, and coronary heart disease: risk is influenced more by education and background than by occupational experiences, in the Bell System. Science 1968; 161:238–246.

26. Antonovsky A. Social class and the major cardiovascular diseases. J Chronic Dis 1968; 21:65–106.

27. Jenkins CD. Recent evidence supporting psychologic and social risk factors for coronary disease [first of two parts]. N Engl J Med 1976; 294:987–994.

28. Holme I, Helgeland A, Hjermann I, Leren P, Lund-Larsen PG. Coronary risk factors in various occupational groups: the Oslo Study. Br J Prev Soc Med 1977; 31:96–100.

29. Marmot MG, Rose G, Shipley M, Hamilton PJS. Employment grade and coronary heart disease in British civil servants. J Epidemiol Community Health 1978; 32:244–249.

30. Rose G, Marmot MG. Social class and coronary heart disease. Br Heart J 1981; 45:13–19.

31. Keil JE, Sandifer SH, Loadholt CB, Boyle E Jr. Skin color and education effects on blood pressure. Am J Public Health 1981; 71:532–534.

32. Jenkins CD. Psychosocial risk factors for coronary heart disease. Acta Med Scand [Suppl] 1982; 660:123–136.

33. Dobson AJ, Gibberd RW, Leeder SR, O'Connell DL. Occupational differences in ischemic heart disease mortality and risk factors in Australia. Am J Epidemiol 1985; 122:283–290.

34. Marmot MG, Adelstein AM, Robinson N, Rose GA. Changing social-class distribution of heart disease. Br Med J 1978; 2:1109–1112.

35. Wing S, Barnett E, Casper M, Tyroler HA. Geographic and socioeconomic variation in the onset of decline of coronary heart disease mortality in white women. Am J Public Health 1992; 82:204–209.

36. Williams RB, Barefoot JC, Califf RM, Haney TL, Saunders WB, Pryor DB, Hlatky MA, Siegler IC, Mark DB. Prognostic importance of social and economic resources among medically treated patients with angiographically documented coronary artery disease. JAMA 1992; 267:520–524.

37. Rogot E, Hrubec Z. Trends in mortality from coronary heart disease and stroke among US veterans; 1954–1979. J Clin Epidemiol 1989; 42:245–256.

38. Rosenman RH, Brand RJ, Jenkins CD, Friedman M, Straus R, Wurm M. Coronary heart disease in the Western Collaborative Group study: final follow-up experience of 8½ years. JAMA 1975; 233:872–877.

39. Matthews KA, Kelsey SF, Meilahn EN, Kuller LH, Wing RR. Educational attainment and behavioral and biologic risk factors for coronary heart disease in middle-aged women. Am J Epidemiol 1989; 129:1132–1144.

40. Jenkins CD. Social environment and cancer mortality in men. N Engl J Med 1983; 308:395–398.

41. Brenner H, Mielck A, Klein R, Ziegler H. The role of socioeconomic factors in the survival of patients with colorectal cancer in Saarland/Germany. J Clin Epidemiol 1991; 44:807–815.

42. Gordon HH, Crowe JP, Brumberg DJ, Berger NA. Socioeconomic factors and race in breast cancer recurrence and survival. Am J Epidemiol 1992; 135:609–618.

43. Mandelblatt J, Andrews H, Kerner J, Zauber A, Burnett W. Determinants of late stage diagnosis of breast and cervical cancer: the impact of age, race, social class, and hospital type. Am J Public Health 1991; 81:646–649.

44. Lebowitz MD. The relationship of socio-environmental factors to the prevalence of obstructive lung diseases and other chronic conditions. J Chronic Dis 1977; 30:599–611.

45. Cobb S, Kasl SV, Chen E, Christenfeld R. Some psychological and social characteristics of patients hospitalized for rheumatoid arthritis, hypertension, and duodenal ulcer. J Chronic Dis 1965; 18:1259–1278.

46. Engel A. National health examination survey: rheumatoid arthritis. Comments. In: Bennett, Wood PHN, eds. Population studies of the rheumatic diseases. Amsterdam: Excerpta Medica, 1968:83–89.

47. Wolfe AM. The epidemiology of rheumatoid arthritis: a review. Part I. Surveys. Bull Rheum Dis 1968; 19:518–523.

48. Pincus T, Callahan LF, Burkhauser RV. Most chronic diseases are reported more frequently by individuals with fewer than 12 years of formal education in the age 18–64 United States population. J Chronic Dis 1987; 40:865–874.

49. Mitchell JM, Burkhauser RV, Pincus T. The importance of age, education, and comorbidity in the substantial earnings losses of individuals with symmetric polyarthritis. Arthritis Rheum 1988; 31:348–357.

50. Callahan LF, Pincus T. Formal education level as a significant marker of clinical status in rheumatoid arthritis. Arthritis Rheum 1988; 31:1346–1357.

51. Callahan LF, Smith WJ, Pincus T. Self-report questionnaires in five rheumatic diseases: comparisons of health status constructs and associations with formal education level. Arthritis Care Res 1989; 2:122–131.

52. Leigh JP, Fries JF. Education level and rheumatoid arthritis: evidence from five data centers. J Rheumatol 1991; 18:24–34.

53. Studenski S, Allen NB, Caldwell DS, Rice JR, Polisson RP. Survival in systemic lupus erythematosus: a multivariate analysis of demographic factors. Arthritis Rheum 1987; 30:1326–1332.

54. Esdaile JM, Sampalis JS, Lacaille D, Danoff D. The relationship of socioeconomic status to subsequent health status in systemic lupus erythematosus. Arthritis Rheum 1988; 31:423–427.

55. Callahan LF, Pincus T. Associations between clinical status questionnaire scores and formal education level in systemic lupus erythematosus. Arthritis Rheum 1990; 33:407–411.

56. Deyo RA, Diehl AK. Psychosocial predictors of disability in patients with low back pain. J Rheumatol 1988; 15:1557–1564.

57. Deyo RA, Tsui-Wu Y-J. Functional disability due to back pain: a population-based study indicating the importance of socioeconomic factors. Arthritis Rheum 1987; 30:1247–1253.

58. Hannan MT, Anderson JJ, Pincus T, Felson DT. Educational attainment and osteoarthritis: differential associations with radiographic changes and symptom reporting. J Clin Epidemiol 1992; 45:139–147.

59. Stewart WF, Lipton RB, Celentano DD, Reed ML. Prevalence of migraine headache in the United States: relation to age, income, race, and other sociodemographic factors. JAMA 1992; 267:64–69.

60. Fisher S. Relationship of mortality to socioeconomic status and some other factors in Sydney in 1971. J Epidemiol Community Health 1978; 32:41–46.

61. Wingard DL, Berkman LF, Brand RJ. A multivariate analysis of health-related practices: a nine-year mortality follow-up of the Alameda County Study. Am J Epidemiol 1982; 116:765–775.

62. Slater C, Carlton B. Behavior, lifestyle, and socioeconomic variables as determinants of health status: implications for health policy development. Am J Prev Med 1985; 1(5):25–33.

63. Snowdon DA, Ostwald SK, Kane RL. Education, survival, and independence in elderly Catholic sisters, 1936–1988. Am J Epidemiol 1989; 120:999–1012.

64. Winkleby MA, Fortmann SP, Barrett DC. Social class disparities in risk factors for disease: eight-year prevalence patterns by level of education. Prev Med 1990; 19:1–12.

65. Helmert U, Herman B, Joeckel K-H, Greiser E, Madans J. Social class and risk factors for coronary heart disease in the Federal Republic of Germany. Results of the baseline survey of the German Cardiovascular Prevention Study. J Epidemiol Community Health 1989; 43:37–42.

66. Kok FJ, Matroos AW, van den Ban AW, Hautvast JGAJ. Characteristics of individuals with multiple behavioral risk factors for coronary heart disease: The Netherlands. Am J Public Health 1982; 72:986–991.

67. Cassel J, Heyden S, Bartel AG, Kaplan BH, Tyroler HA, Cornoni JC, Hames CG. Incidence of coronary heart disease by ethnic group, social class, and sex. Arch Intern Med 1971; 128:901–906.

68. Holme I, Helgeland A, Hjermann I, Lund-Larsen PG, Leren P. Coronary risk factors and socioeconomic status: the Oslo Study. Lancet 1976; 2:1396–1398.

69. Grand A, Grosclaude P, Bocquet H, Pous J, Albarede JL. Disability, psychosocial factors and mortality among the elderly in a rural French population. J Clin Epidemiol 1990; 43:773–782.

70. Jacobsen BK, Thelle DS. Risk factors for coronary heart disease and level of education: the Tromso Heart Study. Am J Epidemiol 1988; 127:923–932.

71. Lammi U-K, Kivela S-L, Nissinen A, Punsar S, Puska P, Karvonen M. Predictors of disability in elderly Finnish men—a longitudinal study. J Clin Epidemiol 1989; 42:1215–1225.

72. Shahtahmasebi S, Davies R, Wenger GC. A longitudinal analysis of factors related to survival in old age. Gerontologist 1992; 32:404–413.

73. Barberger-Gateau P, Chaslerie A, Dartigues J-F, Commenges D, Gagnon M, Salamon R. Health measures correlates in a French elderly community population: the PAQUID study. J Gerontol 1992; 47:S88–S95.

74. Pearce NE, Davis PB, Smith AH, Foster FH. Mortality and social class in New Zealand—I: overall male mortality. NZ Med J 1983; 96:281–285.

75. Pearce NE, Davis PB, Smith AH, Foster FH. Mortality and social class in New Zealand—II: male mortality by major disease groupings. NZ Med J 1983; 96:711–716.

76. Rywik S, Sznajd J, Williams OD, Pajak A, Przestalska-Malkin H, Thomas RP, Kupsc W, Misiowiec P, Irving SH, Magdon M, Wagrowska H, Abernathy JR. Poland and US colaborative study on cardiovascular epidemiology: I. Introduction and baseline findings. Am J Epidemiol 1989; 130:431–445.

77. Sznajd J, Rywik S, Furberg B, Pajak A, Kurjata P, Williams OD, Sznajderman-Ciswicka M, Misiowiec P, Irving SH, Baczynska E, Wagrowska H, Abernathy JR, Czarnecka H, Thomas RP, Konopka M, Morawska I. Poland and US collaborative study on cardiovascular epidemiology: II. Correlates of lipids and lipoproteins in men and women aged 35–64 years from selected Polish rural, Polish urban, and US samples. Am J Epidemiol 1989; 130:446–456.

78. Hollingsworth JR. Inequality in levels of health in England and Wales, 1891–1971. J Health Soc Behav 1981; 22:268–283.

79. Ho SC. Health and social predictors of mortality in an elderly Chinese cohort. Am J Epidemiol 1991; 133:907–921.

80. Mueller CW, Parcel TL. Measures of socioeconomic status: alternatives and recommendations. Child Dev 1981; 52:13–30.

81. Hollingshead AB. Commentary on "The indiscriminate state of social class measurement." Soc Forces 1971; 49:563–567.

82. Duncan OD. A socioeconomic index for all occupations. In: Reiss AJ, Jr, Duncan OD, Hatt PK, North CC, eds. Occupation and social status. Glencoe: Free Press, 1961:109–138.

83. Green L. Manual for scoring socioeconomic status for research on health behavior. Public Health Rep 1970; 85:815–827.

84. Winkleby MA, Jatulis DE, Frank E, Fortmann SP. Socioeconomic status and health: how education, income, and occupation contribute to risk factors for cardiovascular disease. Am J Public Health 1992; 82:816–820.

85. Anderson GF, Erickson JE. National medical care spending. Health Aff 1987; 6(3):96–104.

86. Verbrugge LM. Longer life but worsening health? Trends in health and mortality of middle-aged and older persons. Milbank Mem Fund Q Health Soc 1984; 62:475–519.

87. Auster R, Leveson I, Sarachek D. The production of health: an exploratory study. J Hum Resource 1969; 4:411–436.

88. Feldman JJ, Makuc DM, Kleinman JC, Cornoni-Huntley J. National trends in educational differentials in mortality. Am J Epidemiol 1989; 129:919–933.

89. Rosen S, Taubman P. Changes in the impact of education and income on mortality in the US. In: DelBene L, Scheuren F, eds. Statistical uses of administrative records with emphasis on mortality and disability research. Washington, DC: Social Security Administration, 1979:61–66.

90. Khoury PR, Morrison JA, Laskarzewski P, Kelly K, Mellies MJ, King P, Larsen R, Glueck CJ. Relationships of education and occupation to coronary heart disease risk factors in schoolchildren and adults: the Princeton School District Study. Am J Epidemiol 1981; 113:378–395.

91. Sorel JE, Ragland DR, Syme SL, Davis WB. Educational status and blood pressure: the Second National Health and Nutrition Examination Survey, 1976–1980, and the Hispanic Health and Nutrition Examination Survey, 1982–1984. Am J Epidemiol 1992; 135:1339–1348.

92. Pukkala E, Teppo L. Socioeconomic status and education as risk determinants for gastrointestinal cancer. Prev Med 1986; 15:127–138.

93. Berger MC, Leigh JP. Schooling, self-selection, and health. J Hum Resource 1989; 24:433–455.

94. Shea S, Stein AD, Basch CE, Lantigua R, Maylahn C, Strogatz DS, Novick L. Independent associations of educational attainment and ethnicity with behavioral risk factors for cardiovascular disease. Am J Epidemiol 1991; 134:567–582.

95. Liberatos P, Link BG, Kelsey JL. The measurement of social class in epidemiology. Epidemiol Rev 1988; 10:87–121.

96. Williams DR. Socioeconomic differentials in health: a review and redirection. Soc Psychol Q 1990; 53:81–99.

97. Howard MA, Anderson RJ. Early identification of potential school dropouts: a literature review. Child Welfare 1978; 57:221–231.

98. Fuchs VR. Economics, health, and post-industrial society. Milbank Mem Fund Q Health Soc 1979; 57:153–182.

99. Pincus T. Formal educational level—a marker for the importance of behavioral variables in the pathogenesis, morbidity, and mortality of most diseases? [editorial]. J Rheumatol 1988; 15:1457–1460.

100. Verbrugge LM, Gates DM, Ike RW. Risk factors for disability among US adults with arthritis. J Clin Epidemiol 1991; 44:167–182.

101. Fries JF, Spitz P, Kraines RG, Holman HR. Measurement of patient outcome in arthritis. Arthritis Rheum 1980; 23:137–145.

102. Nicassio PM, Wallston KA, Callahan LF, Herbert M, Pincus T. The measurement of helplessness in rheumatoid arthritis. The development of the Arthritis Helplessness Index. J Rheumatol 1985; 12:462–467.

103. Callahan LF, Brooks RH, Pincus T. Further analysis of learned helplessness in rheumatoid arthritis using a "Rheumatology Attitudes Index." J Rheumatol 1988; 15:418–426.

104. Goeppinger J, Arthur MW, Baglioni AJ Jr, Brunk SE, Brunner CM. A Reexamination of the effectiveness of self-care education for persons with arthritis. Arthritis Rheum 1989; 32:706–716.

105. Callahan LF, Kaplan MR, Pincus T. The Beck Depression Inventory, Center for Epidemiological Studies Depression Scale (CES-D), and General Well-being Schedule Depression Subscale in rheumatoid arthritis: criterion contamination of responses. Arthritis Care Res 1991; 4:3–11.

106. Engle EW, Callahan LF, Pincus T, Hochberg MC. Learned helplessness in systemic lupus erythematosus: analysis using the Rheumatology Attitudes Index. Arthritis Rheum 1990; 33:281–286.

107. U.S. Department of Health, Education and Welfare. (1979) Healthy People: the Surgeon General's report on health promotion and disease prevention. United States Government Printing Office. Washington, D.C.

108. Mullen PD, Laville EA, Biddle AK, Lorig K. Efficacy of psychoeducational interventions on pain, depression, and disability in people with arthritis: a meta-analysis. J Rheumatol 1987; 14(suppl 15):33–39.

109. Bradley LA, Young LD, Anderson KO, Turner RA, Agudelo CA, McDaniel LK, Pisko EJ, Semble EL, Morgan TM. Effects of psychological therapy on pain behavior of rheumatoid arthritis patients: treatment outcome and six-month followup. Arthritis Rheum 1987; 30:1105–1114.

110. Lorig K, Konkol L, Gonzales V. Arthritis patient education: a review of the literature. Patient Educ Couns 1987; 10:207–252.

111. Lorig K. Arthritis self-management leader's manual (revised). Atlanta: Arthritis Foundation, 1984.

112. Lorig K, Seleznick M, Lubeck D, Ung E, Chastain RL, Holman HR. The beneficial outcomes of the arthritis self-management course are not adequately explained by behavior change. Arthritis Rheum 1989; 32:91–95.

113. Lorig K, Chastain RL, Ung E, Shoor S, Holman HR. Development and evaluation

of a scale to measure perceived self-efficacy in people with arthritis. Arthritis Rheum 1989; 32:37–44.

114. Bandura A, Adams NE, Beyer J. Cognitive processes mediating behavioral change. J Pers Soc Psychol 1977; 35:125–139.

14

First-Line Antirheumatic (Anti-Inflammatory) Drugs

Elizabeth A. Kitsis and Steven B. Abramson

New York University Medical Center
and
Hospital for Joint Diseases
New York, New York

I. INTRODUCTION

The Rev. Mr. Edmund Stone of Chipping Norton, Oxfordshire observed that the bark of the willow tree (*Salix alba*) was ''. . .very efficacious in curing anguish and intermitting disorders . . .'' (1). He made this observation in 1763—after treating 50 patients with willow extract—in a letter to the Royal Society in London suggesting that this folk remedy could relieve aches and fever. Salicin, the active component of willow bark, was isolated by Johann Buchner in 1828 at the Pharmacologic Institute of Munich. The compound was further purified, and named salicylic acid in 1838 by Raffaele Piria. Salicylic acid was proposed as a treatment for acute rheumatic fever in 1876, and shortly thereafter as a treatment for chronic polyarthritis (including rheumatoid arthritis), gout, and osteoarthritis.

It was not until 1949 that phenylbutazone, the first compound to be categorized as a nonsteroidal anti-inflammatory drug (NSAID), was introduced. In 1965, indomethacin was observed to inhibit carrageenan-induced inflammation in the rat paw. A large number of medications with similar properties were identified in this manner over the following years.

The NSAIDs, which possess both analgesic and anti-inflammatory properties, have been used to treat a variety of disorders since their discovery. Indeed, NSAIDs have historically been essential therapy for rheumatoid arthritis, having formed the base of the therapeutic pyramid, the traditional paradigm for the treatment of this disease.

In recent years, the recommendation that "NSAIDs be the mainstay of therapy in the treatment of rheumatoid arthritis" (2) has been challenged. This reevaluation is a consequence of the recognition that patients with rheumatoid arthritis have a more guarded prognosis than previously believed. A long-term study of 75 patients with rheumatoid arthritis revealed that 85% of those younger than 65 who were employed at the time of diagnosis stopped working within 9 years (3). Moreover, mortality is increased in patients with rheumatoid arthritis (4,5). Therefore, some have proposed that the pyramid be "inverted" and that therapeutic emphasis be shifted toward the earlier institution of disease-modifying anti-rheumatic drugs (DMARDs). For example, a "step-down bridge" model has been proposed (6). Therapy would begin with a combination of rapidly acting agents (NSAIDs, glucocorticoids), methotrexate, and slower-acting DMARDs. Rapidly acting drugs would be withdrawn after sufficient time had elapsed to permit the DMARDs to have taken effect. This alternative strategy presumes that DMARDs, but not rapidly acting agents, alter the natural course of rheumatoid arthritis. As will be discussed, both presumptions are the subjects of ongoing debate.

Thus, aspirinlike drugs have played a central, and at times exclusive, role in the treatment of rheumatoid arthritis for over a century. Although their place among available antirheumatic therapies is undergoing reevaluation, it is likely that NSAIDs will continue to have an important position in any new therapeutic model for the treatment of patients with chronic articular inflammation of unknown etiology. This chapter will, therefore, review their pharmacokinetics, mechanisms of action, toxicity, and clinical application.

II. PHARMACOLOGY

A. Chemical Properties

The classification of NSAIDs is based on their chemical formulation. Physicochemical differences lead to variable distribution in the body and to variable side effects. Most NSAIDs are organic acids and have a relatively low pK_a; therefore, they may accumulate at sites of inflammation where the pH is commonly acidic (7).

The NSAIDs circulate tightly bound to albumin, with "free" drug representing less than 10% of total plasma concentration. The concentration of an NSAID in synovial fluid is about 60% of the mean plasma concentration, reflecting lower levels of albumin in synovial fluid (8). Synovial fluid concentrations are independent of NSAID half-lives, which vary among drugs (8).

Pharmacokinetically, NSAIDs are nearly completely absorbed. These drugs display minimal first-pass metabolism, with the exceptions of indomethacin, meclofenamate, and sulindac. Most NSAIDs are converted to inactive metabolites in the liver and excreted primarily in the urine. Selected NSAIDs, such as nabumetone and sulindac, are administered as prodrugs and acquire the capacity to inhibit prostaglandin synthesis only after conversion to active metabolites in the liver. Most sulindac is excreted in inactive form in the urine. It has been suggested that these properties result in less gastrointestinal or renal toxicity from nabumetone and sulindac, respectively (9,10). However, clinical studies have not unequivocally confirmed such assertions.

B. Mechanisms of Action

The Vane Hypothesis

It is generally accepted that, at least in part, NSAIDs act by inhibiting prostaglandin synthesis, as demonstrated by Sir John Vane (11). Most NSAIDs block the enzyme prostaglandin H (PGH) synthase (12). The PGH synthase acts both as a cyclooxygenase that converts arachidonic acid to prostaglandin G_2, and as a peroxidase that converts prostaglandin G_2 to H_2.

The inhibition of prostaglandin production by NSAIDs may explain several clinical effects of these drugs. For example, prostaglandin-mediated erythema and edema, hallmarks of inflammation, are inhibited by NSAIDs. Local reduction of prostaglandins by NSAIDs may also account for their analgesic properties, although central mechanisms probably contribute as well. In addition, cyclooxygenase blockade may account for several side effects of NSAIDs, such as bronchospasm, peptic ulceration, platelet dysfunction, decreased glomerular filtration, and hypertension. The pathogenesis of NSAID-induced central nervous system disturbances, interstitial nephritis, and hepatitis is unclear; however, these effects do not appear to be caused by prostaglandin inhibition.

Nonprostaglandin Effects

The Vane hypothesis that NSAIDs exert anti-inflammatory effects exclusively by blocking prostaglandin synthesis is confounded by the observation that non-acetylated salicylates are poor inhibitors of the PGH synthase (13), but are as effective as other NSAIDs in their anti-inflammatory effects (14). Consistent with a lack of prostaglandin inhibition, nonacetylated salicylates do not inhibit platelet function and appear to have less gastrointestinal toxicity than other NSAIDs (15).

It is increasingly clear that NSAIDs have other pharmacological actions unrelated to their capacity to inhibit the enzyme PGH synthase (Table 1). For example, NSAIDs also promote T-cell proliferation and interleukin-2 (IL-2) production (16), uncouple oxidative phosphorylation (17), exert effects on the metabolism of cartilage and bone (18–20), inhibit anion movements in renal tubule cells, and induce heat-shock proteins in *Drosophila* species, none of which depend on prostaglandin inhibition. These agents may also modulate gene

Table 1 NSAID Effects That Are Not Due to the Inhibition of PGH Synthase

Inhibit proteoglycan synthesis by articular cartilage (18–21)
Inhibit message expression of PGH synthase (21)
Inhibit peripheral inflammation by central action (22)
Enhance T-cell proliferation and interleukin-2 production (16)
Inhibit neutrophil activation (28,29)

transcription. For example, recent work by Wu et al. (21) suggests that both aspirin and sodium salicylate inhibit interleukin 1-induced PGH synthase gene expression in cultured endothelium. This effect was not observed with indomethacin and was, therefore, believed to be independent of direct functional inhibition of PGH synthase.

Another possible site of action of NSAIDs involves the central nervous system. Catania et al. (22) recently demonstrated that aspirin and sodium salicylate inhibited edema, induced in the mouse ear by topical application of picryl chloride, when injected into the lateral cerebral ventricle. This was not a consequence of systemic effects of the drug, since systemic administration of comparable doses were ineffective. It was also unlikely that these effects were attributable to inhibition of prostaglandin synthesis, since the central administration of indomethacin at concentrations that were anti-inflammatory when injected intraperitoneally had no effect. This suggests that salicylates also act centrally to inhibit inflammatory in the periphery.

Further evidence that the inhibition of prostaglandins by NSAIDs may not fully explain their pharmacological effects is provided by reports that prostaglandins possess not only proinflammatory but also anti-inflammatory properties. In vivo, prostaglandins of the E series prevent the development of glomerulonephritis in NZB/NZW F_1 hybrid mice (23), inhibit the development of adjuvant arthritis in rats (24), and suppress the reverse passive Arthus reaction in rats (25). These effects may be partially mediated by inhibition of neutrophil activation. In vitro, prostaglandins of the E series and prostacyclin (prostaglandin I_2) inhibit the activation of platelets and mononuclear cells, as well as neutrophils (26–29). In addition, prostaglandin E_1 augments the inhibitory effects of NSAIDs on neutrophil activation (30).

A large body of evidence suggests that at least part of the anti-inflammatory effect of NSAIDs is due to their capacity to inhibit neutrophil activation, a property unrelated to effects on cyclooxygenase (31). A variety of other anti-inflammatory agents also exert inhibitory effects on neutrophils, including methotrexate (32), colchicine, and D-penicillamine (33). Similar to NSAIDs, these agents probably work by several mechanisms.

Is the overall inhibitory effect of NSAIDs on neutrophil activation clinically significant in patients with rheumatoid arthritis? Although various cells contribute to the initiation and propagation of the immune response in rheumatoid synovium (including neutrophils, macrophages, T lymphocytes, endothelial cells, fibroblasts, and synoviocytes), the neutrophil appears to play an important role in joint inflammation (34). Synovial fluid samples from rheumatoid arthritis patients are rich in neutrophils (35). It has been suggested that rheumatoid joint inflammation results from phagocytosis of rheumatoid factor–gamma globulin complexes by neutrophils, with subsequent release of their lysosomal enzymes and complement activation (36,37). Thus, inhibition of neutrophil activation by NSAIDs may diminish the inflammatory response characteristic of rheumatoid arthritis.

Additional studies have evaluated the effects of NSAIDs on the synthesis of proteoglycans by articular chondrocytes. Naproxen sodium, in contrast with salicylate, did not inhibit glycosaminoglycan synthesis by organ cultures of femoral condylar cartilage (19). This topic was reviewed by Brandt (20), who observed that articular cartilage degeneration in animal models is accelerated by aspirin administration. However, there is no evidence in humans that nonsalicylate NSAIDs, which do not inhibit synthesis of proteoglycans in experimental models, are "chondroprotective." Administration of NSAIDs inhibited joint swelling, but did not suppress matrix depletion of proteoglycan in murine antigen-induced arthritis (38). Steroids administered orally or locally, however, normalized chondrocyte proteoglycan synthesis.

III. CLINICAL ASPECTS OF FIRST-LINE THERAPY

A. Efficacy

The efficacy of antirheumatic therapy can be defined in terms of symptomatic relief and disease modification. Symptomatic relief has been measured by a variety of outcome variables, such as patient's global pain assessment, patient's evaluation of disease activity, physician's evaluation of disease activity, and joint count. It has been concluded from available studies that aspirin and other NSAIDs can lead to improvement in each of these variables in patients when compared with placebo (39). From existing literature, the use of multiple endpoints within a given study and different endpoints across studies may make the interpretation of results difficult. From a metanalysis of 130 placebo-controlled NSAID trials, Gotzsche (40) recommended recording only the patient's global assessment of effect, pain, and morning stiffness as effect variables. With these comments in mind, the following studies of NSAID efficacy are of some interest.

Although NSAIDs, in general, may effectively improve symptoms of rheumatoid arthritis, response rates to different NSAIDs may vary. The similarities and differences of NSAIDs have been reviewed recently in detail (41). Although aspirin is the prototype NSAID, it appears to be equally as effective as, but less well tolerated than, other drugs of this class (42). Huskisson et al. (43) studied

90 patients with rheumatoid arthritis in a double-blind, crossover trial comparing naproxen, ibuprofen, ketoprofen, and fenoprofen. Although naproxen and fenoprofen were slightly more effective than the other two drugs, and side effects were less common with naproxen and ibuprofen, there was significant diversity in individual response to each NSAID, despite minimal differences in disease activity.

Another double-blind, crossover study evaluated the same drugs after aspirin treatment, except for the substitution of tolmetin for ketoprofen (44). There was no significant difference in measurements of efficacy among the four drugs, although patients and physicians ranked the drugs in the same order of preference: naproxen, ibuprofen, fenoprofen, tolmetin, and aspirin.

Similar findings were reported by Wasner et al. (45). These investigators evaluated six NSAIDs, using a six-way multiple crossover design. They found minimal differences in response to each agent; however, patients had strong preferences for one drug over another, and no single agent was consistently preferred. In addition, the best predictor of drug preference was the number of pills required per day. Other factors that were suggested to have influenced patient preference included pill size, shape, effectiveness, and toxicity. An alternative explanation for the lack of correlation between response rate and individual patient preference is that comparative NSAID trials are fraught with methodological inadequacies (46).

In a study evaluating the use of NSAIDs in 15 rheumatology private practices, the median number of NSAIDs used was 15, with the most extensively used drug being taken by a mean of 21% of patients (47). This suggests that a variety of NSAIDs are used by private rheumatologists to treat patients with RA, a finding that might be relevant when determining the number of NSAIDs available within a formulary.

The foregoing studies evaluated short-term efficacy. The long-term efficacy of NSAID therapy is less clear. Available studies rarely exceeded 2 years and, more often, spanned 6 months. They also did not routinely analyze radiographic progression, functional status, or mortality rate, endpoints of interest in determining the effect of treatment on a chronic disease. In one of the largest and longest studies, 1220 patients with a variety of joint diseases (719 of whom had rheumatoid arthritis) who were taking flurbiprofen were followed for up to 5 years (48). Radiographic changes were not monitored, but there was a statistically significant improvement in functional capacity (except in elderly patients) up to 18 months after instituting treatment. This improvement was seen with all diseases studied.

A study of 116 patients, which analyzed the duration of NSAID use as an indirect index of combined efficacy and toxicity, reported that naproxen was used significantly longer than ibuprofen, sulindac, indomethacin, piroxicam, or tolmetin (49). Another drug survival study reported that at the end of 2 years, approximately 80% of patients remained on therapy with naproxen and diclo-fenac, whereas only 30% remained on therapy with indomethacin (50). Of note, more than 90% of these patients were also taking DMARDs.

A similar study of the long-term use of DMARDs reported that fewer than 10% of 154 patients with rheumatoid arthritis who were started on a regimen of hydroxychloroquine, gold, D-penicillamine, or azathioprine continued to take those agents at the end of 3 years (51). Most withdrawals were due to adverse reactions. A review of 60 published studies of DMARDs identified 17 that monitored radiographic changes for both experimental and control groups. This review concluded that only two of these studies (one of gold and one of cyclophos-phamide) documented inhibition of radiographic progression (52). Thus, al-though NSAIDs may be of limited practical long-term use and have minimal or, at best, questionable influence on the course of rheumatoid arthritis, drug survival data suggest that DMARDs do not appear to add a dramatic advantage (for further discussion of the role of DMARDs in rheumatoid arthritis, see Chap. 15).

The deliberate semantic distinction made between NSAIDs and the so-called disease-modifying antirheumatic drugs implies that the former do not influence the long-term course of rheumatoid arthritis, whereas the latter do. Is this implication justified? Although NSAIDs have not been proved to modify the course of rheumatoid arthritis, several studies have reported that patients who clinically respond to NSAIDs demonstrate a decrease in erythrocyte sedimenta-tion rate, C-reactive protein, and rheumatoid factor levels, as well as a decrease in the number of circulating activated T cells (53–55). Thus, it appears that NSAIDs may have more of an immunomodulatory effect than traditionally thought.

B. Toxicity

The NSAIDs are the most widely used medications in the world (56). Therefore, it is not surprising that they account for a large percentage of reported side effects experienced by patients taking medications. Twenty-one percent of adverse drug reactions reported to the Food and Drug Administration (FDA) in the United States, and 25% reported to the Committee on Safety of Medicines in the United Kingdom were attributed to NSAID use (57).

Gastrointestinal Toxicity

The NSAIDs are associated with multiple untoward events, involving the gastro-intestinal tract, liver, kidney, central nervous system, blood, integument, and possibly cartilage. Gastrointestinal side effects constitute their major toxicity. The NSAID-induced gastropathy in patients with rheumatoid arthritis has been estimated to account for 20,000 hospitalizations, at a cost of approximately 200 million dollars, and for 2600 deaths per year (58,59). Multivariate analysis of

2747 patients with rheumatoid arthritis followed at five ARAMIS centers identified older age, previous gastrointestinal complaints associated with NSAID use, previous hospitalization for NSAID gastropathy, steroid use, and level of disability as risk factors for serious NSAID-associated side effects (60).

A study comparing elderly patients hospitalized for peptic ulcer disease or upper gastrointestinal bleeding with elderly controls noted that use of nonaspirin NSAIDs was associated with an increased risk for serious gastrointestinal disease, that the risk correlated with dose, and that it was greatest in the first month of administration of drug (61). At least two additional studies have suggested that elderly patients are at greatest risk for fatal upper gastrointestinal bleeding or perforation (62,63), although another study reported no correlation between age and fatal gastrointestinal complications of NSAID administration (64).

The gastrointestinal problems associated with NSAID therapy include dyspepsia, esophagitis, gastritis, gastric erosion, and peptic ulcer disease. A specific gastrointestinal syndrome associated with NSAID use has been described, consisting preponderantly of endoscopically identified antral, prepyloric gastric lesions (59). However, the clinical significance of NSAID-induced gastrointestinal complications detected by endoscopy is uncertain. Gastrointestinal symptoms resulting in discontinuation of NSAID use occur in 2–10% of patients with rheumatic diseases; however, in one study, up to 40% of patients were reported to have asymptomatic erosions, ulcers, bleeding, or anemia (65). In another report, peptic ulcer disease or erosions, or both, were identified in 53% of 47 rheumatoid arthritis patients who had upper gastrointestinal endoscopies, many of whom were asymptomatic and did not have occult fecal blood loss (66). Moreover, pathological evidence of gastritis was documented in 85% of 52 patients with rheumatoid arthritis receiving NSAIDs (67). Gastritis was more likely to be symptomatic if it occurred in association with *Helicobacter* (*Campylobacter*) *pylori* infection.

Lesions occurring in association with NSAID use may result in gastrointestinal hemorrhage. Although the risk of gastrointestinal bleeding is clearly increased by the use of NSAIDs, the magnitude of this increase is unclear, and may range from 1.6- to 14-fold (68). Aspirin and other NSAIDs were implicated in 15–60% of hospital admissions for acute gastrointestinal bleeding (65).

A comparison of gastrointestinal complications reported to the Food and Drug Administration for eight NSAIDs over 12 years determined the highest rates of complications for piroxicam, tolmetin, and sulindac (69). However, such data may reflect reporting bias on the part of physicians. For example, a more recent review of the literature did not clearly indicate a higher risk of gastrointestinal toxicity with any particular NSAID (70).

The gastrointestinal toxicities of NSAIDs are mediated by several mechanisms. Inhibition of prostaglandin synthesis decreases esophageal sphincter tone and increases gastric acid production. This may result in esophageal reflux and consequent dyspepsia or esophagitis. Increased gastric acid production, decreased production of gastric mucus and bicarbonate, and inhibition of gastric mucosal cell proliferation predispose patients taking NSAIDs to the development of gastritis and peptic ulcer disease (15). Inhibition of platelet aggregation may exacerbate gastrointestinal bleeding.

Renal Toxicity

The reported incidence of significant renal side effects from NSAIDs is low. For example, in a study of 65,000 NSAID-treated outpatients, none were hospitalized for kidney disease associated with NSAID therapy (71). Similarly, there was no difference in the incidence of azotemia in a large group of hospitalized patients started on an NSAID regimen, when compared with patients who were not begun on such a regimen.

Nephrotoxicity can be caused by several mechanisms (72). Normally, prostaglandin E_1 and prostacyclin do not influence renal function. However, these prostanoids may become vital to the maintenance of renal function under conditions of decreased renal blood flow and increased catecholamine and angiotensin II levels (73). Thus, although normal subjects experience minimal and reversible nephrotoxicity from NSAIDs, patients who are hypovolemic or who have chronic renal insufficiency may develop significant inhibition of renal blood flow and resultant slowing of the glomerular filtration rate by inhibition of renal prostaglandin synthesis. These effects may result in fluid retention and edema. Severe reduction in medullary circulation may lead to papillary necrosis.

Other risk factors for renal insufficiency from NSAIDs include advanced age, cirrhosis with ascites, nephrotic syndrome, congestive heart failure, diuretic use, and evidence of renal vascular disease (74). NSAID-treated patients with diabetes, azotemia, and those taking potassium-sparing diuretics, angiotensin-converting enzyme inhibitors, or β-adrenergic blockers may develop hyperkalemia.

Acute renal failure with the nephrotic syndrome may occur in association with NSAID treatment (fenoprofen, indomethacin, tolmetin, naproxen; 74). This reaction is idiosyncratic. Unlike classic drug-induced allergic nephritis, it is uncommonly associated with eosinophilia, eosinophiluria, fever, or rash. Acute interstitial nephritis, without nephrotic range proteinuria, has been associated with naproxen, mefenamic acid, tolmetin, phenylbutazone, and zomepirac.

It has been suggested that sulindac has less nephrotoxicity than other NSAIDs because it is metabolized to an inactive form by the kidney (10). However, this assertion has been challenged by other studies that have reported nephrotoxicity associated with sulindac, especially in patients in high-risk groups who receive the drug at high dosages (75).

Hematological Toxicity

Nonaspirin NSAIDs may produce a bleeding diathesis by inhibiting platelet activation and aggregation through reversible cyclooxygenase inhibition (76).

Aspirin irreversibly acetylates platelet cyclooxygenase; platelets, which lack nuclei, cannot replenish dysfunctional cyclooxygenase. Thus, the anticoagulant effect of aspirin persists for 7–10 days, until a new generation of unaffected platelets is produced. The nonacetylated salicylates, which have negligible inhibitory effects on cyclooxygenase and, therefore, minimal effects on platelet aggregation, may be useful in situations for which the risk of bleeding is high.

The NSAIDs are rarely associated with blood dyscrasias, although agranulocytosis, aplastic anemia, and thrombocytopenia have been reported. These complications have been most commonly associated with indomethacin and phenylbutazone therapy, and occur with greater frequency in women older than 60 years of age (77).

Other Toxicity

Reversible, asymptomatic transaminitis occurs occasionally with nonaspirin NSAIDs (2.9%) and more often (5.4%) with aspirin in patients with rheumatoid arthritis (78). Risk factors for hepatotoxicity include rheumatoid arthritis, systemic lupus erythematosus, age, azotemia, prolonged duration of treatment, high dosages, and the use of several drugs. Liver disease may be more severe and, occasionally fatal, when accompanied by hyperbilirubinemia and a prolonged prothrombin time (79). Phenylbutazone and diclofenac, in particular, have been associated with particularly severe and sometimes fatal hepatotoxicity. This occurs more often in older patients and may take the form of cholestatic or granulomatous hepatitis (80).

A variety of skin rashes have been reported in association with NSAID use, including fixed drug eruptions, morbilliform rashes, photosensitivity, urticaria, vesiculobullous eruptions, serum sickness, exfoliative erythroderma, erythema multiforme, toxic epidermal necrolysis, and Stevens–Johnson syndrome. Rashes are most common with sulindac, meclofenamate, and piroxicam. The most severe cutaneous reactions are associated with phenylbutazone and oxyphenbutazone (81).

Patients taking ibuprofen, tolmetin, or sulindac may develop aseptic meningitis. This syndrome occurs more often in patients with systemic lupus erythematosus, and is characterized by fever, headache, stiff neck, and occasionally conjunctivitis, facial edema, and pruritus. Cerebrospinal fluid abnormalities include elevated protein concentrations and lymphocytosis (82–84).

Other central nervous system side effects associated with NSAID treatment are more common in the elderly. They include headache (particularly with indomethacin), confusion, drowsiness, dizziness, syncope, and seizures. Ibuprofen and naproxen may cause memory loss, cognitive dysfunction, loss of concentration, insomnia, irritability, and paranoia.

Anaphylactoid reactions have occurred in association with several NSAIDs, particularly tolmetin and zomepirac. Zomepirac was withdrawn from the market because of this problem (81).

Hypersensitivity reactions to NSAIDs are most common in patients with the triad of asthma, nasal polyps, and vasomotor rhinitis (85). Inhibition of cyclooxygenase diverts arachidonic acid metabolism to the lipoxygenase pathway, with increased production of leukotrienes C_4 and D_4 and resulting bronchospasm (Fig. 1). The use of nonacetylated salicylates (which do not effectively inhibit cyclooxygenase) in patients with aspirin-induced asthma was suggested by Szczeklik et al. (86,87), based on their study of 23 asthmatic patients. Choline magnesium trisalicylate 3000 mg/day po administered for 1 week produced no adverse respiratory symptoms and no significant changes in pulmonary function tests. As expected, administration of the drug did not lower serum thromboxane levels, despite therapeutic serum salicylate levels.

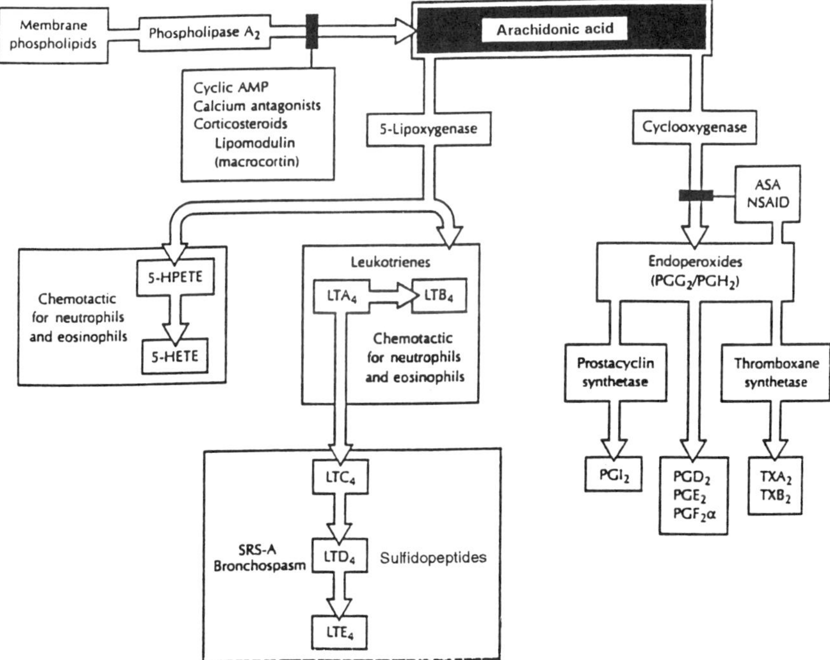

Fig. 1 Arachidonic acid: pathogenic mechanism for aspirin intolerance. SRS-A, LTC_4, LTD_4, AND LTE_4 are produced in increased quantities in the presence of cyclooxygenase inhibitors, such as aspirin and other nonsteroidal anti-inflammatory drugs. Aspirinlike drugs also reduce the production of PGI_2 and PGE_2, which are bronchodilators. Elevated AMP levels, calcium antagonists, and glucocorticoids are potent inhibitors of arachidonic acid liberation. LT, leukotriene; PG, prostaglandin; SRS-A, slow-reacting substance of anaphylaxis.

C. Interaction With Other Agents

Tonkin and Wing (88) comprehensively reviewed the interactions of NSAIDs with other drugs (Table 2). The NSAIDs have been implicated in the displacement of other acidic drugs from albumin. However, the dose-dependent displacement of warfarin, an acidic drug tightly bound to albumin, does not appear to alter the anticoagulant effect. It should be noted, though, that NSAIDs (particularly aspirin) inhibit platelet function and, therefore, are relatively contraindicated in patients taking warfarin.

Phenytoin also is displaced from albumin by NSAIDs. The resulting temporary increase in unbound phenytoin returns to the initial unbound concentration in the presence of normal hepatic function. However, there is a decrease in total plasma concentration of phenytoin; total drug levels are lower at the same unbound concentration. This effect is important in the determination of "therapeutic" drug levels.

Most NSAIDs decrease the renal clearance of lithium, resulting in increased lithium concentrations (88). Consequently, patients taking lithium and NSAIDs should have careful monitoring of lithium levels, especially when beginning or discontinuing NSAID treatment.

D. Prednisone Revisited

Philip Hench was awarded the Nobel Prize in Medicine and Physiology in 1950 for introducing cortisone as a treatment for rheumatoid arthritis and other inflammatory disorders. In fact, the studies of longest duration evaluating an NSAID in rheumatoid arthritis were done in the 1950s, comparing aspirin with prednisone. There were many methodological problems intrinsic to these studies (e.g., unclear disease definition, individualized dosage, lack of blinding); nevertheless, several interesting observations were made. Of four studies comparing aspirin with glucocorticoid therapy, one reported a significant improvement in functional class at the end of 3 years that was equivalent in the two groups (89,90), one observed no improvement (91,92), and two suggested a greater improvement in functional class in prednisone-treated patients (93–95). Evaluation of radiographic progression in three of these studies revealed a trend toward less progression in glucocorticoid-treated patients (90,92,94). A later study by West (96) reported on the long-term course of 74 of the patients evaluated in two trials (94,95). Nine of 39 prednisone-treated patients developed new erosions, whereas new erosions were identified in 32 of 34 analgesic (aspirin or phenylbutazone)-treated patients.

Thus, although the data are flawed and limited, it appears that prednisone, a drug generally considered to be "first-line" or "bridge" treatment, *may* have disease-modifying properties. Several mechanisms of anti-inflammatory action have been demonstrated for this drug (Table 3). Its cost is significantly less than

Table 2 Pharmacodynamic Interactions with NSAIDs

Drug affected	NSAIDs implicated	Effect	Approach to management
NSAID affecting other drug			
Oral anticoagulants	Phenylbutazone Oxyphenbutazone Azapropazone	Inhibition of metabolism of warfarin, increasing anticoagulant effect	Avoid NSAIDs if possible. Careful monitoring where unavoidable (note pharmacodynamic interactions also)
Lithium	Probably all NSAIDs (? except sulindac, aspirin)	Inhibition of renal excretion of lithium, increasing lithium serum concentrations, and increasing risk of toxicity	Use sulindac, aspirin if NSAID unavoidable. Careful monitoring of lithium concentration and appropriate dose reduction
Oral hypoglycemic agents	Phenylbutazone Oxyphenbutazone Azapropazone	Inhibition of metabolism of sulfonylurea drugs, prolonging half-life and increasing risk of hypoglycemia	Avoid this group of NSAIDs if possible; monitor blood sugar closely
Phenytoin	Phenylbutazone Oxyphenbutazone	Inhibition of metabolism of phenytoin, increasing plasma concentration and risk of toxicity	Avoid this group of NSAIDs if possible; if not, intensify therapeutic drug monitoring
	Other NSAIDs	Displacement of phenytoin from plasma protein, reducing total concentration for the same unbound (active) concentration	Careful interpretation of phenytoin total concentration: measurement of unbound concentration may be helpful
Methotrexate	Probably all NSAIDs	Reduced clearance of methotrexate (mechanism unclear), increasing plasma concentration and risk of severe toxicity	Simultaneous dosing is contraindicated. Use of NSAIDs between cycles of chemotherapy is probably safe
Sodium valproate	Aspirin	Inhibition of valproate metabolism, increasing plasma concentration	Avoid aspirin: dose monitoring of plasma concentration if other NSAID used

Table 2 Continued

Drug affected	NSAIDs implicated	Effect	Approach to management
Digoxin	All NSAIDs	Potential reduction in renal function (particularly in very young and very old), reducing digoxin clearance and increasing plasma concentration and risk of toxicity. (No interaction if renal function normal)	Avoid NSAIDs if possible; if not, frequent checks of digoxin plasma concentration and plasma creatinine
Antihypertensive agents β-Blockers Diuretics ACE inhibitors Vasodilators	Indomethacin Other NSAIDs (? except sulindac)	Reduction of hypotensive effect, probably related to inhibition of renal prostaglandin synthesis (producing salt and water retention) and vascular prostaglandin synthesis (producing increased vasoconstriction)	Avoid all NSAIDs in treated hypertensive patients if possible; if not, use sulindac preferentially. May need additional antihypertensive therapy
Diuretics	Indomethacin Other NSAIDs (? except sulindac)	Reduction in natriuretic and diuretic effects; exacerbate congestive cardiac failure	Avoid NSAIDs in patients with cardiac failure; use sulindac; monitor clinical signs of fluid retention
Anticoagulants	All NSAIDs	Gastrointestinal tract mucosal damage, together with inhibition of platelet aggregation, increasing risk of GI bleeding in patients taking anticoagulants	Avoid all NSAIDs if possible
Hypoglycemic agents	Salicylate (high-dose)	Potentiation of hypoglycemic effects (mechanism unknown)	Monitor blood sugar level
Combination with increased risk of toxicity Diuretics			

General	All NSAIDs	Combination associated with increased risk of hemodynamic renal failure	Avoid combination if possible
Triamterene	Indomethacin	Potentiation of nephrotoxicity, including in subjects with normal renal function	Combination contraindicated
Potassium-sparing	All NSAIDs	Potassium retention and hyperkalemia	Avoid combination: monitor K^+
Aminoglycosides	All NSAIDs	Reduction in renal function in susceptible individuals, reducing aminoglycoside clearance and increasing plasma concentration	Close plasma concentration monitoring and dose adjustment
Antacids	Indomethacin ? Other NSAIDs	Variable effects of different preparations: Aluminum-containing antacids reduce rate and extent of absorption of indomethacin Sodium bicarbonate increases rate and extent of absorption of indomethacin	No action required unless marked reduction in absorption results in poor response to NSAID; dose may need to be increased in this case
Probenecid	Probably all NSAIDs	Reduction in metabolism and renal clearance of NSAIDs and acylglucuronide metabolites that are hydrolyzed back to parent drug	May be used therapeutically to increase the response to a given dose of NSAID
Barbiturates	Phenylbutazone ? Other NSAIDs	Increased metabolic clearance of NSAID	May require higher doses of phenylbutazone
Caffeine	Aspirin	Increased rate of absorption of aspirin	No action required
Cholestyramine	Naproxen and probably other NSAIDs	Anion exchange resin binds NSAIDs in gut reducing rate (? and extent) of absorption	Separate dosing times by 4 h; may need higher than expected dose of NSAID
Metoclopramide	Aspirin	Increased rate and extent of absorption of aspirin in patients with migraine	May be used therapeutically

ACE, angiotensin-converting enzyme; GI, gastrointestinal.
Source: Ref. 8.

Table 3   Mechanisms of Anti-inflammatory Actions of Glucocorticoids

Stabilization of lysosomes (94,95)
Redirection of lymphocyte traffic (96–102)
Induction of protein synthesis (e.g., lipocortins; 103–106)
Inhibition of phospholipases (103)
Inhibition of metalloprotease and cyclooxygenase synthesis
Inhibition of secretion of cytokines (107–114)
Inhibition of expression of adhesion molecules on endothelial cells (115)

NSAIDs, and it may be administered once a day. For these reasons, some investigators have proposed the use of low-dose glucocorticoids for patients with rheumatoid arthritis, especially the elderly.

However, the consequences of long-term, low-dose prednisone therapy are unknown. The effect of low-dose prednisone on bone density, a major concern, has not been well defined (97–99). Recent reports suggest that a dose-dependent osteopenia is observed at doses above 5 mg/day of prednisone (100). The adverse effects of chronic low-dose prednisone on cataract formation and soft-tissue (tendon and ligament) integrity are additional considerations to be evaluated. These issues must be weighed against the documented toxicity of NSAIDs in some patients. Hence, the risk/benefit ratio of low-dose prednisone versus NSAIDs in the treatment of rheumatoid arthritis remains controversial. Until more data are available concerning the potential remittive properties and long-term adverse effects of low-dose glucocorticoid treatment, its primary role should be as bridge therapy, or first-line treatment for patients at high risk for complications from NSAIDs.

IV. CONCLUSION

The NSAIDs remain the agents traditionally recommended as first-line treatment for rheumatoid arthritis, whether used alone or in combination with glucocorticoids, methotrexate, or DMARDs. There has been a reevaluation of the role of prednisone in the treatment of rheumatoid arthritis.

Guidelines for selecting a particular NSAID should be based on individual patient needs and differences in properties of NSAIDs. In patients at high risk for bleeding, nonacetylated salicylates are preferable. These agents might also be cautiously prescribed for patients with asthma, nasal polyps, and allergic rhinitis, although confirmatory trials documenting safety for this indication are desirable. Phenylbutazone and indomethacin should be avoided in the elderly because of their increased risk of hepatotoxicity and central nervous system side effects, respectively. Indeed, in view of its bone marrow toxicity, phenylbutazone is rarely indicated. Patients with systemic lupus erythematosus should generally not be given ibuprofen, because of the risk of aseptic meningitis. Since compliance is always a primary consideration, NSAIDs that can be administered less often, such as piroxicam or naproxen, are preferable. Finally, although a clear biological explanation is lacking, patients who do not improve after an adequate trial of one NSAID might benefit from another.

REFERENCES

1. Weissmann G. Aspirin. Sci Am 1991; 1:84–90.
2. Katz WA. Rheumatoid arthritis. In: Roth SH, Calabro JJ, Paulus HE, Willkens RF, eds. Rheumatic therapeutics. New York: McGraw-Hill, 1985:3–18.
3. Pincus T, Callahan LF, Sale WG, Brooks AL, Payne LE, Vaughn WK. Severe functional declines, work disability, and increased mortality in seventy-five rheumatoid arthritis patients studied over nine years. Arthritis Rheum 1984; 27:864–872.
4. Abruzzo JL. Rheumatoid arthritis and mortality. Arch Rheum 1982; 25:1020–1023.
5. Pincus T, Callahan LF, Vaughn WK. Questionnaire, walking time and button test measures of functional capacity as predictive markers for mortality in rheumatoid arthritis. J Rheumatol 1987; 14:240–251.
6. Wilske KR, Healey LA. Challenging the therapeutic pyramid: a new look at treatment strategies for rheumatoid arthritis. J Rheumatol 1990; 17(suppl 25):4–7.
7. Cummings NA, Nordby GL. Measurement of synovial fluid pH in normal and arthritic knees. Arthritis Rheum 1966; 9:47–56.
8. Day RO, Graham GG, Williams KM. Pharmacokinetics of non-steroidal anti-inflammatory drugs. Baillieres Clin Rheumatol 1988; 2:363–393.
9. Dandona P, Jeremy JY. Nonsteroidal anti-inflammatory drug therapy and gastric side effects. Does nabumetone provide a solution? Drugs 1990; 40(suppl 5):16–24.
10. Bunning RD, Barth WF. Sulindac: a potentially renal sparing nonsteroidal antiinflammatory drug. JAMA 1982; 248:2864.
11. Vane JR. Inhibition of prostaglandin synthesis as a mechanism of action for aspirin-like drugs. Nature 1971; 231:232–235.
12. Kulmacz RJ. Topography of prostaglandin H synthase: antiinflammatory agents and the protease-sensitive arginine 253 region. J Biol Chem 1989; 254:14136–14144.
13. Abramson S, Korchak H, Ludewig R, et al. Modes of action of aspirin-like drugs. Proc Natl Acad Sci USA 1985; 82:7227–7231.
14. Altman RD. Neutrophil activation: an alternative to prostaglandin inhibition as the mechanism of action for NSAIDs. Semin Arthritis Rheum 1990; 19:1–5.
15. Scheiman JM, Elta GH. Gastroduodenal mucosal damage with salsalate versus aspirin. Results of experimental models and endoscopic studies in humans. Semin Arthritis Rheum 1990; 29:121–127.
16. Flescher E, Fossum D, Gray PJ, Fernandes G, Harper MJ, Talal N. Aspirin-like drugs prime human T cells. Modulation of intracellular calcium concentrations. J Immunol 1991; 146:2553–2559.

17. Miyahara JT, Karler R. Effect of salicylate on oxidative phosphorylation and respiration of mitochondrial fragments. Biochem J 1965; 97:194–198.

18. Palmoski MJ, Brandt KD. Effects of salicylate and indomethacin on glycosaminoglycan and prostaglandin E_2 synthesis in intact canine knee cartilage ex vivo. Arthritis Rheum 1984; 27:398–403.

19. Brandt KD, Albrecht M. Effect of naproxen sodium on the net synthesis of glycosaminoglycans and protein by normal canine articular cartilage in-vitro. J Pharm Pharmacol 1990; 42:738–740.

20. Brandt KD. The mechanism of action of nonsteroidal antiinflammatory drugs. J Rheumatol 1991; 27(suppl):120–121.

21. Wu KK, Sanduja R, Tsai AL, Ferhanoglu B, Loose-Mitchell DS. Aspirin inhibits interleukin 1-induced prostaglandin H synthase expression in cultured endothelial cells. Proc Natl Acad Sci USA 1991; 88:2384–2387.

22. Catania A, Arnold J, Macaluso A, Hiltz ME, Lipton JM. Inhibition of acute inflammation in the periphery by central action of salicylates. Proc Natl Acad Sci USA 1991; 88:8544–8547.

23. Zurier RB, Damjanov I, Sayadof DM, Rothfield NF. Prostaglandin E_1 treatment of NZB/NZW F_1 hybrid mice. Arthritis Rheum 1977; 20:1449–1456.

24. Zurier RB, Quagliata F. Effect of prostaglandin E_1 on adjuvant arthritis. Nature 1971; 234:304–306.

25. Kunkel SL, Thrall RS, Kunkel RG, McCormick JR, Ward PA, Zurier RB. Suppression of immune complex vasculitis in rats by prostaglandin. J Clin Invest 1979; 64:1525–1527.

26. Tateson JE, Moncada S, Vane JR. Effects of prostacyclin (PGX) on cyclic AMP concentrations in human platelets. Prostaglandins 1977; 13:389–399.

27. Weissmann G, Dukor P, Zurier RB. Effect of cyclic AMP on release of lysosomal enzymes from phagocytes. Nature 1971; 231:131–135.

28. Abramson SB, Korchak H, Ludewig R, et al. Modes of action of aspirin-like drugs. Proc Natl Acad Sci USA 1985; 82:7227–7231.

29. Abramson SB, Weissmann G. The mechanisms of action of nonsteroidal antiinflammatory drugs. Arthritis Rheum 1989; 32:1–9.

30. Kitsis EA, Weissmann G, Abramson SB. The prostaglandin paradox: additive inhibition of neutrophil function by aspirin-like drugs and the prostaglandin E_1 analog misoprostol. J Rheumatol 1991; 18:1461–1465.

31. Abramson SB, Cherksey B, Goode D, et al. Nonsteroidal antiinflammatory drugs exert differential effects on neutrophil function and plasma membrane viscosity. Inflammation 1990; 14:11–30.

32. Sperling RI, Coblyn JS, Larkin JK, Benincaso AI, Austen KF, Weinblatt ME. Inhibition of leukotriene B_4 synthesis in neutrophils from patients with rheumatoid arthritis by a single oral dose of methotrexate. Arthritis Rheum 1990; 33:1149–1155.

33. Auer DF, Ng JC, Seawright AA. Superoxide production by stimulated equine polymorphonuclear leukocytes: inhibition by anti-inflammatory drugs. J Vet Pharmacol Ther 1990; 13:59–66.

34. Kitsis EA, Weissmann G. The role of the neutrophil in rheumatoid arthritis. Clin Orthopaed Relat Res 1991; 265:63–72.

35. Hollingsworth JW, Siegel ER, Creasey WA. Granulocyte survival in synovial exudate of patients with rheumatoid arthritis and other inflammatory joint diseases. Yale J Biol Med 1992; 289:

36. Hollander JL, McCarty DJ Jr, Astorga G, Castro-Murillo E. Studies on the pathogenesis of rheumatoid joint inflammation. Ann Intern Med 1965; 62:271.

37. Ruddy S, Austen KF. The complement system in rheumatoid synovitis: an anlysis of complement component activities in rheumatoid synovial fluids. Arthritis Rheum 1970; 13:713.

38. Van den Berg WB. Impact of NSAID and steroids on cartilage destruction in murine antigen induced arthritis. J Rheumatol 1991; 27:122–123.

39. Harris JR. Management of rheumatoid arthritis. In: Kelley WN, Harris JR, Ruddy S, Sledge C, eds. Textbook of rheumatology. Philadelphia: WB Saunders, 1989:982–992.

40. Gotzsche PC. Sensitivity of effect variables in rheumatoid arthritis: a meta-analysis of 130 placebo controlled NSAID trials. J Clin Epidemiol 1990; 43:1313–1318.

41. Brooks PM, Day RO. Nonsteroidal antiinflammatory drugs—differences and similarities. N Engl J Med 1991; 24:1716–1725.

42. Heller CA, Ingelfinger JA, Goldman P. Nonsteroidal anti-inflammatory drugs and aspirin—analyzing the scores. Pharmacotherapy 1985; 5:30–38.

43. Huskisson EC, Woolf DL, Balme HW, Scott J, Franklyn S. Four new anti-inflammatory drugs: responses and variations. Br Med J 1976; 1:1048–1049.

44. Gall EP, Caperton EM, McComb JE, et al. Clinical comparison of ibuprofen, fenoprofen, calcium, naproxen and tolmetin sodium in rheumatoid arthritis. J Rheumatol 1982; 9:402–407.

45. Wasner C, Britton MC, Kraines G, Kaye RL, Bobrove AN, Fries JF. Non-steroidal anti-inflammatory agents in rheumatoid arthrtis and ankylosing spondylitis. JAMA 1981; 246:2168–2172.

46. Day RO. Variability in response to NSAIDs. Agents Action 1985; 17:15–19.

47. Pincus T, Callahan LF. Clinical use of multiple nonsteroidal antiinflammatory drug preparations within individual rheumatology private practices. J Rheumatol 1989; 16:1253–1258.

48. Sheldrake FE, Webber JM, Marsh BD. A long-term assessment of flurbiprofen. Curr Med Res Opin 1977; 5:106–116.

49. Luggen ME, Gartside PS, Hess EV. Nonsteroidal antiinflammatory drugs in rheumatoid arthritis: duration of use as a measure of relative value. J Rheumatol 1989; 16:1565–1569.

50. Wifnands M, Riel PV, Hof MV, Gribnau F, Putte LV. Long-term treatment with nosteroial antiinflammatory drugs in rheumatoid arthritis: a prospective drug survival study. J Rheumatol 1991; 18:184–187.

51. Thompson PW, Kirwan JR, Barnes CG. Practical results of treatment with disease-modifying antirheumatic durgs. Br J Rheumatol 1985; 24:167–175.

52. Iannuzzi L, Dawson N, Zein M, Kushner I. Does drug therapy slow radiographic deterioration in rheumatoid arthritis? N Engl J Med 1983; 309:1023–1028.

53. Cush JJ, Jasin HE, Johnson R, Lipsky PE. Relationship between clinical efficacy and laboratory correlates of inflammatory and immunologic activity in rheumatoid

arthritis patients treated with nonsteroidal antiinflammatory drugs. Arthritis Rheum 1990;

54. Cush JJ, Lipsky PE, Postlethwaite AE, Schrohenloher RE, Saway A, Koopman WJ. Correlation of serological indicators of inflammation with effectiveness of nonsteroidal anti-inflammatory drug therapy in rheumatoid arthritis. Arthritis Rheum 1990; 33:19–28.

55. Goodwin JS, Ceuppens JL, Rodriguez MA. Administration of nonsteroidal anti-inflammatory agents in patients with rheumatoid arthritis: effects on indexes of cellular immune status and serum rheumatoid factor levels. JAMA 1983; 250:2485–2488.

56. Roth SH. Arthritis therapy today: progress and pitfalls. Med Times 1989; Dec:

57. Langman MJS. Ulcer complications and nonsteroidal antiinflammatory drugs. Am J Med 1988; 84(suppl 2A):15–19.

58. Fries JF, Miller SR, Spitz PW, Williams CA, Hubert HB, Bloch DA. Toward an epidemiology of gastropathy associated with nonsteroidal antiinflammatory drug use. Gastroenterology 1989; 96:647–655.

59. Fries JF, Miller SR, Spitz PW, Williams CA, Hubert HB, Bloch DA. Identification of patients at risk for gastropathy associated with NSAID use. J Rheumatol 1990; 17(suppl 20):12–19.

60. Fries JF, Williams CA, Bloch DA, Michel BA. Nonsteroidal anti-inflammatory drug-associated gastropathy: incidence and risk factor models. Am J Med 1991; 91:213–222.

61. Griffin MR, Piper JM, Daugherty JR, Snowden M, Ray WA. Nonsteroidal anti-inflammatory drug use and increased risk for peptic ulcer disease in elderly persons. Ann Intern Med 1991; 114:257–263.

62. Collier DStJ, Pain JA. Nonsteroidal anti-inflammatory drugs and peptic ulcer perforation. Gut 1985; 26:359–363.

63. Guess HA, West R, Strand HM, et al. Fatal upper gastrointestinal hemorrhage or perforation among users and nonusers of nonsteroidal anti-inflammation drugs in Saskatchewan, Canada, 1983. J Clin Epidemiol 1988; 41:35–45.

64. Carson JL, Strom BL, Morse ML, et al. The relative gastrointestinal toxicity of the nonsteroidal anti-inflammatory drugs. Arch Intern Med 1987; 147:1054–1059.

65. Butt JH, Barthel JS, Moore RA. Clinical spectrum of upper gastrointestinal effects of nonsteroidal anti-inflammatory drugs. Am J Med 1984; 84(suppl 2A):5–14.

66. Semble E, Turner R, Wu W. Clinical and genetic characteristics of upper gastrointestinal disease in rheumatoid arthritis. J Rheumatol 1987; 14:692–699.

67. Upadhyay R, Howatson A, McKinlay A, Danesh BJZ, Sturrock RD, Russell RI. *Campylobacter pylori* associated gastritis in patients with rheumatoid arthritis taking nonsteroidal antiinflammatory drugs. Br J Rheumatol 1988; 27:113–116.

68. Strom BL, Taragin MI, Carson JL. Gastrointestinal bleeding from nonsteroidal anti-inflammatory drugs. Agents Action 1990; 29:27–38.

69. Rossi AC, Hsu JP, Faich GA. Ulcerogenicity of piroxicam: an analysis of spontaneously reported data. Br Med J 1987; 294:147–150.

70. Strom BL, Taragin MI, Carson JL. Gastrointestinal bleeding from nonsteroidal anti-inflammatory drugs. Agents Actions 1990; 29:27–38.

71. Fox DA, Jick H. Nonsteroidal anti-inflammatory drugs and renal disease. JAMA 1984; 251:1299–1300.

72. Lifschitz MD. Renal effects of non-steroidal anti-inflammatory agents. J Lab Clin Med 1983; 102:313–324.

73. DiBona GF. Prostaglandins and nonsteroidal anti-inflammatory drugs. Effects on renal hemodynamics. Am J Med 1986; 80(suppl 1A):12.

74. Clive DM, Stoff JS. Renal syndromes associated with nonsteroidal antiinflammatory drugs. N Engl J Med 1984; 310:563–572.

75. Brater DC, Anderson S, Baird B, Campbell WB. Sulindac does not spare the kidney. Clin Pharmacol Ther 1984; 35:269.

76. Burch JW, Stanford N, Majerus PW. Inhibition of platelet prostaglandin synthetase by oral aspirin. J Clin Invest 1978; 61:314–319.

77. Paulus HE. Government affairs: FDA Arthritis Advisory Committee meeting. Arthritis Rheum 1985; 28:450.

78. Paulus HE. Government affairs: FDA Arthritis Advisory Committee meeting. Arthritis Rheum 1982; 25:1124.

79. Benson GD. Hepatotoxicity following the therapeutic use of antipyretic analgesics. Am J Med 1983; 75(suppl):85.

80. Benjamin SB, Ishak KG, Zimmerman HJ, Grushka A. Phenylbutazone liver injury: a clinical–pathologic survey of 23 patients and review of the literature. Hepatology 1981; 1:255.

81. O'Brien WM, Bagby GF. Rare adverse reactions to nonsteroidal antiinflammatory drugs. J Rheumatol 1985; 12:13.

82. Wibener HL, Littman BH. Ibuprofen-induced meningitis in systemic lupus erythematosus. JAMA 1978; 239:1062–1064.

83. Ruppert GB, Barth WF. Tolmetin-induced aseptic meningitis. JAMA 1981; 245:67–68.

84. Von Regn CF. Recurrent aseptic meningitis due to sulindac. Ann Intern Med 1983; 99:343–344.

85. Szczeklik A. Antipyretic analgesics and the allergic patient. Am J Med 1983; 75:82.

86. Szczeklik A, Nizankowska E, Dworski R. Choline magnesium trisalicylate in patients with aspirin-induced asthma. Eur Respir J 1990; 3:535–539.

87. Szczeklik A. Aspirin-induced asthma: new insights into pathogenesis and clinical presentation of drug intolerance. Int Arch Allergy Appl Immunol 1989; 90:70–75.

88. Tonkin AL, Wing LM. Interactions of nonsteroidal antiinflammatory drugs. Baillieres Clin Rheumatol 1988; 2:455–481.

89. Joint committee of the Medical Research Council and Nuffield Foundation. A comparison of cortisone and aspirin in the treatment of early cases of rheumatoid arthritis. Br Med J 1954; 1223–1227.

90. Joint committee of the Medical Research Council and Nuffield Foundation. A comparison of cortisone and aspirin in the treatment of early cases of rheumatoid arthritis. Br Med J 1955; 695–700.

91. Empire Rheumatism Council. Multi-centre controlled trial comparing cortisone acetate and acetyl salicylic acid in the long-term treatment of rheumatoid arthritis: results up to one year. Ann Rheum Dis 1955; 14:353–370.

92. Empire Rheumatism Council. Multi-centre controlled trial comparing cortisone acetate and acetyl salicylic acid in the long-term treatment of rheumatoid arthritis: results of three years' treatment. Ann Rheum Dis 1957; 16:277–288.

93. Joint committee of the Medical Research Council and Nuffield Foundation. A comparison of cortisone and prednisone in the treatment of rheumatoid arthritis. Br Med J 1957; 199–202.

94. Joint committee of the Medical Research Council and Nuffield Foundation. A comparison of prednisone with aspirin or other analgesics in the treatment of rheumatoid arthritis. Ann Rheum Dis 1959; 18:173–188.

95. Joint committee of the Medical Research Council and Nuffield Foundation. A comparison of prednisolone with aspirin or other analgesics in the treatment of rheumatoid arthritis. Ann Rheum Dis 1960; 19:331–337.

96. West HF. Rheumatoid arthritis: the relevance of clinical knowledge to research activities. Abstr World Med 1967; 41:401–417.

97. Sambrook PN, Eisman JA, Yeates MG. Osteoporosis in rheumatoid arthritis: safety of low dose corticosteroids. Ann Rheum Dis 1986; 45:950–953.

98. Sambrook PN, Cohen ML, Eisman JA. Effects of low dose corticosteroids on bone mass in rheumatoid arthritis: a longitudinal study. Ann Rheum Dis 1989; 48:535–538.

99. Gluck OS, Murphy WA, Hahn TJ, Hahn B. Bone loss in adults receiving alternate day glucocorticoid therapy. Arthritis Rheum 1981; 24:892–898.

100. Buckley L, Leib E, Cooper S. Effects of low dose corticosteroids on bone mineral density in patients with rheumatoid arthritis. ACR 1992; (abstr):20.

101. Weissmann G, Thomas L. Studies on lysosomes. II. The effect of cortisone on the release of acid hydrolases from a large granule fraction of rabbit liver induced by an excess of vitamin A. J Clin Invest 1963; 42:661–669.

102. Bangham AD, Standish MM, Weissmann G. The action of steroids and streptolysin on the permeability of phospholipid structures to cations. J Mol Biol 1965; 13:253–259.

103. Samuels HH, Tomkins GM. Relation of steroid structure to enzyme induction in hepatoma tissue culture cells. J Mol Biol 1970; 52:57–74.

104. Fauci AS, Dale DC. The effect of hydrocortisone on the kinetics of normal human lymphocytes. Blood 1975; 46:235–243.

105. Fauci AS, Dale DC. The effect of in vivo hydrocortisone on subpopulations of human lymphocytes. J Clin Invest 1974; 53:240–246.

106. Fauci AS, Dale DC, Balow JE. Glucocorticosteroid therapy: mechanisms of action and clinical considerations. Ann Intern Med 1976; 84:304–315.

107. Fauci AS. Human bone marrow lymphocytes. I. Distribution of lymphocyte subpopulations in the bone marrow of normal individuals. J Clin Invest 1975; 56:98–110.

108. Dale DC, Fauci AS, Guerry DIV, Wolff SM. Comparison of agents producing a neutrophilic leukocytosis in man. Hydrocortisone, prednisone, endotoxin, and etiocholanolone. J Clin Invest 1975; 56:808–813.

109. Parrillo JE, Fauci AS. Mechanisms of glucocorticoid action on immune processes. Annu Rev Pharmacol Toxicol 1979; 19:179–201.

110. Blackwell GJ, Flower RJ, Nijkamp FP, Vane JR. Phospholipase A_2 activity of guinea-pig isolated perfused lungs: stimulation, and inhibition by anti-inflammatory steroids. Br J Pharmacol 1978; 62:79–89.

111. Di Rosa M, Flower RJ, Hirata F, Parente L, Russo-Marie F. Anti-phospholipase proteins. Prostaglandins 1984; 28:441–442.

112. Larsen C, Zachariae C, Mukaida N, et al. In: Cytokines and lipocortins in inflammation and differentiation. New York: Wiley–Liss, 1990:419–431.

113. Flower RJ. Background and discovery of lipocortins. Agents Action 1986; 17:255–262.

114. Bochner BS, Rutledge BK, Schleimer RP. Interleukin 1 production by human lung tissue. II. Inhibition by anti-inflammatory steroids. J Immunol 1987; 139:2303–2307.

115. Djaldetti R, Rishman P, Shtatlender V, Sredni B, Djaldetti M. Effect of dexamethasone on IL-1 and IL-3-LA release by unstimulated human mononuclear cells. Biomed Pharmacother 1990; 44:515–518.

116. Kirnbauer R, Kock A, Neuner P, et al. Regulation of epidermal cell interleukin-6 production by UV light and corticosteroids, J Invest Dermatol 1991; 96:484–489.

117. Chensue SW, Terebuh PD, Remick DG, Scales WE, Kunkel SL. In vivo biologic and immunohistochemical analysis of interleukin-1 alpha, beta and tumor necrosis factor during experimental endotoxemia. Kinetics, Kupffer cell expression, and glucocorticoid effects. Am J Pathol 1991; 138:395–402.

118. Zuckerman SH, Shellhaas J, Butler LD. Differential regulation of lipopolysaccharide-induced interleukin 1 and tumor necrosis factor synthesis: effects of endogenous and exogenous glucocorticoids and the role of the pituitary–adrenal axis. Eur J Immunol 1989; 19:301–305.

119. Knudsen PJ, Dinarello CA, Strom TB. Glucocorticoids inhibit transcriptional and post-transcriptional expression of interleukin 1 in U937 cells. J Immunol 1987; 139:4129–4134.

120. Dinarello CA, Mier JW. Lymphokines. N Engl J Med 1987; 317:940–945.

121. Beutler B, Cerami A. The biology of cachectin/TNF—a primary mediator of the host response. Annu Rev Immunol 1989; 7:625–655.

122. Cronstein BN, Kimmel SC, Levin RI, Martiniuk F, Weissmann G. A mechanism for the antiinflammatory effects of corticosteroids: the glucocorticoid receptor regulates leukocyte adhesion to endothelial cells and expression of ELAM-1 and ICAM-1. Proc Natl Acad Sci USA 1992; (in press).

15

Second-Line Antirheumatic Therapies

David T. Felson

Boston University School of Medicine
Boston, Massachusetts

I. INTRODUCTION

In the traditional pyramid approach to treatment of rheumatoid arthritis, failure of first-line therapy consisting of nonsteroidal anti-inflammatory drugs (NSAIDs) or salicylates leads to the inauguration of treatment with second-line drugs. In the past, when this approach to therapy was widely accepted and when all the drugs in the second-line drugs category appeared to have slow onset of action and effects on immunological function, rather than inflammation, the category made sense. Furthermore, some second-line drugs appeared to retard radiological progression of disease and, therefore, were thought of as either remission-inducing or disease-modifying antirheumatic drugs (DMARDs).

However, the pyramid approach to treatment has been challenged (1), and ''second-line'' drugs may actually be used very early in treatment (i.e., as first-line agents). Furthermore, some newer members of this category, especially methotrexate, have a rapid onset of action and also may affect inflammatory mediators such as leukotrienes (2). The mechanism of action of second-line drugs is uncertain, raising doubt about whether they should all be classified together. Finally, the studies of Pincus (3) and Wolfe (4) suggest that patients taking these drugs experience long-term deterioration in function and probably radiological progression. Therefore, their role as remission-inducing or even disease-modifying has been thrown into doubt. This chapter will consist of an evaluation of the comparative efficacy and toxicity of commonly used second-line drugs in rheumatoid arthritis, even though the concept that there is a category of second-line drugs may become increasingly obsolete. Nonetheless, the drugs to be evaluated here, including methotrexate, auranofin, injectable gold, penicillamine, sulfasalazine, and azathioprine, will continue to be widely used in the treatment of rheumatoid arthritis, irrespective of how their use is conceptualized. One second-line drug, cyclosporine, will not be reviewed here. Cyclosporine, which has documented efficacy in rheumatoid arthritis, has not become widely used, in part, because it causes renal impairment, which may become irreversible with continued use.

From quantitative synthesis of data from clinical trials, this chapter presents a critical review of which second-line drugs perform best from the perspectives of efficacy and toxicity. Because the clinical trial perspective is short-term and rheumatoid arthritis is a chronic disease, the successful use of these drugs over the long-term will also be reviewed. Lastly, there will be an evaluation of how to evaluate potential new second-line drugs to compare them with those currently available and determine if new candidates offer advantages in therapy.

II. COMPARATIVE EFFICACY OF SECOND-LINE DRUGS

Of the second-line drugs currently available to treat rheumatoid arthritis (RA), all have been more effective than placebo in clinical trials. However, little is known of their relative efficacy, for clinical trials containing head-to-head comparisons of these agents have, in general, failed to document differences between these drugs. Failure to detect differences between drugs in a clinical trial does not necessarily mean that clinically important differences do not exist. However, comparing two effective drugs requires a larger sample size than testing an effective drug against placebo, and it demands attention to clinical trial methods that will maximize the ability to detect differences between effective drugs. One way of detecting small differences when individual trials have failed to detect them is to perform a metanalysis, in which one quantitatively synthesizes data from multiple trials to enhance statistical power. The work presented here is derived from a metanalysis of second-line drug clinical trials (5,6).

We looked for all clinical trials in which second-line drugs were used to treat rheumatoid arthritis. This search included both MEDLINE searches and bibliographic reviews. We restricted our metanalysis to clinical trials of adults, at least 18 years and older, of whom at least 90% had rheumatoid arthritis. Patients must have been assigned to treatment regimens by either random or quasirandom processes; historically controlled trials were excluded. We studied the following drugs, choosing minimally effective doses from literature review: antimalarial drugs, including hydroxychloroquine at a dosage of at least 200 mg/ day and chloroquine at a dose of at least 250 mg/day; injectable gold at a dose of 50 mg/week; auranofin at a dose of at least 6 mg/day; D-penicillamine at a dose of at least 500 mg/day; methotrexate either orally or parenterally at a dose of at least 7.5 mg/week; and sulfasalazine at a dose of at least 2 g/day. We also defined placebo controls as those taking either a true placebo or a trivial dose of effective drug ($< 5\%$ of the minimum effective dose). We required that the duration of the clinical trial be at least 2 months, since many second-line drugs are not effective before this time.

To perform the metanalysis we required numerical values for the tender joint count (or Ritchie articular index), erythrocyte sedimentation rate (ESR), or grip strength or a combination thereof. We had found that these three outcome measures were especially sensitive and nonredundant in measuring improvement in RA clinical trials (7). For each trial, we identified the treatment arm of interest and extracted those data, taking the treatment group out of its trial. For example, for a placebo-controlled trial of injectable gold and auranofin, we analyzed the three treatment arms: injectable gold, auranofin, and placebo. Also, we chose the interval closest to 6 months of therapy for analysis.

From the trial reports, we also extracted information on other factors related to outcome, including mean age, disease duration, initial tender joint count, length of study, year of publication, percentage receiving corticosteroids, and so on. We determined that those factors relevant for efficacy were different for each efficacy variable. For example, for grip strength, the longer the disease duration of the treatment group, the less change occurred in grip strength. For joint count, the initial tender joint count and whether the evaluator was blinded or not affected the amount of improvement in tender joint count experienced by patients in the trial. For ESR, there were no factors that affected improvement other than drug treatment. We also computed a combined effect size improvement, called the composite treatment effect, which was based on the standardized improvements in tender joint count, ESR, and grip strength.

We found 79 trials, which contained 147 treatment groups studying second-line drugs. A total of 6518 patients entered the trials and 4904 completed them. The mean number of patients per treatment group was approximately 34.

Figure 1 shows the composite treatment effect for each drug studied; the effect being a combination of improvement in tender joint count, grip strength, and ESR, each of which is adjusted for factors that affect its change. Results suggest that there are four strong second-line drugs in rheumatoid arthritis, injectable gold, methotrexate, D-penicillamine, and sulfasalazine. Two drugs are intermediate in efficacy, antimalarial drugs and azathioprine. Auranofin is weaker than the other second-line drugs, with the difference between auranofin and the four strong drugs highly significant ($p < 0.0001$). All drugs were significantly more efficacious than placebo.

Regardless of which outcome measures were used, most were consistent in rankings, with methotrexate and sulfasalazine scoring among the strongest drugs. Auranofin also was the weakest of the drugs for almost all outcome measures. However, since azathioprine has little effect on ESR, including ESR

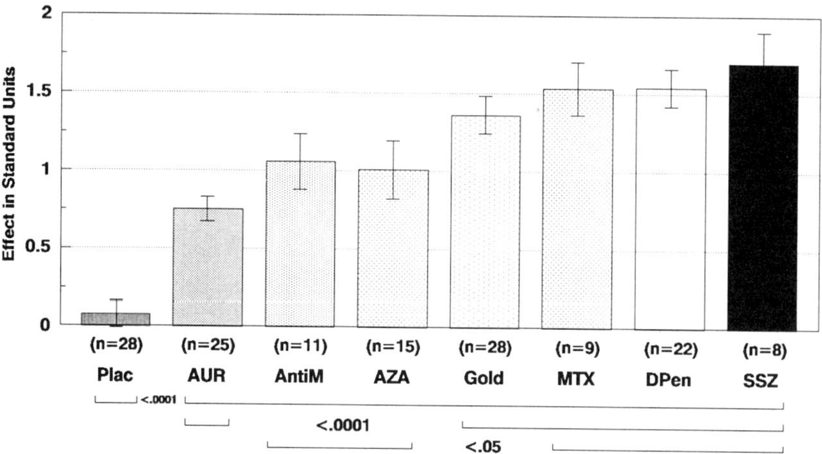

Fig. 1 Standard composite treatment effect. Composite of grip strength (adjusted for disease duration and trial length), tender joint count (adjusted for initial TJC and blinding), and ESR.

in efficacy assessment may bias results against it. Azathioprine, in fact, tied for third among second-line drugs in improvement in tender joint count.

Although our analysis combined data on hydroxychloroquine and chloroquine, clinical trial results, in fact, suggested that chloroquine was more effective than hydroxychloroquine (Fig. 2). Although these two drugs have never been directly compared in a clinical trial, the average improvement experienced by patients receiving chloroquine was consistently higher than that of patients taking hydroxychloroquine, even though the dosage of hydroxychloroquine used in clinical trials was often much higher.

Because we did not find significant differences between some drugs, especially the four most potent, we performed a power analysis to investigate how large a study would be needed to detect significant differences (Table 1). Differences between drugs are expressed in "effect size" units, the same units as the composite outcome measure (see Fig. 1). To demonstrate a difference between any of the strong drugs (an effect size difference of 0.10), a two-drug comparative trial should contain 3000 patients, 1500 per drug. To detect a difference between a stronger and weaker second-line drug, such as methotrexate and auranofin, a difference of approximately 0.30, a two-drug comparative trial should contain 340 patients. These numbers contrast with the average size of treatment groups in trials, 34 patients.

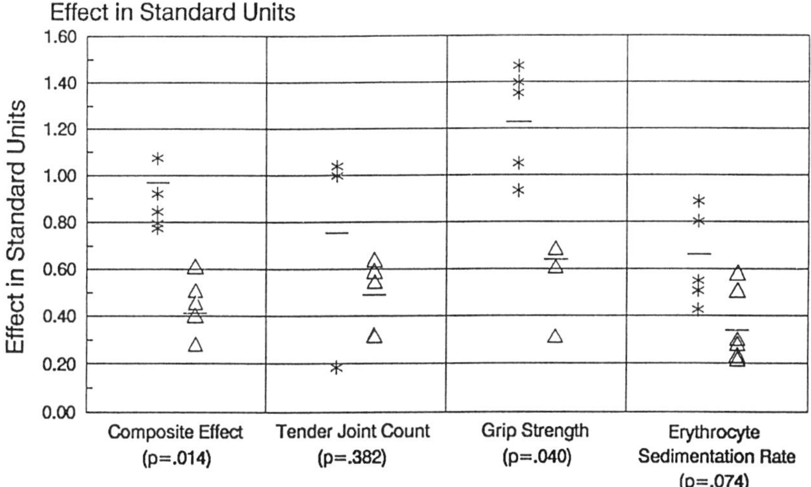

Fig. 2   Antimalarials: hydroxychloroquine (Δ) vs chloroquine (*). (From Ref. 5.)

III. COMPARATIVE TOXICITY OF SECOND-LINE DRUGS

We extended our metanalysis to evaluate the toxicity of second-line drugs, using data from clinical trials. *Toxicity* was defined as side effects severe enough to lead to dropout from a trial. The other methods of the metanalysis were essentially the same as in the efficacy study. By using a toxicity index developed by Fries et al. (8) and modifying it slightly to include information on mild laboratory toxicities (e.g., abnormal liver functions tests, proteinuria), we rated each toxicity for its severity. The toxicity index weights such side effects as renal failure higher than others, such as nausea or skin rash.

Injectable gold had the highest overall toxicity rate when measured by the toxicity index (Fig. 3). Its toxicity rate was significantly higher ($p < 0.001$) than all other drugs and than placebo. Antimalarial drugs had a low toxicity rate, significantly lower than methotrexate, sulfasalazine, and D-penicillamine.

Because the choice of drugs in clinical practice is often motivated by the fear of very serious toxicity and less by the expected risk of modest side effects, we separately analyzed severe toxicities, which we defined, in general, as organ-related side effects (e.g., renal failure, heavy proteinuria, thrombocytopenia). For severe toxicity (Fig. 4), we found nearly comparable rates among D-penicillamine and gold-treated patients, a result that suggests that life-threatening toxicities for gold and penicillamine are similar in frequency. The rate of serious

Table 1 Trial Size Needed to Detect Differences in Efficacy Between Second-Line Drugs Used to Treat Rheumatoid Arthritis[a]

	Actual difference in efficacy (in standardized effect units)				
	0.10[b]	0.20	0.30[c]	0.40	0.50
2-drug comparative trial					
No. per drug	1500	400	170	96	62
No. per trial	3000	800	340	192	124
3-drug comparative trial					
No. per drug	1300	325	143	80	52
No. per trial	3900	975	429	240	156

[a]Power = 80%, α = 0.05 (2-sided).
[b]Approximate difference between drugs in the stronger group of slow-acting drugs (methotrexate, injectable gold, D-penicillamine, sulfasalazine).
[c]Approximate difference between auranofin and each drug in the stronger group of slow-acting drugs.
Source: Ref. 5.

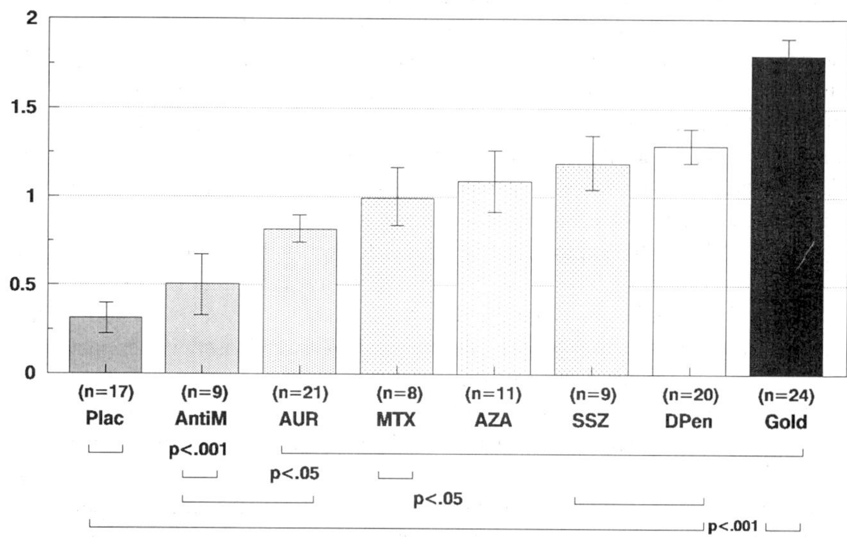

Fig. 3 Toxicity index. Modified Fries index, adjusted for disease duration and length of study.

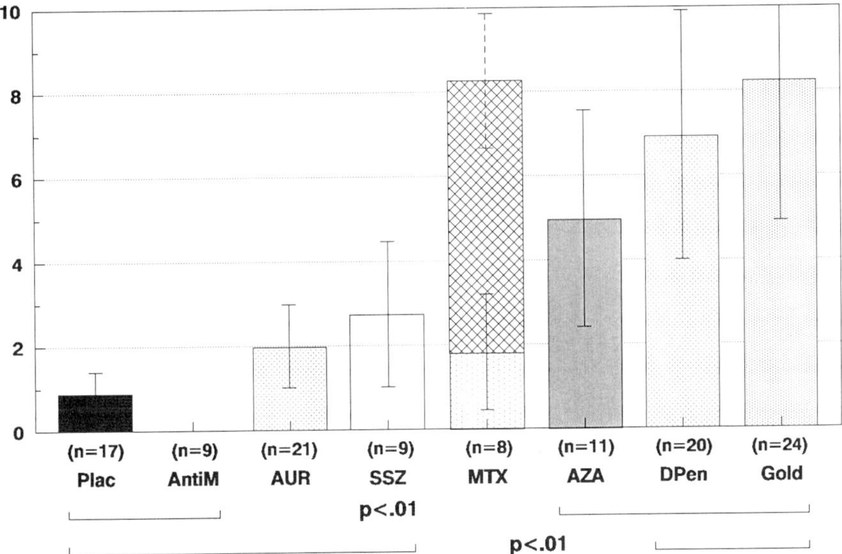

Fig. 4 Severe toxicity (%).

adverse events in patients receiving methotrexate was equivocal because of the variability in rates across clinical trials. If one considers as severe toxicity, liver function abnormalities that reach twice normal, then the rate of methotrexate-induced severe toxicity may be comparable with that of injectable gold. If, on the other hand, liver function tests elevated to twice normal do not necessarily lead to drug discontinuation and are not thought of as severe side effects, then the severe toxicity rate for methotrexate may be low, comparable with that of sulfasalazine or auranofin. Note that no patient in clinical trials suffered severe side effects while receiving antimalarial drugs. In general, few patients in clinical trials experience severe toxicity, and the rarity of these events in trials limits the prognostication of severe toxicity rates.

IV. EFFICACY–TOXICITY TRADE-OFFS

The preferred drugs to treat any condition should provide maximal efficacy, with the least toxicity. From the efficacy and toxicity data provided by the metanalysis, we compared second-line drugs to assess which drugs provide the most efficacy with the least side effects. Barring other considerations (e.g., cost, convenience), these should be the first choice among second-line drugs.

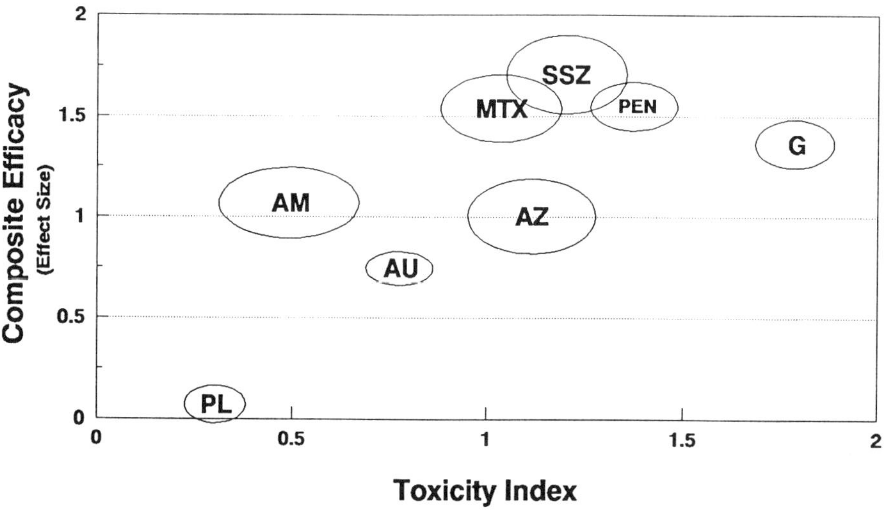

Fig. 5   Composite efficacy vs toxicity index. (From Ref. 6.)

When we plotted composite efficacy against toxicity (Fig. 5), three drugs—
methotrexate, sulfasalazine, and antimalarials—fell closest to the left upperhand
corner and, therefore, provided the maximal efficacy for the least toxicity. Among
the four strong drugs, methotrexate and sulfasalazine have comparable toxicity,
although methotrexate's may be slightly less. Among the weak second-line drugs,
antimalarial drugs have much less toxicity. Other perspectives, using different
definitions of efficacy and toxicity, yielded essentially the same answer: the
two drugs that provide the best trade-offs in terms of efficacy and toxicity are
methotrexate and antimalarial drugs and, in many circumstances, sulfasalazine
comes in a close third.

V.   LONG-TERM STUDIES OF SECOND-LINE DRUGS

Clinical trials in rheumatoid arthritis take a short-term perspective, usually 6
months to a year, whereas rheumatoid arthritis is a long-term chronic disease.
Clinical trials may paint a short-term rosy picture of disease, whereas the patients'
functional status and their joints may deteriorate over the long-term (3). Therefore, to fully evaluate second-line drugs, one must add the long-term view.

One potential reason for the progressive course of rheumatoid arthritis is
that patients, on average, do not continue to take second-line drugs over a long
period. Regardless of the drug, most patients have discontinued it by 5 years of
therapy, if not earlier. One way of comparing the attractiveness of different

second-line drugs is to evaluate which ones patients tend to continue taking the longest. Successful long-term use is a function of drug efficacy, drug safety, convenience of use, and costs.

Clinic-based studies have revealed much about the long-term use of second-line drugs. Nonetheless, these studies are often fraught with methodological problems. The success of long-term use may be systematically underestimated because patients in clinics are started on a drug regimen at different times, and some of the more recently enrolled patients may not have been followed long enough for their ultimate duration of use to be measured accurately. The number of very long-term users is usually underestimated, and the median duration of use may be, also. Loss to follow-up is a major component of any long-term study, and it may often occur when patients, frustrated with continuing symptoms (or with drug ineffectiveness), change doctors. Lastly, although long-term studies separate out patients who have discontinued for lack of efficacy from those who have discontinued from side effects, the two may not be so easily separated. A minor side effect may precipitate drug discontinuation faster if the patient is not experiencing benefit from the drug.

The use of injectable gold, one of the first second-line drugs in rheumatoid arthritis, serves as the paradigm for successful short-term use, followed by long-term discontinuation of treatment. Injectable gold therapy has a high rate of side effects that lead to drug discontinuation. Sambrook et al., for example (9), reported that, by 1 year, 48% of patients had discontinued gold therapy, mostly because of side effects. The number of patients who continue to take injectable gold 4 or 5 years after beginning therapy is depressingly low, reported at 16% (10), 28% (11), and 39% (12). The proportion of patients continuing therapy may be increasing (13), in part, because physicians may be learning to ''disregard discrete and doubtful side effects'' when they have more experience with the drug.

Auranofin has a lower rate of serious side effects than injectable gold, but stoppage rates on auranofin are also high, with discontinuations occurring because of ineffectiveness as often as from side effects. Approximately 50–60% of patients remain on auranofin after 1 year (14).

Patients treated with D-penicillamine also tend to discontinue its use over a long time. Approximately 40% withdraw during the first year (15,16). Fewer than half the patients begun on penicillamine therapy continued to take it 2 years later (16). The main reason for withdrawal is side effects.

Although sulfasalazine performed well in our metanalysis results, successful long-term therapy with the drug is not standard. Two studies have documented an approximately 50% discontinuation rate at 1 year of treatment (17,18). Discontinuations were approximately equally due to side effects and lack of efficacy.

Long-term side effects are unusual in patients receiving antimalarial drugs. Nonetheless, because of both side effects and inefficacy, 50% of patients starting antimalarial therapy have discontinued it by 12–14 months (19), although more experience by physicians with the drug may lower the termination rate to approximately 30% after 15 months of treatment (20).

Because azathioprine has not been widely used in rheumatoid arthritis, little is known about whether prolonged therapy with it is successful.

Methotrexate may be the second-line drug that patients are able to continue taking the longest. In one study (21), 71% of patients continued to take the drug after 1 year of treatment. Several studies have suggested that 50% of patients remain on methotrexate therapy 5 years after starting the drug (21–23), and recent reports (23,24) suggest that many patients continue the drug up to 8 years after initiation. Unfortunately, adverse effects may continue to occur throughout therapy, leading to punctuated discontinuations of the drug (25).

Wolfe et al. (4) (Fig. 6a) found that patients treated with methotrexate remained taking the drug significantly longer than patients treated with other second-line drugs, including hydroxychloroquine, injectable gold, auranofin, and D-penicillamine. The median time on methotrexate therapy was 4.25 years versus 1.72 years for gold, 1.59 years for auranofin, 1.82 years for penicillamine, and 2.01 years for hydroxychloroquine. In a similar study evaluating which drugs patients continued to take over time, Wijnands et al. in Holland (26) (see Fig. 6b), in a study that did not include methotrexate, reported no significant difference in time on therapy with hydroxychloroquine, penicillamine, sulfasalazine, and injectable gold. Fifty percent of patients had discontinued hydroxychloroquine at 1 year, whereas only 30% had discontinued penicillamine or sulfasalazine (see Fig. 6). These two studies reported similar results with high rates of discontinuation for commonly used second-line drugs.

Patients may remain on second-line drug therapy longer if their disease is mild (26) and continue to take their first second-line drug longer than they do drugs started after their first one has failed. Also, the profiles of side effects are different for different second-line drugs. If a given patient has a propensity for gastrointestinal problems or kidney disease, then the toxicity profiles ought to be taken into account in choosing the particular drug. Diarrhea is very common in patients treated with auranofin, whereas altered taste occurs frequently in D-penicillamine-treated patients. Oral ulcers occur with several second-line drugs, but may be most common among patients treated with methotrexate (27). Hepatotoxicity occurs most often in patients treated with methotrexate. Rash can complicate therapy with many second-line drugs, but may be most prevalent in patients treated with gold preparations (injectable and oral) and those treated with D-penicillamine. Upper gastrointestinal side effects, including nausea, vomiting, and upper abdominal pain, occur with most second-line drugs, although the highest rates are seen in patients treated with auranofin, methotrexate, and azathioprine (27).

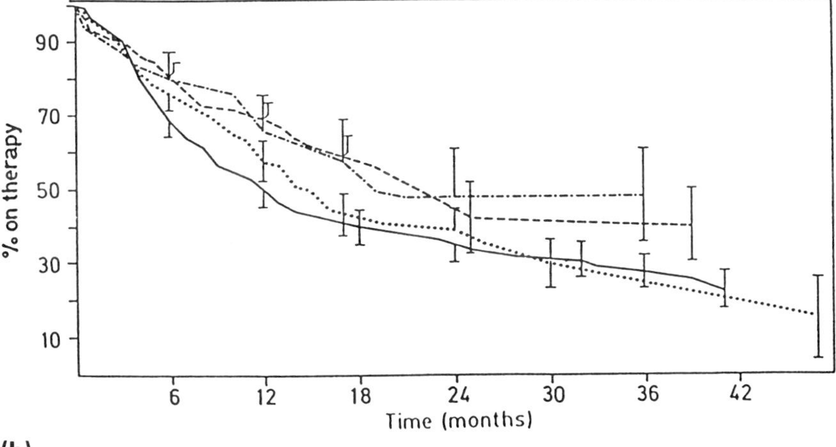

Fig. 6   (a) Product limit (Kaplan–Meier) cumulative survival analysis for SAARD. Difference in cumulative survival is significant at the 0.001 level in Mantel-Cox and Breslow tests. (b) Probability of treatment termination due to efficacy or toxicity. Estimated proportion ($\pm$ SE) of patients on hydroxychloroquine (———), sulfasalazine (------), aurothioglucose (....), and D-penicillamine (-•-•) treatment over time. (From Refs. (a) 4 and (b) 26.)

VI. THE FUTURE

Our current stable of second-line drugs is likely to expand. In addition, nonsteroidal drugs will be increasingly compared with the second-line drugs evaluated here. Our current methods of assessing and comparing second-line drugs are inadequate for the task of precisely differentiating the relative efficacy and toxicity of these drugs. In addition, we will never be able to adequately evaluate the relative efficacy of combination second-line drug therapy in rheumatoid arthritis without more attention to the methodology of drug evaluation. After all, comparative trials of second-line drugs in rheumatoid arthritis have, in general, shown no significant differences between them. Our metanalysis has suggested that these drugs may have substantial and clinically important efficacy differences. These differences should be detectable if more attention is paid to the sensitivity to change of disease activity measures and new trial standards are developed.

There are several current problems. First, rheumatoid arthritis clinical trials often contain an excessive number of disease activity or outcome measures that are used to evaluate drugs. It is not unusual to see 15 primary efficacy measures and, with this number of measures, significant results can occur by chance. A smaller list of standard measures would be more appropriate. Additionally, many of the currently used measures are not sensitive to change (e.g., walking time, digital joint circumference, and functional class) and could be discarded without much loss of information about drug efficacy. Other outcomes measures are redundant (e.g., tender joint count and tender joint score). Ideally, rheumatoid arthritis trials should assess a limited set of disease activity measures to evaluate efficacy. These measures should be standard across all trials and should be measured in a uniform way. Failure to standardize trials makes it difficult to compare drugs across trials. Since the list of drugs already available is long and differentiating between two drugs requires a large expensive clinical trial, it is unlikely that all drug comparisons of interest will be performed. Therefore, comparisons of drug performance across trials are needed and will be facilitated by trial standardization.

Despite all the outcomes measured in rheumatoid arthritis trials, there is no widely accepted method of determining whether a patient has improved. A single, agreed on definition of clinical improvement in a trial would help immeasurably in our ability to compare drugs.

Measurement of disease activity measures that are susceptible to observer variability, such as tender joint count, should be standardized. Standardization means that these measures are assessed the same way in all trials and that observers agree on the specifics of measurement before the trial begins. Rigorous standardization of measurement decreases the amount of noise in the measurement and enhances the ability to detect change or differences between drugs. Recent studies (28) have convincingly shown that the disease activity measures

Table 2 The ACR Core Set of Outcome Measures for RA Clinical Trials and Specific Ways to Assess Each Outcome Measure

Assessment	Method of assessment[a]
Tender joint count	ARA tender joint count, an assessment of 28–68 joints. The joint count should be done on physical examination as a joint score in which several different aspects of tenderness are assessed by examiner pressure and joint manipulation and then the information on various types of tenderness collapsed into a single tender vs nontender dichotomy.
Swollen joint count	The ARA joints swollen joint count 28–66. Joints are classified as either swollen or not swollen.
Patient pain	A horizontal visual analog scale (customarily 10 cm) or Likert scale assessment of current patient pain was recommended.
Patient global assessment	A global assessment by patients of how their arthritis is doing. One example that was acceptable is from the AIMS instrument, ''Considering all the ways your arthritis affects you, mark X on the scale for how well you are doing.'' What should follow is an anchored horizontal visual analog scale (usually 10 cm). A Likert scale response is also acceptable.
Physician global assessment	A horizontal visual analog (usually 10 cm) or Likert scale measure of the physician's assessment of the patient's current disease activity.
Physical disability	Any patient self-assessed instrument that has been validated, has reliability, has been proved to be sensitive to change in RA trials and that measures physical function in RA patients is acceptable. Instruments that have been demonstrated to be sensitive in RA trials include the AIMS, the HAQ, the Quality (or Index) of Well Being, the MHIQ, and the MACTAR.
Acute-phase reactant	ESR or CRP

[a]ESR, erythrocyte sedimentation rate; CRP, C-reactive protein.

used in rheumatoid arthritis trials can be measured with more precision if preliminary standardization of measurement is undertaken.

Because they incorporate information on several outcome measures at once, indexes of disease activity may improve the ability to detect drug differences in trials. Many disease activity indexes are available, and the American College of Rheumatology (ACR) and the international community are currently seeking a consensus on whether to use them and which one(s) to recommend for use.

The ACR, in conjunction with the international rheumatology community, recently proposed a core set of disease activity measures to be employed in all rheumatoid arthritis trials. These measures were developed with attention to whether they met five different types of validity: construct validity, face validity or credibility, content validity or comprehensiveness, criterion validity (whether outcomes predict or correlate with gold standard measures of rheumatoid arthritis outcomes such as death, disability, or radiographic damage), and discriminant validity or sensitivity to change. Focusing especially on criterion and discriminant validity and trying to create a set of outcomes that have overall comprehensiveness or content validity, the ACR committee chose the following seven measures as core measures to be used in all rheumatoid arthritis trials: tender joint count, swollen joint count, patient pain assessment, patient global assessment, physician global assessment, self-assessed physical disability, and an acute-phase reactant. In addition, radiographs are recommended for RA trials of 1 year or more duration in which the therapeutic agent is being tested as a DMARD. For each of these outcomes (except radiographic), specific methods of assessment were recommended (see Table 2) in the hope that similar techniques will be used across trials. The ACR committee considers the specific methods of assessment as preliminary choices, selected, in part, because of their current widespread use. It is possible that, in the future, alternative methods may become more efficient, easier to to standardize, or more sensitive to change, at which point, the recommended modes of measurement of these ACR outcomes may be altered. The use of these activity measures does not exclude use of other measures. It is hoped that, with the widespread acceptance of the ACR core measures, trials can become more uniform in the way they assess disease activity. Furthermore, the set of disease activity measures may be useful in long-term observational studies, including clinic-based investigations.

VII. CONCLUSIONS

A comparison of the efficacy and toxicity of second-line drugs in rheumatoid arthritis suggests that the two drugs with the best efficacy–toxicity trade-offs are methotrexate and antimalarial drugs. Methotrexate is one of the strongest currently available second-line drugs and, of these, has a relatively low adverse effects rate. Antimalarial drugs, on the other hand, are not among the strongest drugs available, but are quite safe. Long-term observational studies suggest that patients started on a methotrexate regimen remain on it, on average, much longer than other second-line drugs.

In the future, new methods must be developed to evaluate drugs in rheumatoid arthritis. Second-line drugs will increasingly be compared with newer drugs, with biological agents, with combination therapy, and with other second-line drugs. Uniformity of trials and standard ways of measuring outcomes within trials should be adopted if we are to successfully choose among new agents and improve the care of rheumatoid arthritis patients.

REFERENCES

1. Wilske KR, Healey LA. Remodeling the pyramid—a concept whose time has come. J Rheumatol 1989; 16:565–567.
2. Sperling RI, Coblyn JS, Larkin JK, Benincase AI, Austen KF, Weinblatt ME. Inhibition of leukotriene B_4 synthesis in neutrophils from patients with rheumatoid arthritis by a single oral dose of methotrexate. Arthritis Rheum 1990; 33:1149–1155.
3. Pincus T. Rheumatoid arthritis: disappointing long-term outcomes despite successful shot-term clinical trials. J Clin Epidemiol 1988; 41:1037–1041.
4. Wolfe F, Hawley DJ, Cathey MA. Termination of slow acting antirheumatic therapy in rheumatoid arthritis: a 14-year prospective evaluation of 1017 consecutive starts. J Rheumatol 1990; 17:994–1002.
5. Felson DT, Anderson, JJ, Meenan RF. The comparative efficacy and toxicity of second-line drugs in rheumatoid arthritis. Results of two metaanalyses. Arthritis Rheum 1990; 33:1449–1461.
6. Felson DT, Anderson JJ, Meenan RF. Using short-term efficacy/toxicity tradeoffs to select second-line drugs in rheumatoid arthritis: a meta-analysis of published clinical trials. Arthritis Rheum 1992; 35:1117–1125.
7. Anderson JJ, Felson DT, Meenan RF, Williams HJ. Which traditional measures should be used in rheumatoid arthritis clinical trials? Arthritis Rheum 1989; 32:1093–1099.
8. Fries JF, Spitz PW, Williams CA, et al. A toxicity index for comparison of side effects among different drugs. Arthritis Rheum 1990; 33:121–130.
9. Sambrook PN, Browne CD, Champion GD, Day RO, Vallance JB, Warwick N. Terminations of treatment with gold sodium thiomalate in rheumatoid arthritis. J Rheumatol 1982; 9:932–934.
10. Rosenthal M. Loss of efficacy and antirheumatic drugs in rheumatoid arthritis. J Rheumatol 1980; 7:1141–1142.
11. Ferraccioli GF, Salaffi F, Nervetti A, Manganelli P. Long-term outcome with gold thiosulphate and tiopronin in 200 rheumatoid patients. Clin Exp Rheumatol 1989; 7:577–581.
12. Pullar T, Hunter JA, Capell HA. Second line therapy in rheumatoid arthritis. A four-year prospective study. Clin Rheumatol 1985; 4:133–142.
13. Bendix G, Bjelle A. Outcome of parenteral gold therapy in RA patients: a comparison between two periods using life-table analysis. Br J Rheumatol 1991; 30:407–412.
14. Williams HJ, Dahl SL, Ward JR, Karg M, Willkens RF, Meenan RF, Altz-Smith M, Clegg DO, Mikkelsen WM, Kay DR, Weinstein AR, Guttadauria M, Paulus HE, Kaplan SB. One-year experience in patients treated with auranofin following completion of a parallel, controlled trial comparing auranofin, gold sodium thiomalate, and placebo. Arthritis Rheum 1988; 31:9–14.
15. Williams HJ, et al. Toxicity of longterm low dose D-penicillamine therapy in rheumatoid arthritis. J Rheumatol 1987; 14:67–72.
16. Hill HFH. Treatment of rheumatoid arthritis with penicillamine. Semin Arthritis Rheum 1977; 6:361–388.
17. Amos RS, Pullar T, Bax DE, Situnayake D, Capell HA, McConkey B. Sulphasalaz-

ine for rheumatoid arthritis: toxicity in 774 patients monitored for one to 11 years. Br Med J 1986; 293:420–423.

18. Jones E, Jones JV, Woodbury FL. Response to sulfasalazine in rheumatoid arthritis: life table analysis of a 5-year followup. J Rheumatol 1991; 195–198.

19. Richter JA, Runge LA, Pinals RS, Oates RP. Analysis of treatment terminations with gold and antimalarial compounds in rheumatoid arthritis. J Rheumatol 1980; 153–159.

20. Husain Z, Runge LA. Treatment complications of rheumatoid arthritis with gold, hydroxychloroquine, D-penicillamine, and levamisole. J Rheumatol 1980; 7:825–830.

21. Alarcon GS, Tracy IC, Blackburn WD Jr. Methotrexate in rheumatoid arthritis. Toxic effects as the major factor in limiting long-term treatment. Arthritis Rheum 1989; 32:671–676.

22. Sany J, Anaya JM, Lussiez V, Couret M, Bombe B, Daures JP. Treatment of rheumatoid arthritis with methotrexate: a prospective open longterm study of 191 cases. J Rheumatol 1991; 18:1323–1327.

23. Weinblatt ME, Weissman BN, Holdsworth DE, Fraser PA, Maier AL, Falchuk KR, Coblyn JS. Long-term prospective study of methotrexate in the treatment of rheumatoid arthritis. 84-month update. Arthritis Rheum 1992; 35:129–137.

24. Kremer JM, Phelps CT. Long-term prospective study of the use of methotrexate in the treatment of rheumatoid arthritis. Arthritis Rheum 1992; 35:139–144.

25. Furst DE, Erikson N, Clute L, Koehnke R, Burmeister LF, Kohler JA. Adverse experience with methotrexate during 176 weeks of a longterm prospective trial in patients with rheumatoid arthritis. J Rheumatol 1990; 17:1628–1635.

26. Wijnands MJH, Van't Hof MA, Van Leeuwen MA, Van Rijswijk MH, Van de Putte LBA, Van Riel PLCM. Long-term second-line treatment: a prospective drug survival study. Br J Rheumatol 1992; 31:253–258.

27. Singh G, Fries JF, Williams CA, Zatarain E, Spitz P, Bloch DA. Toxicity profiles of disease modifying antirheumatic drugs in rheumatoid arthritis. J Rheumatol 1991; 18:188–194.

28. Bellamy N, Anastassiades TP, Buchanan WW, Davis P, Lee P, McCain GA, Wells GA, Campbell J. Rheumatoid arthritis antirheumatic drug trials. 1. effects of standardization procedures on observer dependent outcome measures. J Rheumatol 1991; 18:1893–1900.

16

Long-Acting Drug Combinations in Rheumatoid Arthritis
Updated Overview

Peter Tugwell

University of Ottawa, Ontario, Canada

Maarten Boers

University Hospital Maastricht, The Netherlands

I. INTRODUCTION

We recently completed a review of combination therapy in rheumatoid arthritis (RA) (1). Since its publication, several new trials have been published, testifying to the increased interest in this type of treatment. For the purpose of this chapter, we have updated the review to explain three major approaches: sequential addition, started concurrently and both maintained, and step-down bridge.

II. METHODS

A. Study Identification

To locate the primary studies of interest, the MEDLINE database was searched on CD-ROM from September 1989 (the closing date of the previous review) to August 1992 using the MeSH headings: "arthritis, rheumatoid"; and "drug therapy, combination." Three key articles (2–4) were used to conduct a manual search of Science Citation Index from 1989 up to date.

The bibliographies of all retrieved articles were scrutinized for additional studies. The first author of studies published only in abstract were contacted. Such studies were eligible for inclusion if a full manuscript was available. Titles and abstracts (when available) from the computer printouts were screened by one author (MB), and any article in English, French, German, or Dutch that appeared potentially relevant was retrieved.

B. Study Selection

Included studies had to meet all of the following criteria:

1. Population: Patients with RA (old or new ARA criteria)
2. Intervention: Concurrent therapy with at least two antirheumatic drugs
3. Outcome measures: Severity of RA, measured by at least three of the following: joint count, joint score, pain, physician or patient global assessment, morning stiffness, grip strength, 50-ft ([1]15-m) walking time, erythrocyte sedimentation rate. In addition, toxicity related to treatment had to be reported.
4. Methodological criteria: Prospective cohort or randomized comparison of treatment modalities, of which at least one had to be a combination of long-acting antirheumatic drugs, and at least one a single drug. Systemic corticosteroids were also counted as long-acting antirheumatic drugs.

C. Data Extraction

First, the quality of the studies and, thus, the strength of evidence was score on a 3-point scale on the basis of two primary criteria: randomization and blinding. Accordingly, strong evidence came from randomized, double-blind studies; moderately strong evidence came from studies that were randomized, but open or partially blinded (for example, a study with only blinded outcome assessment); and weak evidence came from all other studies. This score specified the maximum strength of evidence we felt a study could yield. A second set of criteria, modified from Sackett et al., was then applied (5). These were (a) adequate outcome assessment; (b) adequate description of study patients; (c) adequate description of the therapeutic maneuver; (d) complete accounting of study patients in the results. To obtain the final "quality" score, 1 point was subtracted from the initial score for each of these criteria not met.

Data extracted from the studies included baseline patient characteristics, study and concomitant treatment, outcome measures, and details on toxicity and withdrawals. *Active disease*, an entry criterion in most studies was compared with our definition: presence of six or more swollen joints, plus two of three related conditions. These conditions were the following: nine or more tender joints, morning stiffness ≥ 45 min, and erythrocyte sedimentation rate 28 mm/ h or more. When only six swollen joints or two of the conditions were specified, the presence of active disease in the study patients was scored as "maybe."

D. Analysis

Analysis was limited to studies yielding moderate or strong evidence. For the outcome measures reported most frequently, the evidence to support an additional effect of combination therapy over single-drug therapy was summarized. Studies with more than two treatment groups present special problems because of the large number of possible comparisons between groups. Evidence that any single antirheumatic drug is more effective than another is scarce. Therefore, for each outcome measure we treated all drugs as equal, averaged the results of the single-drug groups, and compared this mean result with that of the combination group. Where possible, results of statistical tests comparing the effect of the different treatments were calculated or recalculated using the reported data. The results are reported here together with the results of the trials yielding moderate or strong evidence in the previous review (1).

III. RESULTS

The searches yielded a total of 44 titles of studies, reviews, and editorial comments, of which 14 were retrieved. Together with the previous review, this brings the totals to 385 titles scanned, 64 retrieved, and 12 included for review.

Five randomized trials met our inclusion criteria: all were double-blind (6–10). The excluded titles included reviews and letters, and studies comparing unspecified drugs or drugs not known to be antirheumatic drugs.

A. Methodological Assessment

Three of the five trials were of high quality (Table 1) (6,7,8). These trials lost no ''quality points'' on the secondary criteria. Two other trials, studying the addition of methylprednisolone to antirheumatic therapy were also randomized, double-blind (9,10). These studies suffered from flaws in the secondary criteria, and were thus considered as yielding weak evidence (see Table 1). The study by Wong et al. (9) reported the outcome only in a nonvalidated summary index and acute-phase reactants. The disease and its therapy were insufficiently documented, and no intent-to-treat analysis was done. The study by Hansen et al. (10) had very little documentation of toxicity or treatment history. Comparability of treatment groups at baseline was unclear. Finally, documentation of treatment reallocation and dropout during the trial was unclear. Further results of these trials are not included in this report.

In the included studies, coadministration of systemic and intra-articular corticosteroids, as well as lack of compliance monitoring led to a potential for bias. None of the blinded trials employed a separate observer for toxicity, making unblinding possible when a side effect specific for one of the drugs occurred. In practice this was probably not much of a problem, given that several specific side effects (e.g., proteinuria, retinopathy) were noted in patients not receiving the active drug.

Table 1 Methodological Assessment[a]

Author (Ref.)	Scott (11)	Smyth (12)	Gibson (13)	Corkill (6)	Williams (7)	Willkens (8)	Wong (9)	Hansen (10)
Primary criteria								
random allocation	Yes	Yes	Yes	Yes	Yes	Yes	Yes	Yes
Blinding:								
Patient	Yes	Yes	No	Yes	Yes	Yes	Yes	Yes
Outcome assessor	Yes	Yes	Yes	Yes	Yes	Yes	Yes	Yes
Secondary criteria								
Adequate outcome assessment	Yes	Yes	Yes	Yes	Yes	Yes	Maybe	Maybe
Clinically relevant								
outcomes	Yes	Yes	Yes	Yes	Yes	Yes	No	Yes
Objective definitions	Yes	Yes	Yes	Yes	Yes	Yes	Yes	Yes
Minimized observer								
variation	No	Yes	Yes	Yes	Yes	No	Yes	Yes
Toxicity	Yes	Yes	Yes	Yes	Yes	Yes	Yes	Maybe
Summary index[b]	Yes	No	No	Yes	Yes	Yes	Yes	No
Patient function assessment	No	Yes	No	Yes	No	Maybe*	No	No
Adequate patient description	Yes	Maybe	Yes	Yes	Yes	Yes	Maybe	Maybe
Demographics	Yes	No	Yes	Yes	Yes	Yes	Yes	Yes
Previous, current severity	Yes	Maybe	Yes	Yes	Yes	Yes	Maybe	Yes
Previous, current								
medication	Yes	Yes	Maybe	Maybe	Yes	Maybe	Maybe	Maybe

Groups comparable at baseline	Yes	Maybe*	Yes	Yes	Yes	Yes	Yes	Maybe
Adequate description of therapeutic maneuver	Yes	Yes	Yes	Yes	Yes	Yes	Yes	No
Potential for bias in maneuver[c]	Small	Moderate	Large	Moderate*	Small	Moderate	Small	Moderate
Patients accounted for (%)[d]	100	100	97	100	100	100	100	100
Patients in efficacy analysis (%)	58	100	92	95*	63	76	70	47
Attempt to analyze withdrawals	No	No withdrawals	Yes*	Yes	Yes	Yes	No	Yes
Conclusion: strength of evidence	Strong	Moderate	Moderate	Strong	Strong	Strong	Weak	Weak
Comments		Comparability: RA less severe in placebo group?	Most withdrawals followed to the end of the study	Unequal group sizes; contamination in placebo group only intent-to-treat		Results of Health Assessment Questionnaire (HAQ) not reported	See text	See text

[a]Asterisks in columns refer to the comments in the same column.

[b]Summary index: attempt to summarize various disease measures into one score or outcome (e.g., "remission").

[c]Potential for bias in maneuver is small when blindness, contamination, cointervention, and compliance are adequately addressed, and moderate when three of the above are adequately addressed.

[d]A patient is accounted for when fate is specified (e.g., "early withdrawal", "lost to follow-up").

B. Baseline Characteristics

The total of six (three "old," three "new") included trials yielding moderate or strong evidence form a heterogeneous group (Tables 2 and 3). The size of the trials ranged from 29 to 335 patients entered, and the number of treatment groups from two to three. The duration of the trials ranged from 24 to 52 weeks. In all trials a substantial proportion of patients had been treated previously with other antirheumatic drugs (Tables 2 and 3). Although it was stated in all trials that the disease was "active," only two met our definition.

Reporting of concomitant medication was far from complete: usually, no mention was made of other antirheumatic drugs during the trial, although presumably these were not given. Specifically, systemic steroids were the subject of investigation in two trials, allowed as concomitant medication in two other trials, excluded in one, and not mentioned in two. Intra-articular steroids were allowed in three trials, excluded in one, and not mentioned in two.

Table 2 Characteristics of the Three Trials Yielding (Moderately) Strong Evidence[a]

Author, yr (Ref.)	Scott, 1989 (11)	Smyth, 1975* (12)	Gibson, 1987 (13)
Patients entered	101	29	72
Definite RA	Yes	Yes	Yes
Duration of disease (yr, mean)	2	Not stated	2.0 (median)
Minimum duration (mo)	3	24	2
Previous antirheumatic drugs[b]	Yes*	Yes	Yes*
≥6 swollen joints and 2 of 3 active disease criteria[c]	No	No*	No*
Class IV patients excluded	Not stated	Yes	Not stated
Treatment groups (no. per group)	1. Gold + HCQ (52) 2. Gold + placebo (49)	1. Prednisone + cyclophosphamide (13) 2. Prednisone + placebo (16)	1. CQS + dpen (26) 2. CQS alone (20) 3. dpen alone (26)
Dosage intensity	Normal	Low	Normal
Regimen (oral unless stated)[d]	gold: 20 × 50 mg/wk, 50 mg/2 w IM thereafter; HCQ: 400 mg/d for 6 months, 200 mg/d thereafter	Prednisone: continuing pretrial dose (3–5 mg/d) Cyclophosphamide: 75 mg/d	CQS: 200 mg/d dpen: 250 mg/d increased monthly by 125 mg to max 750 mg/d

Table 2 Continued

Author, yr (Ref.)	Scott, 1989 (11)	Smyth, 1975* (12)	Gibson, 1987 (13)
Not allowed	Any antirheumatic drug in last 3 mo	Gold in last 6 mo; phenylbutazone, salycic acid in last 2 mo	Previous treatment with HCQ or dpen
Concomitant drugs allowed			
NSAIDs	Yes	No	Yes
Systemic steroids	No	In trial	Not stated
Intra-articular steroids	No	Not stated	Yes
Duration of trial (wk)	52	26	52
Comments	27 patients previously treated with antirheumatic drugs. Active disease defined as: stiffness >30 min, ≥3 swollen joints, ESR >30 mm	Part of a larger, uncontrolled study All had "active synovitis" for 2 yr	11 patients had been treated with gold All patients had "conventional indications for second-line therapy"

[a]Asterisks in columns refer to the comments in the same column. Strength of evidence: see Table 1.
[b]Antirheumatic drugs include systemic steroids, but exclude nonsteroidal antiinflammatory drugs.
[c]Active disease: ≥6 swollen joints plus 2 of the following: 9 or more swollen joints; ≥ 45 min morning stiffness; erythrocyte sedimentation rate ≥28 mm maybe: only ≥ 6 joints or 2 related conditions.
[d]Gold: sodium aurothiomalate; HCQ: hydroxychloroquine; dpen: D-penicillamine; CQS: chloroquine sulfate.

C. Analysis of Efficacy

In our original review, we noted that the analysis of efficacy was hard to interpret owing to multiple comparisons, the lack of post-hoc power assessments, and the handling of withdrawals. The new studies handled these points well. Reporting on withdrawals was complete, and both efficacy and intent-to-treat analyses were present. Multiple comparisons were still performed, although the authors recognized the danger and included a primary endpoint, either in the form of "substantial improvement" or as a summary index. However, before being

Table 3 Characteristics of the New Trials Yielding Strong Evidence[a]

Author, yr (Ref.)	Corkill, 1990 (6)	Williams, 1992 (7)	Willkens, 1992 (8)
Patients entered	59	335	209*
Definite RA	Yes	Yes	Yes
Duration of disease (yr, mean)	5.7	5.4	8.0 (median)
Minimum duration (mo)	Not stated	6	12
Previous antirheumatic drugs[a]	Yes	Yes	Yes*
Active disease[d]	No	Yes	Yes
Class IV patients excluded	Not stated	Yes	No (1% in class IV)
Treatment groups (no. per group)	1. Gold + MP (35) 2. Gold + placebo (24)	1. MTX + AUR (106) 2. MTX + placebo (114) 3. AUR + placebo (115)	1. MTX + AZA (69) 2. MTX + placebo (67) 3. AZA + placebo (73)
Dosage intensity	Gold: normal MP: low	Low-normal	Combination: normal* Single: high*
Regimen (oral unless stated)	Gold: 1 × 10 mg, 20 × 50 mg/wk, 50 mg/mo IM therafter; MP: 120 mg IM 0,4,8 wk	MTX: 7.5 mg/wk (3 × 2.5 mg) AUR: 6 mg/d (2 × 3 mg)	AZA: 50 mg/d, increase q 6 wk to 100, 150 mg/d until response or toxicity MTX: 5 mg/wk, increase to 15 mg/wk comb: 50/5, increase to 100/7.5
Not allowed	Gold Steroids in last 2 mo	Never: study drugs, gold, dpen, imm. suppr; last 2 mo: antimal, steroids	Study drugs taken for > 12 wk; any antirheumatic drug in last month; total lymphoid irradiation
Concomitant drugs allowed			
NSAIDs	Not stated	Yes	Yes
Systemic steroids	In trial	Yes*	Yes*

Table 3 Continued

Author, yr (Ref.)	Corkill, 1990 (6)	Williams, 1992 (7)	Willkens, 1992 (8)
Intra-articular steroids	Not stated	One dose	One dose
Duration of trial (wk)	24	48	24
Comments		patients were allowed a stable dose of prednisone, ≤ 10 mg/d	212 entered, 3 never started therapy all had received gold (IM/oral) or dpen % on hi-dose: single, 33%; comb, 14% patients were allowed a stable dose of prednisone, $\leq$ 10 mg/d

[a]Asterisks in columns refer to the comments in the same column. Strength of evidence: see Table 1.
[b]Antirheumatic drugs include systemic steroids, but exclude nonsteroidal anti-inflammatory drugs.
[c]Active disease: ≥ 6 swollen joints plus 2 of the following: 9 or more swollen joints; $\geq$ 45 min morning stiffness; ESR $\geq$ 28 mm; maybe: only $\geq$ 6 joints or 2 related conditions.
[d]Gold: sodium aurothiomalate; MP: methylprednisolone; MTX: methotrexate; AUR: auranofin; AZA: azathioprine; dpen: D-penicillamine.

widely implemented, such index need to be validated and acceptable—such is not true at present (ref OMERACT). Williams et al. included a post-hoc power assessment (7).

Of the three new studies, one suggested a marked short-term benefit for low-dose intramuscular methylprednisolone added to intramuscular gold, and two suggested no benefit of two methotrexate-containing combination strategies over the single drugs: one combination containing auranofin, the other containing azathioprine (see Table 4). In the first study, three doses of 120-mg methylprednisolone, given in a period of 8 weeks, substantially reduced disease activity in several measures, an effect visible until week 12, but gone at week 24 (see Table 4). Contamination in the placebo group (i.e., several dropouts receiving corticosteroid therapy, sometimes in-hospital) may have prevented the difference remaining visible at week 24. The summary index showed the same difference, but with more consistency and power. There was an imbalance in the number of patients allocated to the treatment groups that was not completely explained, leading to small numbers in the placebo arm, especially at the end of the study. Toxicity was higher in the combination group, but dropout rates were not signifi-

Table 4 Results of the New Trials Yielding Strong Evidence[a]

Author (Ref.)	Corkill (6)			Williams (7)			Willkens (8)		
Comparison	Gold ± MP[b]			MTX ± AUR, AUR alone[b]			MTX ± AZA, AZA alone[b]		
Improvement in outcome measures	Additional effect of combination at 12 wk	at 24 wk	Compared with single drug (*p* values)	Additional effect of combination	Compared with single drug (*p* value)		Additional effect of combination	Compared with single drug (*p* value)	
Ritchie index/joint count	+[c]	0	*<0.05, NS*[d]	0	NS		0	NS	
Morning stiffness	—	—	—	0	NS		0	NS	
Grip strength	+	0	*<0.05, NS*	0	NS		0	NS	
Health Ass. Questionnaire	+	0	*<0.05, NS*	—	—		—	—	
ESR[b]	+	0	*<0.05, NS*	0	NS		0	NS	
Rate of X-ray worsening	—	0	*NS*	—	—		—	—	
Summary index	+	0	*<0.01, NS*	0	NS		0	NS	
% patients improved	—	—	—	0	NS		0	NS	
Group (*n*)	gold + MP (35)	gold (24)		MTX + AUR (106)	MTX (114)	AUR (115)	MTX + AZA (69)	MTX (67)	AZA (73)
Withdrawals (total)	13	11		39	39	46	18	5	28
Lack of efficacy	1	3		2	8	15	0	2	5
Toxicity	11	6		22	17	16	16	3	22
Other reasons	1	2		15	14	15	2	0	1
Problems	Placebo groups: small number of patients left; some dropouts received steroids			Many dropouts owing to "other" reasons					
Strength of evidence	Strong			Strong			Strong		
Conclusions for value of combination	Short-term benefit, possibly increased toxicity			No real difference in efficacy and toxicity			Suggests effects similar to MTX; intermediate toxicity		
Comments							AZA was least effective and most toxic; MTX toxicity very low		

[a]Asterisks in columns refer to the comments in the same column. Strength of evidence: see Table 1.
[b]ESR: erythrocyte sedimentation rate; gold: sodium aurothioglucose; MP: methylprednisolone; NS: not significant; MTX; methotrexate; AUR: auranofin; AZA: azathioprine.
[c]+, combination works better than single drug; 0, no difference.
[d]All results that could not be recalculated are in italics.

cantly different. Despite its relatively small sample size, this is the first study to lend strong support for low-dose steroid induction therapy.

In the second study, methotrexate and auranofin were given in their normal starting dose, but no increases were allowed (see Table 4) (7). Auranofin showed a lag time to effect, but scored only slightly (not significantly) lower on most outcomes than did methotrexate and the combination (see Table 4). The combination scored best, and auranofin worst in dropouts, because of lack of effect. Toxicity was slightly more pronounced in the combination group. The authors speculate that the relatively low dosing may be responsible for these results. In all groups, there was a relatively large dropout owing to "other reasons." The results of this large 1-year study "rehabilitate" auranofin as an effective drug, but do not support the use of this drug in combination with methotrexate.

In the third study, methotrexate and azathioprine were given in a low dose, with increments after 6 week intervals until response or toxicity occurred (see Table 4) (8). The highest increments were given in the single-drug groups. Response was defined as a 15% improvement compared with baseline in three of four key activity measures at week 6, and 30% at weeks 12 and 18. Azathioprine was less effective than methotrexate or the combination, but the differences failed to reach statistical significance (see Table 4). In the combination group, 14% had two dose increases to the highest level; in the single groups, this was 33 and 34%. Because the last increase in the combination group was in fact sham, it might be concluded that the drugs had some additive effects. Azathioprine had a significantly higher dropout rate for toxicity than methotrexate or the combination. Methotrexate as a single drug had a very low dropout rate for toxicity. This half-year study yielding strong evidence does not support the use of the combination.

Of the three old studies providing strong or moderately strong evidence, the first suggested an additional improvement of 10% for a combination of parenteral gold and hydroxychloroquine over and above the improvement of 50% given by gold alone, with somewhat higher toxicity in the combination group (Table 5) (11). The second study suggested additional benefit of unknown magnitude for adding low-dose cyclophosphamide to the regimen of patients already taking prednisone, with low toxicity (see Table 5) (12). The third study failed to show any benefit of D-penicillamine plus chloroquine sulfate over either drug alone, but with enhanced toxicity of the combination (see Table 5) (13).

IV. DISCUSSION

Since our previous review, three new high-quality studies have been added. Two other potentially useful studies were hard to interpret owing to flaws in the report. Methotrexate has now been studied in combination with auranofin and azathioprine. Neither of the combinations seem to offer any real advantage over

Table 5 Results of the Three Trials Yielding (Moderately) Strong Evidence[a]

Author (Ref.)	Scott (20)		Smyth (21)		Gibson (23)[e]	
Comparison	Gold ± HCQ[b]		Prednisone ± cyclophosphamide		CQS ± dpen, dpen alone[b]	
Improvement in outcome measures	Additional effect of combination*	Compared with single drug (*p* value)	Additional effect of combination	Compared with single drug (*p* value)	Additional effect of combination	Compared with single drug (*p* value)
Ritchie index/joint						
count	+[c]	NS	+	<0.01	0	*NS*[d]
Morning stiffness	+	NS	—	—	0	*NS*
Grip strength	+	NS	+	0.05<p<0.10	0	*NS*
ESR	+	NS	0	*NS**	0	*NS*
Rate of x-ray						
worsening	+	NS	—	*NS**	+	NS*
Summary index	+	*p<0.05*[d]	—	—	—	—
% patients						
improved	—	—	—	—	—	—
	Combination	Single	Combination	Single	Combination	Single

Withdrawals (total)	25	17	0?	0?	8	5
Lack of efficacy	2	5	0	0	1	2
Toxicity	18	10	0	0	6	3
Other reasons	5	2	0	0	1	0
Problems	None		None		2 patients lost to follow up, 2 unaccounted	
Strength of evidence	Strong		Moderate		Moderate	
Conclusion for value of combination	Suggests increased efficacy and toxicity		Suggests increased efficacy with low toxicity		Suggests only increased toxicity*	
Comments	Magnitude: if single drug improves outcome by 50%, combination adds 10% Authors tested differences between groups in absolute scores, not improvements		Magnitude unknown: only changes from baseline, not baseline itself reported		X-ray worsening: χ^2 of subgroup of 59 pt with complete radiographs Significantly more side effects not warranting discontinuation ($p = 0.02$)	

[a]Asterisks in columns refer to the comments in the same column. Strength of evidence: see Table 1.
[b]gold: sodium aurothiomalate; HCQ: hydroxychloroquine; CQS: chloroquine sulfate; dpen: d-penicillamine; NS: not significant.
[c]+, combination works better than single drug; 0, no difference.
[d]All results that could not be recalculated are in italics; α level is 0.05.
[e]Recalculations of Gibson data: the single drug groups are pooled and compared with the combination group.

methotrexate as a single drug. The third study shows that relatively low doses of intramuscular corticosteroid therapy can speed the improvement obtainable with intramuscular gold. This last report is interesting because it documents the increased sensitivity to change of an index that aggregates several measures into one score. This particular index, a variation of the Mallya and Mace index (ref) needs further validation. However, we feel that it is the way to progress in future studies in RA, for which head-to-head comparisons of active drugs and their combinations are likely to result in smaller, yet important differences.

This experience can be added to the previous experience, in which a modest case could be made for intramuscular gold and hydroxychloroquine, but not for D-penicillamine and chloroquine sulfate. Cyclophosphamide is a drug of last resort owing to its potential for toxicity, despite its efficacy alone or in combination with low-dose prednisone.

In sum, the field is wide open for further studies of combination therapy. Because of several meticulously performed studies, some promising combinations can be fine-tuned, and others put aside.

ACKNOWLEDGMENT

The authors would like to acknowledge the technical assistance given by A. Spoorenberg.

REFERENCES

1. Boers M, Ramsden M. Longacting drug combinations in rheumatoid arthritis: a formal overview. J Rheumatol 1991; 18:316–324.
2. McCarty DJ, Carrera GF. Treatment of intractable rheumatoid arthritis with combined cyclophosphamide, azathioprine and hydroxychloroquine. JAMA 1982; 248:1718–1723.
3. Bunch TW, O'Duffy D, Tompkins RB, O'Fallon WM. Controlled trial of hydroxychloroquine and D-penicillamine singly and in combination in the treatment of rheumatoid arthritis. Arthritis Rheum 1984; 27:267–276.
4. Neumann V, Hopkins R, Dixon J, Watkins A, Bird H, Wright V. Combination therapy with pulsed methylprednisolone in rheumatoid arthritis. Ann Rheum Dis 1985; 44:747–751.
5. Sackett D, Haynes B, Tugwell P. Deciding on the best therapy. In: Clinical epidemiology. A basic science for clinical medicine, 2nd ed. Boston: Little Brown, 1991:193.
6. Corkill M, Kirkham BW, Chikanza IC, Gibson T, Panayi GS. Intramuscular depot methylprednisolone induction of chrysotherapy in rheumatoid arthritis: a 24-week randomized clinical trial. Br J Rheumatol 1990; 29:274–279.
7. Williams HJ, Ward JR, Reading JC, et al. Comparison of auranofin, methotrexate, and the combination of both in the treatment of rheumatoid arthritis. A controlled clinical trial. Arthritis Rheum 1992; 35:259–269.

8. Willkens RF, Urowitz MB, Stablein DM, et al. Comparison of azathioprine, methotrexate, and the combination of both in the treatment of rheumatoid arthritis. A controlled clinical trial. Arthritis Rheum 1992; 35:849–856.

9. Wong CS, Champion G, Smith MD, et al. Does steroid pulsing influence the efficacy and toxicity of chrysotherapy? A double-blind, placebo-controlled study. Ann Rheum Dis 1990; 49:370–372.

10. Hansen TM, Kryger P, Elling H, et al. Double blind placebo controlled trial of pulse treatment with methylprednisolone combined with disease modifying drugs in rheumatoid arthritis. Br Med J 1990; 301:268–270.

11. Scott DL, Dawes PT, Tunn E, Fowler PD, Shadforth MF, Fisher J, Clarke S, Collins M, Jones P, Popert AJ, Bacon PA. Combination therapy with gold and hydroxychloroquine in rheumatoid arthritis: a randomized, placebo-controlled study. Br J Rheumatol 1989; 28:128–133.

12. Smyth CJ, Bartholomew BA, Mills DM, Steigerwald JC, Strong SJ, Recart S. Cyclophosphamide therapy for rheumatoid arthritis. Arch Intern Med 1975; 135:789–793.

13. Gibson T, Emery P, Armstrong RD, Crisp AJ, Panayi GS. Combined D-penicillamine and chloroquine treatment of rheumatoid arthritis—a comparative study. Br J Rheumatol 1987; 27:279–284.

17

The Application of Biotechnological Advances to the Treatment of Rheumatoid Arthritis

Arthur F. Kavanaugh

The University of Texas Southwestern Medical Center at Dallas, and Department of Veterans Affairs Medical Center at Dallas, Dallas, Texas

Peter E. Lipsky

Harold C. Simmons Arthritis Research Center and The University of Texas Southwestern Medical Center at Dallas, Dallas, Texas

I. INTRODUCTION

In recent years, the pathophysiology of rheumatoid arthritis (RA) has become elucidated more clearly (1–3). A large body of data suggest that T cells, and in particular CD4$^+$ helper T cells, subserve a pivotal etiological role in the generation and propagation of the immunologically driven inflammation of RA (Table 1) (4–6). As reviewed in detail in Chapter 1, evidence supporting the role of T cells in RA derives from analysis of the phenotype of cells infiltrating the rheumatoid synovium (7–26), delineation of the cellular basis of animal models of inflammatory arthritis (27,28), and studies of therapeutic interventions that affect T-cell function (29–43). Evidence suggesting that CD4$^+$ T cells play a predominant role in RA comes from the documentation that these are the preponderant cells in the rheumatoid synovium (44–48), genetic studies that establish an association of RA with the expression of specific class II major histocompatibility complex (MHC) molecules (49–62), and anecdotal reports of the attenuation of

Table 1 The Role of T Cells in Rheumatoid Arthritis

Pro

    Synovial tissue infiltrated with T cells

    Synovial T cells express activation markers

    HLA-DR association of RA

    Improvement in RA with elimination of T cells or suppression of T-cell function

        Thoracic duct drainage

        Total lymphoid irradiation

        Lymphocytapheresis

        Cyclosporine

        Anti-T-cell mAb

    Improvement noted after HIV infection

Con

    Small quantities of T-cell-derived cytokines recovered from rheumatoid synovium

    Diminished responsiveness of synovial T cells

established RA in patients who become infected with human immunodeficiency virus (HIV) (63). In view of the complexity of intercellular interactions inherent in the immune response, it is likely that non-T cells also play a contributory role in the immunologically driven inflammation of RA (64). Nevertheless, the available data are most consistent with the conclusion that antigen-reactive $CD4^+$ T cells play the central etiological and regulatory role in the orchestration of synovial inflammation.

Although an understanding of the pathophysiology of RA has evolved considerably, progress in its treatment has been less dramatic. The therapeutic agents currently used in RA, despite their ability to ameliorate symptoms temporarily in a subset of patients, do not impinge on the long-term outcome in most RA patients (3,65–67). This recognition, coupled with an increasing appreciation of the adverse reactions associated with these medications (68,69), has stimulated the development of new therapeutic approaches more specifically aimed at identifiable pathophysiological events in RA. Because T cells perform such a central role in RA, much of the developmental focus of immunomodulatory biological therapies for RA has been directed toward T-cell-driven immune responses. It is anticipated that such therapies might modulate the immunologically driven inflammatory reactions and, thereby, have an impact on the progression of disease.

II. APPROACHES

To achieve the goal of interfering with immunologically driven inflammatory responses, several integral components of the immune response may potentially be targeted (Figs. 1 and 2). During the generation of effective immune responses,

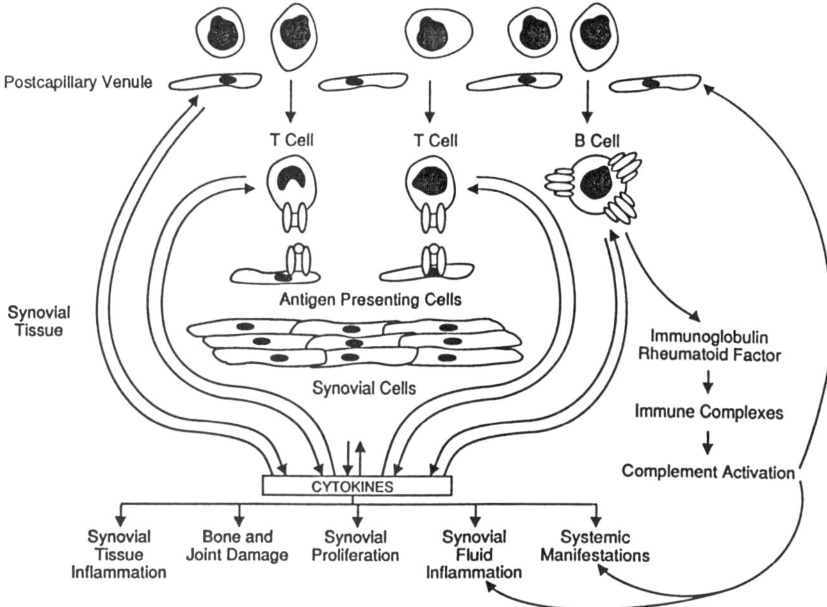

Fig. 1 The pathogenesis of rheumatoid arthritis.

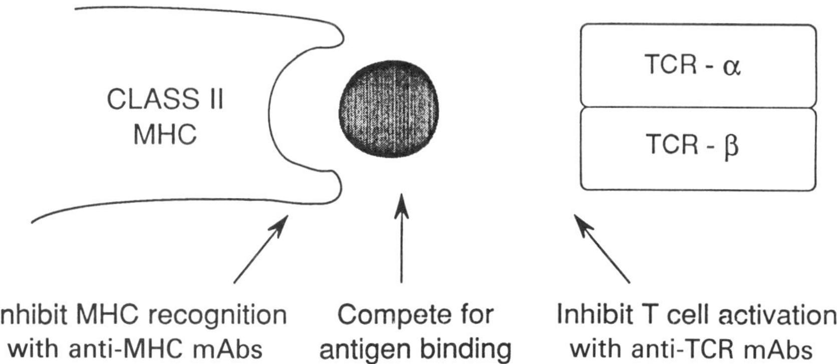

Fig. 2 Interfering with the function of autoreactive T lymphocytes in RA.

Although an understanding of the pathophysiology of RA has evolved considerably, progress in its treatment has been less dramatic. The therapeutic agents currently used in RA, despite their ability to ameliorate symptoms temporarily in a subset of patients, do not impinge on the long-term outcome in most RA patients (3,65–67). This recognition, coupled with an increasing appreciation of the adverse reactions associated with these medications (68,69), has stimulated the development of new therapeutic approaches more specifically aimed at identifiable pathophysiological events in RA. Because T cells perform such a central role in RA, much of the developmental focus of immunomodulatory biological therapies for RA has been directed toward T-cell-driven immune responses. It is anticipated that such therapies might modulate the immunologically driven inflammatory reactions and, thereby, have an impact on the progression of disease.

II. APPROACHES

To achieve the goal of interfering with immunologically driven inflammatory responses, several integral components of the immune response may potentially be targeted (Figs. 1 and 2). During the generation of effective immune responses, a relevant antigen must be presented to T cells by antigen-presenting cells (APC). If the antigen presentation is inhibited, an immune response might not be generated. Alternatively, if the process is partially impeded (e.g., if antigen if presented appropriately, but without the requisite costimulatory signals), tolerance to the particular antigen may develop. Therefore, potential targets of immunomo-

Table 2   Approaches to Target T Cells in Rheumatoid Arthritis

Specific
    Inhibit function of antigen-specific T cells
        mAb directed against specific TCR
        mAb directed against specific HLA-DR epitopes
        Specific blocking peptides
        TCR vaccination
Semispecific
    Inhibit function of specific T-cell subsets
        mAb to CD4
        mAb to ''memory'' T cells
        mAb to IL-2R; IL-2 toxin conjugates
Nonspecific
    Inhibit function of all T cells
        Pan T-cell-directed mAb
        mAb to MHC class II molecules (nonspecific epitopes)

dulatory therapy in RA prominently include those cell surface molecules and secreted cytokines critical to the generation of immune responses (70,71).

A. SPECIFIC THERAPY

Appropriate targets of T-cell–specific immunological intervention would include the MHC molecules that bind antigen and the T-cell receptors (TCRs) that recognize antigen. Such intervention could be accomplished by several means. For example, peptides could be generated that competed with the arthritogenic antigen(s) for presentation by MHC molecules to the T-cell receptor (70–72). Alternatively, monoclonal antibodies (mAb) might be directed against the T-cell receptor of the arthritogenic clones of T cells or at the specific portions of the relevant class II MHC molecules that putatively bind the arthritogenic peptides. Another plausible method is T-cell receptor vaccination. This could involve identification, collection, alteration, and reinfusion of arthritogenic T cells from an individual host (73,74). Alternatively, vaccination might be accomplished using fragments of the specific T-cell receptors of the arthritogenic T cells (75).

The efficacy of approaches such as these has been demonstrated in various animal models of autoimmune disease. One concern that might affect the extrapolation of these types of therapy to human disease is that efficacy is usually predicated on the introduction of arthritogenic antigens and therapeutic agents in close temporal association. Therapy initiated at longer time intervals following induction of disease is generally less successful at modifying the disease. Since the clinician is most commonly faced with the treatment of patients with established RA, the anticipated success of such specific therapies would not be certain. On the other hand, since maintenance of long-term T-cell memory has been suggested to require continued antigenic exposure (76), it is possible that therapy might be able to interfere with this process and, thereby, provide some benefit, even during the course of established disease.

The main obstacle to the use of specific immunomodulatory therapy in RA is that, unlike the animal models alluded to previously, the relevant etiopathogenic antigen or antigens remain undefined. Despite decades of intensive investigation using various investigative techniques, no single agent has been unequivocally implicated in the pathogenesis of RA. More recently, investigators have employed molecular biological techniques to approach this question by attempting to identify T-cell receptors expressed by arthritogenic clones of T cells. In certain animal models of autoimmune disease, such as collagen-induced arthritis, restricted use of T-cell receptor genes has been demonstrated (77). Early studies in humans with RA, using restriction length polymorphism (RFLP) analysis, demonstrated little if any oligoclonal utilization of T-cell receptors by T cells in synovial tissue and fluid of the majority of RA patients (78–81). Even when RFLP analysis demonstrated evidence of oligoclonal T-cell receptor β-chain utilization in synovial samples, no consistent pattern could be identified in different patients (82,83). More recently, investigators have assessed the repertoire of T-cell variable region gene family utilization by such T cells directly by employing the polymerase chain reaction (PCR). Several reports have demonstrated restricted T-cell receptor V_β gene family utilization by T cells isolated from the rheumatoid synovium (84–87). However, the specific V_β families found to be overexpressed have varied among the studies. In addition, other reports have not found such biased V_β gene utilization (88–91). Thus, whether T cells expressing particular T-cell receptors are present uniformly at the sites of rheumatoid inflammation and, by implication, subserve a relevant etiopathic role remains to be proved. The final resolution of this question may await the development of a universally agreed on technology for the recovery and analysis of synovial T cells (91). The absence of documented etiological antigen(s) or arthritogenic T-cell clones now precludes widespread use of specific therapies for RA.

B. Semispecific Therapy

Semispecific therapies would interfere with the function of broader subsets of T cells. Potentially, by including within the targeted T-cell subset most or all arthritogenic T cells, such therapy could have significant influence on T-cell-driven inflammation. To induce and propagate synovial inflammation in RA, subsets of T cells must be localized at the inflammatory site and must be stimulated to express their individual functions. Therefore, potential targets for semispecific intervention would include differentiation markers, expressed by relevant subsets of T cells, and molecules expressed by activated T cells. The latter would include cytokine receptors and cell surface molecules relevant for intercellular interactions. In addition, since the growth and differentiation of activated T cells involves the capacity to respond to various cytokines, blocking the activity of these immunoregulatory molecules could have an immunomodulatory effect limited to activated T cells. Although these therapies are not antigen-specific, by targeting relevant T-cell subsets that include antigen-specific T cells, it is likely that these approaches might modulate the chronic inflammatory response and, accordingly, cause long-term clinical benefit.

C. Nonspecific Therapy

Nonspecific biological immunomodulatory therapies are those that nonselectively affect T cells. This might be achieved directly, for example, by using an mAb recognizing an epitope on all T cells or, indirectly, by altering the function of other cell types that regulate T-cell function. By analogy to procedures or medications with T-cell-depleting or modulating effects, such therapies would be expected to achieve some benefit. However, by affecting T-cell function in a nonspecific manner, these approaches would have the greatest likelihood of being associated with infections and neoplastic side effects characteristic of other nonspecific immunosuppressive therapies.

III. MECHANISMS

Several types of molecules might potentially be used for biological therapy in RA. Currently, the most frequently employed agents have been antibodies. Although earlier investigators had used polyclonal antibodies, more recently most groups have taken advantage of monoclonal antibody (mAb) technology to target relevant antigens specifically. The mAbs have several advantages as therapeutic agents, not the least of which is that unlimited quantities of uniform antibodies, with a single specificity, can be generated. Efficacy of any particular mAb would depend on several variables. This includes the characteristics of the targeted antigen, such as its cell surface density and tissue distribution, as well as characteristics of the mAb, including its fine specificity, avidity, and heavy chain isotype. The exact mechanism(s) by which therapeutic mAbs exert effects on targeted cells or molecules has not been completely delineated. Among the potential mechanisms are (a) blocking, or steric hindrance of the function of the target antigen; (b) cytotoxicity to the cell expressing the target antigen, either by complement activation or cellular mechanisms; and (c) modulation of the function of the cell by binding to an antigen capable of transducing intracellular signals. The ability to enact such mechanisms depends on the function of the Fc piece of the mAb which, in turn, is governed by the subclass of antibody (immunoglobulin heavy chain isotype).

An additional potential cytotoxic mechanism, independent of immunoglobulin isotype, involves the addition of a cellular toxin to the mAb. This takes advantage of the general structure of certain bacterial and plant toxins. The toxins consist of two distinct disulfide bond-linked polypeptides. One peptide governs the specificity of the binding of intact toxin, whereas the other causes cytotoxicity, usually by inhibition of protein synthesis (92,93). By employing biochemical or molecular biological techniques, the toxic peptide part of the toxin can be linked to an mAb. In this manner, cells specifically targeted by the mAb can be eliminated by the action of the toxin. Investigators have used these techniques to couple mAbs with such toxins as ricin, diphtheria toxin, and pseudomonal exotoxin.

Most mAbs used, heretofore, have been mouse antibodies. The efficacy of these mAbs has been hampered predominantly by three problems: (a) variable ability of the mouse Fc piece to interact with human cellular Fc receptors and accomplish the effector functions noted in the above; (b) diminished serum half-life; and (c) adverse reactions related to the development of human antimouse antibodies (HAMA). These problems could conceivably be obviated by using

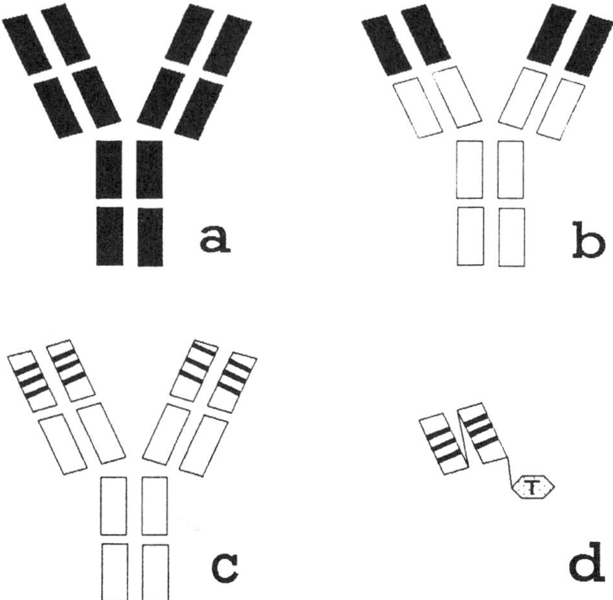

Fig. 3 Modifications of murine mAb used in the therapy of RA. Immunoglobulin molecules are shown with murine components in black, and human components in white. (a) Murine mAb; (b) Chimeric mAb, with variable regions from a murine mAb combined with constant regions from a human antibody to form an intact antibody. (c) Humanized or CDR-engrafted mAb, with only the CDR from a murine mAb combined with the remainder of a human antibody. (d) Immunoglobulin fragment. The variable region of a chimeric mAb, and therefore the binding specificity, is combined with a cellular toxin. The toxin replaces the constant portion of the antibody as an effector molecule (T).

human antibodies. Although human antibodies may be available by a variety of techniques in the future (94,95), the difficulty in generating human mAbs with high-avidity specificities of interest has dictated that for the foreseeable future, most mAbs will be generated in mice.

One potential means of decreasing the immunogenicity of murine mAbs while retaining effector function is by treating the mAbs with chemicals, such as polyethylene glycol (PEG), that increase the half-life and decrease the immunogenicity of proteins, without compromising their functions (96). In addition, by molecular techniques, hybrid mAbs can be created that have the binding specificity of the mouse mAb and the effector functions of a human antibody. There are several strategies to accomplish this (Fig. 3) (97). The simplest approach involves the combination of variable regions, which determine antigen specificity, from a murine antibody with the constant region of a human antibody. These chimeric antibodies would be expected to be less immunogenic than mouse mAbs, and more efficient at executing Fc-dependent functions. An even more elegant construct employs only the hypervariable or complementarity-determining regions (CDR) from the murine mAb. This "humanized" or "CDR-engrafted" antibody would be expected to be even less immunogenic than the chimeric mAb. However, the host could still potentially make anti-idiotypic antibodies to these mAbs. Other modifications of mAbs have generated additional potential therapeutic agents. Single-chain antigen-binding proteins are derived by isolating variable region fragments. These molecules lack any Fc-related function, but may be linked with other molecules, such as toxins. This generates not only effector molecules with pharmacokinetic properties distinct from intact immunoglobulin molecules, but also obviates untoward events related to interactions of mAbs with the Fc receptors of nontargeted cells. The rapid elimination of these molecules and, hence, their very short serum half-lives, might impede their widespread applicability. A variety of mAbs have been employed as immunomodulatory agents in the treatment of RA as well as other conditions, including renal, heart, and liver allograft transplants. The greatest amount of experience to date has been with anti-CD3 mAbs, which are widely used to treat allograft rejection (98). Many of the adverse reactions attributable to mAb administration have been nonlife-threatening and reversible. A frequent constellation of symptoms, the so-called cytokine release syndrome, consists preponderantly of symptoms such as fever, headache, and nausea. It is suggested that one mechanism underlying this symptom complex is the intravascular release of cytokines, especially tumor necrosis factor alpha (TNF-α) (99–101). Such symptoms usually abate, even with continued administration of mAb, or can be effectively prevented by corticosteriods. Interestingly, the occurrence of these symptoms seems to relate to the particular mAb used and may not occur with all murine mAbs, even those with the same target specificity (101). More serious adverse reactions relate to the ability of these mAbs to induce immediate hypersensitivity reactions. Although most patients treated with murine mAbs do develop HAMA, such reactions have fortunately occurred infrequently.

A variety of peptides have also been employed to affect T-cell-directed inflammatory responses. These small, soluble peptide molecules have, in common, the ability to bind and affect the function of a variety of cell surface molecules, including adhesion receptors, cytokine receptors, and MHC molecules. Examples of such peptides would include fragments of cytokines, soluble forms of cell surface receptors, and antigenic peptides. Occasionally, these have been naturally occurring peptides, rather than synthetic molecules. Many additional soluble inhibitors could conceivably be created. The potential mechanisms of action of these soluble molecules would include competitive or noncompetitive inhibiton for ligand and modulation of ligand function or expression. By employing biochemical or molecular biological techniques, it is also possible to link these molecules, for example, to a cellular toxin or to the Fc fragment of a human antibody. Each of these techniques would be expected to enhance the efficacy of the peptide molecules. In addition, soluble peptides can be linked to domains of immunoglobulin molecules, permitting the formation of immunoglobulinlike dimers, which would increase the avidity of the molecules for their targets, as well as increasing the biological half-life. Variables that would be germane to the expected efficacy of these soluble molecules and, hence, their usefulness would be their tissue distribution, their life, and their ability to antagonize specific components of the immune response.

IV. TARGETS

A. Major Histocompatibility Complex Molecules

It has been convincingly demonstrated that there is a relation between the expression of certain class II MHC gene products and both the development as well as the severity of RA (60–62). Thus, a large body of work has shown that there is a strong association between RA and the presence of DR4 or DR1 in different ethnic groups (49,51,56). More specifically, the development of RA appears to be associated with a specific epitope of the third hypervariable region of the DR β-chain which is conserved in the susceptibility-associated alleles *DRB10401* (formerly known as the *DW4* allele of DR4), *DRB10404* (formerly *DW14*), *DRB10405* (formerly *DW15*), *DRB10406* (formerly *DW16*), and *DRB10101* (formerly *DR1*) (32). The MHC molecules play a pivotal role in the generation of immune responses by virtue of their ability to bind antigenic fragments and present them to T cells. Furthermore, MHC molecules play a critical role in the shaping of the T-cell repertoire in the thymus. Given the connection between RA and these specific class II MHC gene products, these MHC molecules may be appropriate targets for specific immunomodulatory therapy. The methods by which interference with the function of class II MHC molecules has been attempted include (a) administration of polyclonal and monoclonal anti-MHC antibodies; (b) induction of anti-MHC molecules by anti-idiotypic mAb; and (c) use of peptide fragments to bind to MHC molecules and competitively inhibit the binding of potentially pathogenic peptides.

Antibodies directed against class II MHC antigens have been used successfully in several forms of class II-associated autoimmune diseases in animals (102). Notable examples are experimental allergic encephalomyelitis (EAE), diabetes mellitus, and lupuslike disease in mice. Importantly, such therapy was quite efficacious, but only when antibodies were given in close approximation to the time of immunization with relevant antigens or before the onset of established disease. Treatment of established disease was much less effective, and prolonged therapy was required.

In humans, polyclonal antibodies with specificity directed against class II MHC molecules were among the first forms of antibody therapy used for RA. With antibodies eluted from pooled placental tissue that had been shown indirectly to possess some anti-MHC class II activity, Sany et al. treated over 80 RA

Table 3 Monoclonal Antibodies Used in the Treatment of Rheumatoid Arthritis

Target	mAb	Isotype	Patients	Dose	Clinical effect[a]	HAMA[b]	Ref.
CD4	VIT4	Mouse IgG2a	3	10 mg/d × 7 d	Yes	100%	112
	MT-151	Mouse IgG2a	32	10–200 mg/d × 3–7 d	55%	40%	112, 115, 117
	BL4	Mouse IgG2a	7	20–40 mg/d × 10 d	Yes	57%	116
	B-F5	Mouse IgG1	20	10–30 mg/d × 10 d	55%	50%	118, 119, 121, 126
	16H5	Mouse IgG1	10	0.3 mg/kg/d × 7 d	60%	60%	122
	cM-T412	Chimeric human IgG1	33	10–200 mg/kg/d × 1–7 d	45%	n/a	123–125
CD5	CD5+	Mouse IgG1 + ricin A chain	76	0.2–0.33 mg/kg/d × 5 d	74%	100%	127
CD7	RFT2	Mouse IgG2a	6	12 mg × 1d, 6 mg × 13 d	33%	100%	128
	SDZ-CHH-380	Chimeric human IgG1	10	4–20 mg/d × 2 d	60%	n/a[c]	129
CDw52	Campath-1H	Humanized IgG1	8	4–8 mg/d × 10 d	88%	n/a	130

[a]Clinical efficacy, percentage of patients improving as defined by any evaluation criteria used by the authors.
[b]HAMA, human antimouse antibiodies, as reported by the authors.
[c]n/a, not applicable.

patients in an uncontrolled trial (103,104). The treatment was well tolerated, and clinical efficacy was noted in about half the patients. Of note, relatively large amounts of antibody were administered at relatively frequent intervals (1500 mg given 7 days of each month for several months). Whether anti-MHC activity of the antibodies explained the apparent efficacy remains unclear, since control immunoglobulin preparations also induced some improvement in treated patients.

The mechanism whereby anti-class II MHC antibodies exert their immuno-modulatory effects are unknown. Among the potential mechanisms are (a) interference with T-cell–APC interactions by blocking restriction sites on APC; (b) alterations in T-cell recirculation; (c) death of APC; (d) inhibition of class II expression on target organs; and (e) activation of suppressor T cells (105). In addition to administration of mAb against class II molecules, investigators have attempted to induce the endogenous production of such antibodies by immunization with anti-idiotypic antibodies. Such an approach would have the theoretical advantage of obviating the necessity for repeated administration of exogenous antibody. In a phase I study of six RA patients, Fiocco et al. (106) used an anti-idiotypic antibody generated in mice by immunization with an anti-HLA-DR/DP mAb. Anti-idiotypic responses to the immunizing mAb were noted in four patients. Three patients experienced a 50% clinical improvement, lasting at least 6 months after three injections of 500 μg of mAb over 13–18 months. No adverse sequelae were noted.

An additional means of inhibiting the function of class II MHC molecules, namely, blockade with competitive peptides, has recently been established as an alternative to treatment with anti-class II mAb (107–109). In EAE, coadministration of competitor peptides with the encephalitogenic peptide results in attenuation of the disease. The mechanism of action of these peptides has not been clearly defined, and may be different for various peptides. In some cases, competitive inhibition for antigen binding to MHC molecules has been suggested. Other mechanisms, however, including generation of regulatory T cells and antagonism at the level of antigen–MHC interactions with the T-cell receptor, have been suggested (109,110).

B. T-Cell-Associated Molecules

CD4

CD4$^+$ helper T cells play a crucial role in the etiopathogenesis of RA; therefore, they are an appropriate target for immunomodulatory intervention. One means to accomplish this is by use of mAbs directed against CD4. Potential mechanisms whereby these mAbs might be expected to exert a beneficial effect could potentially include (a) the eradication of CD4$^+$ cells, (b) alteration in the recirculation of CD4$^+$ cells, and (c) modification of the function of CD4$^+$ T cells. The CD4 molecule is also present on other cell types, including eosinophils and monocytes.

Therefore, it is conceivable that anti-CD4 mAbs might exert an immunomodulatory effect by actions on these cell types as well. Several anti-CD4 mAbs, including murine as well as one chimeric mAb, have been used by various groups of investigators in the treatment of advanced RA that had been refractory to other therapies (111–126). In general, the results obtained in these various uncontrolled trials may be summarized as follows (Table 3): Following administration of mAb, there was a uniform reduction in the numbers of circulating CD4$^+$ T cells. This was usually transient, with numbers of CD4$^+$ cells returning to normal within 24 h. However, in some patients and in chimpanzees, a prolonged depression of the number of circulating CD4$^+$ cells has been noted (114,120). In most cases, in vitro T-cell function is depressed only transiently during treatment. Clinical response, as evidenced by a variety of measurements, was achieved in approximately half of the treated patients. Clinical benefit was usually transient, with relapse of symptoms commonly observed within several months. In several patients, a more prolonged clinical effect has been reported. However, absence of significant clinical efficacy has also been observed. Interestingly, despite improvements in indexes such as joint pain, morning stiffness, and tender joint count, serological markers of disease activity, such as the erythrocyte sedimentation rate (ESR) and C-reactive protein (CRP) levels were less likely to demonstrate improvement. Adverse effects related to therapy were usually mild and reversible, most frequently fever. Approximately half of the patients developed antibodies to mouse protein. However, they were usually low titer and did not preclude retreatment. When patients were retreated, efficacy was comparable with that achieved during the initial course of therapy. Currently, more extensive clinical trials are in progress. The results of these studies will more clearly delineate the role of anti-CD4 antibodies in RA.

CD5

The CD5 molecule was originally chosen as a therapeutic target in RA because it is expressed both on T cells as well as the subset of B cells that have been shown to produce autoantibodies in the mouse. However, it has been suggested that the immunomodulatory effect of anti-CD5 mAb may depend on only its effect on T cells. In an uncontrolled study, using an anti-CD5 mAb that was conjugated to the A chain of the ricin toxin, 76 patients with refractory RA were treated (127). More than half of the treated patients showed a beneficial clinical response that persisted in a few patients. Adverse reactions were mostly cutaneous exanthema or constitutional symptoms. Most patients exhibited a marked transient decrease in the number of circulating CD3$^+$CD5$^+$ cells. Although clinical benefit tended to abate after several months, a significant number of patients were successfully retreated. Of note, almost all patients developed significant titers of HAMA as well as antiricin antibodies. Despite this, serious reactions at retreatment were infrequent.

CD7

Another T-cell surface marker that has been the target of immunotherapy in RA is CD7. This molecule is present on most T cells and is expressed to a greater extent on T cells that have been activated, although its expression is down-regulated on memory T cells as well as on T cells found in the rheumatoid synovium. Administration of a murine mAb to CD7 in an uncontrolled study resulted in a transient depletion of CD7 T cells from the circulation (128). Clinical improvement was not substantial, with only two of six treated patients demonstrating a transient clinical improvement. In another study, a chimeric antibody composed of a murine anti-CD7 mAb and a human IgG1 was used in ten patients with RA (129). Clinical improvement was modest, with six patients demonstrating transient improvement in joint scores. No patients developed anti-globulin antibodies after this single course of therapy. Interestingly, an anti-CD7 mAb had been shown to exert immunosuppressive effects in vitro, and had been used successfully in renal allograft recipients. This suggests that mechanisms other than transient alteration in circulating lymphocyte populations may be of importance in the efficacy of anti-T-cell mAbs in RA. Notably, cells in the rheumatoid synoviun express decreased amounts of CD7, suggesting that they may not be affected by the mAb treatment.

CDw52

Another target of immunomodulatory therapy of RA has been CDw52, a glyco-protein present on lymphocytes as well as on some monocytes. In one study, using a humanized mAb to CDw52, eight patients with severe RA were treated (130). Treatment resulted in a substantial and persistent reduction in circulating lymphocytes, in particular $CD4^+$ T cells. Clinical efficacy was noted in seven of the eight treated patients, although relapse was uniform. Although no antiglobulin antibodies were found after the first course of therapy, anti-idiotypic antibodies were found in three of four retreated patients. These results indicate that even though humanized mAb are less immunogenic than murine mAb, their therapeutic use may elicit an immune response that could affect efficacy.

C. Adhesion Receptors

Adhesion receptors represent a potentially important target for immunomodulatory therapy in RA. By binding their specific counterreceptors, cell surface adhesion receptors mediate cell–cell interactions, thereby governing several processes critical to the immune response (131). Of particular importance to the pathogenesis of RA, this includes the migration of all lineages of leukocytes across the vascular endothelium into sites of inflammation, and immunoregulatory interactions between T cells and antigen-presenting cells. Several studies that used blocking mAbs have evaluated the effect of inhibition of adhesion receptor function in various inflammatory processes (reviewed in 132). In a variety of models of acute inflammation, various mAbs have effectively attenuated the inflammatory response. Because of the role of T cells in the pathogenesis of RA, adhesion molecules utilized by T cells may be a particularly attractive target. Although T cells possess a repertoire of adhesion receptors, several studies have demonstrated a predominant role for lymphocyte function-associated antigen-1 (LFA-1), which binds to its ligands intercellular adhesion molecules-1, 2, and 3 (ICAM-1,2,3) (133).

Interference with LFA-1–ICAM interactions by mAb administration has been successful in the therapy of several animal models of inflammation. This has included ischemia–reperfusion injury, inflammatory asthma, renal allograft rejection, and experimental arthritis (134–138). In addition, tolerance to a cardiac allograft in mice was achieved by simultaneously using mAbs to ICAM-1 and LFA-1 (139). Currently, studies are in progress to evaluate the efficacy of anti-ICAM-1 mAb in patients with RA (140).

In addition to blocking mAb, the function of adhesion receptors may be inhibited by soluble forms of their counterreceptors. These soluble molecules, which are sometimes present in detectable amounts in normal serum, might subserve a competitive and inhibitory role in the inflammatory response. Soluble forms of the adhesion receptors P-selectin and the murine homologue of L-selectin, have been successfully employed to attenuate neutrophil adhesion and accumulation at inflammatory sites (141,142). Salient characteristics of soluble forms of adhesion receptors, such as their tissue distribution, serum half-life, and ability to interact with effector systems could be altered by creating hybrid molecules. For example, soluble adhesion receptors have been coupled to IgG, thereby altering their serum half-life and their potential therapeutic effect (142). Soluble forms of adhesion receptors and their counterreceptors may be an important form of anti-inflammatory therapy in the future.

D. Cytokines

Cytokines exert various effector functions in both normal homeostasis and in the development of immune and inflammatory responses (143). Because these small protein mediators perform an integral role in the initiation and propagation of immune responses, they serve as targets for immunomodulatory therapy. Furthermore, in autoimmune systemic inflammatory disorders, such as RA, there may be an imbalance in the relative quantities of specific cytokines synthesized at sites of inflammation. Such "cytokine dysregulation" has been suggested to be an important contributory pathophysiological mechanism and, therefore, an appropriate target for therapeutic modulation. In patients with RA, mRNAs encoding numerous cytokines, including interleukin (IL)-1α, IL-1β, IL-2, IL-6, IL-8, granulocyte–macrophage colony-stimulating factor (GM-CSF), G-CSF, TNF-α, TNF-β, inteferon (IFN)-γ, platelet-derived growth factor (PDGF), and transforming growth factor (TGF)-β, have been detected in cells recovered from the inflamed synovium (144). Cytokines considered to play an especially prominent role in rheumatoid inflammation are IL-1, IL-6, and TNF-α (143). In addition, because T cells play a prominent role in RA, IL-2 is an additional cytokine target.

There are several potential mechanisms whereby the function of a particular cytokine might be altered (145,146). These include (a) antibodies directed against the cytokine itself, (b) soluble cytokine receptors, (c) cytokine receptor antagonists, and (d) administration of cytokines with opposing functions from the target cytokine. Interestingly, although Abs to cytokines and soluble cytokine receptors are considered to be inhibitory, it has also been suggested that, in addition, they may function as potentiators of cytokine function, perhaps physiologically. Thus, antibodies directed at cytokines, including IL-1 and TNF-α, have been described in normal individuals as well as in those with inflammatory diseases (145). Similarly, soluble TNF receptors have increased the serum half-life of TNF (147). Molecules such as these have been hypothesized to subserve a potentiating or chaperon role, helping to deliver cytokines to appropriate sites. Interfering with the function of these molecules could, paradoxically, exert an immunosuppressive effect. An understanding of the complex networks in which various cytokines function and their interactions is, as yet, incomplete. Therefore, therapeutic interventions that substantially alter the function of these molecules could have unanticipated results for the maintenance of homeostasis as well as various facets of the immune response. Moreover, the apparent redundancy in cytokine action suggests that targeting any individual cytokine may not effect significant alterations in a chronic inflammatory disease, such as RA.

Cytokines themselves may also be used as immunomodulatory tools. One method would be the administration of cytokines possessing effects that might antagonize the function of another target cytokine. Another means of employing cytokines would be to use the specificity of a cytokine for its receptor to target cells expressing the cytokine receptor. If coupled with effector molecules, such as toxins, this would presumably achieve results similar to targeting with anticytokine receptor mAbs.

Interleukin-1

A considerable body of literature has documented the pivotal role of IL-1 as a proinflammatory molecule. The actions of this cytokine extend beyond its influence on the immune system and inflammatory responses, however, and include various other physiological and metabolic effects. Of particular importance in the pathophysiology of RA may be the ability of IL-1 to induce the synthesis of collagenase and other neutral proteases; to up-regulate the expression of adhesion receptors on endothelial cells and, thereby, alter leukocyte traffic; and to cause constitutional symptoms such as fever and anorexia (143). An important role for IL-1 in RA is further supported by several lines of evidence. Thus, although studies looking for the presence of IL-1 in synovial fluid have yielded variable results, several studies provide evidence that cells within the inflamed synovium actively synthesize IL-1 (reviewed in 143,144). Furthermore, injection of IL-1 into the joints of experimental animals can cause inflammatory arthritis. Finally, several therapies directed at IL-1 have been effective in attenuating some forms of inflammation.

Immunomodulatory therapy targeting IL-1 may be theoretically approached in various ways. Much work has focused on the naturally occurring IL-1 receptor antagonist (IL-1Ra) (145,146,148–150). This molecule binds to the IL-1 receptor (IL-1R) on various target cells, but transduces no stimulatory signal and, thereby, acts as a competitive inhibitor in the binding of endogenous IL-1. Interleukin-1Ra has been effectively used in the inhibition of several IL-1-mediated events. Of note, however, inhibition usually required a 10- or 100-fold molar excess of IL-1Ra (148–150). In addition to the ability of IL-1Ra to inhibit IL-1-dependent cellular effects in vitro, this molecule has been used to inhibit IL-1-driven in-flammatory events in vivo. Administration of IL-1Ra abated the synovial leuko-cyte aggregation in response to intra-articular IL-1 (150). Moreover, an IL-1 inhibitor successfully abrogated synovial inflammation, in a dose-dependent fashion, when administered to Lewis rats with adjuvant arthritis (151). In mice, IL-1Ra was able to attenuate the inflammation associated with collagen arthritis (145). The complete spectrum of effects of IL-1Ra in altering experimental models of arthritis remains unclear, however. Thus, IL-1Ra administration did not effectively inhibit antigen-induced arthritis in mice, whereas it did protect against the inhibition of cartilage proteoglycan synthesis (152). The experience with IL-1Ra in RA patients has been limited. In one placebo-controlled study of 25 patients given six different doses, IL-1Ra was effective in a dose-dependent manner (153). Open-label treatment of 15 patients over 28 days similarly showed dose-dependent improvement in joint count, ESR, and CRP.

Tumor Necrosis Factor

Similar to IL-1, TNF has been suggested to play an important role in the patho-physiology of RA, based on both its spectrum of effects as an immunoregulatory and proinflammatory molecule as well as the various metabolic and physiological changes it induces. Thus, intra-articular administration of TNF causes an influx of inflammatory cells (143). In addition, well-described actions of TNF include not only chemotaxis for leukocytes, but also fever and cachexia. As a target of immunotherapy, the function of TNF may be interfered with by several means. In one report, collagen-induced arthritis in mice was attenuated with either monoclonal or polyclonal anti-TNF antibodies (154). Additional potential thera-pies that could interfere with the function of TNF are the soluble forms of TNF receptor proteins. These molecules, which have been recovered from the normal serum of normal persons and in increased amounts in patients with various inflammatory diseases, are cleaved from the surface of several cell types. Because they compete with cell surface TNF receptors, they have been shown to inhibit several TNF-mediated processes (155). Furthermore, soluble forms of the TNF receptor are able to abrogate the effects of TNF in vivo (e.g., endotoxic shock). These molecules might be potential therapeutic alternatives in the treatment of RA. However, as has been suggested for anticytokine antibodies, soluble forms of the TNF receptors might serve a potentiating role for the activity of TNF by inhibiting its degradation (147). Their usefulness as inhibitors of inflammation would depend on several variables, including concentration of soluble receptor, concentration of cytokine, and clearance of cytokine from the local inflammatory site.

Interleukin-2

Interleukin-2 is a potential target for immunomodulation of T-cell-mediated diseases. As it is produced exclusively by activated T cells, and mediates its effects by interacting with specific high-affinity receptors (IL-2R) expressed on T cells only when they are activated, interference with the function of this molecule is relatively selective. However, the activity of IL-2 is not specific for T cells, since IL-2Rs are also expressed by monocytes and B cells, and the function of each of these cells can be altered by IL-2. Because, within the synovium of patients with RA, it has been demonstrated that the relative percentages of T cells that are activated and that express IL-2R are greater than those in contols, IL-2 may be a useful target in the treatment of RA. Furthermore, because cyclosporine inhibits IL-2 production, the established usefulness of cyclosporine in patients with RA offers additional support for a role of IL-2 in this disease process (41–43).

There are two primary approaches that have been used in targeting activated T cells that express IL-2 receptors: (a) mAbs or mAb fragments, which are directed against Il-2R and may be linked to effector molecules, such as toxins; and (b) the IL-2 molecule itself linked to toxins (156). Campath 6, an mAb directed against the IL-2R, was administered to three patients with RA (157). All three showed clinical improvement following the 10-day course of 25 mg/ day; however, the response lasted less than a month in one patient and 3 months in the remaining two. Combinations of anti-IL-2R with pseudomonal exotoxin (PE) have been synthesized, and have shown efficacy in T-cell malignancies. In addition, two fusion toxins, one combining PE with a fragment of anti-IL-2R mAb single-chain antigen-binding protein, anti-Tac[Fv]–PE-40, and another combining IL-2 with the toxic domain of diphtheria toxin (DAB_{486}-IL-2) have been synthesized. The former has been successfully used to treat adjuvant arthritis in rats (158). The latter has been used in animal models and has also been administered to patients with refractory RA (159). Thirteen patients were treated with two different doses administered over a 7-day course, and four patients demonstrated a > 50% response.

Interferon Gamma

Interferon gamma (IFN-γ) is a T-cell-derived cytokine that has profound effects on the immunoregulatory function of antigen-presenting cells as well as other cell types. It has both enhancing as well as inhibitory effects on the immune response, depending on the system investigated. IFN-γ has been used in the treatment of RA, among other autoimmune diseases. In one report, a statistically significant improvement was noted in patients treated with IFN-γ compared with those given placebo (160). A 5-year prospective trial also demonstrated benefit in treated patients after the first year. However, there was a progressive dropout in subsequent years because of lack of efficacy (161). Furthermore, a double-blind, controlled study showed no significant benefit (162). The efficacy of IFN-γ in RA remains to be established.

V. CONCLUSION

The treatment of RA is evolving. Previously used empiric therapies, which addressed the disease in a nonspecific manner, may be replaced by a variety of therapies that target discrete parts of the immunologically driven inflammatory process in RA. As the pathophysiology of RA becomes more clearly delineated, there is the expectation that biotechnical advances may allow additional forms of therapeutic intervention that are even yet more specific to the disease process. As alluded to above, if either the etiopathogenic agent(s) or the arthritogenic clones of T cells can be identified, specific types of therapy would be conceivable using contemporary technology. In addition, it may be reasonably expected that advances achievable in the future would further refine our therapeutic armamentarium. Many prospective therapies might be expected to employ the rapidly developing techniques of molecular biology (163). The expression of certain genes, for example, may be modulated by use of antisense nucleic acids. In the treatment of RA, modulation of cytokine activity or production in this manner might be efficacious. Furthermore, gene manipulation may allow an even more drastic alteration of cell function. For example, the ability of arthritogenic T cells to migrate into inflammatory sites or to engage heterotypic intercellular immunological-potentiating reactions may be altered by targeting the genes for cytokines, cell surface adhesion molecules, HLA-DR, the TCR, or other moieties. These types of therapy might allow the reestablishment of immunological homeostasis. As therapies for RA become more refined and more specific, it might be possible to speak of truly disease-modifying drugs for this disease.

REFERENCES

1. Benedek TG. A century of American rheumatology. Ann Intern Med 1987; 106:304–312.

2. Rose HM, Ragan C, Pearce E, Lipman MO. Differential agglutination of normal and sensitized sheep erythrocytes by sera of patients with rheumatoid arthritis. Proc Soc Exp Biol Med 1948; 68:1–6.

3. Harris ED. Rheumatoid arthritis; pathophysiology and implications for therapy. N Engl J Med 1990; 322:1277–89.

4. Kingsley G, Pitzalis C, Panayi GS. Immunogenetic and cellular immune mechanisms in rheumatoid arthritis: relevance to new therapeutic strategies. Br J Rheumatol 1990; 429:58–64.

5. Kingsley G, Panayi G, Lanchbury J. Immunotherapy of rheumatic diseases— practice and prospects. Immunol Today 1991; 12:177–179.

6. Strober S, Holoshitz J. Mechanisms of immune injury in rheumatoid arthritis: evidence for the involvement of T cells and heat-shock protein. Immunol Rev 1990; 118:233–255.

7. Froland SS, Natvig JB, Busby G. Immunological characterization of lymophocytes in synovial fluid from patients with rheumatoid arthritis. Scand J Immunol 1973; 2:67–73.

8. Sheldon PJ, Papamichail M, Holborow EJ. Studies on synovial fluid lymphocytes in rheumatoid arthritis. Ann Rheum Dis 1974; 33:509–514.

9. Utsinger PD. Synovial fluid lymphocytes in rheumatoid arthritis. Arthritis Rheum 1975; 18:595–602.

10. Van Boxel JA, Paget SA. Predominantly T-cell infiltrate in rheumatoid synovial membranes. N Engl J Med 1975; 293:517–520.

11. Loewi G, Lance EM, Reynolds J. Study of lymphoid cells from inflamed synovial membranes. Ann Rheum Dis 1975; 34:524–528.

12. Burmester GR, Yu DTY, Irani AM, Kunkel HG, Winchester RJ. Ia$^+$ T cells in synovial fluid and tissue of patients with rheumatoid arthritis. Arthritis Rheum 1981; 24:1370–1376.

13. Forre O, Dobloug JH, Natvig JB. Augmented numbers of HLA-DR positive T lymphocytes in the synovial fluid and synovial tissue of patients with rheumatoid arthritis and juvenile rheumatoid arthritis. Scand J Immunol 1982; 15:227–271.

14. Fox RI, Fong S, Sabharwal N, Carstens SA, Kubg PC, Vaughan JH. Synovial fluid lymphocytes differ from peripheral blood lymphocytes in patients with rheumatoid arthritis. J Immunol 1982; 128:351–356.

15. Kluin-Nelemans HC, van der Linden JA, Gmelig-Meyling FH, Scheurman HJ. HLA-DR positive T lymphocytes in blood and synovial fluid in rheumatoid arthritis. J Rheumatol 1984; 11:272–279.

16. Salmon M, Bacon PA, Symmons DP, Blann AD. Transferrin receptor bearing cells in the peripheral blood of patients with rheumatoid arthritis. Clin Exp Immunol 1985; 62:346–352.

17. Poulter LW, Duke O, Panayi GS, Hobbs S, Raftery MJ, Janossy G. Activated T lymphocytes of the synovial membrane in rheumatoid arthritis and other arthropies. Scand J Immunol 1985; 22:683–689.

18. Hemler ME, Glass D, Coblyn JS, Jacobson JG. Very late activation antigens on rheumatoid synovial fluid T lymphocytes. Association with stages of T cell activation. J Clin Invest 1986; 78:696–676.

19. Jahn B, Burmester GR, Gramatzki M, Weseloh G, Stock P, Kalden JR. Intraarticular T lymphocytes in monoarticular and oligoarticular inflammatory joint

diseases. Normal subset distribution and less numbers of activated T cells indicate major differences as compared to rheumatoid arthritis. J Rheumatol 1986; 13:254–259.

20. Goto M, Miyamoto T, Nishioka K. 2 Dimensional flow cytometric analysis of activation antigens expressed on the synovial fluid T cells in rheumatoid arthritis. J Rheumatol 1987; 14:230–236.

21. Jahn B, Burmester GR, Stock P, Rohwer P, Kalden JR. Functional and phenotypical characterization of activated T cells from intra-articular sites in inflammatory joint diseases: possible modulation of the CD3 antigen. Scand J Immunol 1987; 26:745–749.

22. Pitzalis C, Kingsley G, Lanchbury JS, Murphy J, Panayi GS. Expression of HLA-DR, DQ, and DP antigens and interleukin-2 receptor on synovial fluid T lymphocyte subsets in rheumatoid arthritis: evidence for "frustrated" activation. J Rheumatol 1987; 14:662–668.

23. Nakao H, Eguchi K, Kawakami A, Migita K, Otsubo T, Ueki Y, Shimomura C, Tezuka H, Mastsunaga M, Maeda K, Nagataki S. Increment in Tac positive cells in peripheral blood from patients with rheumatoid arthritis. Arthritis Rheum 1989; 16:907–913.

24. Smith MD, Roberts-Thompson PJ. Lymphocyte surface marker expression in rheumatic diseases: evidence for prior activation of lymphocytes in vivo. Ann Rheum Dis 1990; 49:81–85.

25. Potocnik AJ, Kinne R, Menninger H, Zacher J, Emmrich F, Kroczek RA. Expression of activation antigens on T cells in rheumatoid arthritis patients. Scand J Immunol 1990; 31:213–217.

26. Hirose T, Goto M, Okumura K. HLA-DR, DQ, and DP antigen expression in synovial fluid T lymphocytes in rheumatoid arthritis: cell cycle analysis of HLA-DP positive cells. J Rheumatol 1990; 17:18–25.

27. Holoshitz J, Naparstek Y, Ben-Nun A, Cohen IR. Lines of T lymphocyte induce or vaccinate against autoimmune arthritis. Science 1983; 219:56–59.

28. Holoshitz J, Matitiau A, Cohen IR. Arthritis induced in rats by cloned T lymphocytes responsive to mycobacteria but not to collagen type II. J Clin Invest 1984; 73:211–222.

29. Dumont AE, Mayer DJ, Mulholland JH. The suppression of immunologic activity by diversion of the thoracic duct. Ann Surg 1964; 160:373–383.

30. Wegelius O, Laine V, Lindstrom B, Kockars M. Fistula of the thoracic duct as immunosuppressive treatment in rheumatoid arthritis. Acta Med Scand 1970; 187:39–54.

31. Paulus HE, Machleder HI, Levine S, Yu DTY, MacDonald NS. Lymphocyte involvement in rheumatoid arthritis: studies during thoracic duct drainage. Arthritis Rheum 1977; 20:1249–1262.

32. Ueo T, Tanaka S, Tominaga Y, Ogawa H, Sakurami T. The effect of thoracic duct drainage on lymphocyte dynamics and clinical symptoms in patients with rheumatoid arthritis. Arthritis Rheum 1979; 22:1405–1412.

33. Karsh J, Klippel JH, Plotz PH, Decker JL, Wright DG, Flye MW. Lymphapheresis in rheumatoid arthritis. Arthritis Rheum 1981; 24:867–873.

34. Wilder RL, Decker JL. T-inducer lymphocytes, leukapheresis and the pathogenesis of rheumatoid arthritis. Clin Exp Rheumatol 1983; 1:89–91.

35. Emery P, Smith GN, Panayi GS. Lymphacytapheresis—a feasible treatment for rheumatoid arthritis. Br J Rheumatol 1986; 25:40–43.

36. Kotzin BL, Strober S, Engleman EG, Calin A, Hoppe RT, Kansas GS, Terrell CP, Kaplan HS. Treatment of intractable rheumatoid arthritis with total lymphoid irradiation. N Engl J Med 1981; 305:969–976.

37. Trentham DE, Belli JA, Anderson RJ, Buckley JA, Goetzl EJ, David JR, Austen KF. Clinical and immunological effects of fractionated total lymphoid irradiation in refractory rheumatoid arthritis. N Engl J Med 1981; 305:976–982.

38. Strober S, Tanay A, Field E, Hoppe RT, Calin A, Engleman EG, Kotzin B, Brown BW, Kaplan HS. Efficacy of total lymphoid irradiation in intractable rheumatoid arthritis. Ann Intern Med 1985; 102:441–449.

39. Nüsslein HG, Herbst M, Manger BJ, Gramatzki M, Burmester GR, Fritz H, Sauer R, Kalden JR. Total lymphoid irradiation in patients with refractory rheumatoid arthritis. Arthritis Rheum 1985; 28:1205–1210.

40. Gaston JSH, Strober S, Solvera JJ, Gandour D, Lane N, Schurman D, Hoppe RT, Chin RC, Eugui EM, Vaughan JH, Allison AC. Dissection of the mechanisms of immune injury in rheumatoid arthritis using total lymphoid irradiation. Arthritis Rheum 1988; 31:21–29.

41. Dougadas M, Awada H, Amor B. Cyclosporin in rheumatoid arthritis: a double-blind placebo controlled study in 52 patients. Ann Rheum Dis 1988; 47:127–133.

42. Yocum E, Klippel JH, Wilder RL. Cyclosporine A in severe, treatment refractory rheumatoid arthritis. Ann Intern Med 1988; 109:863–869.

43. Weinblatt ME, Coblyn JS, Fraser PA. Cyclosporin: a treatment of refractory rheumatoid arthritis. Arthritis Rheum 1987; 30:11–17.

44. Duke O, Panayi GS, Janossy G, Poulter LW. An immunohistological analysis of lymphocyte subpopulations and their microenvironment in the synovial membranes of patients with rheumatoid arthritis using monoclonal antibodies. Clin Exp Immunol 1982; 49:22–30.

45. Kurosaka M, Ziff M. Immunoelectron microscopic study of the distribution of T cell subsets in rheumatoid synovium. J Exp Med 1983; 158:1191–1210.

46. Goto M, Miyamoto T, Nishioka K, Uchida S. T cytotoxic and helper cells are markedly increased, and T suppressor and inducer cells are markedly decreased, in rheumatoid synovial fluids. Arthritis Rheum 1987; 30:737–745.

47. Pitzalis C, Kingsley G, Murphy J, Panayi G. Abnormal distribution of the helper–inducer and suppressor–inducer T-lymphocyte subsets in the rheumatoid joint. Clin Immunol Immunopathol 1987; 45:252–265.

48. Cush JJ, Lipsky PE. Phenotypic analysis of synovial tissue and peripheral blood lymphocytes isolated from patients with rheumatoid arthritis. Arthritis Rheum 1988; 31:1230–1239.

49. Stastny P. Mixed lymphocyte culture typing cells from patients with rheumatoid arthritis. Tissue Antigens 1974; 4:572–579.

50. McMichael AJ, Sasazuki T, McDevitt HO, Payne RO. Increased frequency of HLA-Cw3 and HLA-Dw4 in rheumatoid arthritis. Arthritis Rheum 1977; 20:1037–1042.

51. Panayi GS, Wooley P, Batchelor JR. Genetic basis of rheumatoid disease: HLA antigens, disease manifestations and toxic reactions to drugs. Br Med J 1978; 2:1326–1328.

52. Stastny P. Association of the B-cell alloantigen DRw4 with rheumatoid arthritis. N Engl J Med 1978; 298:869–873.

53. Schiff B, Mizrachi Y, Orgad S, Yaron M, Gazit E. Association of HLA-Aw31 and HLA-DR1 with adult rheumatoid arthritis. Ann Rheum Dis 1982; 41:403–407.

54. Goronzy J, Weynand CM, Fathman CG. Shared T cell recognition sites on human histocompatibility leukocyte class II molecules of patients with seropositive rheumatoid arthritis. J Clin Invest 1986; 77:1042–1053.

55. Zoschke D, Segall M. Dw subtypes of DR4 in rheumatoid arthritis: evidence for a preferential association with Dw4. Hum Immunol 1986; 118–124.

56. Woodrow JC. Analysis of the HLA association with rheumatoid arthritis. Dis Markers 1986; 4:7–12.

57. Wordsworth BP, Lanchbury JSS, Sakkas LI, Welsh KI, Panayi GS, Bell JI. HLA-DR4 subtype frequencies in rheumatoid arthritis indicate that *DRB1* is the major susceptibility locus within the HLA class II region. Proc Natl Acad Sci USA 1989; 86:10049–10053.

58. Gregersen PK, Silver J, Winchestre RJ. The shared epitope hypothesis: an approach to understanding the molecular genetics of susceptibility to rheumatoid arthritis. Arthritis Rheum 1987; 30:1205–1213.

59. McDermott M, McDevitt H. The immunogenetics of rheumatic diseases. Bull Rheum Dis 1988; 38:1–10.

60. Dalton TA, Bennett JC. Autoimmune disease and the major histocompatibility complex: therapeutic implications. Am J Med 1992; 92:183–188.

61. Singal DP, Green D, Reid B, Gladman DD, Buchanan WW. HLA-D region genes and rheumatoid arthritis (RA): importance of DR and DQ genes in conferring susceptibility to RA. Ann Rheum Dis 1992; 51:23–28.

62. McCusker CT, Reid B, Green D, Gladman DD, Buchanan WW, Singal DP. HLA-D region antigens in patients with rheumatoid arthritis. Arthritis Rheum 1991; 34:192–197.

63. Bijlsma JWJ, Derksen RWHM, Huber-Bruning O, Borleffs JCC. Does AIDS cure rheumatoid arthritis? Ann Rheum Dis 1988; 47:350–352.

64. Firestein GS, Zvaifler NJ. How important are T cells in chronic rheumatoid synovitis? Arthritis Rheum 1990; 33:768–773.

65. Kavanaugh AF, Lipsky PE. Gold, penicillamine, antimalarials, and sulfasalazine. In: Gallin JI, Goldstein IM, Snyderman R, eds. Inflammation: basic principles and practice, 2nd ed. New York: Raven Press, 1992: 1083–1101.

66. Kushner I. Does aggressive therapy of rheumatoid arthritis affect outcome? J Rheumatol 1989; 16:1–4.

67. Wolfe F. 50 years of antirheumatic therapy: the prognosis of rheumatoid arthritis. J Rheumatol 1990; 17(suppl):24–32.

68. Situnayake RD, Gringulis KA, McConkey B. Long term treatment of rheumatoid arthritis with sulphasalazine, gold, or penicillamine: a comparison using life-table methods. Ann Rheum Dis 1987; 46:177–183.

69. Felson DT, Anderson JJ, Meenan RF. The comparative efficacy and toxicity of second-line drugs in rheumatoid arthritis: results of two metaanalyses. Arthritis Rheum 1990; 33:1449–1461.

70. Adorini L, Barnaba V, Bona C, Celada F, Lanzavecchia A, Sercaz E, Suciu-Foca

N, Wekerle H. New perspectives on immunointervention in autoimmune diseases. Immunol Today 1990; 11:383–386.

71. Feldmann M, June CH, McMichael A, Maini R, Simpson E, Woody JN. T-cell-targeted immunotherapy. Immunol Today 1992; 13:84–85.

72. Lamont AG, Sette A, Fujinami R, Colon SM, Miles C, Grey HM. Inhibition of experimental autoimmune encephalomyelitis induction in SJL/J mice by using a peptide with high affinity for I-As molecules. J Immunol 1990; 145:1687–1695.

73. Lider O, Karin N, Shinitzky M, Cohen IR. Therapeutic vaccination against adjuvant arthritis using autoimmune T lymphocytes treated with hydrostatic pressure. Proc Natl Acad Sci USA 1987; 84:4577 4580.

74. Lider O, Reshef T, Beraud E, Ben-Nun A, Cohen IR. Anti-idiotypic network induced by T cell vaccination against experimental autoimmune encephalomyelitis. Science 1988; 239:181–183.

75. Vandenbark AA, Hashem G, Offner H. Immunization with a synthetic T cell receptor V-region peptide protects against experimental autoimmune encephalomyelitis. Nature 1989; 341:541–544.

76. Beverley PCL. Is T-cell memory maintained by crossreactive stimulation? Immunol Today 1990; 11:203–205.

77. Haqqi TM, Anderson GD, Banerjee S, David CS. Resticted heterogeneity in T-cell antigen receptor V_β gene usage in the lymph nodes and arthritic joints of mice. Proc Natl Acad Sci USA 1992; 89:1253–1255.

78. van Laar JM, Miltenburg AMM, Verdonk M-JA, Bernstein BH, de Vries RRP, van den Elsen PJ, Breedveld FC. Analysis of T-cell receptor β-chain gene rearrangements in patients with rheumatoid arthritis. Arthritis Rheum 1990; 33(suppl 9):S56.

79. Savill CM, Delves PJ, Kioussis D, Walker P, Lydyard PM, Colaco B, Shipley M, Roitt IM. A minority of patients with rheumatoid arthritis show a dominant rearrangement of T cell receptor β chain genes in synovial lymphocytes. Scand J Immunol 1987; 25:629–636.

80. Duby AD, Sinclair AK, Osborne-Lawrence SL, Zeldes W, Kan L, Fox DA. Clonal heterogeneity of synovial fluid lymphocytes from patients with rheumatoid arthritis. Proc Natl Acad Sci USA 1989; 86:6206–6210.

81. Cush JJ, Duby AD, Lightfoot E, Lipsky PE. The search for oligoclonal T cells in rheumatoid synovium. Arthritis Rheum 1990; 33(suppl 9):S16.

82. Stamenkovic I, Stegagno M, Wright KA, Krane SM, Amento EP, Colvin RB, Duquesnoy RJ, Kurnick JT. Clonal dominance among T-lymphocyte infiltrates in arthritis. Proc Natl Acad Sci USA 1988; 85:1179–1183.

83. Funkhouser SW, Concannon P, Charmley P, Vredevoe DL, Hood L. Differences in T cell receptor restriction fragment length polymorphisms in patients with rheumatoid arthritis. Arthritis Rheum 1992; 35:465–471.

84. Marguerie C, Lunardi C, So AK. Selectivity of T-cell receptor variable region gene usage by rheumaoid arthritis T-cells. Arthritis Rheum 1991; 34(suppl 10):S38.

85. Aelion JA, Endres RO, Stuart JM, Kang AH, Spinella DG. Clonal diversity and T-cell receptor gene expression of activated T-cells in the rheumatoid synovium. Arthritis Rheum 1991; 34(suppl 10):S38.

86. Chen P-F, Li Y-D, Suzuki R, Berman L, Platsoucas CD. Identification of T-cell antigen receptor (TCR) gene segments employed by IL2-expanded T-cell lines

derived from lymphocytes infiltrating the synovial membrane (SM) of patients with rheumatoid arthritis (RA). Arthritis Rheum 1991; 34(suppl 10):S39.

87. Paliard X, West SG, Lafferty JA, Clements JR, Kappler JW, Marrack P, Kotzin BL. Evidence for the effects of a superantigen in rheumatoid arthritis. Science 1991; 253:325–329.

88. Stabach PR, Sampieri A, Clive JM, Padula SJ. Lack of oligoclonality of T cell receptor (TCR) beta chain gene sequences in rheumatoid arthritis. Arthritis Rheum 1991; 34(suppl 10):S38.

89. Williams WV, Fang O, Demarco D, Zurier RB, VonFeldt JM, Weiner DB. Molecular heterogeneity of T cell receptors in rheumatoid synovium. Arthritis Rheum 1991; 34(suppl 10):S175.

90. Jenkins RN, Meek K, Lipsky PE. T cell receptor (TCR) variable (V) region gene usage in rheumatoid arthritis (RA). Arthritis Rheum 1991; 34(suppl 10):S176.

91. Steinmetz M, Uematsu Y. Heterogeneity of T cell repertoires in human autoimmune disease. Br J Rheumatol 1991; 30(suppl 2):24–27.

92. Olsnes S, Sandvig K, Petersen OW, van Deurs B. Immunotoxins—entry into cells and cellular mechanisms. Immunol Today 1989; 10:291–295.

93. Cobb PW, LeMaistre CF, Jackson LA. Clinical evaluation of immunotoxins. Cancer Bull 1991; 43:233–239.

94. Borrebaeck CAK. Human mAbs produced by primary in-vitro immunization. Immunol Today 1988; 9:355–359.

95. Carlsson R, Martensson C, Kalliomaki S, Ohlin M, Borrebaeck CAK. Human peripheral blood lymphocytes transplanted into SCID mice constitute an in vivo culture system exhibiting several parameters found in a normal humoral immune response and are a source of immunocytes for the production of human monoclonal antibodies. J Immunol 1992; 148:1065–1071.

96. Lang GM, Milton AD, Emmrich F, Kierek-Jaszczuk D, Sehon AH. Induction of tolerance to xenogenic anti-CD4 antibodies in relation to treatment of rheumatoid arthritis (RA). J Allergy Clin Immunol 1992; 89(part 2):289.

97. Mayforth RD, Quintans J. Designer and catalytic antibodies. N Engl J Med 1990; 323:173–178.

98. Chatenoud L, Bach J-F. Monoclonal antibodies to CD3 as immunosuppressants. Semin Immunol 1990; 2:437–447.

99. Chatenoud L, Legendre C, Ferran C, Bach JF, Kries H. Corticosteroid inhibition of the OKT3-induced cytokine-related syndrome—dosage and kinetics prerequisites. Transplantation 1991; 51:334–338.

100. Horneff G, Krause A, Emmrich F, Kalden JR, Burmester GR. Elevated levels of circulating TNF-α, IFN-γ, and IL-2 in systemic reactions induced by anti-CD4 therapy in patients with rheumatoid arthritis. Cytokine 1991; 3:266–267.

101. Zlabinger GJ, Stuhlmeier KM, Eher R, Schmaldienst S, Klauser R, Vychytil A, Watschinger B, Traindl O, Kovarik J, Pohanka E. Cytokine release and dynamics of leukocyte populations after CD3/TCR monoclonal antibody treatment. J Clin Immunol 1992; 12:170–177.

102. Vladutiu AO. Treatment of autoimmune diseases with antibodies to class II major histocompatibility complex antigens. Clin Immunol Immunopathol 1991; 61:1–17.

103. Sany J. Treatment of rheumatoid arthritis by antibodies directed against class II MHC antigens. Scand J Rheumatol 1988; 76(suppl):289–295.

104. Combe B, Cosso B, Clot J, Bonneau M, Sany J. Human placenta-eluted gamma-globulins in immunomodulating treatment of rheumatoid arthritis. Am J Med 1985; 78:920–928.

105. Shoenfeld Y, Ferrone S, Bombardieri S. New aspects in the treatment of immu-nomediated diseases. Clin Exp Rheumatol 1991; 9:663–673.

106. Fiocco U, Cozzi L, Cozzi E, Fagiolo U, Ferrone S. Treatment of rheumatoid arthritis by murine antiidiotypic monoclonal antibodies to a syngeneic anti-HLA class II monoclonal antibody. Br J Rheumatol 1991; 30(suppl2):90.

107. Sakai K, Zamvil SS, Mitchell DJ, Hodkinson S, Rothbard JB, Steinman L. Preven-tion of experimental allergic encephalomyelitis with peptides that block interaction of T cells with major histocompatibility complex protein. Proc Natl Acad Sci USA 1989; 86:9470–9474.

108. Adorini L. Peptide interactions with MHC class II molecules. Br J Rheumatol 1991; 30(suppl 2):10–13.

109. Wraith DC. The use of class II MHC binding peptides in immunotherapy. Br J Rheumatol 1991; 30(suppl 2):14–16.

110. De Magistris MT, Alexander J, Coggeshall M, Altman A, Gaeta FCA, Grey HM, Sette A. Antigen analog–major histocompatibility complexes act as antagonists of the T cell receptor. Cell 1992; 68:625–634.

111. Herzog C, Walker C, Pichler W. Monoclonal anti-CD4 in arthritis. Lancet 1987; 2:1461–1462.

112. Herzog C, Walker, Miller W, Rieber P, Reiter C, Riethmüller G, Wassmer P, Stockinger, Madic O, Pichler W. Anti-CD4 antibody treatment of patients with rheumatoid arthritis: I. Effect on clinical course and circulating T cells. J Autoim-mun 1989; 2:627–642.

113. Walker C, Herzog C, Rieber P, Riethmüller G, Muller W, Pichler W. Anti-CD4 antibody treatment of patients with rheumatoid arthritis: II. Failure to demonstrate inhibitory signals by anti-CD4 antibody binding to CD4 cells. J Autoimmun 1989; 2:643–649.

114. Burmester GR, Horneff G, Emmrich F, Kalden JR. Immunomodulatory treatment of rheumatoid arthritis with an anti-CD4 (anti-helper T cell) monoclonal antibody. Arthritis Rheum 1990; 33:S25.

115. Wassmer P, Neidhart M, Hintermann U, Reiter C, Rieber P, Riethmüller G, Fehr K, Wagenhauser G. Therapy of rheumatoid arthritis with CD4 monoclonal antibodies. Arthritis Rheum 1990; 33:S153.

116. Goldberg D, Chatenroud L, Morel P, Boitard C, Revillard J-P, Bertoye P, Bach J-F, Menkes C-J. Preliminary trial of an anti-CD4 monoclonal antibody (MoAb) in rheumatoid arthritis (RA). Arthritis Rheum 1990; 33:S153.

117. Reiter C, Kakavand B, Rieber EP, Schattenkircher M, Riethmüller G, Krüger K. Treatment of rheumatoid arthritis with monoclonal CD4 antibody M-T151. Arthri-tis Rheum 1991; 34:525–535.

118. Wendling D, Wijdenes J, Racadot E, More-Fourier B. Therapeutic use of monoclonal anti-CD4 antibody in rheumatoid arthritis. J Rheumatol 1991; 18:325–327.

119. Racadot E, Wijdenes J, Wendling D, Girard A, Lienard A, Peters A. Immunologic follow-up of 13 patients with rheumatoid arthritis treated by anti-CD4 monoclonal antibodies. Br J Rheumatol 1991; 30(suppl 2):88.

120. Jonker M, Slingerland W, Treacy G, Pak KY, Wilson E, Tam S, Daddona PE, LoBuglio AF, Riethmüller G, Iuliucci D. Anti-CD4 treatment with chimeric monoclonal antibody results in prolonged CD4$^+$ cell depression. Br J Rheumatol 1991; 430(suppl 2):87.

121. Wendling D, Didry C, Wijdenes J, Racadot E, Morel-Fourier B, Clot J, Brochier J, Andary M, Portales P, Liautard J, Combe B, Sany J. Bicentric open study of the treatment of rheumatoid arthritis with monoclonal CD4 antibody, clinical and immunological results. Br J Rheumatol 1991; 30(suppl 2):87.

122. Horneff G, Burmester GR, Emmrich F, Kalden J. Treatment of rheumatoid arthritis with an anti-CD4 monoclonal antibody. Arthritis Rheum 1991; 34:129–40.

123. Moreland LW, Bucy RP, Pratt PW, Khazeli MB, LoBuglio AF, Ghrayeb J, Daddona P, Sanders ME, Kilgariff C, Riethmüller G, Koopman WJ. Use of a chimeric anti-CD4 monoclonal antibody in refractory rheumatoid arthritis. Arthritis Rheum 1991; 34(suppl):S49.

124. van der Lubbe PA, Reiter C, Riethmüller G, Sanders ME, Breedland FC. Treatment of rheumatoid arthritis (RA) with chimeric CD4 monoclonal antibody. Arthritis Rheum 1991; 34(suppl):S89.

125. Reiter C, van der Lubbe PA, Breedvald FC, Daddona P, Krüger K, Kakavand B, Riethmüller G. Chimeric monoclonal CD4 antibody cM-T412 induces a long lasting CD4 cell depletion in rheumatoid arthritis (RA) patients. Arthritis Rheum 1991; 34(suppl):S91.

126. Didry C, Portales P, Andary M, Brochier J, Combe B, Clot J, Sany J. Treatment of rheumatoid arthritis (RA) with monoclonal anti-CD4 antibodies. Clinical results. Arthritis Rheum 1991; 34(suppl):S92.

127. Strand V, Lipsky PE, Cannon G, Calabrese L, CD5 plus RA investigators group. Treatment of rheumatoid arthritis with an anti-CD5 immunoconjugate: final results of phase II studies. Arthritis Rheum 1991; 34(suppl):S91.

128. Kirkham BW, Pitzalis C, Kingsley GH, Chikanza IC, Sabharwal S, Barbatis C, Grahame R, Gibson T, Amlot PL, Panayi GS. Monoclonal antibody treatment in rheumatoid arthritis: the clinical and immunological effects of a CD7 monoclonal antibody. Br J Rheumatol 1991; 30:459–463.

129. Kirkham BW, Thien F, Pelton BK, Pitzalis C, Amlot P, Denman AM, Panayi GS. Chimeric CD7 monoclonal antibody therapy in rheumatoid arthritis. J Rheumatol 1992; 19:1348–1352.

130. Isaacs JD, Watts RA, Hazleman BL, Hale G, Keogan MT, Cobbold SP, Waldmann H. Humanised monoclonal antibody therapy for rheumatoid arthritis. Lancet 1992; 340:748–752.

131. Springer TA. Adhesion molecules of the immune system. Nature 1990; 346:425–433.

132. Carlos TM, Harlan JM. Membrane proteins involved in phagocyte adherence to endothelium. Immunol Rev 1990; 114:5–28.

133. de Fougerolles AR, Springer TA. Intercellular adhesion molecule 3, a third adhesion counter-receptor for lymphocyte function-associated molecule 1 on resting lymphocytes. J Exp Med 1992; 175:185–190.

134. Vedder NB, Fouty BN, Winn RK, Harlan JM, Rice CL. Role of neutrophils in generalized reperfusion injury associated with resuscitation from shock. Surgery 1988; 81:939–949.

135. Wegner CD, Gundel RH, Reilly P, Haynes N, Letts LG, Rothlein R. Intercellular adhesion molecule-1 (ICAM-1) in the pathogenesis of asthma. Science 1990; 247:456–460.

136. Cosimi AB, Conti D, Delmonico FL, Preffer FI, Wee S-L, Rothlein R, Faanes R, Colvin RB. In vivo effects of monoclonal antibody to ICAM-1 (CD54) in nonhuman primates with renal allografts. J Immunol 1990; 144:4604–4611.

137. Jasin HE, Lightfoot E, Kavanaugh A, Rothlein R, Faanes B, Lipsky PE. Successful treatment of antigen-induced arthritis in rabbits with monoclonal antibodies to leukocyte adhesion molecules. Arthritis Rheum 1990; 33(suppl):S34.

138. Iigo Y, Takashi T, Tamatani T, Miyasaka M, Higashida T, Yagita H, Okumura K, Tsukada W. ICAM-1-dependent pathway is critically involved in the pathogenesis of adjuvant arthritis in the rat. J Immunol 1991; 147:4167–4171.

139. Isobe M, Yagita H, Okumura K, Ihara A. Specific acceptance of cardiac allograft after treatment with antibodies to ICAM-1 and LFA-1. Science 1992; 255:1125–1127.

140. Kavanaugh AF, Nichols LA, Lipsky PE. Treatment of refractory rheumatoid arthritis with an anti-CD54 (intercellular adhesion molecule-1, ICAM-1) monoclonal antibody. Arthritis Rheum 1992; 35(suppl)S43.

141. Gamble JR, Skinner MP, Berndt MC, Vadas M. Prevention of activated neutrophil adhesion to endothelium by soluble adhesion protein GMP140. Science 1990; 249:414–418.

142. Watson SR, Fennie C, Lasky LA. Neutrophil influx into an inflammatory site inhibited by a soluble homing receptor-IgG chimera. Nature 1991; 349:164–167.

143. Lipsky PE, Davis LS, Cush JJ, Oppenheimer-Marks N. The role of cytokines in the pathogenesis of rheumatoid arthritis. Springer Semin Immunopathol 1989; 11:123–162.

144. Kroemer G, Martinez-A. Carlos J. Cytokines and autoimmune disease. Clin Immunol Immunopathol 1991; 61:275–295.

145. Arend WP, Malyak M, Smith MF, Janson RW. The biological role of naturally-occurring cytokine inhibitors. Br J Rheumatol 1991; 30(suppl 2):49–52.

146. Durum SK, Quinn DG, Muegge K. New cytokines and receptors make their debut in San Antonio. Immunol Today 1991; 12:54–57.

147. Aderka D, Engelmann H, Maot Y, Brakebusch C, Wallach D. Stabilization of the bioactivity of tumor necrosis factor by its soluble receptors. J Exp Med 1992; 175:323–329.

148. Arend WP, Dayer J-M. Cytokines and cytokine inhibitors or antagonists in rheumatoid arthritis. Arthritis Rheum 1990; 33:305–315.

149. Arend WP. Interleukin 1 receptor antagonist; a new member of the Interleukin 1 family. J Clin Invest 1991; 88:1445–1451.

150. Smith RJ, Chin JE, Sam LM, Justen JM. Biologic effects of an interleukin-1 receptor antagonist protein on interleukin-1-stimulated cartilage erosion and chondrocyte responsiveness. Arthritis Rheum 1991; 34:78–83.

151. Barak V, Mahajna N, Okon E, Peritt D, Flechner I, Yanai P, Halperin T, Treves AJ. Reduction or elimination of rheumatoid arthritis by an IL-1 inhibitor. Br J Rheumatol 1991; 30(suppl 2):84.

152. van de Loo FAJ, Arntz OJ, Otterness IG, van der Berg WB. Protection against

cartilage proteoglycan biosynthesis by antiinterleukin 1 antibodies in experimental arthritis. J Rheumatol 1992; 19:348–356.

153. Lebsack ME, Paul CC, Bloedow DC, Burch FX, Sack MA, Chase W, Catalano MA. Subcutaneous IL-1 receptor antagonist in patients with rheumatoid arthritis. Arthritis Rheum 1991; 34(suppl):S45.

154. Williams RO, Feldmann M, Maini RN. Anti-tumor necrosis factor (TNF) treatment inhibits the progression of established collagen-induced arthritis. Arthritis Rheum 1991; 34(suppl):S67.

155. Engelmann H, Novick D, Wallach D. Two tumor necrosis factor-binding proteins purified from human urine. Evidence for immunological cross-reactivity with cell surface tumor necrosis factor receptors. J Biol Chem 1990; 265:11974–11978.

156. Waldmann TA, Pastan IH, Gansow OA, Junghans RP. The multichain interleukin-2 receptor: a target for immunotherapy. Ann Intern Med 1992; 116:148–160.

157. Kyle V, Coughlan RJ, Tighe H, Waldmann H, Hazleman BL. Beneficial effect of monoclonal antibody to interleukin 2 receptor on activated T cells in rheumatoid arthritis. Ann Rheum Dis 1989; 48:428–460.

158. Case JP, Lorberboum-Galski H, Lafyatis R, FitzGerald D, Wilder RL, Pastan I. Chimeric cytotoxin IL-2-PE40 delays and mitigates adjuvant-induced arthritis in rats. Proc Natl Acad Sci USA 1989; 86:287–291.

159. Sewell KL, Trentham DE. Improvement in refractory rheumatoid arthritis by interleukin-2 receptor targeted therapy. Arthritis Rheum 1991; 34(suppl):S89.

160. Lemmel EM, Gaus W, Hofschneider PH. Multicenter double-blind trial of interferon-γ versus placebo in the treatment of rheumatoid arthritis. Arthritis Rheum 1991; 34:1621—1622.

161. Cannon GW, Emkey RD, Denes A, Cohen SA, Wolfe F, Saway PA, Jaffer AM, Weaver AL, Cogen L, Fay AM. Prospective five year follow-up of recombinant interferon-gamma in rheumatoid arthritis. Arthritis Rheum 1991; 34(suppl):S91.

162. Cannon GW, Pincus SH, Emkey RD, et al. Double-blind trial of recombinant gamma-interferon versus placebo in the treatment of rheumatoid arthritis. Arthritis Rheum 1989; 32:964–673.

163. Gutierrez AA, Lemoine NR, Sikora K. Gene therapy for cancer. Lancet 1991; 339:715–721.

18

Clinical Implications of the Relative Therapeutic Toxicity of Medications Used to Treat Rheumatoid Arthritis

James F. Fries

Stanford University School of Medicine
Palo Alto, California

I. INTRODUCTION

The traditional therapeutic progression in rheumatoid arthritis was based on the concept of the therapeutic pyramid (1,2). The pyramid, in turn, was based on three underlying assumptions: (a) rheumatoid arthritis is frequently a benign or even self-limited disease, (b) aspirin and the nonsteroidal anti-inflammatory drugs (NSAIDs) are therapeutic alternatives with very low toxicity, and (c) disease-modifying antirheumatic drugs (DMARDs) are too toxic to be widely deployed, even granting that they are the most effective agents. With these three assumptions, the philosophy of the therapeutic sequence was to first use aspirin or nonsteroidal anti-inflammatory drugs, with the expectation that this therapy would suffice for most patients, to employ DMARD therapy in those who failed to satisfactorily respond, and finally to employ experimental therapy for those patients who were still under inadequate control.

Each of these assumptions was incorrect. First, rheumatoid arthritis, as defined by evolving criteria sets, is most certainly not a benign disease. As thoroughly documented in this volume, it results in a doubling of standardized mortality ratios, and death occurs 10 years or more prematurely on average (3–5). It results in progressive substantial disability in 90% or more of patients (5). Second, NSAID therapy has frequent and severe toxicity, particularly secondary to gastric ulcer, and results in frequent hospitalization and not infrequently in fatal complications (6–8). Third, DMARD therapy, on the other hand, encom-

403

passes a range of toxicities, and overall toxicity is roughly equivalent to the toxicity of NSAIDs (9,10).

With these major changes in the underlying data on which the logic of therapy must be based, and with the additional observation that prior therapeutic progression recommendations did not sufficiently alter the progressive disability of rheumatoid arthritis (11,12), it is mandatory that we rethink the therapeutic progression. In this chapter we briefly review recent data, developed in substantial part by The Arthritis Rheumatism and Aging Medical Information System (AR-AMIS) and consider the implications of these data; particularly, the new data on the comparative toxicity of specific therapeutic alternatives on the definition of a new therapeutic progression for management of rheumatoid arthritis.

II. THE TOXICITY INDEX

For the past several years, the ARAMIS postmarketing surveillance program has been developing methodology to approach a central question of therapeutic intervention: Which drugs are most toxic, and by how much? We have developed and reported on a toxicity index that counts and weighs symptoms, laboratory side effects, and hospitalizations, both by side effect type and severity, and computes these into a single index number representing the toxicity of a particular medicine; this number is adjusted statistically for differences in length of time on different drug therapeutic regimens and for differences in characteristics of patients receiving different drugs (13). Studies have consisted of analyses of many thousands of courses of DMARD, NSAID, and prednisone therapy in 2747 patients with rheumatoid arthritis over approximately 8000 patient years of observation. Patients are studied prospectively and longitudinally. All patients have rheumatoid arthritis, and five data bank centers have contributed data. Two of these centers (Santa Clara County and Saskatoon) represent community-based populations, two centers (Wichita and Phoenix) represent private rheumatological practices, and one center (Stanford) represents a university referral practice. Data available consist of routine clinical information, demographics, diagnoses, symptoms, physical signs, laboratory findings, therapy employed, and data each 6 months from the Health Assessment Questionnaire (HAQ) detailing disability, symptoms, side effects, and economic effect. Development, validation, and methodology of the toxicity index has been separately reported, as has utilization of the methodology in analysis of the comparative toxicity of NSAIDs and DMARDs. Hospitalizations are individually abstracted from discharge summaries, and deaths from discharge summaries, and death certificates. Deaths in patients lost to follow-up are identified by use of the National Death Index.

The toxicity index includes components of symptoms, laboratory tests, and hospitalizations. Events resulting in hospitalization or death are attributed to a drug if the attending physician made that attribution, and if no such attribution was made, they are fractionally attributed on the basis of the relative risk of the event while patients are receiving a class of medications, compared with the relative risk of the event while not receiving this class of medications. If more than one potential contributing drug is present, as for example, with the upper gastrointestinal hemorrhage associated with both prednisone and an NSAID, attribution is further fractionally allocated between the potential offending agents. Symptoms are additionally categorized as mild, moderate, or severe, and scores weighted accordingly. Units for the toxicity index are scored per year of exposure to the agent.

Hospitalization records and death certificates for all events occurring during each 6-month reporting period are reviewed to determine the relation of hospitalizations and death to drug use. Discharge summaries are supplemented by ARAMIS clinical data and HAQ data. To be attributed, events have to be either directly attributed by a physician to a specific drug, to a specific drug and a clinical problem, or likely to be drug-related, based on a known relation (previously reported in the literature) between a class of drugs and a particular set of symptoms or complications. Thus, any toxic event, no matter how rare, can be attributed if the physician attending the patient believes the drug to be responsible, whereas in the absence of physician notation, a probable drug relation can be counted as well, but only if the relation between drug and event is established. The algorithms may be readily applied by trained abstractors in most instances and, in ambiguous situations, records are further reviewed by an ARAMIS physician who makes the final judgment (13).

The toxicity index is computed as the sum of symptom side effects, laboratory side effects, and hospital days. Symptom side effect weights range from 0 to 10 and are multiplied by the severity factor, 0.5 for mild, 1.0 for moderate, and 1.5 for severe. The same procedure is employed for laboratory side effects. The number of hospital days is multiplied by the weighting factor for a hospital day (8.4) and fractionated according to the rules described in the foregoing.

Since some side effects tend to occur early in the course of treatment (e.g., rash), others late (e.g., osteoporosis), and others relatively evenly over time (gastrointestinal hemorrhage), toxicity index values and standard errors are computed for 6-month periods of exposure (for the first 6-month period, second and third 6-month periods, and so on) for each drug and then combined. Raw scores are statistically adjusted by standardization, as described later, using age, race, sex, duration, disease severity, new start versus continuing therapy, comorbidity, presence of concurrent therapy, and other variables. Sensitivity analyses using several alternative weighing systems have been performed.

Regression trees were used to develop strata for standardization, following the procedures of Bloch and Segal and using the computer program CART (14). Regression trees were constructed for the first period, the second and third periods, periods four through eight, and periods nine and above. A similar list of classifying variables was obtained for each set of periods. Each regression tree first split either on disability or comorbidity, and these variables appeared in all trees. Additional variables selected included age, duration, and number of swollen joints. Since we are not able to distinguish patients who were started on therapy with a drug in the first observation period from those who had begun taking the drug before our observation, we repeated the standardized analyses on those who were not taking the drug at first observation period, but subsequently began treatment. The variables appearing in these regression trees were closely similar to those already described. Strata developed by these techniques were used to develop standardized toxicity index scores. The hypothesis for analysis is that there is no difference in standardized toxicity index scores between drugs; thus, the alternative hypotheses are two-sided. The test statistic is based on the normal approximation to the distribution of differences between the standardized toxicity index values.

III. DATA

Table 1 summarizes results describing gastrointestinal toxicity with NSAIDs. The number of hospitalizations for upper gastrointestinal (GI) problems, generally gastric hemorrhage, is more than of 1%/year at all centers, and the best estimate of yearly excess risk is 1.3%. The relative risk of such an event while taking an NSAID compared with while not taking the NSAID is 5.2 (7). This percentage cumulates over time to a risk of 5% to over 60% for individual patients. Nationally, there are approximately 30,000 excess hospitalizations for GI complications in rheumatoid arthritis annually.

Table 2 tabulates death from gastrointestinal causes in patients with rheumatoid arthritis compared with those deaths expected in a normal population. Whether individual data from a single ARAMIS center (Saskatoon) are considered (3), or all deaths at all ARAMIS centers (7), or the aggregated literature values from other studies (5), there are approximately twice as many gastrointesti-

Table 1 Gastrointestinal (GI) Hospitalization in Rheumatoid Arthritis

Number of patients studied	2747
Person-years of observation	9525
Person-years on NSAIDs	6741
Number of GI hospitalizations	116
Number of these taking NSAIDs	107
Relative risk while taking NSAIDs	5.2:1
Rate per year while taking NSAIDs (%)	1.6
Excess rate while taking NSAIDs (%)	1.3

Source: Data from five ARAMIS data bank centers.

Table 2 Gastrointestinal Deaths in Rheumatoid Arthritis

Investigator (ref.)	Observed deaths	Expected deaths
Mitchell et al. (1986)	15	8
Pincus et al. (1986)	96	45
ARAMIS (1991)	17	8
Excess rate = 0.11% per year of disease		

nal deaths as expected, and the excess GI mortality rate per year of disease is approximately 1:1000. Over the course of illness, the excess GI mortality approximates 3%, and there are an estimated 2600 deaths annually in the United States.

Table 3 presents the toxicity indices for NSAIDs (9). There is a range of three- to fourfold in toxicity between the most toxic and least toxic NSAIDs. Of prescription NSAIDs, when employed in rheumatoid arthritis, salsalate, ibuprofen, and naproxen are the least toxic, and ketoprofen, tolectin, meclofenamate, and indomethacin are the most toxic. Enteric-coated aspirin also performed well, in large part owing to relatively low doses employed in actual practice.

Table 4 shows a similar display of relative toxicity for the DMARDs (10). A wide range of toxicities is seen here, ranging from a benign profile and score for hydroxychloroquine to higher values for methotrexate, azathioprine, auranofin, and the reference drug prednisone. Comparing data for NSAIDs (see Table 3) with DMARDs (see Table 4), interesting conclusions emerge. All data were obtained from the same patients over the same time period, with statistical adjustment for time taking the drug and for characteristics of patients receiving

Table 3 Relative Toxicity of NSAIDs

Drug	Number of courses	Mean	Standard error	Rank
Salsalate	121	1.28 ±	.34	(1)
Ibuprofen	503	1.94 ±	.43	(2)
Naproxen	939	2.17 ±	.23	(3)
Sulindac	511	2.24 ±	.39	(4)
Piroxicam	790	2.52 ±	.23	(5)
Fenoprofen	161	2.95 ±	.77	(6)
Ketoprofen	190	3.45 ±	1.07	(7)
Meclofenamate	157	3.86 ±	.66	(8)
Tolmetin	215	3.96 ±	.74	(9)
Indomethacin	386	3.99 ±	.58	(10)

Source: Data from five ARAMIS data bank centers; standardized toxicity index scores.

Table 4 Relative Toxicity of DMARDs

Drug	Number of courses	Mean	Standard error	Rank	Hospitalization component
Hydroxychloroquine	639	1.38 ±	.15	(1)	0.00
Intramuscular gold	659	2.27 ±	.17	(2)	0.15
D-Penicillamine	496	3.38 ±	.36	(3)	0.99
Methotrexate	660	3.82 ±	.35	(4)	1.02
Azathioprine	190	3.92 ±	.39	(5)	0.83
Auranofin	409	5.25 ±	.32	(6)	0.00

Source: Data from five ARAMIS data bank centers; standardized toxicity index scores.

specific therapies. The overlap of toxicities between NSAIDs and DMARDs is much more pronounced than are the differences. Hydroxychloroquine would be a very nontoxic NSAID, whereas the most toxic NSAIDs exhibit overall toxicity similar to DMARDs such as methotrexate and azathioprine. Each of the results reported in the foregoing holds when the overall drug experience or only new starts are analyzed, and holds at five clinical centers with greatly differing patient selection characteristics. As a caveat, therapy in our series of patients was prescribed by experienced physicians with appropriate monitoring to detect early toxicity, and toxicity might have been greater if regular monitoring had not been performed.

IV. IMPLICATIONS

The old form of the therapeutic pyramid is dead, and cannot be rationally defended in view of the new data. The initial premises were incorrect. Rheumatoid arthritis is a serious disease, with substantial mortality; NSAIDs are not benign therapy; and DMARDs, used with appropriate monitoring, are of acceptable toxicity. To improve long-term outcome in rheumatoid arthritis it is necessary, although probably not always sufficient, that DMARD therapy be begun early in the course of disease and that a DMARD-based strategy be regularly followed throughout the course. Clinical observations suggest that it is unusual for a single DMARD to be sufficient over an entire 20- to 30-year duration of illness. This implies that there is a rational therapeutic progression by which one might employ DMARDs and combinations of DMARDs sequentially through the course of illness. Determination of the optimal sequence of treatment and the relative role of individual DMARDs is a major research challenge. Currently, there are many opinions, but few firm data.

In some ways this challenge raises questions analogous to those of the old ''pyramid,'' since physicians must remain sensitive to minimization of overall treatment toxicity. Comparative data on efficacy of different DMARDs is as yet fragmentary, although studies are underway that may provide better data in this area over the next several years. The metanalysis of published DMARD trials presented by Felson and colleagues provides one glimpse at comparative efficacy (15), although there are problems with metanalysis techniques. In this study auranofin was found less effective, and methotrexate, intramuscular gold, antimalarials, and sulfasalazine more effective. General clinical experience is also relevant, and there is general clinical consensus, for example, that methotrexate is among the most effective of DMARDs, perhaps together with intramuscular gold, and that hydroxychloroquine and auranofin are perhaps less effective.

V. THE THERAPEUTIC PROGRESSION

Although most authors currently addressing questions of therapeutic strategy in rheumatoid arthritis urge early intervention with DMARDs (16,17), the question of ''how early'' remains unanswered. An early justification for the old pyramid was that rheumatoid arthritis might be a self-limited illness in some circumstances, and that, in particular, with disease of very short duration, the possibility of spontaneous remission was substantial. Thus, if one treated with a disease-modifying drug too early in the course, the patient might go into remission, and this remission might be falsely attributed to the action of the drug, rather than to the natural history of the illness. It was argued that spontaneous remissions could occur quite frequently in the first months of disease, but that after perhaps 1 year of sustained progressive disease, such remissions were infrequent.

We believe, in contrast, that rheumatoid arthritis is a serious disease that must be treated seriously from the very outset of illness, and that this treatment imperative outweighs any problems with interpretation of complete remissions that might result from immediate DMARD treatment. Consider the following argument:

In the comparative DMARD experience reported earlier, two drugs, hydroxychloroquine and auranofin, were not associated with serious toxicity requiring hospitalization or resulting in death, although auranofin had a very frequent occurrence of annoying, but reversible, side effects, principally diarrhea. If a patient with an illness consistent with rheumatoid arthritis is seen very early in the course, such as after 3–6 weeks duration, we believe that laboratory tests, including hemoglobin, sedimentation rate, latex fixation titer, and antinuclear antibody, should be drawn, and DMARD treatment immediately begun, usually with hydroxychloroquine because of its favorable safety record. Over the next several weeks as hydroxychloroquine tissue levels rise toward therapeutic levels, both the diagnosis and the severity of the rheumatoid arthritis will generally become apparent. Should the patient go into complete remission, the possibility of a spontaneous remission is present, and the initial medication may be discon-

Table 5 A Preliminary New Therapeutic Progression For Management
of Rheumatoid Arthritis

Level 1 (early disease)	
Hydroxychloroquine	Low toxicity, low serious toxicity, moderate efficacy
Auranofin	High toxicity, low serious toxicity, modest early efficacy
Sulfasalazine	Probable low toxicity, low serious toxicity, moderate efficacy
Level 2 (early progressive)	
Methotrexate	Moderate toxicity, moderate serious toxicity, major efficacy
Intramuscular gold	Moderate toxicity, moderate serious toxicity, major efficacy
D-Penicillamine	Moderate toxicity, moderate serious toxicity, moderate efficacy
Level 3 (continued progressive, failure of prior therapy)	
Empiric combinations	MTX-OH-chloroquine, others
Azathioprine	Moderate toxicity, moderate serious toxicity, efficacy in late disease
Level 4 (experimental)	
Cyclosporine, total lymphoid irradiation, others	
Other therapy	
Acetaminophen, aspirin, NSAIDs, self-management courses, physical therapy, exercise programs, splints, surgery, and other modalities of treatment used as required	

tinued, after a period of some months to ensure consolidation of the remission.
If the remission had been spontaneous, then the patient will remain asymptomatic,
and if it was related to drug therapy, then the disease will again become active.
The cost of thereby treating some cases of viral or other arthritides that were
destined to be self-limited is only the cost of a few months of hydroxychloroquine
therapy, which is a low cost both in dollars and in toxicity. The reward, on the
other hand, may be substantial.

A similar initial strategy could be undertaken with auranofin, with the
proviso that there will be frequent early drug discontinuations owing to diarrhea,
or treatment might be initiated with sulfasalazine, which also appears to have a
benign safety profile, although data are not yet established. Combination therapy
with these ''minor DMARDs'' also appears quite free of serious toxicity.

One might, therefore, consider a new therapeutic progression (Table 5) not
unlike, in some senses, the old therapeutic pyramid. At the first level, for early
treatment, would be hydroxychloroquine, auranofin, or sulfasalazine. These can
be used as single agents or in combination. At the second level, with early
progressive disease refractory to the first treatments, intramuscular gold, metho-

trexate, and probably D-penicillamine might be employed, in some individuals. With progressive disease, the progression to level 3 might well occur in the first 6 months of illness.

Level 3, with continued progressive disease, or with escape from previously effective therapy, might be managed with combinations of methotrexate and hydroxychloroquine, particularly if there had been signs of hepatic enzyme elevation with methotrexate; hydroxychloroquine has been shown to reduce the transaminitis associated with methotrexate therapy (18). Azathioprine, in our data, shows particular promise as a later agent in management of rheumatoid arthritis and may find particular use later in the course. A variety of other drugs and combinations of drugs may also be employed.

Level 4, consisting of experimental or not well-established therapies, might include cyclosporine, a number of new agents under development, total lymphoid irradiation, or other modalities. In prospective clinical trials such new agents should often be studied at earlier stages of illness, but in clinical practice, unless a new agent is manifesting extraordinary promise, we believe that its use conservatively should be deferred in favor of thoughtful deployment of agents of proved effectiveness.

Treatment does not consist solely of DMARD use, but this is the basis of medical therapy. Acetaminophen, aspirin, and NSAIDs may be employed as therapeutic adjuncts, with the primary goal of symptomatic relief. Arthritis self-management courses are a proved adjunct. Exercise programs, physical therapy, occupational therapy, and other modalities may be of benefit. Surgery will sometimes be required, despite optimal medical management.

We are skeptical that early use of multiple drug treatment, patterned after lymphoma chemotherapy, will result in prolonged complete remissions, despite speculations to the contrary (19). With lymphoma, the individual drugs employed in combination were capable, by themselves, of inducing remissions that persisted after cessation of treatment; this is not frequently true in rheumatoid arthritis. Data supporting the usefulness of such an aggressive multiple drug approach have not yet been presented, nor has toxicity been defined.

The sequential DMARD strategy is shown schematically in Fig. 1. The course of illness under the treatment progression of the past 20 years is shown as the upper curve. Over this period, disability has progressed inexorably in most patients. Therapy with DMARD was first initiated some 6–8 years into the course, and maintained for an average of only 15% of the course. Given this circumstance, we believe it has not been reasonable to maintain that our treatments have no long-term effectiveness. They have been given too late and too little. We now have an enlarged repertoire of DMARDs, and a strategy based on their sequential employment is readily practical.

The new assumptions are that (a) DMARD therapy is the foundation of management of rheumatoid arthritis, (b) that a single DMARD is unlikely to sufficiently control disease throughout a prolonged course, (c) that sequential

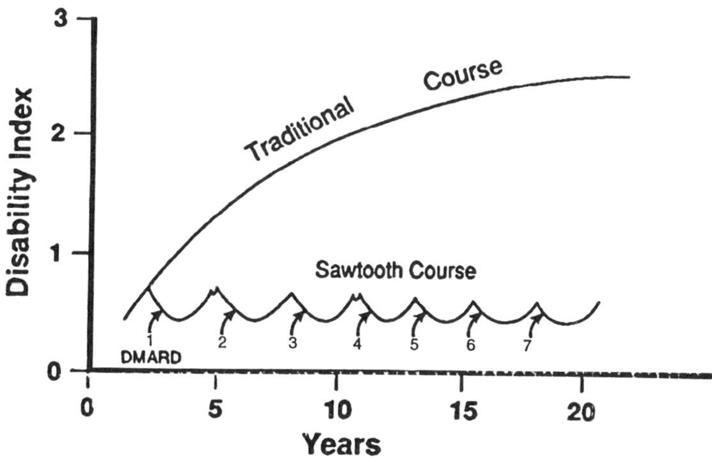

Fig. 1 The consecutive DMARD (sawtooth) strategy: Under traditional treatment regimens, the average patient with rheumatoid arthritis develops substantial disability over time, as shown by the upper line. The sawtooth strategy differs by (a) early use of DMARDs, (b) continuous use of DMARDs, alone or in combination, (c) regular monitoring of disability levels, (d) intensification or change in therapy when disability levels exceed a preestablished ceiling. (From Ref. 16.)

deployment of different DMARDs and combinations of DMARDs will be required, (d) that progression of disability needs to be regularly monitored using now-established techniques, such as the Health Assessment Questionnaire (HAQ) so that the decision about loss of effectiveness of an agent may be made early and appropriate therapeutic change initiated before irreversible joint destruction has occurred. With these measures, with the aid of additional agents coming on line and with additional data on relative efficacy and toxicity (20), we have the potential ability to effectively alter the long-term outcome of rheumatoid arthritis.

ACKNOWLEDGMENT

This work was supported by a grant from the National Institutes of Health to ARAMIS (Arthritis Rheumatism and Aging Medical Information System) (AM21393), and was modified from a paper presented to the conference "Combination Therapy in the Treatment of Rheumatoid Arthritis," St. Thomas, February 1992. The author would like to acknowledge the contributions of Daniel A. Bloch, Catherine A. Williams, and Dena R. Ramey.

REFERENCES

1. Kelley WN, Harris ED Jr, Ruddy S, Sledge CB, eds. Textbook of rheumatology, 2d ed. Philadelphia: WB Saunders, 1985:979–987.

2. Hess EV, Luggen ME. Remodeling the pyramid—a concept whose times has not yet come. J Rheumatol 1989; 16:1–4.

3. Mitchell DM, Spitz PW, Young DY, Bloch DA, McShane DJ, Fries JF. Survival, prognosis, and causes of death in rheumatoid arthritis. Arthritis Rheum 1986; 29:706–714.

4. Wolfe F, Kleinheksal SM, Cathey MA, Hawley DJ, Spitz P. Antecedents of mortality in rheumatoid arthritis (RA): a study of 1405 patients with RA in a community setting [abstr]. Arthritis Rheum 1991; 34(suppl 9):S48.

5. Pincus T, Callahan LF, Sale WG, et al. Severe functional declines, work disability, and increased mortality in seventy-five rheumatoid arthritis patients studied over nine years. Arthritis Rheum 1984; 27:864–872.

6. Fries JF, Miller SR, Spitz PW, Williams CA, Hubert HB, Bloch DA. Toward an epidemiology of gastropathy associated with nonsteroidal antiinflammatory drug use. Gastroenterology 1989; 96:647–655.

7. Fries JF, Williams CA, Bloch DA, Michel BA. Nonsteroidal antiinflammatory drug-associated gastropathy: incidence and risk factor models. Am J Med 1991; 91:213–222.

8. Gabriel SE, Bombardier C: NSAID induced ulcers: an emerging epidemic? J Rheumatol 1990; 17:1–4.

9. Fries JF, Williams CA, Bloch DA. The relative toxicity of nonsteroidal antiinflammatory drugs. Arthritis Rheum 1991; 34:1353–1360.

10. Fries JF, Williams CA, Bloch DA. The relative toxicity of disease modifying antirheumatic drugs (DMARDs) [abstr]. Arthritis Rheum 1991; 34(suppl 9):S54.

11. Kushner I. Does aggressive therapy of rheumatoid arthritis affect outcome? [editorial]. J Rheumatol 1989; 16:1–4.

12. Scott DL, Symmons DPM, Coulton BL, Popert AJ. Long-term outcome of treating rheumatoid arthritis: results after 29 years. Lancet 1987; 1:1108–1111.

13. Fries JF, Spitz PW, Williams CA, Bloch DA, Singh G, Hubert HB. A toxicity index for comparison of side effects among different drugs. Arthritis Rheum 1990; 33:121–130.

14. Breiman L, Freidman J, Olshen R, Stone C. Classification and regression trees. Belmont CA: Wasworth, 1984:93–129.

15. Felson DT, Anderson JJ, Meenan RF. The comparative efficacy and toxicity of second-line drugs in rheumatoid arthritis: results of two meta-analyses. Arthritis Rheum 1990; 33:1449–1461.

16. Fries JF. Reevaluating the therapeutic approach to rheumatoid arthritis: the "sawtooth" strategy. J Rheumatol 1990; 17(suppl 27):12–15.

17. Pincus T, Callahan LF. Remodeling the pyramid or remodeling the paradigms concerning rheumatoid arthritis—lessons from Hodgkin's disease and coronary artery disease. J Rheumatol 1990; 17:1582–1585.

18. Fries JF, Singh G, Lenert L, Furst DE. Aspirin, hydroxychloroquine, and hepatic enzyme abnormalities with methotrexate in rheumatoid arthritis. Arthritis Rheum 1990; 33:1611–1619.

19. Wilske KR, Healey LA. Remodeling the pyramid—a concept whose time has come. J Rheumatol 1989; 15:565–567.

20. Fries JF. Toward an understanding of patient outcome measurement. Arthritis Rheum 1983; 26:697–704.

19
Physical Therapy in Rheumatoid Arthritis

Antoine Helewa

*University of Western Ontario
London, Ontario, Canada*

Hugh A. Smythe

*University of Toronto and
Wellesley Hospital
Toronto, Ontario, Canada*

I. INTRODUCTION

Physical therapy (PTy) is an essential treatment strategy for patients with rheumatoid arthritis (RA). Any patient with RA must receive PTy at one time or another, regardless of disease stage or severity. It is exposure to PTy as a health discipline that is important, not necessarily any of its individual modalities in isolation. Best results are achieved when PTy is delivered as a package, tailored to the patient's needs, and encompassing elements of disease education, counseling, assessment, treatment, and independence in activities of daily living. In managing RA, physical therapists (PTs) function as members of a larger team of physicians and arthritis health professionals, whose overall objective is to enhance the patient's quality of life. More specific PTy objectives involve controlling disease activity, reducing pain, correcting deformities, restoring or improving function, or preventing future episodes of pain and dysfunction.

The PTy techniques used in RA consist chiefly of analgesic modalities and therapeutic exercise to mobilize joints, strengthen muscles, and enhance endurance and fitness. The literature relating to the efficacy and cost-effectiveness of PTy programs demonstrate that RA patients generally benefit from this therapy; however, serious methodological problems (discussed later in this chapter) do exist, and many research questions must be asked using experimental design.

A. Physical Therapy Referrals

In making therapeutic choices, health professionals must first consider whether a procedure will do more good than harm, or whether carrying out a particular procedure is better than doing nothing, or better than doing something else. They must consider the cost of a test or treatment procedure relative to its effectiveness. Since PTy, by its nature, can be highly technical and is labor-intensive, the length, intensity, and frequency of an individual treatment program, compared with a less expensive alternative, must be considered.

The number of PTs who specialize in arthritis is woefully inadequate, considering the current prevalence and incidence of the arthritides. In North America, there were about 83,000 licensed PTs in 1991; of these, only 250 (a fraction of 1%) were members of the Arthritis Health Professional Association (AHPA), and not all members are specialized in treating arthritis. It is not known how many PTs specialize in arthritis, but are not members of the AHPA. The spinoffs from this apparent shortage of arthritis specialists are worrisome, especially the profession's inability to generate an adequate number of leaders and role models in arthritis education, research, and specialized practice. Therefore, it is not surprising to find that much of PTy practice in arthritis is not based on good evidence, in spite of repeated challenges by health scientists, arthritis professionals, and rheumatologists (1,2). A new vision of the role and scope of PTy in arthritis is needed, as consumer-led changes in patterns of practice and other public expectations will increase the pressure on PTs to evaluate new and old management strategies using randomized experimental design.

Although under certain North American jurisdictions, RA patients may have direct access to PTy, they are usually referred to PTy by physicians. The treatment setting varies according to the patient's needs and the availability of PTy services. Patients with aggressive, uncontrolled polyarthritis are likely to be treated on an inpatient basis in a tertiary care center, progressing to outpatient PTy or home PTy. Those with less severe disease activity or with early disease will most likely receive treatment in hospital-based settings, community-based settings, or in their own homes.

Before referring an RA patient to PTy, a physician should ask the following questions: (a) What are my treatment objectives? (b) Are these objectives feasible in that clinical setting? (c) Is the setting accessible to the patient?

Formulating objectives is a standard procedure in clinical practice and, since PTy is only one aspect of the patient's overall treatment, a statement of PTy-specific objectives by the physician will help crystallize the overall treatment plans. As PTy is provided in different settings, it is important that a disabled RA patient not be referred to a setting that is not accessible, a setting with limited resources, or a setting to which travel is difficult. For such patients, their own home could be the best setting for treatment.

Like physicians, PTs may vary in their skills while caring for RA patients. Ideally, PTs who treat RA patients should be trained to conduct detailed assessments and formulate appropriate treatment plans that are based on experience and critical appraisal of the literature. However, the current shortage of arthritis specialists (physicians and PTs alike), means that some RA patients will receive less than ideal care. In contemplating a referral to PTy, a physician should provide a provisional medical diagnosis, concomitant conditions or complications of the disease or its treatment, the physician's objectives with an explanation of how the referral will benefit the patient, medical or surgical procedures performed or planned, and the date of next medical appointment. Notably absent from this list is the need for a physician to prescribe the PTy procedures or their dosage. Although some physicians continue to prescribe PTy out of habit or conviction, they would do well to remember that PTs, like physicians, are legally accountable. Furthermore, the science-based university training prepares PTs to critically appraise these treatment procedures before applying them to a patient. It is incumbent on the PT and the physician to communicate and discuss their treatment plans to ensure that all therapeutic procedures are compatible and lead to the best possible outcome.

B. Elements of Physical Therapy

A popular definition of PTy in the 1950s was ''therapy by physical means.'' *Physical* in this sense refers to elements and forces within the human body (e.g., exercise and movement) or natural forces outside the body, such as temperature, water, and electricity. This definition is very limiting, as it describes only some of the therapies PTs provide, not the overall package. It is widely known that other groups with or without adequate training (e.g., untrained assistants supervised by physicians, athletic trainers, kinesiologists, and chiropractors) provide treatment modalities identified with PTy. As many PTy modalities are not licensed acts, some are even provided by fringe practitioners; therefore, an up-to-date definition of PTy would encompass not only the provision of modalities, but elements of assessment, treatment determination, education, and prevention.

Three basic tenets form the core of PTy practice for RA patients. Physical therapy should (a) help nature restore normal physical function (e.g., therapeutic exercise for atrophied muscle); (b) ensure that the natural-healing process and symptoms do not themselves become a source of disability (e.g., scarring, contracture, pain, degenerative changes); (c) develop preventive strategies that will prevent further deterioration of function.

The PTy modalities are seldom applied singly, but usually with something else, such as cold packs, therapeutic exercise, and disease education, or in association with other therapies, such as anti-inflammatory or analgesic drugs. Most electrotherapeutic modalities have no specific effects on disease processes, but are used as adjuncts to therapeutic exercise, which is at the core of what most PTs do. Therapeutic exercise is also the modality that PTs perform better than any other group, and it constitutes over 70% of PTs' clinical education.

Therefore, PTy is the total of all its elements, not just heat, massage, ultrasound, or exercise alone. As will be discussed later in this chapter, most of these passive modalities, when applied alone (except therapeutic exercises), do not confer clinically important benefits.

II. ASSESSMENT

The accurate measurement of disease activity and treatment response is an essential component of overall management. The techniques must be quantitative, so that numbers can be produced; objective, so that observer impressions do not affect measurement; sensitive to differences in disease severity; reliable, in that the instrument is free from defect; and reproducible in the hands of different observers. The method should also be fast, safe, comfortable, easy to apply, and inexpensive. Physical therapists should obtain complete information relating to medical history and physical findings from the referring source; if that information is not available, PTs should conduct a complete workup.

A. Inflammation

Present curricula prepare PTs to evaluate the patient's level of function by recording range of joint movement, muscle strength, and effects of disability on activities of daily living (3). Contributing to dysfunction may be persistent joint activity, deformities, systemic manifestations, concurrent diseases, or problems of motivation, all of which may vary. To design an appropriate management program, a PTy evaluation must incorporate, in varying degrees, elements of all these problems. For example, hand exercises for an RA patient with 20 active hand joints would be different from exercises for a patient with two or three active joints. For the former, control of disease activity and gentle hand exercises are needed, whereas exercises for the latter can be more vigorous for the uninvolved joints and gentler to the active joints. Therefore, recognizing regional or systemic disease activity is as important for the physical therapist as it is for the physician prescribing drugs, or for that matter, any other member of the treatment team. Although information on disease activity is normally included by a referring rheumatologist, such evaluation cannot be done well by other physicians with little training in rheumatology and who have a relatively small number of patients with RA at any one time. In contrast, PTs are full-time professionals in musculoskeletal diseases, and a significant proportion of their basic training lends itself well to acquiring specialized skills in assessing disease activity. Studies conducted by our group demonstrate this point (3–5).

Quantitative measures of disease activity would be identical with those used by rheumatologists and in clinical trials, and would include a count of active joints, grip strength, duration of morning stiffness, erythrocyte sedimentation rate, pain using a visual analog scale, and function. Therefore, every patient's program becomes a minitherapeutic trial, permitting PTs and other members of the treatment team, to tailor their therapeutic strategies to the patient's disease status.

B. Impairments

The PT-specific assessments involve the measurement of disease impairments, especially loss of movement range, muscle weakness, and dysfunction.

Range of Movement

The measurement of joint stiffness is obtained by measuring the range of movement (ROM) in degrees or centimeters distance between designated points. Degrees are measured by using a simple goniometer, a gravity goniometer, or an electronic goniometer. Regardless of instrument type, studies have repeatedly shown that interobserver variation in goniometry tends to be high, making the goniometer an unreliable tool in the hands of different observers; however, intraobserver variability was low (6,7). In a disease characterized by joint effusions, subluxation, or contractures, all of which can singly or in combination alter the normal alignment of articular surfaces, special care must be taken when performing these tests; nevertheless, goniometric techniques can provide a broad indication of change and continue to be in general clinical use for specific joints, such as the knees or elbows. Measures of spinal mobility, such as finger tip to floor distances, using a simple flexible tape or rigid ruler, have been shown to be valid and reproducible when compared with other methods (8,9). As ROM measurements are affected by diurnal variation, observers, and the technique used, repeat measurements should be taken at the same time of day and by the same observer using a standardized technique.

Muscle Strength

Muscle strength measurements, using a variety of techniques and instruments, tend to be more reliable than goniometry. For RA patients, a single maximal isometric contraction is commonly employed, using a hand-held dynamometer. Of the devices available, only the modified sphygmomanometer (10–12) has been validated on RA patients. It can be adapted at little cost, applied quickly, and is comfortable and safe for patients with joint dysfunction. Although the Medical Research Council (MRC) scale is commonly used, it is inappropriate for patients with RA (10).

Function

In the past decade, several functional measures have been developed as indexes of overall function (13), or to assess regional problems, such as hand and arm function (14). The former are usually used to evaluate the effects of a new therapy within the context of a clinical trial and, rarely, as clinical treatment measure. Valid and reproducible clinical measures of function that are PTy-specific have not been developed; however, numerous functional assessment tools are available, including self-administered questionnaires.

III. PHYSICAL THERAPY MANAGEMENT OF RHEUMATOID ARTHRITIS

A. Overview

Because polypharmacy is now accepted as essential to a successful outcome for most patients with active RA, physical and other rehabilitation therapies should also be an integral part of the polytherapies for RA. Each drug and each therapy should play a specific role in a well-orchestrated approach to harmonic management of the disease (2).

We now know a great deal more about drug management of RA, owing to extensive research dollar investments by the drug industry and other traditional sources of support. In contrast, support from all sources for PTy research in arthritis in Canada did not reach 300,000 dollars in 1991. By extrapolation, comparative figures for the United States would not exceed 3 million dollars. In contrast with drug research in arthritis, this amounts to a fraction of 1%. Why the difference? Two interrelated issues come to mind. First, physicians, in spite of their interest in PTy and the general recognition of its role in managing RA, are chiefly preoccupied with the areas of practice with which they are most familiar: drug and surgical therapy. Second, the rehabilitation therapies are not well-known; therefore, they do not attract much public and corporate attention. Consequently, PTs are attempting to fill a credibility gap. As PTs lack the power base and infrastructure from which medicine can draw, the task is slow and arduous.

B. Objectives

Important criteria for a successful PT management program for RA are an accurate diagnosis, effective medical–surgical management, and the use of quantitative assessment techniques of disease activity, impairment, and dysfunction. Generally, the objectives of PTy are to control pain, increase and maintain joint mobility and muscle strength, maintain cardiopulmonary fitness, protect joints, conserve energy, and preserve function. These objectives are not influenced by disease stage or severity, but the technique used and intensity of application vary with each patient. For example, if an RA patient is referred early after onset (a rare occurrence), these objectives would be accomplished through disease education and emphasis on self-management and the long-term prevention of joint destruction and deformity.

To accomplish these objectives, PTs use a variety of treatment techniques, singly or in combination. Central to all these techniques is the judicious application of therapeutic exercise, tailored to the patient's needs. Most other techniques used are primarily adjuncts to therapeutic exercise and include heat, cold, and electrical muscle stimulation. Table 1 provides a summary of the techniques

Table 1 Summary of Physical Therapy Techniques for Rheumatoid Arthritis

Modality	Effects	Objective	Comments
Analgesics			
Cold	Inhibits nerve conduction	Control pain and muscle spasm	Best for active joints[a] Applied to muscles in spasm (flexors)
Heat	Increases nerve conduction	Control pain and muscle spasm	Best for chronic joints Applied to muscles in spasm (flexors)
TENS	Inhibits nerve conduction	Control pain	Limited to one or two sites
Facilitatory			
Electrical muscle stimulation or ice massage	Facilitatory	Preserve or restore muscle strength	Precedes strengthening exercises
Therapeutic exercise			
Mobilizing	Elasticity of joint and soft-tissue structures	Preserve or restore joint range	Active joint: exercise to pain tolerance
Strengthening (isometric/ isotonic)	Facilitatory	Preserve or restore muscle strength	Active joint: submaximal isometric
Conditioning (aerobic)	Muscle endurance, cardiopulmonary fitness	Preserve or restore physical fitness	Low-impact or water aerobics

[a]Exercise should not be applied to joints anesthetized by cold.

Table 2   General Principles in Physical Therapy Management
of Rheumatoid Arthritis

1. Treatment plans must be based on an accurate diagnosis and assessment of disease activity and dysfunction.
2. The selection of treatment techniques and dosage specifications must be supported by scientific evidence. If this evidence is unavailable, then the treatment and dosage should make biological sense. Careful assessment and periodic review of treatment results is essential.
3. Treatment techniques should be brief and simple to apply (preferably by the patient) and adapted for home use.
4. Treatment techniques should be pain-free and safe. If joint swelling or pain lasts 2 h or more after treatment, the therapy should be reviewed or its intensity reduced.
5. Therapeutic exercise has many objectives and is central to PT management; all other techniques are largely treatment adjuncts.
6. Strategies to improve patient compliance, in addition to principles 3 and 4, should be based on patient instruction about the disease and its treatment.

commonly used in the treatment of RA, listed by objective and physiological effects sought. Table 2 outlines general principles to follow when planning a treatment program.

C. Analgesic Physical Therapy

In general, pain-relieving PTy modalities do not provide long-term pain relief, but rather a decrease in pain, lasting 1 or 2 h in most cases. Since it is difficult to achieve analgesia in any form when the disease is active, physical therapy's pain-relieving modalities are most useful following successful anti-inflammatory therapy, as a warm-up to therapeutic exercise, or preceding activities of daily living. Two forms of analgesia are used: thermal and electrical stimulation.

Thermal Modalities

The two most commonly used pain-relieving techniques (and by consensus, the most sensible) are the application of simple hot or cold packs to painful sites. As heat can increase molecular activity, causes vasodilatation, and increases nerve conduction, it can increase pain in active joints. In contrast, cold, which has opposite physiological effects, would be more beneficial when applied to active joints. Cold is known to increase the pain threshold by directly reducing the activity of pain-conducting fibers and receptors, by alleviating muscle spasm, and by supplying competitive sensations as suggested by the gate control theory (15,16). The anti-inflammatory effects of cold are mediated through vasoconstriction, reducing hyperemia (17), as well as direct effects on abnormal metabolic processes by reducing the activity of collagenase in the inflammatory reaction (18). Finally, cold decreases muscle spasm secondary to joint disease by reducing the activity of muscle spindle receptors and their 1A afferent fibers (19,20). In contrast, the application of ice cubes in short strokes over a muscle belly can stimulate muscle response by facilitating α motor neurones discharge and is most effective when applied to muscles inhibited by pain and swelling (21,22). For example, in treating a rheumatoid knee with moderate synovitis, a cold pack would be applied to the skin overlying all knee flexors (usually in spasm) for 15–20 min. This is followed with ice massage, given in short strokes for 1 min, to the knee extensors, presumably in a state of reflex inhibition, followed by active isotonic–isometric exercise to the knee to increase ROM and muscle strength.

Hot or cold packs are usually applied for 15–20 min, the material wrapped in a damp towel to permit even conduction of thermal energy. Ice should never be applied directly to the skin (ice massage excepted), nor should the weight of a limb or torso rest on the pack, as this may burn the cold, anesthetized skin. A practical homemade hot pack can be made by putting a wet facecloth in a plastic freezer bag and heating it in a microwave oven for 1 min. The heated pack is then wrapped in a damp towel and applied to the affected area for 15–20 min. If pain and swelling in a joint is severe, cold may be applied for 10 min to the skin overlying the target joint. As this will result in cold anesthesia, immediate exercise to already inflamed but anesthesized structures may cause more harm than good and should be avoided. Damaged but inactive joints can benefit from direct application of heat to the joint surface or muscles in spasm.

In patients with acute synovitis, the two modalities are not interchangeable because they have opposite physiological effects. However, an uncontrolled study of patients with chronic RA of the knee showed that there was no difference in pain or stiffness resulting from heat and ice packs after 5 weeks of treatment (23). In another study of 24 RA patients (30 active knee joints in all), 15 knees were allocated at random to an ice treatment group or to a control group. All patients were stabilized on bed rest for 1 week, and both groups received therapeutic exercise during the experimental period. After 5 days of therapy, there was no difference between the groups in joint circumference or skin temperature measured by thermography (24). The small sample size and, therefore, the possibility of a type II error, as well as the application of therapeutic exercises to active knee joints may have contributed to these results. In another randomized study of 18 RA subjects with shoulder pain, hot packs and ice were compared; all subjects received exercise. No differences between groups were noted, but the sample size was inadequate (25).

Another form of heat used in the past was melted paraffin wax at 48°C applied to hands and feet. Wax application at home can be cumbersome and time-consuming for the RA patient and could cause a fire unless the wax is heated in a double boiler. A safer alternative is to apply mineral oil to the hands, wear rubber dish-washing gloves and soak in hot water from the tap for 5–10 min.

On the surface, these studies would suggest that heat and ice are interchangeable and that patient preference should determine the choice between these two modalities. A closer look shows that each study was fraught with methodological problems, such as lack of control groups and small sample sizes. Therefore, the question of the interchangeability of hot and cold treatments has not been properly addressed.

An earlier randomized clinical trial of 131 RA and osteoarthritis (OA) patients showed no difference in range of movement, walking, and stair-climbing time between patients who received exercise and one of short-wave diathermy (SWD), sham short-wave diathermy, or infrared and electrical muscle stimulation. The authors conclude that the improvement seen in all patient groups was almost certainly a result of the other treatments offered, plus the encouragement obtained (26). A recent study showed that SWD can raise the intra-articular temperature by 2.4°C and thereby cause harm (27).

In light of this danger and the fact that SWD is more expensive, can aggravate joint pain, and can cause slow-healing skin burns if not applied carefully, there is consensus that SWD does not offer any advantages over hot packs (28,29). Furthermore, these modalities cannot be applied at home as part of a self-management program.

There are no controlled studies of ultrasound on RA patients, and very few on patients with regional pain syndromes. The lack of well-performed controlled studies leads to uncritical and inappropriate application of a treatment method that may at times be harmful and an unnecessary expense (17).

Electrical Stimulation Modalities

Analgesic electrical stimulation consists largely of transcutaneous electrical nerve stimulation (TENS) and, to a lesser extent, interferential currents.

The use of TENS stimulates endorphin release in the spinal cord because of increased simulation of large myelinated nerve fibers, which tend to override the nociceptive inputs from unmyelinated C and small myelinated A delta fibers (30,31). Although it is commonly used for regional intractable pain and can be applied by the patient at home, for RA patients with multiple joint problems and generalized pain, TENS is impractical and time-consuming, as there may be a half dozen sites that require stimulation. It is popular among patients and PTs because of its portability and relatively low cost.

Of the 25 randomized trials of TENS published, only 2 were conducted on RA patients. The first was double-blind and involved 32 patients allocated to active TENS and placebo TENS to the wrist, but maintained on "anti-inflammatory analgesics" (32). Resting pain and gripping pain were measured by a visual analog scale. The experimental group fared better in both measures of pain, and this difference was statistically significant; however, the observation period lasted only 3 weeks, had no follow-up, and sample size estimates were not given. The second randomized trial was also double-blind and involved 33 patients allocated to TENS or placebo TENS. There was no difference between the two groups; however, the small sample size raises the specter of a type II error (33).

The remaining 24 studies, for other conditions, show conflicting results, with half showing that TENS is no better than placebo (17). In view of this, the evidence suggests that TENS continues to be a controversial modality, and its effects need to be further researched. For patients with regional pain problems, it can provide short-term relief.

Interferential currents are a special modification of middle-frequency currents (> 1000 Hz), which tend to avoid the sensory disadvantage of lower-frequency currents such as TENS (80–120 Hz) by passing through the skin without being felt (17). Interferential current, similarly to TENS, is an impractical therapy for the RA patient and has the same disadvantages of ultrasound and diathermy in terms of the high cost of these devices (over 20,000 dollars), which the patient can receive only in a clinical setting. There are no published reports of the efficacy of interferential therapy in RA.

D. The Value of Rest

Total bed rest for RA patients is rarely prescribed, as it can lead to deconditioning. Patients generally do not enjoy enforced inactivity and are easily bored, become depressed, and frequently do not adhere to strict bed rest. Younger patients fear that muscle wasting and weakness, and prolongation of their hospital stay may threaten income or job security (34). The prohibitive cost of hospitalization to patients and third-party payers makes total bed rest unattractive in today's climate of cost constraints. Two randomized clinical trials comparing total bed rest with activity showed no significant overall anti-inflammatory effect on the bed rest groups, and the benefits shown were marginal (34,35). This is not to be confused with hospitalization for RA for which inpatient therapy was shown to be superior to intensive outpatient therapy (36). As RA can put a tremendous strain on both physical and emotional resources, bed rest for 1–2 h once or twice daily may prevent fatigue and improve recuperation (37,34). Local rest to painful joints can be achieved through supportive devices such as splints, insoles, neck collars, and joint protection techniques. A recent randomized clinical trial of the effects of occupational therapy (OT) on RA patients using these techniques, showed statistically significant and clinically important differences in function favoring the OT group (38).

E. Therapeutic Exercise

Exercise therapy serves many purposes in the treatment of RA, and usually only one purpose is achieved optimally by any specific exercise (2). For example, range of motion exercises are no substitute for strengthening exercises, and these are no substitute for conditioning exercise. The main objectives of therapeutic exercises are to preserve motion or restore lost motion, increase muscle strength and endurance, provide cardiovascular conditioning, enhance a feeling of well-being, and provide active recreation. For patients with controlled disease, but residual impairments, it is by far the most important aspect of their therapy; however, exercise is given at all stages of RA and is tailored to suit the patients' disease state.

Muscle atrophy and weakness is a common feature of RA, and is caused by a variety of pathological processes, steroids, reflex inhibition, and disuse. Movement loss and immobility may also lead to fixed contractures of periarticular and intrarticular soft tissue structures, through shortening of collagen, which may also cause loss of articular structures. The application of therapeutic exercise, therefore, is central to the rehabilitation of these patients (39–41).

Exercise is either dynamic or static. Contractions may be *isometric*, during which the muscle length does not change, no joint movement occurs, only muscle tension is generated; *isotonic*, during which muscle length changes, joint movement takes place, and force is generated; or *isokinetic*, during which the limb moves through joint range while in contact with a rate-limiting device, such as a dynamometer, generating torque (42). A shortening reaction in an isotonic or isokinetic contraction is referred to as *concentric action*, and a lengthening reaction as *eccentric action*.

Exercise can be passive (performed by PTs or outside force), assisted active (by patient with help), active (by patient alone), or resisted active (resisted by PTs or outside force).

Three types of exercise by objective will be reviewed: mobilizing exercise to maintain or restore joint movement, exercise to maintain or restore muscle strength, and conditioning exercise.

Mobilizing Exercise

The objectives of mobilizing exercises are to increase mobility, and flexibility and to relieve stiffness.

Thermal modalities should be applied before a session of mobilizing exercises. Cold is the modality of choice for active joints, and moist heat may be used for inactive joints; however, if an RA patient has ten or more joints that should be mobilized, the application of hot or cold packs to each is impractical. In this event, a warm shower or a swim in a warm pool is recommended before the exercise session. Some of the exercises can be performed in a shower or in a pool.

Active joints should be moved gently through the possible range by the patient or with outside assistance. Three repetitions, once or twice daily, are recommended. As joint activity decreases, the joints should continue to be moved as before, but through full range, with possible assistance at the end of the range, to ensure that shortened joint structures and tendons are fully stretched. Special techniques to inhibit resistance to movement, according to Sherrington's principles of reciprocal inhibition, may be taught to the patient or performed by the PT. The technique involves taking the joint through available active range. As resistance of tight structures is encountered, a maximal isometric contraction of the tight muscles (antagonists) is elicited, followed by voluntary relaxation of these tight muscles, and then by active movement in the desired range (43). For example, if knee extension is limited, this could, in part, be a result of spasm and tightening of knee flexors. Since knee extension is the desired movement, the patient is asked to extend the knee fully; at the limit of range (e.g., say 20° short of full extension), a maximal isometric contraction of knee flexors is obtained for 5 s, followed by voluntary relaxation of knee flexors; and then by active knee extension using the quadriceps. This sequence can be repeated four to five times with isometric resistance to flexors applied by the patient, an operator, or an object such as the surface of a plinth or table. Referred to as "hold relax," this technique is familiar to all PTs, and the principles can be adapted for any painful joint with movement limitations. A sensation of full muscle stretch accompanies this technique, and it should be pain free.

Muscle groups and joints targeted for mobilizing exercises are shown in Table 3.

Table 3 Muscle and Joints Targeted for Strength Training and Stretching

	Muscle group	
Joints	Strengthen	Stretch (ROM)
Head and neck	Extensors, retractors	All muscle groups[a]
Scapulo/humeral	Scapular retractors and depressors	Scapular protractors and elevators
	Shoulder flexors, abductors, and rotators	Shoulder adductors and rotators
Elbows	All muscle groups	All muscle groups
Forearm, wrist, and hands	Supinators, pronators, adductors and abductors of wrist and fingers, flexor and extensors of wrist and fingers	Supinators, pronators
		Wrist and finger flexor and adductors
		Hand intrisincs
Hips	Abductors, extensors, rotators	Flexors, rotators, and adductors
Knee	Extensors, flexors	Flexors (hamstrings, gastrocnemius)
Foot and ankle	All muscle groups	All muscle groups
Trunk	Flexors, extensors	All muscle groups

[a]Contraindicated in subluxed atlantoaxial joints.

Strengthening Exercise

Muscle atrophy from disuse and reflex inhibition is a common feature of RA. Consequent loss of muscle strength and endurance ensues, limiting certain activities of daily living. Therefore, therapeutic exercise designed to increase strength and endurance is an essential component of RA management. The muscles should not be exercised to fatigue, and any resistance offered to isotonic contraction must be just submaximal. Active joints should not be put through many repetitions. Movement should not be resisted, and muscles acting on active joints should be exercised isometrically for both strength and endurance. The exercises should not cause harm; pain that lasts over 1 h after an exercise session or results in joint swelling is an indication of excessive exercise, especially if symptoms increase overnight.

An isometric muscle contraction is obtained when the subject is asked to contract one or more muscles while the limb or part is held in a static position. The usual command is "Tighten these muscles while holding your leg in that position to the count of 6 s, then let go."

One study of RA patients showed that three maximal isometric contractions of the quadriceps, in full extension and at 90° flexion, held for 6 s, produced a 27% increase in strength in the exercised leg and 17% in the quadriceps of the contralateral limb (44). Although isometric training improves performance of isotonic tasks, clinically important improvements have also been noted for both types of tasks, regardless of type of contraction (45).

After joint activity decreases and sufficient strength is attained by isometric exercise, isotonic contractions can be introduced, using low resistance and a few repetitions. Isotonic exercise must be tailored to the patient with RA and consider factors related to age, severity, strength, and interests of the patient (46). One session a day is recommended, increasing the number of repetitions and resistance to tolerance. Muscle groups and joints targeted for strengthening exercises are shown in Table 3.

Conditioning Exercise

Conditioning exercise through endurance training can have two major purposes: (a) to improve the maximal aerobic power (i.e., to increase the maximal mechanical power output that can be maintained aerobically); (b) to increase aerobic capacity (i.e., to increase the capacity to sustain a given work load for a longer time) (17).

Patients with RA are often restricted in their general physical activities by pain or fear of pain, disability, fatigue, and a belief (encouraged by some health professionals) that strenuous physical activities do more harm than good. These restrictions lead to lower physical work capacity, low muscle strength, and low cardiovascular capacity and endurance (47). Over the last two decades, the value of rest as a way to control disease activity has been increasingly challenged by people who recommend early activity and fitness training (48,49). These trends are also seen in other disease categories, such as cardiovascular and respiratory diseases, as a valuable part of rehabilitation therapy. A number of factors may be responsible for this new approach, chiefly early control of disease activity through aggressive drug management so that the need for rest and joint protection is diminished, the increased costs of hospitalization, and greater public preoccupation with physical fitness. More critical, however, are the recent findings that RA patients have a low level of cardiopulmonary fitness and that conditioning exercises to improve physical endurance help these patients resume optimal activities of daily living (50).

A study of 37 RA patients randomized to receive a standard program of strength training and ROM exercises (control) or the standard program plus bicycle training and gradual strengthening (experimental), showed that after a 6-week stay inhospital, experimental patients performed significantly better on a walk test, stair-climbing, and oxygen consumption rate (VO_2), without exacerbating their arthritis (50). A retest of these patients 6 months after discharge showed that those who continued with the experimental program maintained their level of fitness, suggesting that continued training is important to maintain benefits obtained in the first 6 weeks (51).

A cohort analytic study of 23 RA patients, who received a physical training program for home use or physical training in groups, were compared with a matched group of equal size and disease severity, who received standard outpatient treatment (48). Patients trained for 4–8 years. Those in the active group had fewer radiographic changes in their joints, a higher fitness level, and a lower Lansbury joint index. Also, the training group had fewer sick days and hospital days, and received fewer sickness benefits. These differences were all statistically significant ($p < 0.05$). As patients were not randomized into groups, it is likely that selection biases may have crept into the study.

A more recent study of 120 RA and OA patients, allocated at random to a program of aerobic walking, or aerobic aquatic, or range of motion group (control). At 12 weeks, the aerobic walking and aquatic groups showed significant improvement in aerobic capacity, 50-ft ([1] 15-m) walking time, depression, anxiety, and physical activities compared with the control group (49); however, there were no differences in measures of disease activity among the three groups.

Well-controlled RA patients may participate in aerobic exercises, such as swimming, bicycling, walking, low-impact aerobic dance, and water aerobics (46). Water activities in a relatively warm pool have the added advantage of increasing mobility, strength, endurance, as well as aerobic capacity.

An aerobic exercise program should progress slowly, starting at 5–10 min, and progressing to 45 min, performed three to four times a week (46). The sessions would start with a 10-min warmup, consisting of gentle stretches, followed by 20–30 mins of aerobic exercise, and a 10-min cool-down period of gentle stretches to prevent postexercise muscle soreness (46).

Activities, such as walking, swimming, and gardening, are useful forms of conditioning exercise and have a higher recreational value for some patients, compared with a structured aerobic-training program.

IV. RESEARCH QUESTIONS

There are more questions that can be asked about PTy methods in RA than there are answers. Physical therapists recognize this deficit, and an increasing number strive to seek answers using valid scientific methods; however, in terms of scientific personnel and research support, the current infrastructure remains weak, as evidenced in the low proportion of PTs specializing in arthritis and the meagre funding currently available to them.

Therefore, a greater number of PTs must be recruited to specialize in the management of the arthritides, and within that group (in association with academic centers) greater efforts are needed to address important research questions. Improved research proposals by PTs will no doubt make them more competitive for research grant funding from existing agencies; however, dedicated funds are also needed to increase the pool of research dollars available to PTs.

The PTy literature related to RA indicates that the quality of research articles published is low in terms of design architecture. The number of randomized clinical trials of PTy methods is very small, and among these, there are several methodological problems. Very little of the research cited includes statistically derived estimates of appropriate sample sizes to control for type II errors. Primary outcome measures for testing the primary hypothesis are usually not prespecified and are not always physical therapy-specific. When multiple measures are used, the investigators tend to choose the outcome that best suits their hypothesis. Although statistical significance is reported, the clinical importance of their results is not discussed. Finally, many studies do not account for all patients studied, making it difficult to distinguish between an intent-to-treat analysis (efficacy) and an effectiveness analysis. Cost-effectiveness studies are not cited.

Better-designed, randomized trials are needed to address a multitude of research questions relating to the effect of PTy programs generally e.g., health services research and the effect of specific intervention for specific problems, and clinically based research. Also, PTy-specific valid outcome measures must be developed to evaluate the effect of PTy for specific interventions.

REFERENCES

1. Vignos PJ. Physiotherapy in rheumatoid arthritis. J Rheumatol 1980; 7:269–271.
2. Sweezey RL. Rheumatoid arthritis: the role of the kinder and gentler therapies. J Rheumatol 1990; 17(suppl 25):8–13.

3. Helewa A, Smythe HA, Goldsmith CH, Groh J, Thomas MC, Stokes BA, Sugarman J. The total assessment of rheumatoid polyarthritis: evaluation of a training program for physiotherapists and occupational therapists. J Rheumatol 1987; 14:87–92.

4. Smythe HA, Helewa A, Goldsmith CH. "Independent assessor" and "pooled index" as techniques for measuring treatment effects in rheumatoid arthritis. J Rheumatol 1977; 4:144–152.

5. Smythe HA, Helewa A, Goldsmith CH. Failure of rheumatoid patients to respond to therapy directed by family physicians. Ann R Coll Physicians Can 1979; 12:96.

6. Rothstein JM, Miller PJ, Roettger RF. Goniometric reliability in a clinical setting: elbow and knee measurements. Phys Ther 1983; 63:1611–1615.

7. Watkins MA, Riddle DL, Lamb RL, Personius WJ. Reliability of goniometric measurements and visual estimates of knee range of motion obtained in a clinical setting. Phys Ther 1991; 71:90–96.

8. Miller M, Lee P, Smythe HA, Goldsmith CH. Measurement of spinal mobility: new skin contraction technique compared with established methods. J Rheumatol 1984; 11:507–511.

9. Stokes BA, Helewa A, Goldsmith CH, Groh JD, Kraag GR. Reliability of spinal mobility in ankylosing spondylitis patients. Physiother Can 1988; 40:338–344.

10. Helewa A, Goldsmith CH, Smythe HA. The modified sphygmomanometer—an instrument to measure muscle strength: a validation study. J Chronic Dis 1981; 34:353–361.

11. Helewa A, Goldsmith CH, Smythe HA. Patient, observer and instrument variation in the measurement of strength of shoulder abductor muscles in patients with rheumatoid arthritis using a modified sphygmomanometer. J Rheumatol 1986; 13:1044–1049.

12. Andrews AW. Hand held dynamometry for measuring muscle strength. J Hum Muscle Perform 1991; 1:35–50.

13. Liang MH, Larson MG, Cullen KE, et al. Comparative measurement efficiency and sensitivity of five health status instruments for arthritis research. Arthritis Rheum 1985; 28:542–547.

14. Phillips CA. Rehabilitation of the patient with rheumatoid hand involvement. Phys Ther 1989; 69:1091–1098.

15. Melzack R, Wall PD. Pain mechanisms: a new theory. Science 1965; 150:971–979.

16. Wall PD, Melzack R. Textbook of pain. New York: Churchill Livingston, 1984.

17. Schlapbach P, Gerber NJ. Physiotherapy: controlled trials and facts, vol 14. Basel: S. Karger, 1991.

18. Harris ED Jr, McCroskery PA. The influence of temperature and fibril stability degradation of cartilage collagen by rheumatoid synovial collagenase. N Engl J Med 1974; 290:1–6.

19. Eldred E, Lindsley DG, Buckwald JS. The effect of cooling on mammalian muscle spindles. Exp Neurol 1960; 2:144–157.

20. Ottoson D. The effects of temperature on the isolated muscle spindle. J Physiol 1965; 180:636–648.

21. Harviken K. Ice therapy in spasticity. Acta Neurol Scand 1962; 38(suppl 3):72–84.

22. Knutsson E, Mattssone E. Effects of local cooling on monosynaptic reflexes in man. Scand J Rehabil Med 1969; 1:126–132.

23. Kirk JA, Kersley GD. Heat and cold in the physical treatment of rheumatoid arthritis of the knee. Ann Phys Med 1968; 9:272–274.

24. Bulstrade S, Clarke A, Harrison R. A controlled trial to study the effect of ice therapy on joint inflammation in chronic arthritis. Physiother Pract 1986; 2:104–108.

25. Williams J, Harvey J, Tannenbaum H. Use of superficial heat versus ice for the rheumatoid arthritic shoulder: a pilot study. Physiother Can 1986; 38:8–13.

26. Hamilton DE, Bywaters EGL, Please NW. A controlled trial of various forms of physiotherapy in arthritis. Br Med J 1959; 1:542–544.

27. Osterveld FGJ, Rasker JJ, Jacobs JWG, Overmars HJA. The effects of local heat and cold therapy on the intra articular and skin surface temperature of the knee. Arthritis Rheum 1992; 35:146–151.

28. Goddard DH, Revell PA, Cason J, Gallagher S, Currey HLF. Ultrasound has no anti-inflammatory effect. Ann Rheum Dis 1983; 42:582–584.

29. Mainardi CL, Walter JM, Spiegel PK, Goldkamp OG, Harris ED Jr. Rheumatoid arthritis: failure of daily heat therapy to affect its progression. Arch Phys Med Rehabil 1979; 60:390–394.

30. Ersek RA. Transcutaneous electrical neurostimulation: a new therapeutic modality for controlling pain. Clin Orthop 1977; 128:314–324.

31. Sjolund B, Terenius L, Eriksson M. Increased cerebrospinal fluid levels of endorphins after electro-acupuncture. Acta Physiol Scand 1977; 100:382–384.

32. Abelson K, Langley GB, Sheppeard H, Vlieg M, Wigley RD. Transcutaneous electrical nerve stimulation in rheumatoid arthritis. NZ Med J 1983; 96:156–158.

33. Langley GB, Sheppeard H, Johnson M, Wigley RD. The analgesic effect of TENS and placebo in chronic pain patients. Rheumatol Int 1984; 4:119–123.

34. Alexander GJM, Hortas C, Bacon PA. Bed rest, activity and the inflammation of rheumatoid arthritis. Br J Rheumatol 1983; 22:134–140.

35. Mills JA, Pinals RS, Ropes MW, Short CL, Sutcliff J. Value of bed rest in patients with rheumatoid arthritis. N Engl J Med 1971; 284:453–258.

36. Helewa A, Bombardier C, Goldsmith CH, Menchions B, Smythe HA. Cost-effectiveness of inpatient and intensive outpatient treatment of rheumatoid arthritis. A randomized, controlled trial. Arthritis Rheum 1989; 32:1505–1514.

37. Lee P, Kennedy AC, Anderson J, Buchanan WW. Benefits of hospitalization in rheumatoid arthritis. Q J Med 1974; 43:205–214.

38. Helewa A, Goldsmith CH, Tugwell P, Bombardier C, Lee P, Smythe HA, Hanes B. The effects of occupational therapy home service on patients with rheumatoid arthritis: a randomized controlled trial. Lancet 1991; 337:1453–1456.

39. Akeson WH, Amiel D, Woo SLY. Immobility effects on synovial joints: the pathomechanics of joint contracture. Biorheology 1980; 17:95–110.

40. Enneking WF, Horowitz ML. The intra-articular effects of immobilization on the human knee. J Bone Joint Surg 1972; 54A:973–985.

41. Tardieu C, Tabary JC, Tabary C, et al. Adaptation of connective tissue length to immobilization in the lengthened and shortened positions in cat soleus muscle. Physiology 1982; 78:214–220.

42. Gerber LH. Exercise and arthritis. Bull Rheum Dis 1990; 39(6):1–9.

43. Voss DE, Ionta MK, Myers BJ. Proprioceptive neuromuscular facilitation—patterns and techniques. Philadelphia: Harper & Row, 1985.

44. Machover S, Sapecky AJ. Effect of isometric exercise on the quadriceps muscle in patients with rheumatoid arthritis. Arch Phys Med Rehabil 1966; 47:737–741.

45. deLateur BJ, Lehmann J, Stonebridge J. Isotonic vs isometric exercise: a double-shift transfer of training study. Arch Phys Med Rehabil 1972; 53:212–217.

46. Semble EL, Loeser RF, Wise CM. Therapeutic exercise for rheumatoid arthritis and osteoarthritis. Semin Arthritis Rheum 1990; 20:32–40.

47. Ekblom B, Lövgren O, Alderin M, Fridström M, Sätterström G. Physical performance in patients with rheumatoid arthritis. Scand J Rheumatol 1974; 3:121–125.

48. Nordemar R, Ekblom B, Zachrisson L, Lundquist K. Physical training in rheumatoid arthritis: a controlled long-term study. I. Scand J Rheumatol 1981; 10:17–23.

49. Minor MA, Hewitt JE, Webel RR, Anderson SK, Kay DR. Efficacy of physical conditioning exercise in patients with rheumatoid arthritis and osteoarthritis. Arthritis Rheum 1989; 32:1396–1405.

50. Ekblom B, Lövgren O, Alderin M, Fridström M, Sätterström G. Effect of short-term physical training on patients with rheumatoid arthritis I. Scand J Rheumatol 1975; 4:80–86.

51. Ekblom B, Lövgren O, Alderin M, Fridström M, Sätterström G. Effect of short-term physical training on patients with rheumatoid arthritis. A six-month follow up study. Scand J Rheumatol 1975; 4:87–91.

20

The Surgical Treatment of Early and Advanced Rheumatoid Arthritis

Matthew H. Liang and Gerold Stucki

*Harvard Medical School
and Brigham and Women's
Hospital, Boston, Massachusetts*

I. INTRODUCTION

Conventional wisdom states that the treatment of rheumatoid arthritis precedes in an orderly sequence, moving from conservative to more aggressive treatment. Recent data suggest, but do not prove by any means that this might be an error. Earlier use of medical, surgical, and rehabilitative treatment may improve outcomes and prevent the insidious decline of patients with established disease, and it has a rationale based on an understanding of the pathogenesis of rheumatoid synovitis.

Total joint arthroplasty, particularly of the hip and knee, has been a major advance in the management of patients with advanced structural damage from rheumatoid synovitis. Future improvements lie in improved patient selection, perioperative management, and in solving the problems of loosening and biomaterial failure. Systematic, standardized long-term outcome assessment is absolutely essential to all of these objectives.

As these salvage procedures improve, better understanding of the basic biology of rheumatoid synovitis or pannus—the primary destructive lesion of rheumatoid arthritis—has stimulated the development of specific biological agents directed at primary immunological events in its pathogenesis, and a major shift in the way medications are used during the course of disease. Instead of building on conservative management and moving on to more aggressive treatment, the classic pyramid approach, there is evidence for, and enhanced interest

435

in, aggressive treatment early in the course of disease. The surgical parallel is the application of synovectomy to earlier-stage disease. This chapter reviews the early and late surgical approaches and important areas for future developments.

II. BIOLOGY OF RHEUMATOID SYNOVITIS

Removal of rheumatoid pannus was first done in 1894 (1), but it was not commonly done until after World War II, when synovectomy was performed by surgical, chemical, or radioisotopic procedures. Why synovectomy has a rational appeal can be appreciated by an understanding of the biology of rheumatoid synovitis.

We know that rheumatoid arthritis (RA) is a chronic immune-mediated disease, the initiation and perpetuation of which are dependent on T-cell responses to unknown antigen(s). As a consequence of T-cell stimulation, T-cell lymphokines, such as interferon gamma (IFN-γ), are released, which then activate monocyte–macrophage cells to release a variety of monokines (interleukin-1; IL-1), tumor necrosis factor (TNF), and other mediators of inflammation, such as granulocyte–macrophage colony-stimulating factor (GM-CSF) and growth factors. Fibroblasts are then activated, endothelial cells proliferate and form new blood vessels, and osteoclasts are activated and erode bone. Rheumatoid synovitis is a complex process, with both destruction and repair occurring simultaneously in the same synovium. Rheumatoid pannus consists of monocytes and lymphocytes from the circulation, and the local proliferation of synovial fibroblasts. Mast cells at the junction of the pannus and the bone and cartilage have an important role in the destructive process. The T cells that infiltrate the synovium are preponderantly of the CD4 helper class, belonging almost entirely to the memory subset, CD44RO. These T cells are primed to react to recall antigens, with the production of T-cell lymphokines, such as IFN-γ and IL-2.

Rheumatoid synovium shows vast differences at a gross and microscopic level; normal tissue is seen next to pannus. Areas of marked synovial cell proliferation, resembling a malignant mesenchymal tumor, with almost no lymphocytes or plasma cells, and with destruction of cartilage and bone, coexist with areas where almost no destruction is apparent (2).

Even more important to appreciate are the changes of rheumatoid synovitis over time. During a proliferative stage, the cell mass, consisting of a single synovial cell type, lacks blood vessels and is short-lived. Most cells die, and the surviving ones "modulate" to fibroblasts, which produce collagen fibers, and the tissue becomes more vascularized (early pannus formation). Thus, the invasive phase of the cells from the synovial tissue occurs before the development of the pannus. It is believed that the process of cell mass invasion and differentiation into pannus can recur.

The inflammatory process is amenable to anti-inflammatory agents, but control of the proliferative synovial cells during the florid, aggressive stage, for which no blood vessels exist, requires a different approach and gives justification to examining approaches to ablate these cells.

In addition to the potential role of synovectomy to reduce or eliminate the aggressive cell mass, establishing normal biomechanics and alignment of individual joints, which should improve function, diminish energy expenditure, and reduce secondary pain syndromes, is another theoretical rationale. Tenosynovectomy allows one to eliminate a physiological bottleneck that may become permanent and alter function in one joint, which influences the mechanics of others in the chain.

III. SURGICAL SYNOVECTOMY

The literature on synovectomy is inconclusive about whether early synovectomy is effective in preventing progression of disease, because the vast experience is in late disease and is based on the crudest assessment (i.e., radiographic) of disease progression. As medications do little in the advanced structurally damaged joint, so too would surgery not be expected to reverse structural damage. In addition, study design flaws, such as heterogeneity of subjects, lack of standardized outcome assessment or the patient's evaluation, absence of comparison groups, lack of information on cotreatment, and other variables known to affect outcomes, do not permit firm conclusions (3).

The literature suggests that synovectomy relieves pain and improves function. With the exception of synovectomies of the elbow and shoulder, there is only a slight influence on the mobility of the operated-on joint. As one would expect, the results depend on the degree of preoperative structural damage. Most studies of synovectomies in larger joints show that the radiographic appearance deteriorates gradually after the surgery.

Early surgical synovectomy is seldom done in the hip joint. This is because of the difficulty of access and the danger of disturbing the blood supply of the femoral head, resulting in vascular necrosis. It is not possible to perform a synovectomy in the depths of the acetabulum without dislocating the joint.

The ankle joint is readily accessible for synovectomy, and a painful synovitis is frequently encountered in the peroneal tendons or the posterior tibial tendon. Occasionally, tenosynovitis of the toe extensors is seen. When the tendon sheaths are markedly affected, there is usually only mild involvement of the joints. Gschwend et al., who reported on a large series of late synovectomy patients, used independent and standardized clinical and radiographic assessment over a 5-year period (4). In 370 finger synovectomies, clinical deterioration was chiefly attributable to an increase number of deformities. Deterioration in the radiographs occurred in about 30% of the cases, most of whom exhibited degenerative and not inflammatory features. Better results with early synovectomy and mono- and pauciarticular cases were observed.

In two controlled studies, with relatively small samples, surgically treated joints were compared clinically and radiographically with joints treated by conservative means during a 3-year period. A British study reported results in knee and metacarpophalangeal (MP) joints (5), and an American study also included proximal interphalangeal (PIP) joints (6,7).

The British study showed no difference in clinical and radiographic criteria between the surgically and nonsurgically treated joints. The American study found nothing to recommend surgical management 3 years postoperatively. In contrast with synovectomy of the MP joints, the British study showed better results in synovectomy of the knee joint for pain, swelling, and radiographic changes. The American study, on the other hand, showed only improvement in knee swelling. In evaluating the usefulness of synovectomy on the basis of radiographs in the knee and finger joints, there is also a striking discrepancy between the findings at operation, with lesions revealed that are not visible radiographically. This may explain why a study by Thompson came to different conclusions concerning the efficacy of MP synovectomy (8).

The European Rheumatoid Arthritis Surgical Society (ERASS) (9) multicenter study reported on results after more than 10 years following synovectomy of various joints. Overall, the American Rheumatism Association (ARA) functional class—a relatively coarse and insensitive measure—and radiographic grade were not affected, but more than 10 years after synovectomy, pain and swelling had diminished remarkably on the surgically treated side, and most patients' assessment of the operation was positive.

IV. CHEMICAL AND RADIATION SYNOVECTOMY

Injection of chemicals or radioisotopes into joints is a useful alternative and perhaps superior to surgical synovectomy in the treatment of chronic unresponsive synovitis. The theoretical and practical advantages include minimal burden for the patient, simplicity of the techniques with less associated risks, ability to reach areas inaccessible to surgery, minimal or no hospitalization, simple rehabilitation, and low cost.

Since 1951, when von Reis introduced osmic acid (10), different chemical agents such as thiotepa (11,12), varicocid (13–15), and cyclophosphamide (16,17) have been tried. Because of side effects or lack of efficacy, only osmic acid and varicocid have been adopted into clinical practice. They have been used especially in younger patients for whom radiation synovectomy might be harmful. The main concern with chemical synovectomy is its potential for damaging cartilage. Radiation synovectomy has similar concerns, with the addition of injury to the subchondral bone marrow, especially in the presence of cartilage damage (18), and of chromosomal damage (19,20).

Radiation synovectomy with [198]Au was introduced by Ansell in 1963 (21). Since then, [198]Au, [90]Y (22), and [169]Er (23) in different preparations have been widely used, especially in Europe. Comparatively less experience is reported with [32]P (24), [186]Re (25), [165]Dy (26) and [166]Ho.

The ideal radionuclide for radiation synovectomy is theorectically a pure β- (electron) emitter or a β-emitter with minimal γ-emission, because of their limited penetration, typically releasing all their energy within 1 cm of tissue or less. It should have a short half-life, to minimize the extra-articular radiation exposure, but one long enough to permit transport from the site of manufacture to the clinic. None of the available nuclides fulfills all these criteria. Gold 198 has considerable γ-emission; [198]Au, ^{90}Y, [186]Re, and especially, [169]Er and ^{32}P, have a long half-life, up to 14.4 days. The half-life of [165]Dy is only 2.3 h, which limits its application. To minimize leakage from the joint, with consequent chromosomal damage, especially in lymphocytes, larger radioactive particles (^{90}Y better than [198]Au) or aggregates (Dy, Y-carriers) are preferred. Bed rest or rigid splinting significantly reduces leakage (27).

Depending on penetration range, Y, Au, P, and Dy have been used for large joints, such as knee, hip, shoulder; Re for the elbow; and Er for the small joints of the hand. Since the thickness of the inflamed synovium differs from patient to patient, the optimal choice of the nuclide and dosage would require arthroscopic or magnetic resonance imaging (MRI) staging (28). If a preinjection of intra-articular steroids, to reduce the thickness of the synovium and the consequently needed energy is used, the MRI needs to be done immediately before radiation synovectomy. An arthroscopic synovectomy combined with a staging arthroscopy could be performed to ablate as much synovium as possible. Other physicians use arthroscopic evaluation and treatment after failure to respond to radiation synovectomy, and in a series of seven patients undergoing a single arthroscopic synovectomy (29), an almost complete success rate has been reported. In contrast a series of 25 patients, who had undergone arthroscopic synovectomy before radiation synovectomy, showed a success rate of 44%, which is similar to the results of a single radiation or surgical synovectomy (30).

In treating synovitis of the wrist, a multicompartment joint for which the entire joint cannot be reached by the injected substance, the operative approach is superior. Where a tenosynovectomy or reconstructive measure is necessary, as often happens in the wrist joint, surgery is also preferred.

In the few controlled studies comparing an active agent with placebo, a significant effect could be shown (23,31–33). The results for specific agents in the few studies comparing chemical, radiation, and surgical synovectomy (34–36) differ considerably. Not controlling for predictors found in univariate analysis, such as disease stage, disease activity, technique used, or lack of sufficient sample size, makes a judgment of the relative value of the different procedures difficult. For pain relief and clinically detected synovitis, the reported results at 1 year are good in about 60%, fair in about 20%, and decline over time to about 20% after 3 years (30). In terms of progression of radiological damage, no benefit has been demonstrated.

Generally, the results obtained with radioisotope synovectomy are superior to those attained with chemical synovectomy (10–15). Early stages of disease fare much better, and better results occur in moderate than in severe synovial hypertrophy, or in very thin synovial layers with extensive effusion and fibrin formation.

V. THE FUTURE

An important role for synovectomy, particularly in early synovitis and repeatedly over the course of the disease, is therefore suggested.

The future use of radiation synovectomy depends on further development of suitable nuclides for different thicknesses of pannus assessed by MRI or arthroscopy. Whether or not steroids should be used intra-articularly before treatment, to reduce the thickness of the inflamed synovium, the required dosage, and the predictors of the outcome have to be established. Since the treatment effect is of limited duration, long-term follow-up, including repeat therapy, should be evaluated. The comparison of radiation and chemical synovectomy with arthroscopic synovectomy as a single or combined procedure should include cost-effectiveness considerations.

More sensitive localization of rheumatoid pannus by MRI with enhancing techniques or arthroscopy could be used to assess their efficacy and to identify the earliest lesions for ablation. Arthroscopy, using laser technology, could conceivably selectively ablate diseased synovium, but doing repeated ablations through needle-bores may be a reality—particularly in critical large weight-bearing joints. Surgical synovectomy has been evaluated only in chronic disease and shows value in only marginally delaying the progression. With aggressive medical therapy and newer techniques to identify early pannus, surgical synovectomy may have even greater value.

VI. TOTAL HIP AND KNEE REPLACEMENT

Total hip and knee replacement are two of the most frequently performed reconstructive procedures in orthopedic surgery (37). Tracking the results of early and late total joint arthroplasty, underscores the phenomenon of late results and complications. Loosening is the primary complication of total joint arthroplasties that have been in place more than a decade. Significant femoral osteolysis has been reported in up to a quarter of cemented total hip replacements (THRs) that require revision surgery, and is also seen in well-fixed cemented and cementless THRs. Because rheumatoid patients are roughly a decade younger than those who receive total joint arthroplasties for degenerative joint disease, long-term consequences need to be understood.

Polyethylene wear has been implicated as the major stimulant of loosening. In animals and humans, particulate debris is generated around loose prostheses from abrasive wear. The cellular response to this debris is made up of macrophages that engulf polyethylene particles and then release prostaglandin E_2, IL-1, tumor necrosis factor, and other cytokines that resorb bone, and is the major cause of hip socket instability (38–41).

Osteolysis occurs preponderantly in the femur and in the acetabulum around cemented and cementless sockets. Acetabular osteolysis incidence is expected to increase in cementless, modular sockets with supplemental screws for fixation. Fretting and wear of the polyethylene liner and screws against the metallic shell can occur, leading to debris generation and subsequent bone resorption.

Debonding of the cement–prosthesis interface and fractures within the cement are the initial events on the femoral side. On the other side, a resorptive membrane, consisting of bioactive macrophages in response to particulate polyethylene debris, starts from the cup periphery at the acetabular bone–cement interface (42,43). When this becomes circumferential, acetabular component-loosening occurs. Improved understanding of these events will enable one to improve biomaterial, prosthetic design, and surgical technique and, one hopes, to improve durability of total joint arthroplasties.

Biological responses to wear debris and bone remodeling around joint implants are being actively investigated. Newer imaging techniques are being developed to evaluate component position and bone density in a more reproducible and standardized fashion. It is crucial to accurately establish the natural history of bone remodeling around implants. Proximal metaphyseal bone resorption caused by stress shielding has been documented with cemented and cementless THRs. The extent of stress shielding is more significant with fully-coated cementless components. It remains to be determined if this will adversely affect the long-term clinical results of these arthroplasty designs.

Pharmacological modalities, such as prostaglandin inhibitors, are being used to see if prosthetic loosening can be arrested or even reversed. Suitable animal models are being developed to study prosthetic loosening and to produce similar membranous tissue around loose implants for cell culture studies.

Hydroxyapatite coating of cementless hip implants has become increasingly popular (44). Initial (2–4 years) clinical experience has been excellent. Thigh pain has been decreased to 4%. Long-term stability of the coating remains suspect. Addition of this coating to the porous surfaces during manufacture is being used to achieve even better osseointegration in the long-term.

Although laboratory investigations are essential, the only way to fully assess the long-term results of total joint arthroplasty is with time. There is an extensive understanding of the long-term results of cemented THR, and it remains the standard against which all newer technology must be compared. Cementless THR offers a greater advantage over cement; but is in evolution, and clinical follow-up has not been sufficient to draw any firm conclusions.

A. Cement Versus Cementless Total Hip Replacement

Much of the current debate over cemented versus cementless THR rests on the theoretical projections of the longevity of both types of fixation (45). The success of cemented THR is well-documented (37). Aseptic loosening incidence ranges between 4 and 15% at up to 15 years of follow-up (35). The overall survival rate of the prosthesis is 85–91% at 15 years, with over 90% of the patients able to maintain good to excellent functional status.

Success of cemented femoral fixation has been improved using contemporary techniques, such as retrograde injection of cement, cleansing of the bony bed with pulsatile lavage, and cement pressurization. Several groups have reported loosening rates of less than 2% at 5 years and 3% at 10 years of follow-up. Cemented cups have also been improved, but to a smaller degree. These improvements were observed equally in both osetoarthritic and rheumatoid patients.

Loosening rates of cemented THR are higher in young, active, obese patients; in patients with osteonecrosis; and following revision surgery. Several reports have shown 10–50% clinical or radiographic failures in patients younger than 50 years of age. Acetabular fixation, in particular, has been inferior to the stem. It has, therefore, been recommended that cementless THR be performed in these high-risk groups. It must be emphasized that medium- to long-term clinical follow-up data are scant in these patients.

Cementless THR is in a state of evolution. Design geometry and biomaterials have been altered more frequently and significantly than the changes that have occurred with cemented THR over the past two decades. These changes, along with modifications in surgical techniques, have made accurate and meaningful assessment of the clinical success or failure difficult.

Cementing techniques that ensure the most intimate cement–bone interdigitation show an improved radiographic appearance and may delay the onset of loosening (46). Most of the effort in improving fixation has been to achieve a permanent interlock using porous coatings, but it has been difficult to avoid gaps around a sizable fraction of the interface. The motions around the interface are due to deformations of the materials, especially trabecular bone, during weight-bearing. Some uncemented total hips and knees, relying on macrointerlock, rather than on porous coating, are slightly less successful than cemented designs, and most of the failures have occurred early, from imprecise fit (47).

There has been concern that bone remodeling will occur with uncemented hip stems owing to the altered stress patterns. Although proximal osteopenia and distal hypertrophy have been observed, they tend to stabilize after a few years. Of the various methods to improve uncemented fixation, perhaps the use of hypdroxapatite (HA) coating is the most significant. Numerous laboratory studies have shown the rapid formation of bone on to HA-coated surfaces, with high shear strength, consistent with the histologically observed direct bone–implant bond.

In the United States, most surgeons favor a microinterlock surface in cementless implants, whereas Europeans favor macrointerlock designs. Although bony ingrowth is extensive in the animal models, human postmortem studies of cementless prostheses are disappointing, with one-third showing no bony ingrowth, one-third showing ingrowth in less than 2% of all available surfaces, and one-third show bony ingrowth in 2–10% of the surfaces. Femoral components generally demonstrated greater bony ingrowth than the acetabular components. Moreover, the degree of bony ingrowth does not appear to correlate with clinical or radiographic status of the hip reconstruction.

For now, it is likely that conventional cemented total hips and total knees will continue to be used for elderly patients. For the hip, more stem sizes will be available, whereas modular femoral heads will encourage the use of midrange ball diameters, which are the best compromise for friction, wear, and stability. For knees, modularity of tibial components and simpler more accurate instrumentation will improve the quality of results. Femoral–tibial geometries with better conformity will replace those with low conformity and excessive laxity, which will reduce wear and instability problems.

In the younger patient, who has a more active lifestyle, improved designs will be required. There are several promising designs in use, with potential benefits over cemented designs. Advances in design methodologies for obtaining early indicators of performance in the patient, should spur the use of uncemented devices. Iterative, finite element analysis for comparing hip stem designs on the basis of bone remodeling change has now been developed. Photoelastic coating and holographic techniques for determining surface strains, and micromotion studies for predicting interface behavior, are being used for design optimization. The RSM method, whereby small beads are inserted into the bone to monitor component–bone motion over time, may well offer an early indicator of long-term performance for a particular design.

There will be an expanded use of hydroxyapatite coating, both with and without porous coating. Other types of coating will receive increasing attention to reduce the egress of metallic ions and protect the surface from wear. Another approach to provide a bioactive surface is of interest because of the finding that growth hormone at an interface can accelerate bone growth and osseointegration. The investigation of polymeric composites, such as polysulfone or polyetherketone reinforced with carbon fibers or polyamide fibers for hip stems, are also promising.

Technology for customizing hip stems to provide a more accurate fit will increase. Close fit results in improved performance; failures are frequently associated with poor fit. Individualized stems, possibly with HA coatings, will find application in femurs with unusual geometries, such as seen in the younger RA patients and in revision arthroplasties.

B. Wear

Fixation was the major concern in the first two decades of experience with THR. As prostheses remain in situ for longer periods, wear of the biomaterial becomes increasingly important. Generation of particulate wear debris, from cement, polyethylene, and metal, and the biological response of the host to these particles, have become a focus of intense investigation over the past few years.

Polyethylene has been an essential part of most artificial joints since their innovation. Wear has been held responsible for secondary loosening by allowing impingement of the femoral neck on the wall of the cup; and products of wear are believed to induce granulomatous reactions at the bone–implant interface (49).

Polyethylene also worked well in the tibial components of semiconstrained knee replacements designed in the 1970s. Insall et al. reviewed the 5- to 9-year results of the total condylar prosthesis and found no radiographic evidence of the metal component penetrating the polyethylene (47).

In most hip and knee designs, thick layers of polyethylene are used, the joint surfaces are nearly congruous, and these large areas of contact permit low load per unit area. In designs with incongruous articulation or a relatively thin layer of polyethylene, excessive wear may occur. The apparent sporadic nature of wear, compared with the many arthroplasties performed, argues against a fundamental defect in design. The occasional instance of excessive wear might be explained by a manufacturing imperfection, a technical error during implantation, or result from misuse of the prosthetic joint.

The more common area of the femoral portion of the total hip replacement results from loosening on the femoral side of the symmetric THR and, in this type of failure, the implant separates from the cement and the cement cracks, but there is no biologically derived change in the contact between the cement and the femur.

Polyethylene wear is a function of the thickness of the material and the size of the femoral head. Metal-backing and large head size reduce plastic thickness, leading to potentially greater wear. Increased clinical cup failures occur in cemented metal-backed components. In patients with small acetabuli, the femoral head selected should be smaller, to maximize plastic thickness. Newer extended-chain polyethylene is supposed to have greater resistance to wear, but no clinical data exist. Bioceramic femoral heads create less friction and, in theory, less plastic wear, but are two to three times the cost of metallic femoral heads.

Metallic wear of the femoral component can occur at the articulating surface or along the stem. Stem wear is generally associated with loosening, whereas articulating surface wear is not. Titanium alloy appears to have poorer wear characteristics as an articulating surface, and Co-Cr alloy is the preferred biomaterial for the femoral head. Porous-coated implants increase surface area of metal, but metal ion release and surface corrosion remain potential concerns.

Newer biomaterials, such as extended-chain polyethylene and ion impregnation of metallic surfaces, are being used to decrease wear at the articulation. Extensive efforts are being made to fabricate femoral components using more flexible nonmetallic biomaterials. Ceramic heads have led to a reduction in socket wear by a factor of almost four, but have not been generally used because of doubt and the cost.

Until now, wear in total knees has been addressed mainly by mobile bearing or sliding meniscus designs. Although they do offer reduced wear and deformation of the plastic, several factors limit their widespread application. If a fixed-bearing design, with moderate to high conformity, is used, wear is not a major problem in older patients. The inherent low stability of mobile bearing designs, requires adequate ligamentous and muscular stability, not always present in patients with advanced RA.

New is not necessarily better in total joint implants, since the long-term results cannot be documented without systematic study and tracking of patients with standardized techniques. The dangers and missed opportunities from not following patients with any implant, recently highlighted by the controversy around silicon breast implants, will, one hopes, stir action in this area.

In sum, much has been achieved since the first joint implant of Sir John Charnley. Experiences anchored in in vitro and clinical studies outline the agenda for the future. Advances in both our understanding of the basic biological events in RA and technical breakthroughs in sensitive, noninvasive, quantitative methods of assessing pannus may make synovectomy a promising technique for the total early aggressive management of RA. Failing that, total joint arthroplasty, with its ever-changing technology promises an effective backup. It, too, promises to improve but it is incumbent on the field to track its results over time to gain understanding of the factors that ensure the best results.

ACKNOWLEDGMENT

Dr. Stucki is a recipient of grants from the Swiss Science National Foundation, the Swiss Rheumatology and Physiatry Association, and the European League against Rheumatism. Supported in part by NIH Grants AR36308 and AR39921.

REFERENCES

1. Mueller W. Zur frage der operativen behandlung der arthritis deformans und des chronischen gelenkrheumatismus. Langenbecks Arch Klin Chir 1984; 47.
2. Fassbender HG. Structural basis of articular cartilage destruction in rheumatoid arthritis. Collagen Relat Res 1983; 3:141.
3. Gschwend N. Synovectomy. In: Kelley WN, Harris Ed Jr, Ruddy S, Sledge CB, eds. Textbook of rheumatology. Philadelphia: WB Saunders, 1989:1934–1961.
4. Gschwend N, Winer J, Böni A. Clinical results of synovectomy in rheumatoid arthritis. Darmstadt: D Steinkopff Verlag, 1977.
5. Arthritis and Rheumatism Council and British Orthopaedic Association. Controlled trial of synovectomy of knee and metacarpophalangeal joints in rheumatoid arthritis. Ann Rheum Dis 1976; 35:437.
6. McEwen C, O'Brian WB. A multicenter evaluation of early synovectomy in the treatment of rheumatoid arthritis. J Rheumatol 1974; 1(suppl):107.
7. Arthritis Foundation Committee on Evaluation of Synovectomy. Multicenter evaluation of synovectomy in the treatment of rheumatoid arthritis. Arthritis Rheum 1977; 20:765.
8. Thompson M, Douglas G, Davison EP. Evaluation of synovectomy in rheumatoid arthritis. Proc R Soc Med 1973; 66:197.
9. Brattstrom et al, Czurda et al, Gschwend et al, Hagena et al, Kinell et al, Hohler et al, Mori et al, Pavlov et al, Thabe et al. Long-term results of knee synovectomy in early cases of rheumatoid arthritis. Clin Rheumatol 1985; 4:19–22.
10. Von Reis G, Swensson A. Intraarticular injections of osmic acid in painful joint affections. Acta Med Scand [Suppl] 1951; 259:27–32.
11. Scherbel AL, Schuchter SL, Weyman SJ. Intra-articular administration of nitrogen mustard alone and combined with corticosteroid for rheumatoid arthritis. Cleve Clin Q 1957; 24:78–89.
12. Vainio K, Julkunen H. Intra-articular nitrogen mustard in treatment of rheumatoid arthritis. Acta Rheum Scand 1960; 6:25–30.
13. Tillmann K. Chemische synovektomie. Orthopäde 1973; 2:10.
14. Häfner R, Truckenbrodt H. Die synoviorthese mit varicocid in der Behandlung der juvenilen chronischen arthritis. Akt Rheumatol 1985; 10:202–205.
15. Niculescu D, Stancuilescu P, Negoescu M, et al. Chemische synovektomie durch Natriumsalze von Fettsäuren. Z Rheumaforsch 1970; 29:27–35.
16. Langkilde M, Rossel I. Intra-articular use of cytostatica. Acta Rheum Scand 1967; 13:92–100.
17. Chlud K, Kotz R, Zeitlhofer J. Die intraartikuläre zytostatikaawendung bei chronischer polyarthritis. Therapiewoche 1972; 22(35):2740.
18. Kerschbaumer F, Pfaller K, Siorpaes R. Neuere aspekte zur radiosynoviorthese des Kniegelenkes—klinische und experimentelle ergebnisse. Akt Rheumatol 1987; 12:143–146.
19. Stevenson AC. Chromosomal damage in human lymphocytes from radio-isotope therapy. Ann Rheum Dis 1973; 32(Suppl):19.
20. Delachapelle A, Oka M, Rekonen A, Ruotsi A. Chromosome damage after intraarticular injections of radioactive yttrium. Ann Rheum Dis 1972; 31:508.

21. Ansell BM, Crook A, Mallard JR, Bywaters EGL. Evaluation of intra-articular colloidal gold Au-198 in the treatment of persistent knee effusions. Ann Rheum Dis 1963; 22:435–439.

22. Delbarre F, Cayla J, Menkes CJ, Aignan M, Roucayrol JC, Ingrand J. La synovior thèse par les radioisotopes. Presse Med 1968; 76:1045.

23. Menkes CJ, Le Go A, Verrier P, Aignan M, Delbarre F. Double-blind study of erbium 169 injection in rheumatoid digital joints. Ann Rheum Dis 1977; 36:254–256.

24. Winston MA, Bluestone R, Cracchiolo A, Blahd WH. Radioisotope synovectomy with ^{32}P-chromic phosphate: kinetic studies. J Nucl Med 1973; 14:886.

25. Delbarre F, Menkes CJ, Aignan M, Roucayrol JC, Ingrand J, Sanchez A. Une nouvelle preparation radioactive pour la synoviorthese: le rhenium 186 colloidal. Advantages par rapport au colloide d'or 198. Nouv Presse Med 1973; 2:1372.

26. Sledge C, Zuckerman J, Zalutsky M, Atcher R, Shortkroff S, Lionberger D, Rose H, Hurson B, Lankenner P, Anderson R, Bloomer W. Treatment of rheumatoid synovitis of the knee with intra-articular injection of dysprosium 165-ferric hydroxide macroaggregates. Arthritis Rheum 1986; 29:153–159.

27. Williams PL, Crawley JCW, Freeman AM, Lloyd DC, Gumpel JM. Feasibility of outpatient management after intra-articular yttrium-90: comparison of two regimens. Br Med J 1981; 282:13–14.

28. Johnson LS, Yanch JC. Absorbed dose profiles for radio-nuclides of frequent use in radiation synovectomy. Arthritis Rheum 1991; 34:1521–1530.

29. Cleland LG, Treganza R, Dobson P. Arthroscopic synovectomy: a prospective study. J Rheumatol 1986; 13:907–910.

30. Stucki G, Bozzone P, Treuer E, Wassmer P, Felder M. Efficacy and safety of radiation synovectomy with yttrium-90. Br J Rheumatol 1993; 32:383–386.

31. Boussina I, Toussaint M, Ott H, et al. A double-blind study of erbium-169 synoviorthesis in rheumatoid digital joints. Scand J Rheumatol 1979; 8:71–74

32. Yates DB, Scott JT, Ramsay N. Double-blind trial of yttrium 90 for chronic inflammatory synovitis of the knee. Ann Rheum Dis 1977; 36:481.

33. Gumpel JM, Matthews SA, Fisher M. Synoviorthesis with erbium-169: a double-blind controlled comparison of erbium-169 with corticosteroid. Ann Rheum Dis 1979; 38:341–343.

34. Gumpel JM, Roles NC. A controlled trial of intra-articular radiocolloids versus surgical synovectomy in persistent synovitis. Lancet 1975; 1:488–489.

35. Nissila M, Anttila P, Hamalainen M, et al. Comparison of chemical radiation and surgical synovectomy for knee joint synovitis. Scand J Rheumatol 1978; 7:225–228.

36. Sheppeard H, Aldin A, Ward DJ. Osmic acid versus yttrium-90 in rheumatoid synovitis of the knee. Scand J Rheumatol 1981; 10:234–236.

37. Harris WH, Sledge CB. Total hip and total knee replacement (first of two parts). N Engl J Med 1990; 323:725–731; 801–807.

38. Herman JH, Sowder WG, Anderson D, Appel AM, Hopson CN. Polymethylmethacrylate induced release of bone-resorbing factors. J Bone Joint Surg 1989; 71A:1530–1541.

39. Murray DW, Rushton N. Mediators of bone resorption around implants. Clin Orthop 1992; 297:295–304.

40. Santavirta S, Konttinen YT, Hoikka V, Eskola A. Immunopathological response to loose cementless acetabular components. J Bone Joint Surg 1991; 73:38–43.

41. Schmarlzried TP, Kwong LM, Jasty M, Sedlacek RC, Haire TC, O'Connor DO, Bragdon CR, Kabo JM, Malcolm AJ, Harris WH. The mechanism of loosening of cemented acetabular components. Clin Orthop 1992; 274:60–78.

42. Goldring SR, Jasty M, Roelke MS, Rourke CM, Bringhurst FR, Harris WH. Formation of a synovial-like membrane at the bone–cement interface. Its role in bone resorption and implant loosening after total hip replacement. Arthritis Rheum 1986; 29:836–842.

43. Goldring SR, Wojno WC, Schiller AL, Scott RD. In patients with rheumatoid arthritis the tissue reaction associated with loosened total knee replacements exhibits features of a rheumatoid synovium. J Orthop Rheumatol 1988; 1:9–21.

44. Walker PS. Joint replacements in the 1990's. Br J Rheumatol 1991; 30:401–404.

45. Mehlhoff MA, Sledge CB. Comparison of cemented interface. Its role in bone resorption and implant loosening after total hip replacement. Arthritis Rheum 1986; 29:836–842.

46. Mulroy RD, Harris WH. The effect of improved cementing techniques on component loosening in total hip replacement. J Bone Joint Surg 1990; 72:757.

47. Rothman RH, Cohn JC. Cemented versus cementless total hip arthroplasty. Clin Orthop 1990; 254:153.

48. Black J. The future of polyethylene. J Bone Joint Surg 1978; 60B:303.

49. Insall JN, Hood RW, Flawn LB, Sullivan BJ. The total knee prosthesis in gonarthrosis: a five to nine year followup of the first 100 consecutive replacements. J Bone Joint Surg 1983; 65A:619–628.

21

Arthritis Patient Education
What We Know,
What Clinicians Can Do

Kate R. Lorig

Stanford University School of Medicine
Palo Alto, California

I. BACKGROUND

Physicians and patients agree that education is an important part of the arthritis treatment regimen. However, traditionally, arthritis patient education, while acknowledged by all as important, has had little systematic implementation. The purpose of this chapter is to (a) set a context for arthritis patient education, (b) give an overview of what is known about arthritis patient education, and (c) to present ideas on how physicians and other health professionals can facilitate quality patient education in an office setting.

Patient education is defined as a set of planned, educational activities designed to improve patients' decision making, health behaviors, and health status. There is nothing in this definition about improving knowledge. Changes in knowledge may be necessary before health behaviors or health status change. However, just because someone has correct knowledge does not mean that he or she will use that knowledge. If all we needed was knowledge, everyone with arthritis would exercise and be totally compliant with medication regimens. Thus, patient education is much more than knowledge change.

The purpose of arthritis patient education is to maintain or improve health, or to slow deterioration. The means by which this occurs are changes in behaviors or mental attitudes, or both. The desired outcomes of patient education are changes in health status, for example, pain, disability, fatigue, joint count, depression, or dependency such as changes in need for health care.

From the foregoing definition, it can be seen that the expectations for arthritis patient education are not very different than those for medical interventions, such as the use of medications or surgery. However, although the use of medications and surgery are well-accepted arthritis treatments, patient education is often relegated to being a "nice extra" or an "unproven treatment".

Twenty years ago arthritis patient education was unproven; this is no longer true. We have more than 100 published studies on the effectiveness of this treatment modality (1–3). Since all of these studies involve patients who are already receiving conventional therapies, the effects of patient education are in addition to those achieved by such therapy. A review of this literature follows later in this chapter. In short, what we know is that arthritis patient education, when properly executed, can increase helpful arthritis behaviors, reduce pain, depression, disability, and joint count, and in some cases reduce health care costs.

In the definition of patient education the word *planned* has a central place. Patient education does not just happen; it is not haphazard. Rather, it is a series of educational activities that are tailored to the needs of the individual patients. Such planned educational interventions can be given in any number of ways. They can be classes or groups, as is done with the Arthritis Self-Help Program (4). They can be a series of booklets and audio tapes, as are used in Bone Up on Arthritis (5). Patient education can also be delivered by means of a computer, as was done by the University of Connecticut program (6). It can also be part of a standard patient–physician interaction. In short, there are many ways to present patient education. In deciding the delivery method, one must look at the learner, resources, and desired outcomes.

With the foregoing brief overview, what follows are sections on what is generally believed about arthritis patient education, what is known about arthritis patient education, and finally what can be done about patient education in clinical practice.

II. WHAT IS GENERALLY BELIEVED ABOUT ARTHRITIS PATIENT EDUCATION

Most clinicians believe that (a) patient education can be beneficial and, at worst, is not harmful; (b) that changes in knowledge generally lead to changes in health behaviors; and (c) that the effects of patient education on health status, if such effects exist, are largely mediated by getting patients to comply with treatment regimens. Although each of these beliefs is partially true, there are some problems.

Patient education, as with every other medical treatment, has the potential for both benefit and harm. Of the more than 100 studies published on the effects of arthritis patient education, all but one suggest that patient education is effective. Let us now examine what is believed about the roles of increased knowledge and compliance.

Most patient teaching is centered around giving patients knowledge about their disease. Although knowledge is necessary before behavior change can occur, knowledge alone is usually insufficient to bring about such change. This is evidenced by the numbers of people who smoke, are overweight, or do not exercise regularly, although knowledge about the detrimental effects of these behaviors is nearly universal. For the purposes of this paper, what differentiates patient teaching from patient education is that the former is aimed at the transfer of knowledge, whereas the latter is aimed at changing health behaviors and affecting health status. Patient teaching gives patients information, whereas patient education gives patients the motivation, skills, and confidence to act on that knowledge. Thus, patient education consists of *content*, or the message to be delivered; and *process*, the means of helping patients to act on that message. More will be said about this later.

Finally, it is generally believed that the effects of health education on health status are the result of improved compliance with treatment regimens. To some extent this is true. Those patients who take their medications as prescribed or do their exercises regularly probably do better than those patients who are less compliant. However, recent evidence from a host of studies suggest that patient education can also have an independent effect on health status (7). For example, in an evaluation of the Arthritis Self-Management Program, subjects increased their frequency of taught behaviors, such as exercise and the practice of cognitive pain management techniques. At the same time their pain and depression were decreased. The expected associations between changes in behavior and changes in pain, however, were not found (8). Self-efficacy, or confidence in one's ability to control pain or depression, was also measured. Unlike changes in behaviors, changes in self-efficacy correlated with changes in health status. People who did the things they were taught were not necessarily those who had less pain and depression. In other words, the course affected health status through mechanisms other than changes in behavior.

From the foregoing examples it can be seen that many of the common beliefs about patient education are, at best, only partially true. These points will be expanded on later in this chapter. First, we will briefly review what is known about arthritis patient education.

III. WHAT IS KNOWN ABOUT ARTHRITIS PATIENT EDUCATION

More than 100 studies have now been published examining the effectiveness of arthritis patient education. These studies have been summarized in several reviews (1–3). One conclusion that can be drawn from the literature is that there are many effective ways of giving patient education. My work and that of others have emphasized group education (9–10). Studies by Goeppinger and her colleagues have emphasized home study, whereas those of Rippey have demonstrated the effectiveness of interactive computer education (5,6). Finally, Weinberger has demonstrated that monthly telephone calls to osteoarthritic patients reduces their pain (11). Although the modes of offering education are very different, all of these studies have demonstrated the effectiveness of arthritis patient education for changing behaviors or health status. Before reviewing these studies we should examine some ways in which arthritis patient education studies are similar to and different from other clinical studies.

There are several similarities. As in most clinical studies, participants are randomized into treatment and control groups. Of the 101 published arthritis patient education studies, 49 or nearly half were randomized trials. As in all clinical studies, participants are volunteers. This characteristic of study participants may differentiate them from the general population of persons with arthritis. However, this differentiation should be no more for participants in patient education studies than for participants in other clinical trials.

Patient education studies differ from most other clinical trials in two important ways. First, there is no washout period; that is, patients are not taken off all medications and other treatments before starting the patient education study. Patient education is tested as an addition to more traditional medical regimens. Therefore, most participants have already received the benefits of traditional therapies. Any changes demonstrated by patients receiving education are benefits above and beyond those received from these therapies. Second, it is impossible to "blind" a patient education study. Participants know that they are receiving education. To control for the placebo and Hawthorne effects, many studies have attention control groups. These are groups of subjects who receive education other than that being tested. The following is a summary of what we have learned about the effectiveness of arthritis patient education.

A. Knowledge

Of the 101 reported studies, 42 examined changes in patients' knowledge about arthritis. Increases in knowledge were found in 90% of these studies. More recent studies have largely dropped knowledge as a study variable.

B. Behaviors

Most recent studies have examined changes in one or more behaviors believed to affect the health status of people with arthritis. Exercise was examined in 25 studies. Of these 84% demonstrated positive changes. A similar pattern was shown for the practice of relaxation, stress management, or cognitive pain management techniques. These were examined in 17 studies, with 88% of these studies demonstrating positive changes. Sixteen studies examined the effects of patient education on compliance, with 81% of the studies demonstrating positive effects. From this brief synopsis it appears that patient education can have positive effects on the practice of behaviors believed to improve the health status of people with arthritis.

C. Health Status

If patient education is to be considered a necessary part of rheumatology treatment, it must demonstrate an effect on health status. A 1981 conference on Outcome Measures in Rheumatological Clinical Trials at McMasters University concluded that pain, disability, joint count, and depression were among the most important endpoints for clinical trials (12). When these important variables have been studied in patient education, changes have been demonstrated. Depression was decreased in two-thirds of the patient education studies that included this variable. Pain was an outcome variable in 43 studies and was decreased in 72% of these. Disability was included in 24 studies and was decreased in 63%, whereas joint count was included in 13 studies and was decreased in 77% of them. These findings suggest that patient education can affect the health status of arthritis patients.

Although there is little question that patient education can affect health status, questions persist about the magnitude of these effects. To examine this question we compared the effects from all the patient education studies between 1988 and 1991 with the effects of 101 drug trials published in the *Journal of Rheumatology* or in *Arthritis and Rheumatism* during these same years (Fig. 1)

Examination of Fig. 1 suggests that the magnitude of changes demonstrated in patient education studies was slightly less, but similar to, the magnitude of changes in drug trials. It should be remembered, however, that these effects of patient education studies occurred in addition to the effects of standard treatment.

Another conclusion that can be drawn from the literature is that the most powerful education has generally consisted of group interventions. Group education has several advantages over one-to-one education. First, it is usually cost-effective. More importantly, group participants act as motivators, social support, models, and problem-solvers for each other. These factors are very important in determining the effectiveness of patient education. More will be said about this later.

In conclusion, it appears that patient education has significant benefits when added to standard medical treatment. In addition, the most powerful forms of education generally occur in group settings.

From the foregoing discussions, it is clear that arthritis patient education can be effective in improving health behaviors and health status, and that these improvements are of sufficient magnitude to be clinically important. It is also

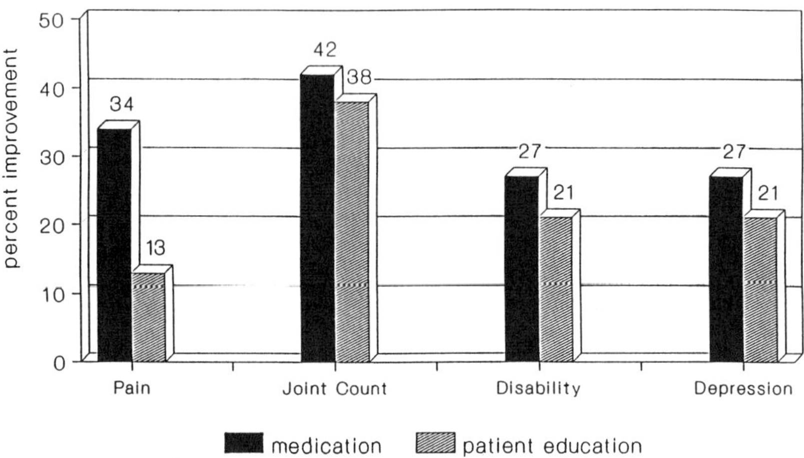

Fig. 1 Comparison of mean changes in health status: patient education and drug studies 1988–1991.

clear that patient education programs are not uniformly effective, and that there is a great deal of variability from one program to another. This raises the question of what accounts for effective arthritis patient education programs. Unfortunately, there are fewer studies on the causes of effects than on the effects themselves. One line of inquiry explored by me and others is that of self-efficacy (13,14). It has been demonstrated that changes in self-efficacy have greater association with changes in health status than do changes in behaviors.

IV. SELF-EFFICACY

Self-efficacy theory states that (a) the strength of belief in one's capability is a good predictor of motivation and behavior; (b) one's self-efficacy beliefs can be enhanced through performance mastery, modeling, reinterpretation of physiological symptoms, and social persuasion; and (c) enhanced self-efficacy leads to improved behavior, motivation, thinking patterns, and emotional well-being. Another way of thinking about self-efficacy it to equate it with confidence. The theory would then state that the more confident one is that he or she can accomplish something, the more likely the goal will actually be achieved.

In examining this definition, several parts need emphasis. First, self-efficacy is behavior-specific. That is, there is no such thing as an efficacious person. Rather, someone may have very high efficacy for walking outside on flat ground, but very low efficacy for being able to control arthritis pain without medication. In this way, self-efficacy differs from two related theories: learned helplessness and locus of control (15,16). Both of these theories refer to relatively enduring personality traits or attitudes, rather than to changeable states and specific behaviors.

Second, self-efficacy deals with perceptions of beliefs that one can accomplish some future behavior. In this way, it is predictive. Efficacy for future performance is a good predictor of actual future performance. Thus, a patient who reports that she is 90% certain that she will take her medications as prescribed is more likely to be compliant than a patient who reports that she is only 50% certain that she will take her medication as prescribed.

Finally, research has demonstrated that it is relatively easy to change self-efficacy, and that changes in self-efficacy are associated with changes in behavior and cognitive symptoms, such as pain and stress. Because of all these characteristics, self-efficacy theory is applicable to arthritis patient education. The following will examine the four specific efficacy-enhancing mechanisms and give examples of how they can be applied in arthritis patient education and clinical settings.

A. Skills Mastery

Probably the most powerful way of enhancing self-efficacy and achieving new behaviors is through skills mastery. This is generally done by breaking skills into small manageable tasks and then making sure that each task is successfully completed. Some of the original work with skills mastery was done with agoraphobics who first walked outside the door, then walked a few steps, then walked to the pavement, and so on. Another example is Alcoholics Anonymous, for which members promise not to drink today only. In achieving skills mastery, each commitment must be clear, relatively simple, and short-term. Thus, in getting arthritis patients to begin a walking program, the health professional should determine what the patient is doing now, or believes himself or herself capable of doing. If this is to walk two blocks, the suggestion to the patient should be that he or she walks two blocks, four times a week and then to increase it by about 20% or a half block each week. The key to skills mastery is mastery. If people are going to become more efficacious in an area, it is important that they are successful in what they are trying to do.

One of the best ways to accomplish mastery is to have patients contract for specific behaviors. It is important that contracting be mostly patient-driven; that is, the patient decides on the behavior. Equally important, there must be an opportunity to give and get feedback and make midcourse corrections. In a class setting, each session might end with a contracting session and each class begin with feedback on individual performance since the last class. Skills mastery is so important that up to 30% of class time may be used profitably in establishing contracts, discussing successes and problems, and providing modifications to behavior change programs.

If education is given in a clinical setting, it is important to set up ongoing feedback mechanisms. This can be done by noting the contract in the chart and asking about it on the next visit. A better mechanism would be to call the patient a week to 10 days after an office visit to receive feedback on the contract and to assist with any problems or misunderstandings that have arisen because of a new treatment.

Earlier we discussed how a patient's confidence can predict future behaviors or outcomes. This confidence or self-efficacy is easy to check, either in a class or clinical setting. Ask the patient, "given a scale of 0 to 10, with 0 being totally uncertain and 10 being totally certain, how certain are you that you will (repeat the patient's contract or directions for carrying out a treatment)?" If the answer is below 7, then the commitment should be reassessed, as there is a good chance the patient will not or cannot follow through. In this case, the next step is to ask the patient "what makes you uncertain? What problems do you foresee?" Then discuss the problems and seek possible solutions. Once the problem-solving is complete, have the client restate the contract or commitment and check it again using the 0–10 scale.

In addition to making short, specific commitments, there are two other activities that assist patients in integrating new activities into their lives. The first is to link any new activity with an ongoing habit. Thus, medications that are to be taken twice a day can be placed next to the toothbrush and taken when teeth are brushed in the morning and at night. Walking should take place at a specific time each day. For example, before reading the morning paper or before watching the evening news. Second, patients can be urged to keep a written record of the new activity. Thus, they can write on a calendar how far or how long they have walked each day or mark off each time they take their medication. If for some reason the activity was not completed, the calendar should contain a notation of why. For example, "visited my sister and forgot to take my medications." These notations can then be used to solve problems as they arise. They also serve as very powerful feedback. For someone who does not believe that she or he can walk at all, to find that she or he has walked 1½ hours during the past week reinforces the fact that walking is possible; it also serves as a motivation to walk even more in the coming week.

B. Modeling

Another excellent way of enhancing efficacy and changing behavior is to provide opportunities for people to see someone else with the same problem coping effectively with it. Modeling is the principle used in the Arthritis Foundation's Arthritis Self-Help Course; the course is taught largely by people with arthritis. It is also one of the reasons that support groups are popular and successful. In choosing models one should look for a person who is as much like the patient as possible. Thus, matching should be done by age, sex, ethnic origin, and socioeconomic status, whenever possible.

Unfortunately, the wrong types of models are often chosen. For want of better words, these are often ''superachievers'' or ''media images.'' The former are people who have had problems and have overcome them in some spectacular manner. An example would be the older woman with two hip replacements who, after hiking all day, chairs the local political party and does Scottish dancing too. The latter is the middle-aged athlete or film star who produces an arthritis exercise video. Although these people can be inspirational, they are not the best models. Their achievements are not relevant or do not seem realistic to most patients. A better model is someone who has a problem and is coping with it on a day-to-day basis. This is a ''coping'' model to whom patients can relate.

There are several ways to use coping models. We have already discussed the use of lay instructors in the Arthritis Self-Help Course. People with arthritis also can be brought into health education classes and arthritis talks to share experiences. In an office practice, newly diagnosed patients or those contemplating surgery can be put in touch with patients like themselves who have had the disease a few years or have had successful surgery. If this is done, it is best to get permission from both the potential ''model'' and the patient. If both agree, have the model call the patient.

Lastly, all patient education media should demonstrate appropriate modeling. Before anything is put on paper, tape, or film, it should be reviewed by a group of patients like the group to whom the media is aimed. This will prevent misunderstandings. There is no such thing as a media-based program that serves all people. However, pieces can be made ''more generic'' by using drawings and examples that include both sexes, varied ages, races, and body types. Unfortunately, many patient education media use models for their photogenic or charismatic qualities, rather than for their ability to act as role models.

C. Reinterpretation of Physiological Signs and Symptoms

For the most part, people who are not mentally or cognitively impaired act in a rational manner. At least, their actions are rational within their own belief system. However, health professionals see many actions that do not seem rational. The job of patient education is to determine why people believe as they do and then, when appropriate, change these beliefs. For example, one of the common arthritis symptoms is fatigue. Patients are usually told to rest or to balance work with rest. This advice is given by professionals and followed by patients based on the belief that the fatigue is caused by the disease and can be relieved by rest. However, the fatigue of arthritis can also be caused by things other than active disease. These include physical deconditioning, poor nutrition, depression, and poor quality sleep. Rest will not help any of these conditions. When patients are given a number of reasons for a symptom, they then have several alternative ways for managing that symptom. In the case of fatigue, rest may be an answer, but so might exercise, improved nutrition, and improved sleep. These latter solutions will never be considered if the patient does not first reinterpret or change his or her beliefs about the cause of fatigue. The rule of thumb is to help patients see that most arthritis symptoms have multiple causes; accordingly, there are many strategies that may be used to manage each symptom.

Another problem is that health professionals sometimes give mixed messages. For example, for years patients were told that osteoarthritis was a wear-and-tear disease. Is it then, little wonder that they were confused when told to exercise? The two statements appear to be in direct conflict.

Determining someone's beliefs about arthritis is not difficult. Questions that are helpful in soliciting beliefs are the following: (a) When you think of arthritis what do you think of? (b) If you start exercising or taking methotrexate what are you afraid might happen? (c) What do you think causes _____________? (d) What is preventing you from _____________? Once a belief has been identified it can be reinterpreted. For example, if a patient says she or he is afraid that taking methotrexate will cause cancer, then the health professional can focus the education on this concern. Here language is important. What is said may not be what is meant. In arthritis we often talk about "joint protection," which means using joints in an appropriate, nonstressful way. However, some patients interpret this as not using their joints. Avoiding jargon and keeping language simple serves everyone's best interests.

D. Persuasion

Persuasion has a long history as an educational technique. It can take many forms, from fear arousal, to social support. One form of persuasion that has been found useful is to urge patients to do slightly more than they are now doing. As with skills mastery, goals should be short-term and realistic. More importantly, they should not be much beyond what the patients believe they can now accomplish. Thus, instead of saying "you could lose 20 pounds if you tried," it would be better to say "you could lose 5 pounds this month." It has also been found that physicians' opinions are highly valued. Therefore, it is best to use a direct message such as "I want you to exercise for 10 min three times a week," rather than "Try to exercise more." Social support has also been shown to be a very important persuasive technique. Thus, for some behaviors, such as eating less and exercise, group programs may be more helpful than having patients try to change behaviors on their own. These groups do not have to be arthritis-specific. Most people with arthritis can participate in any gentle exercise class, and many can benefit from gentle nonimpact aerobic classes. These are often available through recreational departments, adult education, or senior centers. Social support can also be encouraged by urging patients to bring a family member with them to important appointments.

In summary, self-efficacy is a person's belief that he or she can perform some future behavior or use some cognitive strategy such as cognitive pain management. It can be enhanced by skills mastery, modeling, reinterpretation of physiological signs and symptoms, and persuasion. There is growing evidence that the enhancement of self-efficacy is at least one of the mechanisms by which arthritis patient education affects health status.

V. WHAT CAN BE DONE TO INTEGRATE PATIENT EDUCATION INTO CLINICAL PRACTICE?

Although most agree that patient education is an important aspect of good clinical care, it is seldom practiced in a scientific or systematic manner. There are at least three major reasons for this divergence between established standards and usual practice: First, health professionals believe that by giving people information about their condition they are giving good patient education. Second, patient education is seldom taught in medical school or in schools for other health professionals. Although it is generally considered important, it is also one of those skills that one is expected to learn through common sense and observation. Third, the system of daily office practice does not allow time for patient education. The general perception is that good patient education requires talking with patients for relatively long periods. An equally important consideration is that the time used for patient education is not reimbursable. Therefore, the system for scheduling patients, coupled with the lack of preparation and lack of monetary incentive, conspire against the systematic application of patient education. Although arguments can be made for changing the educational, delivery, and payment systems, none of these is controlled by the individual practitioner. Therefore, the focus of the following discussion will be on patient education techniques that can be integrated into practice as it exists today.

1.   One of the most important things a physician can do is to refer patients to established groups, such as those offered by the Arthritis Foundation (AF). These are among the most powerful forms of patient education programs. However, arthritis patient education groups are not limited to those of the Arthritis Foundation. For selected patients, such groups as Weight Watchers, senior citizens' walking clubs, or water aerobics may be very useful. It is not enough to mention these groups in a general way. Rather, be more direct by giving the patient the phone number and, if possible, a contact person. Sometimes preprinted patient education prescription pads are helpful for this purpose. These can be made inexpensively at most instant copy shops.

2.   Time is often lost during a clinical encounter because patients are not able to clearly communicate their problems or changes in their condition. More

time is lost because many patients come with more questions than can possibly be answered in the time allotted for the visit. Both of these problems can be partially solved by having the patient, while waiting for the doctor, write down (a) what they want from the visit, (b) what changes have occurred since the last visit, and (c) the two or three most important questions they want answered today. This information can then be handed to the physician allowing both the patient and physician to better focus the visit and use the available time.

3.   When giving the patient a medication or treatment regimen, ask how this will be carried out. Do not accept the answer ''I will take the pills three times a day.'' Rather, ask when during the day the patient will take the pills. This forces the patient to think about how the new treatment or medication will be integrated into their routine and helps to assure compliance.

4.   Always tell patients how long it will be until they can expect the medication to affect their symptoms. Many patients expect effects in 1 or 2 days. When these are not forthcoming, they stop taking the medication. Unmet expectations are a major cause of medication noncompliance.

5.   As discussed earlier, ask patients how certain they are that they will follow the new treatment, using a scale of 0, not at all certain, to 10, totally certain. Their confidence or self-efficacy for carrying out a treatment is a good predictor of future compliance.

6.   When a patient is hesitant about taking a medication, such as metho-trexate, ask ''what are you afraid might happen?'' or ''what is it about this drug that bothers you?'' Don't give reassurance until you clearly understand the problem.

7.   With a new patient do not try to teach everything at once; rather, be reassuring. ''You have rheumatoid arthritis. Most people with this disease do quite well. We will need to work together to find the best treatment for you.'' Next take some time to answer any specific questions the patient has and then schedule another appointment or time to talk on the phone with the patient in the next week or two. You might also suggest a book or two the patient would find helpful and give the patient the number of the Arthritis Foundation.

Although each first encounter will be different, five points should be re-membered: (a) Do not overwhelm the patient with information, (b) be reassuring, (c) give specific resources where the patient can find out more, (d) answer any immediate questions, (e) be sure that the patient has a specific time to recontact you in the near future.

8.   Be specific with advice. Do not say, ''I want you to exercise.'' This leaves too much room for misinterpretation. Rather, suggest a specific exercise regimen or work one out with the patient. You can also refer the patient to a specific exercise class.

9.   Put a bulletin board in your waiting room on which you post notices of Arthritis Foundation classes and other activities that your patients might find helpful. Assign one of your office staff to keep it current.

10.   When you see patients who are doing well with their disease, ask them if they would be willing to share their experiences with other patients. Keep a list or card file of these patients and when you see a similar patient who could use some help or support ask your "model" patient to call him or her.

11.   Plan a periodic "ask the doctor" session with your patients. Invite all your patients with RA or all your young patients with RA to an hour's meeting. Rather than give a lecture, ask them what they want to talk about. Make a list of the topics and then have the group vote on the three topics of most interest. Talk on these topics. Although this takes more than 60 seconds, it is a way of giving education to a larger group of people in a short time. It serves the additional purpose of helping patients believe that their physician is accessible.

12.   Avoid asking questions that can be answered "yes" or "no." Very often such questions are answered in a way the patient believes the physician would want. The downside of asking open-ended questions is that you may get more information than you want.

VI. SUMMARY

This chapter has attempted to examine four aspects of arthritis patient education; what we believe about arthritis patient education, what we know about arthritis patient education, an examination of one of the mechanisms by which patient education affects health status, and finally some ideas of how patient education can be integrated into clinical practice.

We now have ample evidence that patient education properly applied can be a powerful treatment for arthritis. Unfortunately, most patients are denied these benefits. It is up to physicians and other health professionals to ensure that patients receive the benefits from the full range of treatment options.

REFERENCES

1.   Lorig K, Konkol L, Gonzalez V. Arthritis patient education: a review of the literature. Patient Educ Counsel 1987; 10:207–252.
2.   Mullen PD, Laville E, Biddle AK, Lorig K. Efficacy of psycho-educational interventions on pain, depression, and disability with arthritis adults: a meta-analysis. J Rheumatol 1987; 14:33–39.
3.   Hirano P, Laurent D, Lorig K. Arthritis patient education studies, a review of the literature: 1987–1991, Patient Education and Counseling 1994 (in press).
4.   Lorig K, Lubeck D, Kraines RG, Seleznick M, Holman HR. Outcomes of self-help education for patients with arthritis. Arthritis Rheum 1985; 28:680–685.
5.   Goeppinger J, Arthur MW, Baglioni AJ, Brunk SE, Brunner CM. A reexamination of the effectiveness of self care education for persons with arthritis. Arthritis Rheum 1989; 32:706–716.
6.   Rippey RM, Bill D, Abels M, et al. Computer-based patient education for older persons with osteoarthritis. Arthritis Rheum 1987; 30:932–935.

7. Lorig K, Laurin J. Some notions about the assumptions underlying health education. Health Educ Q 1985; 12:231–243.

8. Lorig K, Seleznick M, Lubeck D, Ung E, Chastain R, Holman HR. The beneficial outcomes of the arthritis self-management course are inadequately explained by behavior change. Arthritis Rheum 1989; 32:91–95.

9. Lorig K, Gonzalez V. The integration of theory with practice: a 12 year case study. Health Educ Q 1992; 19:

10. Lorig K, Holman HR. Arthritis self-management study: a twelve year review. 1992. Health Educ Q 1993; 20:

11. Weinberger M, Tierney WM, Booker P, Katz B. Can the provision of information to patients with osteoarthritis improve functional status? Arthritis Rheum 1989; 23:1577–1583.

12. Decker J. Summary. J Rheumatol 1982; 9:802–806.

13. Bandura A. Self-efficacy: toward a unifying theory of behavior change. Psychol Rev 1977; 84:191–215.

14. Bandura A. Social foundations of thought and action. Englewood Cliffs, NJ: Prentice-Hall, 1986.

15. Seligman M. Helplessness: on depression, development, and death. San Francisco: WH Freeman, 1975.

16. Wallston BS, Wallston KA, Kaplan GD, Maides SA. Development and validation of the health locus of control (HLC) scale. J Consul Clin Psychol 1976; 44:580–585.

22

Data Collection and Utilization
A Methodology for Clinical Practice and Clinical Research

Frederick Wolfe

University of Kansas School of Medicine
Wichita, Kansas

I. DATA COLLECTION: PROMISES AND PROBLEMS

Among the important trends within rheumatology within the last two decades are three: (1) the development of the concept of the longitudinal database to monitor care and outcomes in rheumatology; (2) the development of self-report health status assessment questionnaires, by which outcomes could be assessed and measured; and (3) the emergence of inexpensive personal computers—the modern technology for storage, reporting, and analysis of longitudinal data. The promise of these technologies was that they could apply not only to the academic research center, but also to the clinic, where they might transform rheumatology so that clinicians could make use of the advances in health status questionnaires, and so that they might be able to perform and participate in clinical research (Table 1).

To a large extent, the promises inherent in Table 1 have not been delivered. Health status questionnaires (HSQ) are rarely used in the clinic. Longitudinal databases have not been implemented regularly, except in special circumstances, and computers have, for the most part, been confined to billing and word-processing purposes. Why this is so and whether it may be changed is a matter of interest and form the basis of this chapter.

A. Health Status Questionnaires

Health status questionnaires are instruments that measure items such as functional ability, pain, psychological distress, and such; in extended formats they capture

Table 1 Premises and Promises in Rheumatology: Longitudinal Data Banks, Health Status Questionnaires, and Computers

1. Development of health status assessment questionnaires (HSQ)
    A. Use in patient care for better understanding of patient status
    B. Use in research to better understand disease and outcomes
2. Development of the concept of chronic disease data banks
    A. Longitudinal record keeping for the clinician
    B. Performance of longitudinal research in chronic rheumatic disorders using clinical observations
    C. Performance of longitudinal research in the academic setting
3. Availability of inexpensive computers
    A. Management of patient records in rheumatic disease clinics
    B. Capacity to perform research in a rheumatology clinic setting
    C. Implementing and expediting research in the academic center

information concerning socialization, work ability, and other aspects of life that may be affected by rheumatic diseases. That HSQ are useful in research may be surmised from the fact they are routinely finding their way into drug trials and longitudinal outcome studies (1–3). Recently, the American College of Rheumatology proposed that a functional status instrument be made a part of all clinical trials (4).

But regardless of the setting, HSQ, when used, are almost invariably used *after the fact*. That is, they are used to evaluate, rather than predict, outcomes. In a sense, this seems paradoxical, since studies of HSQ that measure functional disability, pain, and psychological status indicate that they have strong predicative power and clinical value (5). They constitute the best predictors of mortality (5–9), future disability (10), work disability (11,12), psychological status (13), and even length of time on second-line therapies, such as methotrexate (14).

In addition, HSQ are rarely used in the clinic. If, as we believe, rheumatologists are especially good physicians as opposed to technicians, why would such techniques be put aside? We suspect that there are five possible reasons (Table 2). First, a certain amount of the information provided by HSQ can be obtained within the usual rheumatological examination without HSQ. Second, even if handed out in the clinic, HSQ cannot be scored by the clinician in a setting and time frame that is acceptable. Third, HSQ results are not clearly interpretable. Fourth, HSQ data have their most value when they can be compared with previous HSQ data (usually unavailable), and, finally, that the effort/benefit ratio is simply too high.

The Rheumatology Examination: Substituting for a
Health Status Questionnaire
What do rheumatologists do during their examinations of patients with rheumatoid arthritis? Surprisingly, there is little information on this point.

Table 2 Why Health Status Questionnaires (HSQ) Are Not Used In Clinics

1. A portion of the information provided by HSQ can be obtained within the usual rheumatological examination without HSQ.
2. As used in many clinics, data from HSQ are most often available after the physician–patient encounter is completed.
3. Even if handed out in the clinic, HSQ cannot be scored by the clinician in a setting and time frame that is acceptable.
4. HSQ results are not clearly interpretable.
5. HSQ data have their most value when they can be compared with previous HSQ data (usually unavailable).
6. The effort/benefit ratio is too high.

Kirwan and co-workers have shown that when rheumatologists are presented with ''paper patients'' they evaluate such patients differently than when seeing actual patients (15). That is, they say one thing, yet do something quite different. In the Kirwin et al. study, the physicians evaluated the real and paper patients with knowledge of aspirin consumption, erythrocyte sedimentation rate (ESR), erosions, hemoglobin, morning stiffness, patients global assessment, pain score, functional capacity, grip strength, and articular index. But it is almost certain that, in a real setting, physicians almost never have all of these measurements available. Anecdotally, most rheumatologists do not have the results of the ESR before they see patients. It is likely that few (15–25%) perform or record grip strength, pain scores, estimate morning stiffness, or *record* joint counts at the majority of clinical encounters.

It is likely, then, that the key feature of the rheumatologist's examination is the joint examination. As performed in the clinic the clinician gets an estimate of the patient's pain, pain tolerance, and pain threshold. Active and passive range of motion are glimpsed, as is functional ability. One sees the number and severity of tender and swollen joints, as well as the specific joints that are involved and their clinical significance. Aspects of psychological status and coping ability can also be derived from the examination. It seems apparent, then, that the essential aspects of the ordinary rheumatologist–patient encounter are unmeasurable and unrecordable by the physician. The joint count when recorded on paper (or a mannequin) is a poor substitute for what actually happens during the clinical encounter.

Although the foregoing discussion suggests that the course of the regular rheumatological examination yields much momentary detailed and useful information, it has important limitations. Functional disability cannot be quantified; nor is it routinely inquired about. Psychological status can be surmised, but not measured, and pain levels remain unknown to the ordinary rheumatological examination. What information is obtained is not quantifiable, may not be reliable, and cannot be communicated; therefore, it loses its value over time. From year to year the rheumatologist does not have an accurate picture of the patient's progression (or lack of it) or his or her response to therapy; and the physician–patient encounter yields no data useful for research. In contradistinction, HSQ can summarize important aspects of the key physician–patient encounter, since they measure satisfaction, pain, functional ability, and psychological status.

Although HSQs are potentially useful, Kazis et al. found that HSQ failed to influence physician behavior, patient satisfaction, and a number of other objective measures during a 1-year trial (16). Fifty-five percent of physicians found the HSQ "moderately useful . . . primarily in improving [the] doctor–patient relationship." In this study, the results of the HSQ were made available to the physician many days after the patient was seen in the clinic. We believe that *HSQ reports returned well after the patient has left, like ESR and radiographic data available later, are of marginal use to the clinician (although they may be of research use).*

An additional problem with an HSQ is the time required for administration and scoring. Certain instruments can have no place in the clinic. These include the standard version of the [AIMS; Arthritis Impact Measurement Scale AIMS I (17,18) or AIMS II (19) and Sickness Impact Profile; SIP (20)], since the time required for administration (15–30 min) is too long and unacceptable to patients and clinic staff. Simpler instruments such as the MHAQ (21), CLINHAQ (22), and shortened versions of the AIMS (23) have been advocated. They require less than 5 min to complete, but they must be scored by staff, some with calculators or computers. A final problem with HSQ is that the questionnaire results are not always meaningful or intuitive. Research studies may show difference in means that are "significant," but the clinician struggling with the problems of an individual patient, may find it difficult to interpret the results in his patient. Despite urgings (24), there are few users of these simpler instruments and essentially no users of the complex instruments.

In the Clinic, Where Should the Health Status Questionnaire Be Used?

There are two instances where HSQ and other clinical measures may be useful to the practicing rheumatologist. First, in evaluating the individual patient *at the time* of the clinical interview to understand the patient's status and to predict his or her outcome and, second, in performing clinical research. The two settings are somewhat different. In the former, the clinician needs to obtain more useful help and information than he or she gets by standard office techniques with no greater time investment. In the latter, the clinician wants to do clinical research, provided the expense and time commitment is not increased significantly. If structured correctly, both goals can be accomplished simultaneously. We have done both in our practice and propose to detail in the following a methodology of data collection that can be accomplished efficiently and with pleasure.

II. HOW AND WHY WE COLLECT DATA: THE STRUCTURE AND VALIDITY OF LONGITUDINAL RESEARCH AND PATIENT CARE DATABASES

Rheumatic disease data represent more than HSQ. In rheumatoid arthritis, it is common to collect additional data concerning joint examinations, laboratory information, drug therapy, and other. Which data are collected and how they are collected and stored is dependent on the underlying purpose of data collection. In the academic setting, the collection is for research; for the clinician, it is patient care. But, as we have suggested, the most useful data are those that are collected for both purposes simultaneously.

Four types of longitudinal observational databases can be recognized that overlap clinical care with clinical research (Tables 3 and 4).

The *clinical practice (type I)* database represents ordinary rheumatology practice. In this setting, multiple clinical observations and insights are obtained, HSQ may or may not be used, but data are usually not kept in a retrievable way and are generally not reported for research. More importantly, data collection is not standardized and is without an overall protocol. Data obtained may not be reliable or valid. Clinical practice is, in fact, a database, since it collects and retains data in a longitudinal fashion (e.g., in chart notes and flow sheets). Clinical practice is also related to research in many ways. Clinicians gather "clinical experience (i.e., come to conclusions based on observations)"; they use investigational therapy (nonapproved indications); and they conduct N-of-1 type trials (25).

The *clinical research (type II)* database evaluates patients at each clinic visit. In contradistinction to the clinical practice database, data are usually collected in standardized ways, using validated, reliable methods. There is generally an understood protocol, although it may be unwritten (26). The main difference between the clinical practice and the clinical research database is the method of data collection. It can easily be seen that clinical practice can become clinical research by the imposition of standardized, reliable, and valid methods of data collection. Clinic research databases are often incomplete, however, since they are confined to patients seen in the clinic, at the time they are seen in the clinic.

Table 3 Types of Longitudinal Databases and Research

I. *Clinical practice:* Patients are seen during ordinary rheumatology clinic visit; multiple observations are made, but often not recorded; HSQs are rarely used.

II. *Clinical research:* Patients are surveyed at every clinic visit by physical examination, interview, and or questionnaire.

III. *Nonclinic follow-up studies:* Patients are followed outside of clinic setting by questionnaire or interview at fixed interval, often 6–12 months.

IV. *Longitudinal clinical research:* Combined clinical practice and regular nonclinic follow-up studies (II + III).

Table 4 Characteristics of Observational Database Research

	Standardized observations/ protocols	Longitudinal follow-up	Complete data capture
I. Clinical practice	−	+	−
II. Clinical research	+	+	−
III. Nonclinic follow-up studies	+	+	−
IV. Longitudinal clinical research	+	+	+

Nonclinic follow-up studies (type III), reevaluate a cohort in a nonclinic setting. Usually the cohort is derived from those seen at sometime in the clinic. Follow-up can be sporadic or at fixed intervals (often 6–12 months). One advantage to this type of database is that events that occur between clinic visits, in the absence of clinic visits, and across time periods can be identified and quantified. Nonclinic follow-up studies, however, are often incomplete, since they are confined to patients who choose to participate in the follow-up evaluation process.

The *Longitudinal clinical research (type IV)*, is in many ways the best database. It combines the clinical research database with the nonclinic follow-up studies. This model allows the most complete data capture, since persons no longer followed in the clinic may be captured, whereas those followed only in the clinic can also be captured. This methodology, in rheumatology studies, is patterned on the Arthritis, Rheumatism, and Aging Medical Information System (ARAMIS) model (27).

A. Are Longitudinal Observational Data Bases Valid?

Observational studies run the gamut from convenience samples of patients in a clinic through the type IV longitudinal clinical research database described earlier (see Table 4). Clinical databases (type II) are potentially biased by overrepresentation of those with "active disease," who usually have many more clinic visits than those with lesser disease activity. Clinical databases tend to lose patients: those who die, but whose deaths are not known, those who are too ill to travel or to continue to attend the clinic, those who illness may not be responding and have sought care from another clinic, and sometimes those who have improved enough not to require care. Finally, when the time between observations (clinic visits) is long, important events may occur between visits that are lost to the research process. The overrepresentation problem can be overcome at the analysis stage of the research process, and some events occurring between visits can be recovered, but patients lost to the clinic represent an important bias in the type II clinical research.

Nonclinic follow-up studies (type III), particularly when they represent regular follow-up (e.g., 6 month intervals), allow capture of all events between assessments. The evaluations, often carried out by mailed questionnaires or telephone interviews, can be quite detailed; and those with active as well as inactive disease are captured equally well. The main problem with type III databases is that important subsets of patients tend to be underrepresented: The elderly, less educated, poorer, sicker, more psychologically disturbed, and those who are young males. That such biases are important is underscored by the study of RA mortality conducted by the epidemiologist, Erik Allander, where responders (participants) with RA had *less* subsequent mortality than the population at large (28). Allander observed that "The oft-written comment, found in reports, that the 'non-response group did not significantly differ from the rest of the population' is probably nearly always wrong" (28). When rheumatology studies document nonresponders, they almost always differ in important ways from the group being studied, although perhaps not as dramatically as in the Allander mortality study.

The type IV databases, by capturing all patients, come as close as possible to the valid research sample. For the clinician or the researcher with limited funding, the type IV database, requiring contact outside of ordinary clinic activities, can present problems. Regular surveillance by questionnaire (type III) requires personnel and increases study cost. If the number of patients being followed is small, or if only a single disorder is to be assessed, then the additional cost may be small. Clinicians can move from type II to type IV data collection well after the databank is begun, so that insufficient current resources are not restraining.

A second important problem with observational databases is the potential for biased ascertainment. Since observational studies lack blinding, an investigator or clinician might tend to find what he or she expects. For example, if belief in the efficacy of a drug is strong, results of patients using that drug might be better than it actually is. In good clinical and research practice, however, biased ascertainment is a minimal problem, since almost all important data can and should be collected directly from the patient by HSQ and by nonphysician staff members (e.g., grip strength, stiffness, or other) before the patient interview and joint examination. When performed this way, biased ascertainment, except perhaps for the joint examination, is rarely a problem.

A third potential problem with observational studies is that they may lack generalizability when they come from a single clinic. This can be particularly true when treatment decisions are involved. For example, certain clinics might treat patients with early RA with methotrexate (MTX), whereas other clinics might delay the use of the agent for several years. The efficacy of MTX might appear different in the two clinical settings. To overcome such a problem, clinics might choose to pool data. But observational studies have other ways to approach such problems. Because observational studies tend to be large, and because they include many covariates, it is possible to understand and to adjust for factors such as disease duration.

B. Observational Studies Versus Randomized Clinical Trials.

Table 5 describes differences between these two types of studies. The most important features of randomized clinical trials (RCT)—the use of randomization and of control groups—of critical importance in understanding short-term drug efficacy, hampers understanding in assessing long-term outcome in chronic illnesses: it is rarely possible to use controls, particularly placebo controls, beyond a short duration of follow-up (29); and the extrapolation of short-term efficacy of second-line antirheumatic therapy to long-term outcome has led to erroneous conclusions concerning RA (see Introduction Chapter). In addition, although randomization controls for patient differences, it is exactly these covariate differences that are so important in chronic illness. There are several other problems with RCT, including selection and spectrum bias. Most RA patients, for example, are not eligible to participate in RCT because of concomitant therapy, previous therapy, or illness that is too mild or too severe (30,31). Although observational studies lack natural controls groups—limiting short-term comparisons—comparisons between drugs over longer periods are possible and add information concerning efficacy that is not available in RCT. In fact, most of what we know about RA, its treatment, and outcome, has come from observational studies, rather than from RCT (31,32).

Table 5 Observational Studies vs Randomized Clinical Trials

Characteristic	Randomized clinical trials	Observational studies
Focus	Drug	Patient
Duration	Short-term	Long-term
Measures pertinent outcomes	Related to drug	Related to patient (and drug)
Selection bias	Often: most RA patients are ineligible for RCTs	No exclusions
Spectrum bias	Often: patients selected by "activity" criteria	No exclusions
Ascertainment bias	Rare (controlled for by placebo treatment)	Possible for investigator-determined items
Generalizability	Fair–good	Good
Comorbidities	Excluded	Included
Medications	Excluded	Included
Outcomes	Emphasis on pain, swollen-tender joints, ESR, physician and patient "global."	Functional capacity, psychological status, work disability, death, etc; includes joint and laboratory data

C. What Should Be the Content of a Rheumatoid Arthritis Database?

The extent of data collection is largely an individual matter, reflecting the interest and resources of the clinic. Fries has suggested that outcome in rheumatic disease is encompassed by the five Ds: death, disability, discomfort, dollar costs, and drug- or doctor-related adverse reactions (27). Subsumed in this rubric are additional issues such as work disability, psychological issues, and other measures of quality of life. Additionally, clinicians may want to collect specific data about clinical, laboratory, and radiographic abnormalities and outcomes. Table 6 lists a computer database for rheumatic disease (CDRD), based on the ARION-CLINHAQ computer-based system, but supportive of all HSQ. The database version presented here has been shortened to deal primarily with rheumatoid and other forms of inflammatory arthritis. In practice, additional sections, dealing in detail with systemic lupus erythematosus, back pain, and so on, are included. The sections (*Tables*) of the database correspond to convenient data collection, organization, and entry break points. The *Measurements* section, for example, includes all of those "measurements" that are not self-report and that may be done by the physician or staff. Self-report data are listed in the *Questionnaires* section, and joint data in the *Joint module*. The *Fixed demographics* table is used to capture demographic data that are unchanging, whereas the other tables capture data that may change from visit to visit.

The minimal database of Table 6 is simple to collect, largely based on HSQ, and excludes laboratory data. It can be collected in a clinic, with essentially no extra cost to the clinician and researcher. At the moderate level, significantly more information is collected, but at a substantial increase in time and cost, since detailed assessments of demographic, sociodemographic, symptom review, adverse drug reaction, and surgical data require specific efforts to acquire. In this level radiographic and laboratory assessments are scored simply. Many database items will always remain optional. For example, it is not meant that one should collect the Shober test data when such collection would have no relevance. Similarly, the user will usually choose one of the HSQ or HSQ components listed. At the most complex level, extensive, detailed, time-consuming data about all aspects of RA are added. At a minimum, a complete research database should include most of those items labeled moderate.

Table 7 outlines the time and expense involved in data acquisition in the clinic. The cost of data collection, scoring, and entry in the rheumatic disease clinic depends on several factors. Physician-dependent data are always expensive, since physician time is expensive. Physician data (e.g., joint counts and clinical assessments) are also least reliable and most susceptible to bias. Similarly, data that require the hiring of additional people are expensive. The least expensive data, and the most cost-effective data are obtained from the patient directly by means of questionnaires. In the end, beyond the decision to collect

Table 6   A Computer Database for Rheumatic Disease

Table	Minimal	Moderate	Extensive
Fixed demographics	1. Name 2. Date of birth 3. Sex 4. Symptom date 5. Education 6. Ethnic origin	1. Past surgical Hx 2. Mortality data	1. Cause of death 2. Death certificate data
Sociodemographic	1. Marital status	1. Occupation 2. Surgical history 3. Medical history 4. Work disability 5. Employment status	1. Pt. occupation code 2. Spouse occupation 3. Spouse occupation code 4. Income 5. Smoking Hx 6. Alcohol Hx 7. Disability payments 8. Comorbicity importance 9. Hospitalizations 10. Allergies 11. Living arrangements
Symptom review		1. General 2. Skin 3. HEENT 4. Cardiopulmonary 5. GI 6. GU 7. Hematological 8. Neuromuscular	
Physical examination		1. Skin 2. HEENT 3. Chest 4. Heart 5. Abdomen 6. Genitalia 7. Neuromuscular	
Measurements		1. Height, weight 2. Blood pressure 3. Grip strength 4. AM stiffness	1. Other vital signs 2. Pain location

Table 6 (*continued*)

Table	Minimal	Moderate	Extensive
		5. Sleep disturbance 6. Shober tests 7. Chest expansion 8. Occiput to wall	
Questionnaire data	1. CLINHAQ, HAQ or MHAQ 2. Rh. attitudes index 3. VAS pain 4. VAS global severity 5. VAS fatigue 6. VAS GI scale 7. VAS sleep 8. Health status 9. Health satisfaction 10. Work ability 11. AIMS anxiety 12. AIMS depression		1. Other functional instruments 2. Other psychological scales
Joint module	1. Simple joint count 2. Joint swelling	1. Simple joint count or score 2. Simple joint swelling count or score 3. Nodules 4. Nodes 5. Tophi	1. Complex joint count or score 2. Complex joint swelling count or score 3. Joint deformity assessments 4. Epicondylitis 5. Tenosynovitis 6. Straight-leg test 7. Back spasm 8. Shober test 9. Dactylitis 10. Dupuytren's 11. Synovial cyst 12. Bursitis

Table 6 (*continued*)

Table	Minimal	Moderate	Extensive
Radiology data			
		1. Simple assessments of joint space narrowing	1. Complex scoring
		2. Simple assessments of erosions	2. Bone mineral assessments
		3. Simple assessments of degenerative changes	3. CT scan and MRI data
		4. Chondrocalcinosis	
		5. Axial skeletal assessments	
		6. Chest assessments	
Laboratory data			
		1. Simple tests (e.g., CBC, platelets, UA, ESR, RF, FANA)	1. Complex or less frequently performed chemistries
			2. Complex or less frequently performed immunological tests
Treatment data	1. Current therapy		1. Interim therapies
	2. Intra-articular and periarticular injections		2. Trigger point injections
ADR data		1. ADR (brief)	1. ADR (detailed)
RD surgery module		1. Surgery	
Diagnosis and status	1. Diagnosis	1. Non-RD diagnosis	
	2. Pt status in data bank		

Table 7 Time and Expense Estimates of Rheumatic Disease
Data Collection Items

Item	Source[a]	Clinic time/expense
Demographics	Pt-Staff	$+/++$
Symptom data	Pt-Staff	$+$
Functional questionnaire	Pt	$+$
Psychological questionnaire	Pt	$+$
Pain	Pt	$-/+$
Physical examination (e.g., joints)	Staff	$+/++$
Radiograph	MD	$+++$
Laboratory	Staff	$+$
Work disability	Pt-Staff	$++$
Drug use (clinic)	Pt-Staff	$++$
Drug use (complete)	Pt-Staff	$++++$
Rheumatic disease surgery	Pt-Staff	$+++$
Costs/services	Pt-Staff	$++++$
Adverse reactions	Pt-Staff	$++++$
Mortality	Staff	$++++$

[a]Staff refers to physician, nurse, or others who collect data.

data for research and patient, the single most important issue is the time cost and
expense of data collection (see later).

III. PRACTICAL DATA COLLECTION: THE ARION–CLINHAQ AND MHAQ SYSTEMS

For data collection to be successful, it has to be an integral component of ordinary
patient care (Table 8). If the clinic or the physician has to interrupt ordinary care
activities to perform special data collection tasks, then the data collection activities will generally fail. Similarly, if the collection requires extra staff time or
interferes with normal clinic operation, it will become burdensome and is likely
to be resisted or abandoned. To overcome these problems we describe a system
that integrates data collection with clinic care. ARION (*arthritis research information office network*) is a computer system for clinical record-keeping and
rheumatology research in outpatient clinics. The original computer code was
written by the author (FW), and the content of the system was developed by the
author beginning in 1974, modeled on the ARAMIS time-oriented data bank
system (TOD) and the Uniform Data Base for Rheumatic Disease (27). Subse-

Table 8   Rules for Data Collection in the Clinic

1. Data collection must be a component of clinical care, not in addition to it.
2. Collect as much data as possible by patient self-report questionnaires.
3. Make the data collection instrument *the* clinical record.
4. Data collection and computerization must be integrated.
5. Clinic staff, rather than the physician, should be responsible for data collection as part of their ordinary patient care activities.

quent modifications and improvements followed suggestions by Theodore Pincus. The current computer version of ARION was additionally supported by the ACR Committee on Health Care Research (COHCR). It is available to clinicians and investigators at a nominal fee (cost of materials) on request to the author.

Underlying the ARION system is the belief that data acquisition and analysis must be integrated with methods of collection and reporting if efficiency, low cost, and usefulness are to be maintained. As a measure of its success, I have recorded more than 10,000 patients and 60,000 clinic visits as part of my own clinical practice. The MHAQ system, developed by Pincus (21) uses similar questionnaire methodology to record data on flow sheets kept with the patient's record. One advantage of the of MHAQ system is that it can be implemented easily, and does not require immediate access to a computer. Forms for data collection and recording using the MHAQ system are included in Appendix B.

There are several differences and many similarities between the ARION and MHAQ systems. ARION requires the use of a computer, uses the computer for reporting and summarizing the patient's course, can accept large volumes of data for entry, can be used simultaneously by multiple persons on a network, can extract data to statistical subsetting and analysis programs (e.g., MEDLOG, SAS, BMDP, SPSS), and can perform some analyses itself. Both systems are similar in that they use HSQ. The CLINHAQ (22) questionnaires used by ARION are similar to the MHAQ questionnaires (21). Both systems use questionnaires distributed to patients in the clinic, both rely on flow sheets, and both use data collected for the purposes of patient care at the time of the patient–physician interview. Although what follows is mostly about the ARION–CLINHAQ system, both the MHAQ and the ARION–CLINHAQ questionnaires are presented in the chapter appendices.

A key feature of ARION is the production of a computer-generated report following every clinic visit (Fig. 1). The report has two key features. First, it becomes the major part of the clinical record, supplanting the usual record and eliminating most additional records. Updated versions of the printout (updated at each clinic encounter) are always kept in the patient's chart. Second, the report serves as the input document for the next clinic visit. Physicians and other clinic staff record the ordinary patient care observations directly on to the computer

ARION: THE DATABASE FOR RHEUMATIC DISEASE

Churchmouse, Peter	DOB	2/26/34	Marital Married
32 Library Rd	Sex	Male	Current Occ. Tooling Foreman
Wichita, KS 67209	Ethnicity	Caucasian	Lifetime Occ.Tooling Foreman
316-555-0001	Educational Level	12	Disability Payments None

Patkey   3765

Referring MD: J. Doolittle

First Symptom		1/01/81
First Visit No.	1	5/04/82
Last Visit No.	44	9/25/92

HEALTH STATUS	Min	Max	Current	Date	ANTI-RHEUMATIC THERAPY Agent	From	Thru	Current
Height	70.0	70.5		May 82 (First)	Gold (Cum)			
Weight	130	146	135	Dec 85 (Max)	Auranofin	Jan 87	Dec 88	
B. P.	84/50	130/86	114/64	Dec 85 (Max)	Plaquenil			
Joint Count	2	5	2	May 92 (Max)	Penicillamine			
T. P. Count	0	0	0	Sep 92 (Max)	Methotrexate	Sep 89	Dec 90	
Grip	96/86	220/188	178/188	Jan 87 (Min)	Sulfasalazine	Apr 91	Sep 92	2000
A M Stiff	0.0	24.0	0.0	Sep 86 (Max)	Azathioprine			
HAQ Score	.6	2.2	1.2	Dec 90 (Max)	Prednisone	Mar 91	Sep 92	5
Pain Scale	1.1	2.3	1.3	Dec 90 (Max)	Flurbiprofen			
Global	20	70	41	Dec 90 (Max)	Etodolac			
Anxiety	0.0	3.9	1.3	Sep 88 (Max)	Sulindac	<May 82	May 82	
Depression	0.0	2.3	2.0	Sep 88 (Max)	Piroxicam	Aug 84	Dec 85	
					Indomethacin			
LABORATORY DATA					Meclofenamate			
					Ibuprofen	<May 82	<May 82	
RF (Titer)	0	160		Dec 83 (Max)	Fenoprofen			
ANA (Titer)	0	20		Sep 86 (Max)	Naproxen	Jan 86	Jul 88	
ESR (Mm/hr)	10	100	15	Sep 86 (Max)	Ketoprofen			
HgB (Gm/dl)	10.0	13.1	13.1	Jul 88 (Min)	Tolemetin			
WBC (x1000)	4.7	12.1	6.2	Jun 86 (Min)	ASA	Dec 83	Dec 83	
					Salsalate			
					Diclofenac	Sep 88	Sep 92	150
RADIOGRAPHS (R/L)					Nabumetone			

RADIOGRAPHS (R/L)				CURRENT RHEUMATOLOGIC DIAGNOSES
Hand DJD	(0-3)	0 / 0	Sep 92 (Last)	
Hand Narrowing	(0-3)	3 / 3	Sep 92 (Last)	RA
Hand Erosions	(0-3)	3 / 3	Sep 92 (Last)	
Hip Narrowing	(0-3)	3 / 1	Sep 92 (Last)	
Knee Narrowing	(0-3)	3 / 1	Sep 92 (Last)	

COMORBID CONDITIONS			JOINT SURGERY
Hypertension	Myo. Infarct	Other C.V.	
Stroke	Mental Illness	Diabetes	
Cancer	Alcohol/Drug	Kidney	
Lung	Asthma	Sev.Allergy	
Liver/G.B. 6/15/82	Ulcer/G.I. 6/15/75	Neurological	
Fractures	Thyroid	G.U.	

Visit #	36	37	38	39	40	41	42	43	44
Date	17-Dec-90	25-Mar-91	24-Apr-91	30-May-91	18-Jul-91	8-Oct-91	9-Jan-92	13-May-92	25-Sep-92

Fig. 1   ARION: the database for rheumatic disease. The first page contains summary data for important clinical variables, comorbidities, joint surgery, and demographics. Subsequent pages constitute the detailed computerized flow sheet for each individual patient. The last (unused) column on the right is used to enter data for the current patient visit.

VISIT	35	36	37	38	39	40	41	42	43	44		
DATE	Nov5	Dec17	Mar25	Apr24	May30	Jul18	Oct8	Jan9	May13	Sep25		
YEAR	1990	1990	1991	1991	1991	1991	1991	1992	1992	1992		

SELECTED SYMPTOM REVIEW

GENERAL												
Fatigue	1	1	0	0	0	0	0	0	0	0	[ ]	Fatigue
Fever	1	0	0	0	0	0	0	0	0	0	[ ]	Fever
Chills	0	0	0	0	0	0	0	0	0	0	[ ]	Chills
Weight Loss	0	0	0	0	0	0	0	0	0	1	[ ]	Weight_Los
SKIN												
Malar Rash	0	0	0	0	0	0	0	0	0	0	[ ]	Malar_Rash
Psoriasis	0	0	0	0	0	0	0	0	0	0	[ ]	Psoriasis
Digital Ulce	0	0	0	0	0	0	0	0	0	0	[ ]	Digital_Ul
Skin Ulcer	0	0	0	0	0	0	0	0	0	0	[ ]	Skin_Ulcer
Rash	0	0	0	0	0	0	0	0	0	0	[ ]	Rash
Purpura	0	0	0	0	0	0	0	0	0	0	[ ]	Purpura
Alopecia	0	0	0	0	0	0	0	0	0	0	[ ]	Alopecia
Raynauds	0	0	0	0	0	0	0	0	0	0	[ ]	Raynauds
Tight Skin	0	0	0	0	0	0	0	0	0	0	[ ]	Tight_Skin
Urticaria	0	0	0	0	0	0	0	0	0	0	[ ]	Urticaria
Pruritis	0	0	0	0	0	0	0	0	0	0	[ ]	Pruritis
Photosensiti	0	0	0	0	0	0	0	0	0	0	[ ]	Photosensi

HEENT

	1	2	3	4	5	6	7	8	9	10			
Head Pain	0	0	0	0	0	0	0	0	0	0	[	]	Head_Pain
Xeropathy	1	1	1	1	1	1	1	1	1	1	[	]	Xeropathy
Conjunctivit	0	0	0	0	0	0	0	0	0	0	[	]	Conjunctiv
Uveitis	0	0	0	0	0	0	0	0	0	0	[	]	Uveitis
Tinnitus	0	0	0	0	0	0	0	0	0	0	[	]	Tinnitus
Mouth Ulcer	0	0	0	0	0	0	0	0	0	0	[	]	Mouth_Ulce
Dry Mouth	0	0	0	0	0	0	0	0	0	0	[	]	Dry_Mouth
Parotid	0	0	0	0	0	0	0	0	0	0	[	]	Parotid
Taste	0	0	0	0	0	0	0	0	0	0	[	]	Taste
Cold URI	0	0	0	0	0	0	0	0	0	0	[	]	Cold_URI
Sore Throat	0	0	0	0	0	0	0	0	0	0	[	]	Sore_Throa

CARDIO PULMONARY

	1	2	3	4	5	6	7	8	9	10			
Pleurisy	0	0	0	0	0	0	0	0	0	0	[	]	Pleurisy
Angina	0	0	0	0	0	0	0	0	0	0	[	]	Angina
Dyspnea	0	0	0	0	0	0	0	0	0	0	[	]	Dyspnea
Pedal Edema	0	0	0	0	0	0	0	0	0	0	[	]	Pedal_Edem
Cough	0	0	0	0	0	0	0	0	0	0	[	]	Cough
Asthma	0	0	0	0	0	0	0	0	0	0	[	]	Asthma
Hemoptysis	0	0	0	0	0	0	0	0	0	0	[	]	Hemoptysis

GASTROINTESTINAL

	1	2	3	4	5	6	7	8	9	10			
Anorexia	0	0	0	0	0	0	0	0	0	0	[	]	Anorexia
Dysphagia	0	0	0	0	0	0	0	0	0	0	[	]	Dysphagia
Peptic Ulcer	0	0	0	0	0	1	0	0	0	0	[	]	Peptic_Ulc
Abdomin Pain	0	0	0	0	0	0	0	0	0	0	[	]	Abdomin_Pa
Vomiting	0	0	0	0	0	0	0	0	0	0	[	]	Vomiting
Hematemis	0	0	0	0	0	0	0	0	0	0	[	]	Hematemis
Pyrosis	0	0	0	0	1	1	0	0	0	0	[	]	Pyrosis
Diarrhea	0	0	0	0	0	0	0	0	0	0	[	]	Diarrhea
IBS									0	0	[	]	IBS

Fig. 1 Continued

VISIT	35	36	37	38	39	40	41	42	43	44			
DATE	Nov5	Dec17	Mar25	Apr24	May30	Jul18	Oct8	Jan9	May13	Sep25			
YEAR	1990	1990	1991	1991	1991	1991	1991	1992	1992	1992			
Constipation							1	0	1	1	[	]	Constipati
GENITO-URINARY													
Dysuria	0	0	0	0	0	0	0	0	0	0	[	]	Dysuria
Nocturia									0	0	[	]	Nocturia
Urethral Dis	0	0	0	0	0	0	0	0	0	0	[	]	Urethral_D
Stone	0	0	0	0	0	0	0	0	0	0	[	]	Stone
Men Abnor	0	0	0	0	0	0	0	0	0	0	[	]	Men_Abnor
Hematuria	0	0	0	0	0	0	0	0	0	0	[	]	Hematuria
Proteinuria	0	0	0	0	0	0	0	0	0	0	[	]	Proteinuri
NEURO-MUSCULAR													
Convulsions	0	0	0	0	0	0	0	0	0	0	[	]	Convulsion
Muscle Pain	0	0	0	0	0	0	0	0	0	0	[	]	Muscle_Pai
Muscle Weakn	0	0	0	0	0	0	0	0	0	0	[	]	Muscle_Wea
Memory Loss	0	0	0	0	0	0	0	0	0	0	[	]	Memory_Los
Affect Abn	0	0	0	0	0	0	0	0	0	0	[	]	Affect_Abn
Paresthesias	0	0	0	0	0	0	0	0	0	1	[	]	Paresthesi
Carp Tunnel	0	0	0	0	0	0	0	0	0	0	[	]	Carp_Tunne

CLINIC MEASUREMENTS

	35	36	37	38	39	40	41	42	43	44			
Weight	132	134	133	133	134	131	138	136	138	135	[	]	Weight
BP Systolic	94	84	100	114	120	88	90	104	104	114	[	]	BP_Systoli
BP Diastolic	60	66	68	74	80	60	64	64	66	64	[	]	BP_Diastol
Pulse	68	76	76	76	72	64	72	68	68	76	[	]	Pulse

ARTICULAR HX — PAIN

Neck Pain	1	1	0	0	0	0	0	0	0	0	[	]	Neck_Pain
Ch Wall Pain	0	0	0	0	0	0	0	0	0	0	[	]	Ch_Wall_Pa
Thorac Pain	0	0	0	0	0	0	0	0	0	0	[	]	Thorac_Pai
Back Pain	0	0	0	0	0	0	0	0	0	0	[	]	Back_Pain
Joint Pain	1	1	1	1	1	1	1	1	1	1	[	]	Joint_Pain
Heel Pain	0	0	0	0	0	0	0	0	0	0	[	]	Heel_Pain
Gen Pain	1	1	1	0	0	0	0	0	0	0	[	]	Gen_Pain
Night Pain	1	0	1	0	0	0	1	0	0	0	[	]	Night_Pain
Jaw Pain	0	0	0	0	0	0	0	0	0	0	[	]	Jaw_Pain

FUNCTIONAL MEASURES

Sleep Distur	0	0	0	0	0	0	0	0	0	0	[	]	Sleep_Dist
AM Stiffness	0	0	0	0	0	0	.2	0	0	0	[	]	AM_Stiffne
Grip R	118	104	98	144	166	168	160	160	194	178	[	]	Grip_R
Grip L	114	104	88	138	138	156	140	164	154	188	[	]	Grip_L

FUNCTIONAL DATA — QUESTIONNAIRES

Pain Scale	1.8	2.3	1.9	1.3	1.4	1.4	1.3	1.1	1.2	1.3	[	]	Pain_Scale
Patient Pain	1	1	1	1	1	1	1	1			[	]	Patient_Pa
Dressing	2	2	1	1	1	1	1	1	1	1	[	]	Dressing
Arising	2	2	2	1	1	1	1	1	1	1	[	]	Arising
Eating	2	2	2	1	1	1	1	2	1	1	[	]	Eating
Walking	2	2	2	1	1	1	1	1	1	1	[	]	Walking
Hygiene	3	3	3	1	2	2	2	2	2	2	[	]	Hygiene
Reach	2	3	2	1	1	2	2	2	2	1	[	]	Reach
Grip	2	2	2	1	1	1	2	1	2	2	[	]	Grip

Fig. 1 Continued

VISIT	35	36	37	38	39	40	41	42	43	44			
DATE	Nov5	Dec17	Mar25	Apr24	May30	Jul18	Oct8	Jan9	May13	Sep25			
YEAR	1990	1990	1991	1991	1991	1991	1991	1992	1992	1992			
Activity	2	2	2	0	1	1	2	1	1	1	[	]	Activity
HAQ Disabili	2.125	2.25	2	.875	1.125	1.25	1.5	1.375	1.375	1.25	[	]	HAQ_Disabi
ACR Class	2	2	2	2	2	2	2	2			[	]	ACR_Class
Glb Severity	68	70	69	48	50	45	55	39	39	41	[	]	Glb_Severi
Anxiety	2.9	1.6	1.6	0	1.9	1.6	1.6	.3	1.98	1.32	[	]	Anxiety
Depression	1.3	1.6	.6	0	2.3	2.3	.9	1.6	.99	1.98	[	]	Depression
Health Statu									1	2	[	]	Health_Sta
Satisfaction									1	2	[	]	Satisfacti
AbleToWork										4	[	]	AbleToWork
ShortDays										0	[	]	ShortDays
WorkWell										4	[	]	WorkWell
WorkChange										0	[	]	WorkChange

JOINT EXAMINATION

UPPER EXTREMITY

	35	36	37	38	39	40	41	42	43	44			
DIPs	0/0	0/0	0/0	0/0	0/0	0/0	1/1	0/0	0/0	0/0	[	]	DIPs
PIPs	0/0	0/0	0/0	0/0	0/0	0/0	0/0	0/0	0/0	0/0	[	]	PIPs
IP Thumb	0/0	0/0	0/0	0/0	0/0	0/0	0/0	0/0	0/0	0/0	[	]	IP_Thumb
MCPs	0/0	0/0	0/0	0/0	0/0	0/0	0/0	0/0	0/0	0/0	[	]	MCPs
FMC Thumb	1/1	1/1	1/1	1/1	0/0	0/0	0/0	0/0	0/0	0/0	[	]	FMC_Thumb
Wrist	1/1	1/1	1/1	1/1	0/0	1/1	1/1	1/1	1/1	0/0	[	]	Wrist
Elbow	1/1	1/1	1/1	1/1	1/1	0/0	1/1	1/1	1/1	1/0	[	]	Elbow
Shoulder	1/1	1/1	1/1	1/1	0/0	0/0	0/0	0/0	0/0	0/0	[	]	Shoulder

LOWER EXTREMITY

Hip	0/0	0/0	0/0	0/0	0/0	0/0	0/0	0/0	0/0	0/0	[	]	Hip
Knee	0/1	0/1	0/1	0/1	0/1	0/0	0/1	0/1	0/1	0/1	[	]	Knee
Ankle	0/0	0/0	0/1	0/1	0/0	0/0	0/0	0/0	0/0	0/0	[	]	Ankle
Subtalar	0/0	0/0	0/0	0/0	0/0	0/0	0/0	0/0	0/0	0/0	[	]	Subtalar
Tarsal	0/0	0/0	0/0	0/0	0/0	0/0	0/0	0/0	0/0	0/0	[	]	Tarsal
MTPs	1/1	1/1	0/0	0/0	0/0	0/0	0/0	0/0	0/0	0/0	[	]	MTPs
1st MTP	0/0	0/0	0/0	0/0	0/0	0/0	0/0	0/0	0/0	0/0	[	]	1st_MTP
PIP Foot	0/0	0/0	0/0	0/0	0/0	0/0	0/0	0/0	0/0	0/0	[	]	PIP_Foot
DIP Foot	0/0	0/0	0/0	0/0	0/0	0/0	0/0	0/0	0/0	0/0	[	]	DIP_Foot
1stIP Foot	0/0	0/0	0/0	0/0	0/0	0/0	0/0	0/0	0/0	0/0	[	]	1stIP_Foot
Heel									0/0	0/0	[	]	Heel

CENTRAL

SI Joint	0	0	0	0	0	0	0	0	0	0	[	]	SI_Joint
Lumbar Sp	0	0	0	0	0	0	0	0	0	0	[	]	Lumbar_Sp
Thoracic Sp	0	0	0	0	0	0	0	0	0	0	[	]	Thoracic_S
Cervical Sp	0	0	0	0	0	0	0	0	0	0	[	]	Cervical_S

OTHER JOINTS

TMJ	0/0	0/0	0/0	0/0	0/0	0/0	0/0	0/0	0/0	0/0	[	]	TMJ
Sterno Clav	0/0	0/0	0/0	0/0	0/0	0/0	0/0	0/0	0/0	0/0	[	]	Sterno_Cla
Acro Clav	0/0	0/0	0/0	0/0	0/0	0/0	0/0	0/0	0/0	0/0	[	]	Acro_Clav
Costo Chond	0	0	0	0	0	0	0	0	0	0	[	]	Costo_Chon
Sternal	0	0	0	0	0	0	0	0	0	0	[	]	Sternal

PHYSICAL/ANATOMICAL

Jnt Swelling	1	1	1	1	1	1	1	1	1	1	[	]	Jnt_Swelli
Dactylitis	0	0	0	0	0	0	0	0	0	0	[	]	Dactylitis
Tenosynoviti	0	0	0	0	0	0	0	0	0	0	[	]	Tenosynovi

Fig. 1 Continued

VISIT	35	36	37	38	39	40	41	42	43	44			
DATE	Nov5	Dec17	Mar25	Apr24	May30	Jul18	Oct8	Jan9	May13	Sep25			
YEAR	1990	1990	1991	1991	1991	1991	1991	1992	1992	1992			

Nodules	0	0	0	0	0	0	0	0	0	0	[	]	Nodules
Tophi	0	0	0	0	0	0	0	0	0	0	[	]	Tophi
Nodule Other	0	0	0	0	0	0	0	0	0	0	[	]	Nodule_Oth
Heberdens	0	0	0	0	0	0	0	0	0	0	[	]	Heberdens
Bouchard's	0	0	0	0	0	0	0	0	0	0	[	]	Bouchard's
Dupuytren	0	0	0	0	0	0	0	0	0	0	[	]	Dupuytren
Joint Count									5	2	[	]	Joint_Coun

NON-ARTICULAR EXAMINATION DATA

TENDER POINTS

Occiput	0/0	[	]	Occiput
Low C Spine	0/0	[	]	Low_C_Spin
Trapezius	0/0	[	]	Trapezius
Supraspinous	0/0	[	]	Supraspino
2nd Rib	0/0	[	]	2nd_Rib
Lat Epicon	0/0	[	]	Lat_Epicon
Gluteal	0/0	[	]	Gluteal
Trochanter	0/0	[	]	Trochanter
Knee TP	0/0	[	]	Knee_TP
Trapez	3.5/4.3	[	]	Trapez
2ndRib	3.5	[	]	2ndRib
Lat Epi	5	[	]	Lat Epi
Knees	9.0/9.5	[	]	Knees
TP Count	0	[	]	TP_Count

RADIOGRAPHIC EXAMINATION DATA

C Spine(-)		+	[	]	C_Spine(-)
C1-C2 Sub		2	[	]	C1-C2 Sub
Erosions	3	3	[	]	Erosions
Jt Narrowing	3	3	[	]	Jt_Narrowi
Periosti	0	0	[	]	Periosti
DJD	0	1	[	]	DJD
Chondrocalci	0	0	[	]	Chondrocal
Hip Nar		3/1	[	]	Hip_Nar
Knee Nar		3/1	[	]	Knee_Nar
Hand Nar	3/3	3/3	[	]	Hand_Nar
Hand Eros	3/3	3/3	[	]	Hand_Eros
Hand DJD		0/0	[	]	Hand_DJD
R Hip Narrow		3	[	]	R_Hip_Narr
R Hip Osteop		0	[	]	R_Hip_Oste
L Hip Narrow		1	[	]	L_Hip_Narr
L Hip Osteop		0	[	]	L_Hip_Oste
R Knee Nar L		3	[	]	R_Knee_Nar
R Knee Nar M		2	[	]	R_Knee_Nar
R Knee Ost L		1	[	]	R_Knee_Ost
R Knee Ost M		0	[	]	R_Knee_Ost
R Knee Align		1	[	]	R_Knee_Ali
R Knee Scler		2	[	]	R_Knee_Scl
L Knee Nar L		0	[	]	L_Knee_Nar
L Knee Nar M		1	[	]	L_Knee_Nar
L Knee Ost L		0	[	]	L_Knee_Ost
L Knee Ost M		0	[	]	L_Knee_Ost
L Knee Align		1	•[	]	L_Knee_Ali
L Knee Scler		1	[	]	L_Knee_Scl

Fig. 1 Continued

VISIT	35	36	37	38	39	40	41	42	43	44
DATE	Nov5	Dec17	Mar25	Apr24	May30	Jul18	Oct8	Jan9	May13	Sep25
YEAR	1990	1990	1991	1991	1991	1991	1991	1992	1992	1992

LABORATORY-I

HEMATOLOGY

	35	36	37	38	39	40	41	42	43	44	[	]	
WBC	7.5	8	9.8	10.1	8.3	7.5	11.4	6.9	6.6	6.2	[	]	WBC
PCV	35	35	37	41	40	41	38	39	39.5	39.9	[	]	PCV
Hemoglobin	11.4	10.8	11.9	12.5	12.1	13	12.2	12.2	12.9	13.1	[	]	Hemoglobin
Neutrophils	70	67	83	66	2	72	82	64	62	62	[	]	Neutrophil
Bands	4	0	0	0	3	0	3	2	2	2	[	]	Bands
Lymphocytes	24	31	16	34	35	27	14	34	36	36	[	]	Lymphocyte
Monocytes	0	0	0	0	0	0	0	0	0	0	[	]	Monocytes
Eosinophils	2	2	1	0	0	1	1	0	0	0	[	]	Eosinophil
Basophils	0	0	0	0	0	0	0	0	0	0	[	]	Basophils
Platelet	555	555	500	463	409	397	478	410	393	405	[	]	Platelet
RBC Count	4.3	4.3	4.6	5	4.7	4.6	4.3	4.6	4.5	4.49	[	]	RBC_Count
MCV	83	82	80	83	84	88	88	86	87.8	88.8	[	]	MCV
ESR	97	83	45	15	13	10	50	15	22	15	[	]	ESR

URINE

	35	36	37	38	39	40	41	42	43	44	[	]	
Urine PH						5	6	6	6	5	[	]	Urine_PH
Specific Gra						1	1	1	1.015	1.02	[	]	Specific_G
Urine Glucos						0	0	0	0	0	[	]	Urine_Gluc
Urine Protei						0	0	0	0	0	[	]	Urine_Prot
Urine Blood						0	0	0	0	0	[	]	Urine_Bloo
RBC/HPF						0	1	1	1	0	[	]	RBC/HPF
WBC/HPF						0	0	1	0	2	[	]	WBC/HPF

Parameter	1	2	3	4	5	6	7	8	9	10	Field	Variable
Gr Casts						0	0	0	0	0	[ ]	Gr_Casts
WBC Casts						0	0	0	0	0	[ ]	WBC_Casts
RBC Casts						0	0	0	0	0	[ ]	RBC_Casts
Joint Asp	237										[ ]	Joint_Asp
Joint Cells	30000										[ ]	Joint_Cell

LABORATORY-II

Parameter	1	2	3	4	5	6	7	8	9	10	Field	Variable
SGOT	20	20									[ ]	SGOT
Creatinine	1.2	1.1									[ ]	Creatinine

TREATMENT DATA

Parameter	1	2	3	4	5	6	7	8	9	10	Field	Variable
Azulfidine				1500	1500	1500	1500	2000	2000	2000	[ ]	Azulfidine
D Medrol	80										[ ]	D_Medrol
MTX	15	15									[ ]	MTX
Voltaren	150	150	150	150	150	150	150	150	150	150	[ ]	Voltaren
Cytotec						400	200				[ ]	Cytotec
Prednisone			10	10	10	10	10	5	5	5	[ ]	Prednisone
Inj KneeR	30										[ ]	Inj_KneeR
Inj KneeL							30				[ ]	Inj_KneeL
Inj KneeL			30								[ ]	Inj_KneeL

DIAGNOSIS

Parameter	1	2	3	4	5	6	7	8	9	10	Field	Variable
RA	+	+	+	+	+	+	+	+	+	+	[ ]	RA

STATUS

Parameter	1	2	3	4	5	6	7	8	9	10	Field	Variable
Observer	7	7	7	7	7	7	7	7	7	7	[ ]	Observer
Status	0	0	0	0	0	0	0	0	0	0	[ ]	Status

Fig. 1 Continued

printout during the clinical encounter. The data are then keyed into the computer and a new document is produced that contains the additional material. One cycle is complete, and the next ready to begin.

The initial page of the clinic record (printout) summarizes pertinent rheumatology and demographic information about the patient (see Fig. 1). Recorded are the key demographic data and selected rheumatic disease variables. Antirheumatic drugs are listed, together with their dates of administration and termination, and dose for current medications. Comorbidities (and dates) are listed, as are dates and types of articular surgery. One section of this page summarizes the most useful clinical data. For example, for weight, ESR, joint count, radiograph erosion score, and so on, the computer lists (with dates), the greatest, smallest, and current values. At the clinical level such a ''face sheet'' is extremely valuable, since it summarizes the patient's entire clinical course and records his or her current status. From it reports can be dictated, insurance forms completed, or the form itself can be sent to insurance companies.

The following pages of the patient record represent a time-oriented flow sheet (see Fig. 1). The flow sheet is a matrix with the variables of interest lying against the left side of the page, and the data for each visit displayed in columns running left to right across the page. Each column is headed by a visit number and a date. The last column on the right is open, leaving room for the clinician and staff to record current (new) visit data.

The ARION system is designed to allow the clinician or investigator to specify any variables or group of variables he or she chooses for inclusion. Thus the printout can be as simple or detailed as required, and is equally suitable for clinics with specialized interests as it is for general rheumatic disease care. It forms a method for gathering research data, but simultaneously is a useful patient care system. Because the ARION computer system is content-independent, it will work with any HSQ, including, AIMS, HAQ, MHAQ, CLINHAQ, or other.

Although computers have many advantages, someone has to record the data onto the input document and someone has to key in the data into the computer (just as someone has to record detailed notes and observations in noncomputerized systems). ARION is optimized for data entry in several ways. First, it takes advantage of the fact that a significant number of the usual observations in rheumatology are usually ''normal'' (e.g., no telangectasia), and that most observations do not change from visit to visit. For example, most joints active at one visit will be active at the next, just as drugs, such as digoxin or aprazolam, tend to be continued at the same dose from one visit to the next. The ARION system allows clinicians to declare large blocks of observations as ''normal'' or unchanged from their values at the last visit. Similarly, at keypunch time, function keys (F1–F12) permit block entry of normal and unchanged values. For example, if all the current medications and drugs, except one, are continued at the current visit, then a single key stroke enters the unchanged data, requiring the separate entry of only the item that was changed. In general, then, data recording and keypunching are reduced dramatically by only recording "changes" or "nonnormal" observations. To expedite scores of HSQ, the system also provides "calculators" for common health status instruments, such as the AIMS, HAQ, and MHAQ, so that complicated data can be calculated by the computer and automatically entered into the database.

There are other benefits of the ARION system. It presents full documentation of the rheumatology encounter for third-party carriers. By making data entry easy, it can stimulate rheumatologists to record the examinations they actually do, but do not record manually. Finally, the record is clearly formatted so that the dictation of consultation reports and the substantiation of disability are both easily accomplished.

A. Health Status Questionnaires, and Their Integration into the Clinic

As indicated earlier, most clinics and clinicians do not use HSQ (see Table 2). On the other hand, I have found them useful and convenient in a busy clinic. Table 9 describes requirements for use of HSQ in the outpatient clinic. Appendix A describes the CLINHAQ instruments, and Appendix B the MHAQ forms of Pincus. The two-page folded (four sides) CLINHAQ document (see Appendix A) is completed within 5–10 min by all patients. The CLINHAQ represent an adaptation of a variety of instruments designed by others. The first two pages contain the Stanford Health Assessment Questionnaire (HAQ) Disability Index, a measure of functional disability (33), and visual analog scales for pain and global severity. In addition, a pain diagram is included, with additional detail given to the hands. The third page contains the AIMS anxiety and depression scales (34) and estimates of fatigue. On the fourth page, patients are asked about gastrointestinal problems, sleep problems, global health and satisfaction, and work ability. We administer this HSQ to every patient at every clinic visit as

Table 9 What Clinicians Require to Use HSQ in The Clinic

1. They must be short, not use more than minimal staff time, and not disturb the routine of the clinic. Indeed, they must fit in with the routine of the clinic.
2. HSQ must help the physician and staff with record-keeping, not impede it. They must assist in documentation of clinical care.
3. Cost must be minimal.
4. The results must be available at the time the patient is seen.
5. Comparison with previous data and with other patients must be contemporaneous.
6. The results must be intuitive and interpretably simply.
7. The information must not just be additional data. It must be clinically useful.

part of our ordinary patient care. On separate documents (fifth to ninth pages) we record data concerning comorbidity, demographic, work, and disability changes.

In the clinic the CLINHAQ HSQ is the last form the patient completes before seeing the physician. This is preceded by an interview from our clinic nurse. From the ARION clinical record printout, she reviews the symptom review data with the patient, adding new items, verifying old, and making changes when necessary. Drugs and their doses are verified and added. Clinic measures of items, such as blood pressure, weight, grip strength, and morning stiffness, are obtained and entered onto the printout input form. Items that the nurse thinks important, but are not captured in the computerized form, are often written on the database form by the nurse in longhand. The patient then completes the CLINHAQ while waiting for the physician.

When the physician sees the patient, then, all rheumatic disease data have been recorded and the HSQ completed. On the ARION printout are all of the data from previous clinic visits as well as current observations. In our clinic, the nurse (or physician) adds up the HAQ functional disability score and scores the AIMs depression score with a template during the course of the interview. By the use of templates, these operations take a few seconds, and comparisons with previous scores are made simultaneously. The physician also has other powerful measures to review. The sensitive pain and global severity scales are in view, as are data on grip strength, stiffness, and similar items. These data are compared with previous data on the printout page. Finally, in our clinic, but often not in others, laboratory data are obtained as the patient enters the clinic, and are usually available toward the end of the clinical interview and examination. The physician reviews the data, asks more question, performs and records the joint examination, and then discusses course and therapy with the patient. At the end of the encounter, the physician dictates or writes a brief note. This is usually very brief, since all the data are already recorded. Its value is to annotate special problems or clinical decisions. Although we have described the ARION system, almost exactly the same activity takes place using the MHAQ questionnaire system. Pincus et al. administer the MHAQ (Appendix B) in the waiting room and score it before the patient enters the examining room. The data obtained and the use of flowsheets for patients care are otherwise similar.

Is it worthwhile? It has been shown repeatedly that the best data are obtained from patients and staff, and the worse (least reliable) data from physicians. The ARION–CLINHAQ and MHAQ systems shift data collection to the left, obtaining information on the HSQ from patient and minimal cost in time or expense to clinic. Much of the clinical data are screened and recorded by the nursing staff, who thereby become ever increasingly knowledgeable parts of clinic system (colleagues). By virtue of the delegation of a number of tasks, and the reduction in the dictation obligation, the physician has more time, and more time for direct patient interaction. It does not come free. Where are the costs? Although computers cost dollars, hardware is now inexpensive. A computer and its accessories represent less than one-tenth of a nurse's salary. The added expense is in keypunching. We require about 2 h/day to enter ARION data from a busy clinic. We estimate that the trade-off in extra physician time and better clinical records compensates for the cost of keypunching (e.g., extra patients can be seen).

As we have shown, the first five items on Table 9 are accomplished by the ARION–CLINHAQ and MHAQ systems. But interpretability of HSQ data has remained a problem. The AIMS depression scores, for example, are neither normally distributed nor intuitive. The HAQ functional disability scores appear intuitive. For example, a score of 1 means that on the average the patient has difficulty in performing every activity of daily living. Yet it is not clear how "bad" a score 1.16 is and what is the actual meaning of a score of 1.16 as opposed to 1.22. For the AIMS depression data the situation is worse. Not only is the score not intuitive, there have been few data to suggest what any score means (34). For both of these questionnaires, research studies may show how they influence or are influenced by disease, but for the clinician looking at the actual number, the data have been largely uninterpretable. Although these problems are particularly acute for HSQ, they also extend to other common clinic measures. One might similarly ask the "meaning" of and ESR of 29 as opposed to 35 mm/h. Similar questions might be asked about a number of clinic items including grip strength, morning stiffness, pain scales, and such.

We have conducted several investigations aimed at establishing normative data for clinical measurements in RA and other disorders. In RA we used the following methodology. We evaluated 1297 consecutive RA patients seen in our clinic who had at least 2 years of follow-up (35): 16,095 visits (12.4 per patient) were used, with a mean follow-up of 7.2 years. For each patient we calculated an average value for the clinical and HSQ variable of interest. For example, if a patient had 12 HAQ scores over his 7 years of clinic follow-up, we calculated an "average" HAQ score for that patient. We then ranked each patient's score for each clinical variable and determined its relative percentile when compared with all of the 1297 patients (35). The effect of these analyses is to associate "clinical" significance with the actual clinical measurement. The results of these analyses are presented in Table 10. Even though such data may change with time, the use of average scores over 7.2 years (range 0.5–14 years) establishes the percentile ranking as representing the usual course of RA over time. Data such as these have not been available previously. We have also determined the significance of the AIMS depression scores by comparing them with CES-D (34) scores (see Table 10). Thus, in the clinic, patients with a high probability of depression (AIMS depression $\geq$ 4) can be identified quickly. The data presented in Table 10 can be used to "place" patient data. Thus, it is possible to scan the patient's scores and rank the patient in comparison with all other patients with RA for any given measure on Table 10. An overall index of patient severity, the

Table 10 Ranked Average Scores for Clinical and HSQ Variables for 1297 Rheumatoid Arthritis Patients

	Percentiles									
	10th	20th	30th	40th	50th	60th	70th	80th	90th	100th
VAS severity (0–100)	21.2	28.8	34.7	40	45	50	51.2	58.3	67.3	100
VAS pain (0–3)	0.6	0.89	1.11	1.3	1.4	1.6	1.8	2.0	2.3	3.0
HAQ DI (0–3)	0.29	0.54	0.75	0.92	1.10	1.27	1.5	1.75	2.11	3.00
Grip strength (20–300 mm/Hg)	300	191.2	148.5	129.7	114.4	102.3	99.4	80.6	73.3	62.5
ESR (0–150 mm/hr)	11.3	17.4	22.7	27.7	32.5	38	44	52	65	128.3
AM stiffness (hr)	0.2	0.5	0.83	1.1	1.5	2.0	2.5	3.3	5.2	24
Joint count (0–24)	2	3	4	4.7	5.5	6.3	7.2	8.2	10.1	24
Platelets (0–555)	219	249	273	293	315	341	361	397	446	>555
AIMS depression (0–9.9)	0.8	1.2	1.6	1.9	2.3	2.7	3.3	3.9	4.9	9.5
AIMS anxiety (0–9.9)	1.5	2.0	2.6	3.0	3.5	4.1	4.7	5.3	6.1	9.9

Disease Status Index (DSI) (35,36), is computed by taking the rank of each of six measures: VAS patient global, VAS pain, joint count, ESR, grip strength, and HAQ disability index. The sum of the ranking of the six measures divided by 6, yields an overall severity ranking for the patient compared with all other RA patients. With familiarity, then, HAQ and AIMS scores, as well as overall severity placement, become as simple to understand as hemoglobin levels and blood pressures.

The final demand of Table 9 is that data be clinically useful. There is ample evidence that HSQ have important predictive utility (24,37). We believe that the data presented in Table 10 can extend that research usefulness into the clinic. In the clinic we have found the flow sheet record demonstrates trends that are obscured when only single observations are considered.

IV. SUMMARY

The usual real and imagined objections and needs associated with data collection, HSQ, and computerization of rheumatology practice have been noted (see Tables 2, 4, and 9). Our observations suggest that most of these objections were real and important, but can be overcome easily by appropriate instrument use, computerization, and normative data. The HSQ and computers improve patient care and record keeping, probably at minimal cost (they may be less expensive than current methods). In addition the ARION–CLINHAQ and MHAQ systems provide an entry into clinical research for the clinician. Such research capabilities by clinicians is important. Does anyone doubt that if a consortium of data-collecting clinics existed over the last 10 years that answers to question concerning prednisone toxicity and efficacy, the use of multiple drug combinations, and other important questions would have been answered long ago?

APPENDICES

Appendix A

The following forms (pages 495–503) constitute Appendix A: The first is the Clinical Health Assessment Questionnaire (CLINHAQ). The second is the demographic data acquisition sheet used for a ''new'' patient. The third form is the demographic data acquisition sheet for a returning patient. The fourth form is the adverse drug reaction data acquisition form. These forms are used to record functional disability, pain, and global severity, and describe the CLINHAQ instruments.

Appendix B

Four MHAQ questionnaires (pages 504–511) comprise Appendix B: First, the Activities and Lifestyle Index. Second, the Rheumatology Function Flow Sheet.

The third form is the Rheumatoid Arthritis Yearly Evaluation (RAYE). The fourth is the Rheumatology Health Outcome Monitoring form and Physical Function Tests and Joint Examination. These forms help the physician to assess the patient's condition and symptoms.

Clinical Health Assessment Questionnaire (CLINHAQ)

Name____ Date__________ ID#__________

We are interested in learning how your illness affects your ability to function in daily life.

Please check the response which best describes your usual abilities OVER THE PAST WEEK:

	Without Any Difficulty	With Some Difficulty	With Much Difficulty	Unable To Do

DRESSING & GROOMING Are you able to:

-Dress yourself, including shoelaces and buttons?
-Shampoo your hair?

Dressing _____ (184)

ARISING Are you able to:

-Stand up from a straight chair?
-Get in and out of bed?

Arising _____ (175)

EATING Are you able to:

-Cut your meat?
-Lift a full cup or glass to your mouth?
-Open a new milk carton?

Eating _____ (183)

WALKING Are you able to:

-Walk outdoors on flat ground?
-Climb up five steps?

Walking _____ (174)

Please check any AIDS OR DEVICES that you usually use for any of these activities:

_____ Cane (W)   _____ Walker (W)   _____ Built up or special utensils (E)
_____ Crutches (W)   _____ Wheelchair (W)   _____ Special or built up chair (A)
_____ Devices used for dressing (button hook, zipper pull, long handled shoe horn) (D)
_____ Other specify: (____)

Please check any categories for which you usually need HELP FROM ANOTHER PERSON:

_____ Dressing and Grooming   _____ Eating
_____ Arising   _____ Walking

We are also interested in learning whether or not you are affected by pain because of your illness.

How much pain have you had because of your illness IN THE PAST WEEK?

PLACE A MARK ON THE LINE TO INDICATE THE SEVERITY OF THE PAIN

NO PAIN   SEVERE PAIN

Painscal _____ (453)

0   100

We are also interested in learning about the severity of your illness.

Consider ALL THE WAYS THAT YOUR ILLNESS AFFECTS YOU, RATE HOW YOU ARE DOING on the following scale by placing a mark on the line:

VERY WELL   VERY POOR

Global _____ (156)

0   100

OFCEHAQ 93

Please check the response which best describes your usual abilities OVER THE PAST WEEK:	Without Any Difficulty	With Some Difficulty	With Much Difficulty	Unable To Do

HYGIENE Are you able to:

- Wash and dry your body?
- Take a tub bath?
- Get on and off the toilet?

REACH Are you able to:

- Reach and get down a 5 pound object (such as a bag of sugar) from just above your head?
- Bend down to pick up clothing from the floor?

GRIP Are you able to:

- Open car doors?
- Open jars which have been previously opened?
- Turn faucets on and off?

ACTIVITIES Are you able to:

- Run errands and shop?
- Get in and out of a car?
- Do chores such as vacuuming or yardwork?

Hygiene ____ (185)

Reach ____ (172)

Grip ____ (584)

Activity ____ (583)

Please check any AIDS OR DEVICES that you usually use for any of these activities:

____ Bathtub bar (H)	____ Long-handled appliances in bathroom (H)
____ Raised toilet seat (H)	____ Jar opener for jars previously opened (G)
____ Long-handled appliances for reach (R)	____ Other (Specify): __________

Please check any categories for which you usually need HELP FROM ANOTHER PERSON:

| ____ Hygiene | ____ Gripping and opening things |
| ____ Reach | ____ Errands and Chores |

Please indicate all of the locations of your pain **OVER THE PAST WEEK** by shading the *body figures* and the *hands.*

EXAMPLE:

OFFICHAQ.PM4 P2 9/92

Please check the most appropriate answer for each question. Try to answer every question.

	Always	Very Often	Fairly Often	Some-times	Almost Never	Never
1. During the PAST MONTH, how much of the time have you enjoyed the things you do?						
2. During the PAST MONTH, how much of the time have you felt tense or "high strung"?						
3. How much have you been bothered by nervousness, or your "nerves" during the PAST MONTH?						
4. How often during the PAST MONTH, did you find yourself having difficulty trying to calm down?						
5. During the PAST MONTH, how much of the time have you been in low or very low spirits?						
6. How much of the time during the PAST MONTH did you feel relaxed and free of tension?						

	Always	Very Often	Fairly Often	Some-times	Almost Never	Never
7. How much of the time during the PAST MONTH have you felt downhearted and blue?						
8. How often during the PAST MONTH did you feel that nothing turned out for you the way you wanted it to?						
9. How much of the time during the PAST MONTH have you felt calm and peaceful?						
10. During the PAST MONTH, how often did you feel that others would be better off if you were dead?						
11. How much of the time during the PAST MONTH were you able to relax without difficulty?						
12. How often during the PAST MONTH have you felt so down in the dumps that nothing could cheer you up?						

We are interested in knowing about any problems that you may have been having with fatigue.
How much of a problem has fatigue or tiredness been for you IN THE PAST WEEK?
Place a mark on the line below:

0   100

FATIGUE   FATIGUE IS A
IS NO PROBLEM   MAJOR PROBLEM

How much trouble have you had with your stomach (ie, nausea, heartburn, bloating, pain, etc.)
IN THE PAST WEEK?

Place a mark on the line below:

0   100

NO STOMACH   A LOT OF
PROBLEM   STOMACH PROBLEMS

How much of a problem has sleep (ie, resting at night) been for you
IN THE PAST WEEK?

Place a mark on the line below:

0   100

SLEEP   SLEEP IS A
IS NO PROBLEM   MAJOR PROBLEM

In general would you say that your HEALTH NOW is:

_______ Excellent   _______ Good   _______ Fair   _______ Poor

DURING THE LAST 6 MONTHS, if you were:
1. Employed
   OR
2. A Housewife or Househusband, please answer the next four questions:

	All Days 100%	Most Days 70-99%	Some Days 41-69%	Few Days 1-40%	No Days 0%
-How often were you able to work?	____	____	____	____	____
-How often did you have to work a shorter day?	____	____	____	____	____
-How often were you able to do your work as carefully and accurately as you would like?	____	____	____	____	____
-How often did you have to change the way your work was usually done?	____	____	____	____	____

How satisfied are you with your HEALTH NOW?

______ Very satisfied
______ Somewhat satisfied
______ Neither Satisfied nor dissatisfied
______ Somewhat dissatisfied
______ Very dissatisfied

	HAQ	AIMS
0	0.000	
1	.125	
2	.250	
3	.375	
4	.500	
5	.625	
6	.750	0.00
7	.875	.33
8	1.000	.66
9	1.125	.99
10	1.250	1.32
11	1.375	1.65
12	1.500	1.98
13	1.625	2.31
14	1.750	2.64
15	1.875	2.97
16	2.000	3.30
17	2.125	3.63
18	2.250	3.96
19	2.375	4.29
20	2.500	4.62
21	2.625	4.95
22	2.750	5.28
23	2.875	5.61
24	3.000	5.94
25		6.27
26		6.60
27		6.93
28		7.26
29		7.59
30		7.92
31		8.25
32		8.58
33		8.91
34		9.24
35		9.57
36		9.90

Ablewk _______

Shortwk _______

Accuwk _______

Chngwk _______

OFCHAQ93.4

Background and Medical History

NAME____ Date ___________________ ID# ____________

Date of Birth_____________ Age_____ Male_____ Female_____ Height_______ Weight_______

Marital Status: _____Never married _____Divorced _____Widowed _____Remarried after divorce
_____Married _____Separated _____Remarried after death of spouse

With whom do you live? _____Alone _____With Children _____With other relatives or friends
_____With Spouse _____In a retirement home _____In a convalescent center or home

Ethnic Background: _____White _____Asian _____American Indian or Alaskan Native
_____Black _____Hispanic _____Other

Please circle the highest grade that you attended?

1 2 3 4 5 6 7 8   9 10 11 12   13 14 15 16   17+
Grade School   High School   College   Post College   Other _________

Do you smoke cigarettes? Now? Yes _____ No _____ } How many years?_______
In the past? Yes _____ No _____ } How many packs per day? _____

We are interested in finding out if you __now__ have or have had __in the past__, any of the following medical problems, and if you take medication for them. Please indicate the year or age when the condition began and how important the medical problem is in your daily life.

	Have you had any of the following?			When did this condition begin?		Do you take medication for this condition?		How important is this medical problem in your daily life? PLEASE CIRCLE			
	NOW	IN THE PAST	NEVER	THE YEAR WAS	MY AGE or WAS	YES	NO	Not at all	Some-what	Moder-ately	Very
High blood pressure	___	___	___	___ or ___		___	___	0	1	2	3
Heart Attack	___	___	___	___ or ___		___	___	0	1	2	3
Other Heart Condition	___	___	___	___ or ___		___	___	0	1	2	3
Stroke	___	___	___	___ or ___		___	___	0	1	2	3
Mental illness	___	___	___	___ or ___		___	___	0	1	2	3
Depression	___	___	___	___ or ___		___	___	0	1	2	3
Diabetes	___	___	___	___ or ___		___	___	0	1	2	3
Cancer	___	___	___	___ or ___		___	___	0	1	2	3
Alcohol or drug problem	___	___	___	___ or ___		___	___	0	1	2	3
Kidney problem	___	___	___	___ or ___		___	___	0	1	2	3
Lung problem	___	___	___	___ or ___		___	___	0	1	2	3
Cataract	___	___	___	___ or ___		___	___	0	1	2	3
Asthma	___	___	___	___ or ___		___	___	0	1	2	3
Severe Allergies	___	___	___	___ or ___		___	___	0	1	2	3
Liver or gallbladder problems	___	___	___	___ or ___		___	___	0	1	2	3
Ulcers or stomach problems	___	___	___	___ or ___		___	___	0	1	2	3
Neurological problem (*such as Seizures / Parkinson's Disease*)	___	___	___	___ or ___		___	___	0	1	2	3
Fracture of the spine, hip, or leg	___	___	___	___ or ___		___	___	0	1	2	3
Thyroid or endocrine disorder	___	___	___	___ or ___		___	___	0	1	2	3
Problems with prostate (men) or Uterus, ovaries, etc. (women)	___	___	___	___ or ___		___	___	0	1	2	3

BIQ.1 2/93

We are interested in learning about your employment history and income related to your illness.

What is your current occupation? _______________________________

Over your working life what was/is your main occupation? _______________________

Over your spouse's working life, what was/is his/her occupation? _______________________

Do you live on a farm?   _______ Yes   _______ No

Please check your main form of work:

_______ Paid work   _______ Housework   _______ Student

_______ Unemployed   _______ Disabled   _______ Retired   _______ Farmwork

---

What type(s) of health insurance do you have?   Check all that apply.

_______ None   _______ Health Maintenance Organization (HMO)

_______ Medicaid   _______ Private insurance company: (For example: Blue Cross, Blue Shield, Aetna)

_______ Medicare   _______ Medicare disability

Have you received disability payments because of your arthritis or muscle or joint problem?   _______ Yes _______ No

If "YES", please check the source of payments and the year that payments were started.

	Source of payment	Year payments began	Still receiving Yes	No	If No, when stopped
_______	Job	__________	___	___	__________
_______	Workers compensation	__________	___	___	__________
_______	State or local government disability payments	__________	___	___	__________
_______	Social Security disability payments	__________	___	___	__________
_______	Other: __________	__________	___	___	__________

Which income group below comes closest to your total household income in 1993 from ALL SOURCES BEFORE TAXES?

_______ Under $10,000	_______ $40,000-49,999	_______ $80,000-89,999
_______ $10,000-19,999	_______ $50,000-59,999	_______ $90,000-99,999
_______ $20,000-29,999	_______ $60,000-69,999	_______ $100,000 or more
_______ $30,000-39,999	_______ $70,000-79,999	

Occupa _______
Mainocc _______
Spousocc _______
Farm _______
Employ _______

Ins1 _______
Ins2 _______

Dispay _______
Dispay1 _______
Disyr1 _______
Still 1 _______
Dispay2 _______
Disyr2 _______
Still 2 _______
Dispay3 _______
Disyr3 _______
Still3 _______

TOTINCOM _______

Medical Information Update

Name ____ Date ____________ ID# ____________

We are interested in knowing if you have you had any of the following medical problems and if

you have taken medication for these problems since your last visit on _________________.

Please answer each question in Column I by checking the appropriate box to indicate whether you <u>now</u> have,
have had <u>in the past</u> or have <u>never</u> had any of the following medical conditions. For those questions that you
have checked NOW or IN THE PAST in COLUMN I, please complete columns II, III and IV.

	I — Have you had any of the following?			II — Did this condition begin before your last visit?		III — Do you take medication for this condition?		IV — How important is this medical problem in your daily life? PLEASE CIRCLE			
	NOW	IN THE PAST	NEVER	YES	NO	YES	NO	Not at all	Some-what	Moder-ately	Very
High blood pressure	___	___	___	___	___	___	___	0	1	2	3
Heart Attack	___	___	___	___	___	___	___	0	1	2	3
Other Heart Condition	___	___	___	___	___	___	___	0	1	2	3
Stroke	___	___	___	___	___	___	___	0	1	2	3
Mental illness	___	___	___	___	___	___	___	0	1	2	3
Depression	___	___	___	___	___	___	___	0	1	2	3
Diabetes	___	___	___	___	___	___	___	0	1	2	3
Cancer	___	___	___	___	___	___	___	0	1	2	3
Alcohol or drug problem	___	___	___	___	___	___	___	0	1	2	3
Kidney problem	___	___	___	___	___	___	___	0	1	2	3
Lung problem	___	___	___	___	___	___	___	0	1	2	3
Cataract	___	___	___	___	___	___	___	0	1	2	3
Asthma	___	___	___	___	___	___	___	0	1	2	3
Severe Allergies	___	___	___	___	___	___	___	0	1	2	3
Liver or gallbladder problems	___	___	___	___	___	___	___	0	1	2	3
Ulcers or stomach problems	___	___	___	___	___	___	___	0	1	2	3
Neurological problem (*such as Seizures / Parkinson's Disease*)	___	___	___	___	___	___	___	0	1	2	3
Fracture of the spine, hip, or leg	___	___	___	___	___	___	___	0	1	2	3
Thyroid or endocrine disorder	___	___	___	___	___	___	___	0	1	2	3
Problems with prostate (men) or Uterus, ovaries, etc. (women)	___	___	___	___	___	___	___	0	1	2	3

Please Turn Over and Complete the Other Side   OFCHAQ93.5

Since your last visit ....

Have you taken any NEW medications for either arthritic or non-arthritic conditions?

[ ] No   [ ] Yes   If "Yes", please list:

_______________   _______________   _______________

_______________   _______________   _______________

Have you been hospitalized or had surgery for any reason since your last visit?

[ ] No   [ ] Yes   If "Yes", please list:

Reason for Hospitalization or Surgery   Hospital / Location   Date

_______________________   _______________   _______

_______________________   _______________   _______

Have you had any NEW non-arthritis illnesses since your last visit?

[ ] No   [ ] Yes   If "Yes", please list the type of Illness:

____

____

Since your last visit, have you:

[ ] No [ ] Yes   Stopped working?

[ ] No [ ] Yes   Started working?

[ ] No [ ] Yes   Changed jobs? If "yes", what is your current job? _______________

[ ] No [ ] Yes   Reduced work hours?   Current total hours worked per week _____

[ ] No [ ] Yes   Increased work hours?   Current total hours worked per week _____

Have you started to collect disability payments since your last visit?

[ ] No [ ] Yes   If "Yes", please check:

_____ Social Security Disability   _____ State or local government

_____ Job Payments   _____ Workers compensation   _____ Other   DISPAY _______

Have you had a change in your marital status since your last visit?

[ ] No [ ] Yes If "Yes", please put a checkmark to indicate your current marital status:

_____ married   _____ divorced   _____ remarried after divorce   MARITAL _____

_____ separated   _____ widowed   _____ remarried after death of spouse

Have you had a change in your living arrangements since your last visit?

[ ] No [ ] Yes   If "Yes", please put a checkmark to indicate the change:

_____ Live Alone   _____ With Spouse   _____ In a convalescent center

_____ In a retirement home   _____ With family members who help with your care   LVWITH _______

Which income group below comes closest to your total household income in 1993 from ALL SOURCES BEFORE TAXES?

_____ Under $10,000   _____ $40,000-49,999   _____ $80,000-89,999   TOTINCOM _____

_____ $10,000-19,999   _____ $50,000-59,999   _____ $90,000-99,999

_____ $20,000-29,999   _____ $60,000-69,999   _____ $100,000 or more

_____ $30,000-39,999   _____ $70,000-79,999

OFCHAQ93.8

ARION: The Database For Rheumatic Disease

ADVERSE DRUG REACTIONS Medication / Code	DATE (MMDDYY)	S.E. Code	CERTAINTY 1= Possible 2= Probable 3= Certain	IMPORTANCE 1= Minor 2= Moderate 3= Serious 4= Fatal Patient / M.D.	OUTCOME 1= Resolved 2= Continued	ADR RX 1= Untreated 2= Treated	Continuation 1= Continued 2=Continued w/ dose alteration 3=D/C'd not 2° SE 4= D/C'd 2° SE
1.							
2.							
3.							
4.							
5.							
6.							

DRUG OR DOSE CHANGE	CHANGE TYPE	REASON CODE	DOSE	START/ CHANGE DATE	STOP DATE

JOINT SURGERY

R / L Joint Procedure Date	R / L Joint Procedure Date
1.	1.
2.	2.

Change Codes
1. Increased dose
2. Decreased dose
3. Stopped med before patient visit
4. Started med before patient visit

Reason Codes
1. Side Effect
2. Lack of efficacy
3. Cost
4. Personal reasons
5. Have to take too many times per day
6. Forgot to take med

DIAGNOSIS 1 ___________   DIAGNOSIS 4 ___________

DIAGNOSIS 2 ___________   DIAGNOSIS 5 ___________

DIAGNOSIS 3 ___________   DIAGNOSIS 6 ___________

X-RAY CODING

Code		Code	
31	C Spine (-)	30	Met CA
20	C Spine DJD	16	O Porosis
23	C Spine RA	37	Pagets
21	C Fracture	5	Pneumonia
22	C1 C2 - SL	4	RH Lung
44	Calcino	11	S.I. (+) (3)
1	Chest (-)	36	S.I. (+) (1)
8	COPD	40	S.I. Sclero
2	Fibrosis	35	S.I. (-)
6	Heart Enlarg	19	T. Spine DJD
15	Hilar Adenop	32	T. Spine (-)
17	I. Necrosis		
33	LS Spine (-)		
18	LS Spine DJD		

SIDE EFFECTS CODING

Code		Code		Code		Code	
100	**GENERAL**	300	**HEENT**	600	**GI**	613	Liver Symptoms
101	Fatigue	301	Oral dryness	601	Anorexia	614	*Liver (Lab)
102	Fever	302	Taste abnormality	602	Nausea / vomiting	700	**GU**
103	Weight loss	301	Oral pain or burning	603	Dyspepsia	701	Dysuria
104	Weight gain	304	Oral ulcerations	604	Heartburn	702	Nocturia
105	Sweating	305	Ocular erythema	605	Dysphagia	703	Menstrual abn
200	**SKIN**	306	Visual blurring	606	Epigastric distress	704	*Hematuria
201	Rash	307	Hearing problems	607	Ulcer (dx by MD)	705	*Proteinuria
202	Alopecia	400	**CARDIAC**	608	GI Bleeding	706	*BUN / Creatinine
203	Bruising	401	Edema	609	Lower abd pain	707	Impotence
204	Photosensitivity	500	**PULMONARY**	610	'Gas'	800	**CNS**
205	Pruritis	501	Shortness of breath	611	Diarrhea	801	Headache
		502	Asthma	612	Constipation	802	Confusion
803	Memory loss	900	**MUSC / SKEL**	100	**HEMATOLOGIC**		
804	Convulsion	901	Muscle weakness	1001	*Leukopenia		
805	Paresthesias	902	Fracture	1002	*Leukocytosis		
806	Depression	903	Muscle cramps	1003	*Thrombocytopenia		
807	Anxiety						
808	Sleep abnormality						

Activities and Lifestyle Index

The questions below concern your daily activities.
Please try to answer each question, even if you do
not think it is related to you or any condition you
may have. There are no right or wrong answers.
Please answer exactly as you think or feel.

Please check (√) the ONE best answer for your abilities:

1. **AT THIS MOMENT,** are you able to:

	Without **ANY** Difficulty	With **SOME** Difficulty	With **MUCH** Difficulty	**UNABLE** To Do
a. Dress yourself, including tying shoelaces and doing buttons?	___1	___2	___3	___4
b. Get in and out of bed?	___1	___2	___3	___4
c. Lift a full cup or glass to your mouth?	___1	___2	___3	___4
d. Walk outdoors on flat ground?	___1	___2	___3	___4
e. Wash and dry your entire body?	___1	___2	___3	___4
f. Bend down to pick up clothing from the floor?	___1	___2	___3	___4
g. Turn regular faucets on and off?	___1	___2	___3	___4
h. Get in and out of a car?	___1	___2	___3	___4

2. **How do you feel TODAY compared to ONE MONTH AGO?**   *Please check (√) only one.*

___Much better **today** than one month ago

___Better **today** than one month ago

___The same **today** as one month ago

___Worse **today** than one month ago

___Much worse **today** than one month ago

3. **Which of the following best describes you TODAY?** *Please check (√) only one.*

___I can do everything I want to do.

___I can do most of the things I want to do, but have some limitations.

___I can do some, but not all, of the things I want to do, and I have many limitations.

___I can hardly do any of the things I want to do.

4. **How SATISFIED are you with your ability to do your usual activities?**
Please check (√) only one.
___Very Satisfied
___Somewhat Satisfied
___Somewhat Dissatisfied
___Very Dissatisfied

5. **When you get up in the morning, do you feel stiff?**
___Yes   ___No

6. **If you answer "Yes," how long is it until you are as limber as you will be for that day?**

___ minutes or ___ hours

7. **How much pain have you had because of your condition IN THE PAST WEEK?**   Place a mark on the line below to indicate how severe your pain has been:

| NO
PAIN | |——————————————————————| | PAIN AS BAD AS
IT COULD BE |

8. **How much trouble have you had with your stomach or gastrointestinal (GI) tract (including nausea, heartburn, bloating, pain, etc.) IN THE PAST WEEK?**   Place a mark on the line below:

| NO
GI TROUBLE | |——————————————————————| | A LOT OF
GI TROUBLE |

9. **How much of a problem has UNUSUAL fatigue or tiredness been for you OVER THE PAST WEEK?**   Place a mark on the line below:

| FATIGUE IS
NO PROBLEM | |——————————————————————| | FATIGUE IS A
MAJOR PROBLEM |

PLEASE TURN TO THE NEXT PAGE

692-REPORD-183

Please list below all drugs or medicines taken over the last week (include birth control pills, aspirin, and any kind of drug or medicine bought without prescription).

	Name of Drug or Medicine	Dose (If known)	How many per day?	How Helpful is it? A lot / Some / None	Any side effects? No / Yes	If Yes, Is It GI / Skin / Other
1.						
2.						
3.						
4.						
5.						
6.						
7.						
8.						
9.						
10.						

(Please list any others on a separate page)

==

Please check (√) if you have experienced any of the following over the last month:

- Fever
- Change in weight
- Headaches
- Unusual fatigue
- Swollen glands
- Skin rash or hives
- Loss of hair
- Problems with your eyes
- Unusual bleeding or bruising
- Problems with hearing
- Ringing in the ears
- Stuffy nose
- Sores in the mouth
- Dry mouth
- Problems with taste
- Cough
- Pain in the chest

- Shortness of breath
- Smoking cigarettes
- Heart pounding (palpitations)
- Stomach pain or cramps
- Heartburn
- Nausea or vomiting
- Constipation
- Diarrhea
- Dark stools (bowel movement)
- Blood in the stool
- Problems with urination
- Swelling of the ankles
- More than 2 alcoholic drinks a day
- Losing your balance
- Muscle aches or cramps
- Muscle weakness

- Any new health problem
- Any new drug - prescription or not
- Side effects from any drug
- Use of drugs not sold in stores
- Depression - feeling blue
- Anxiety - feeling nervous
- Problems with thinking
- Problems with sleeping
- Sexual problems
- Change in marital status
- Change in your job
- Change in work duties at job
- Quit working or retired
- Applied for disability
- Problems with social activities

==

The statements below concern your personal beliefs. Please circle the number beside each statement that best describes how you feel about the statement. There are no right or wrong answers.

	STRONGLY DISAGREE	DISAGREE	DO NOT AGREE OR DISAGREE	AGREE	STRONGLY AGREE
1. My condition is controlling my life.	1	2	3	4	5
2. I would feel helpless if I couldn't rely on other people for help with my condition.	1	2	3	4	5
3. No matter what I do, or how hard I try, I just can't seem to get relief from my pain.	1	2	3	4	5
4. I am coping effectively with my condition.	1	2	3	4	5
5. It seems as though fate and other factors beyond my control affect my condition.	1	2	3	4	5

It is important to know about all the conditions which may affect your health:

Please circle "YES" or "NO" to indicate whether or not you have ever been told by a doctor that you have...

If you circle "YES" for any condition, please answer the following three questions about that condition:

1. When did this condition begin?
2. Do you take medicine for this condition?
3. How much of a problem is this condition in your daily life?

	Please circle YES or NO	The YEAR was...	My AGE was...	Please circle YES or NO	None of the time	Some of the time	Most of the time	Always
Examples:								
Arthritis	(YES) NO	1975	____	(YES) NO	____	____	✓	____
Thyroid problems	YES (NO)	____	____	YES NO	____	____	____	____
Arthritis	YES NO	____	____	YES NO	____	____	____	____
Hypertension (high blood pressure)	YES NO	____	____	YES NO	____	____	____	____
Heart Attack	YES NO	____	____	YES NO	____	____	____	____
Other heart condition, such as atherosclerosis	YES NO	____	____	YES NO	____	____	____	____
Stomach (peptic, duodenal) ulcer	YES NO	____	____	YES NO	____	____	____	____
Other gastrointestinal (GI) disease, such as ulcerative colitis	YES NO	____	____	YES NO	____	____	____	____
Gallbladder or liver disease	YES NO	____	____	YES NO	____	____	____	____
Kidney problem	YES NO	____	____	YES NO	____	____	____	____
Lung problems, such as bronchitis or emphysema	YES NO	____	____	YES NO	____	____	____	____
Diabetes	YES NO	____	____	YES NO	____	____	____	____
Thyroid problems	YES NO	____	____	YES NO	____	____	____	____
Disabling back pain	YES NO	____	____	YES NO	____	____	____	____
Cancer	YES NO	____	____	YES NO	____	____	____	____
Stroke (cerebrovascular disease)	YES NO	____	____	YES NO	____	____	____	____
Neurological problem, such as Alzheimer's or Parkinson's Disease	YES NO	____	____	YES NO	____	____	____	____
Mental or psychiatric illness	YES NO	____	____	YES NO	____	____	____	____
Alcohol or drug problem	YES NO	____	____	YES NO	____	____	____	____
Gout	YES NO	____	____	YES NO	____	____	____	____
Asthma	YES NO	____	____	YES NO	____	____	____	____
Severe allergies	YES NO	____	____	YES NO	____	____	____	____
Fracture of the spine, hip, or leg	YES NO	____	____	YES NO	____	____	____	____
Blindness or near-blindness	YES NO	____	____	YES NO	____	____	____	____
Osteoporosis (fragile or soft bones)	YES NO	____	____	YES NO	____	____	____	____
Problems with female organs (women) or prostate (men)	YES NO	____	____	YES NO	____	____	____	____

PLEASE TURN TO THE NEXT PAGE

PLEASE FILL IN THE FOLLOWING INFORMATION IN THE SPACES PROVIDED:

___Mr.   ___Mrs.   ___Ms.   ___Miss

Name____
          First   Middle   Last

Street Address____

City_________________________ State_________________ Zip___________

Telephone (Home) (____)________________ Date of Birth _______________
                 AreaCode   Number

        (Work) (____)________________ Sex: ___Female   ___Male
               AreaCode   Number

Race: ___Asian   ___Hispanic   Marital status: ___Single   ___Divorced
       ___Black   ___White   ___Married   ___Widowed
       ___Other   ___Separated

1. What is your current occupation? (If you are not working now, what was your past occupation?)

____

2. At this time, are you? *Please check (✓) all that apply.*
___Working full time
___Working part time
___Homemaker—full time
___Homemaker—need help from others
___Retired
___Student
___Disabled
___Other *(describe)*_______________________

3. Who lives at home with you?
Please check (✓) all that apply.
___Spouse/partner
___Other relatives
___Sons or daughters
___Parents
___I live alone
___Other *(describe)*_______________

4. How many years of school have you attended?
Please circle the number of years of school.
1   2   3   4   5   6   7   8   9   10
11   12   13   14   15   16   17   18   19   20

Today's date___________ Time of day___________ AM PM   Social Security Number ______________________
                                                        (For identification only)

☐ Please check the box if this questionnaire is completed entirely by the patient.
If box is not checked, please indicate who
assisted in completing the questionnaire: _______________________________

Please indicate the name, address, and telephone number of someone who lives at a <u>different</u> address from you, and who will be likely to know your whereabouts if we are unable to reach you:

Name_______________________________ Address_______________________________

Telephone__________________________ Relationship__________________________

****
WE ASK YOU BELOW FOR PERMISSION TO REVIEW YOUR RECORDS FOR MEDICAL RESEARCH:

I will allow information from my medical record in my physician's office and hospitals to be available to the Vanderbilt University Arthritis and Lupus Center. I understand that these records will remain confidential with my doctor and the Vanderbilt University Arthritis and Lupus Center. I understand that my choice will not affect my medical care.

Please put an "X" in **one** box. Thank you!

☐ YES   ☐ NO   Signature_______________________________

Rheumatology Function Flow Sheet PATIENT: Male DOB: 05/30/40 RA Onset 1985

DATE:	03/18/87	05/19/89	05/01/91	12/08/92	02/16/93	03/30/93	06/01/93
ERYTH SED RATE	14	10	17	46	73	27	8
RATINGS BY RHEUMATOLOGIST:							
ARA FUNCTIONAL CLASS	1	1	1	1	2	2	1
CHANGE OVER LAST MONTH	Better	Same	Same	Same	Worse	MBetter	Same
PATIENT SELF-REPORT QUESTIONNAIRE MEASURES:							
ADL SCORE (1-4)	1.0	1.0	1.25	1.63	1.87	1.38	1.25
CHANGE OVER LAST MONTH	Same	Same	Same	Worse	Same	Better	Same
PATIENT GLOBAL(1-4)	2/4	1/4	2/4	2/4	2/4	2/4	2/4
PT SATISFACTION(1-4)	1/4	1/4	2/4	2/4	3/4	2/4	2/4
AM STIFFNESS(Min)		0	0	60	120	60	0
PAIN-VAS SCORE(0-10)	0.3	0.4	0.2	2.2	2.3	0.4	0.3
GI-VAS SCORE(0-10)			0.1	0	0	0	0.1
FATIGUE-VAS(0-10)				0.9	3.1	0.6	0.3
THERAPIES:							
Zero order release aspirin					1600bid	1600bid	1600bid
Prednisone	5qod	0	0	0	3qd	3qd	2.5qd
Piroxicam	20qd	20qd	20qd	20qd	D/C		
Intraarticular Steroids			Elbow Hyd20				
Parenteral Steroids					Kenalog 60		
Folic Acid						1mgqd	1mgqd
Methotrexate					7.5qw	7.5qw	7.5qwk

RHEUMATOLOGY FUNCTION TEST INTERPRETATION: The most important concerns of patients with rheumatic conditions include capacity to perform activities of daily living (ADL), as well as pain, and fatigue. These concerns are assessed quantitatively according to self-report questionnaires, which are highly reproducible, and as useful as any available measure to monitor clinical status and to predict disability and mortality.

RATINGS BY RHEUMATOLOGIST:
ARA FUNCTIONAL CLASS: 1 = No limitations, 2 = Some limitations, 3 = Many limitations, 4 = Disabled
CHANGE OVER LAST MONTH: Much Worse, Worse, Same, Better, Much Better

PATIENT SELF-REPORT MEASURES:
ADL (Activities of Daily Living) SCORE: Capacity to perform usual ADL, scored 1-4:
   1 = Normal, 1.1-1.5 = Mild limitations, 1.6-2.0 = Moderate limitations,
   2.1-3.0 = Severe limitations, 3.1-4.0 = Bed and chair restricted
CHANGE OVER LAST MONTH: Patient impression. Five responses:
   Much better, Better, Same, Worse, Much Worse
PATIENT GLOBAL: Self-report of global status, scored 1-4:
   1 = No limitations, 2 = Some limitations, 3 = Many limitations, 4 = Unable to do most activities
PT SATISFACTION: Satisfaction with capacity to perform daily activities. Four responses:
   1 = Very satisfied, 2 = Satisfied, 3 = Dissatisfied, 4 = Very dissatisfied
AM STIFFNESS: Useful index of inflammatory activity, may be increased up to 15 minutes in patients
   with any type of musculoskeletal problem
VAS: Visual Analog Scales SCORES for **PAIN, GI** (Gastrointestinal) Symptoms, and **FATIGUE:** 0 = No problem,
   < 1.0 = Minimal problem, 1.1-3.0 = Mild problem, 3.1-6.0 = Moderate problem, 6.1-10.0 = Severe problem

RHEUMATOID ARTHRITIS YEARLY EVALUATION (RAYE) (692-RAYE-207)   RA DATABASE

NAME OF PATIENT_____________________________ DOB__________ SS#______________ FORM COMPLETED
                                                                             BY ________________

DATE ______________ NAME OF MD ___________________________ RECORD NO. ________________

ARA CRITERIA FOR RA (CIRCLE "N" OR "Y")

	Ever Present?	If Yes, Present Now?
1. Morning stiffness >1 hour	N Y	N Y
2. Soft tissue swelling of 3 or more joint groups	N Y	N Y
3. Swelling of PIP, MCP or wrist joints	N Y	N Y
4. Symmetrical swelling	N Y	N Y
5. Subcutaneous nodules	N Y	N Y
6. Rheumatoid factor positive	N Y	N Y
Highest titre_______ Date______		
7. Radiograph - Abnormal	N Y	N Y
Erosions	N Y	N Y
Joint space narrowing	N Y	N Y

ARA FUNCTIONAL CLASS (AS OF TODAY)

______ Class I: Complete ability to carry out all usual duties without handicaps.
______ Class II: Adequate for normal activities despite handicap of discomfort or limited motion at one or more joints
______ Class III: Limited only to little or none of duties of usual occupation or self-care
______ Class IV: Incapacitated, largely or wholly bedridden or confined to wheelchair; little or no self-care

EXTRA-ARTICULAR DISEASE (CIRCLE "N" OR "Y")

	Ever Present?	If Yes, Present Now?
1. Malaise or weakness	N Y	N Y
2. Clinical pulmonary disease	N Y	N Y
If "Y": __ Fibrosis __ Nodule __ Other		
3. Raynaud's phenomenon	N Y	N Y
4. Sjogren's syndrome	N Y	N Y
If Yes: Dry eyes	N Y	N Y
Dry mouth	N Y	N Y
5. Clinical pericarditis	N Y	N Y
6. Felty's syndrome. i.e., splenomegaly (SEE WBC)	N Y	N Y
7. Lymphadenopathy	N Y	N Y
8. Carpal tunnel	N Y	N Y
9. Noncompressive neuropathy	N Y	N Y
10. Vasculitis	N Y	N Y
11. Non-vasculitic skin ulcer	N Y	N Y
12. Scleritis	N Y	N Y

COMORBIDITY AND HABITS - HAS PATIENT EVER HAD? (CIRCLE "N" OR "Y") (IF "Y", GIVE YEAR OF ONSET)

Hypertension	N Y	Year _____
Angina pectoris	N Y	Year _____
Myocardial infarction	N Y	Year _____
Peptic ulcer	N Y	Year _____
Other GI ___________	N Y	Year _____
Renal disease	N Y	Year _____
Chronic bronchitis	N Y	Year _____
Diabetes mellitus	N Y	Year _____
Thyroid disease	N Y	Year _____
Chronic back pain	N Y	Year _____
Cancer	N Y	Year _____
Stroke	N Y	Year _____
Psychiatric disease	N Y	Year _____
Abuse alcohol	N Y	Year _____
Smoke cigarettes - ever	N Y	# Pk Yrs _____
currently	N Y	Yr D/C _____
Other ___________	N Y	Year _____
Other ___________	N Y	Year _____
Allergies/Adverse events:	N Y	Year _____

General   Drugs
_________________   _________________
_________________   _________________
_________________   _________________
_________________   _________________

JOINT SURGERY - PLEASE INDICATE # OF SURGERIES IF NONE, CHECK ______

	# of Synovectomies	# of Joint Replacements	# Other	Total #
Hands	_____	_____	_____	_____
Knees	_____	_____	_____	_____
Hips	_____	_____	_____	_____
Other:	_____	_____	_____	_____
	_____	_____	_____	_____
	_____	_____	_____	_____
	_____	_____	_____	_____
	_____	_____	_____	_____

MOST RECENT LABORATORY FINDINGS (GIVE RESULT AND DATE)

Westergren Sed Rate	Result _____	Date _______
C-Reactive Protein	Result _____	Date _______
Hematocrit	Result _____	Date _______
White blood count	Result _____	Date _______
Other____________	Result _____	Date _______

RHEUMATOID ARTHRITIS YEARLY EVALUATION (RAYE) (692-RAYE-208)   MEDICATION REVIEW

PATIENT _________________________________ VUH # _________ DX _________ ONSET _____ DATE _______

Name of Drug or Medicine	If never taken, please check (✓)	If taken in past or now, please indicate:			Efficacy[1]	Toxicity[2]	If discontinued, reason[3]
		Mo/Yr begun	Mo/Yr discontinued	Taking at this time (✓)			
Aspirin (plain)	____	____	____	____	__________	__________	__________
Aspirin (other) (Circle one: Ascriptin™, Ecotrin™, Anacin™, Bufferin™, etc.) (If >1 or other, list below.)	____	____	____	____	__________	__________	__________
non-acetylated salicylate (Circle one: salsalate, Disalcid™, Salflex™, Trilisate™) (If >1, list below.)	____	____	____	____	__________	__________	__________
Easprin™ or Zorprin™ (Circle one)	____	____	____	____	__________	__________	__________
ibuprofen (Circle one: Motrin™, Advil™, Medipren™, Nuprin™.) (If >1, or other, list below.)	____	____	____	____	__________	__________	__________
Naprosyn™ (naproxen)	____	____	____	____	__________	__________	__________
Clinoril™ (sulindac)	____	____	____	____	__________	__________	__________
Feldene™ (piroxicam)	____	____	____	____	__________	__________	__________
Indocin™ (indomethacin)	____	____	____	____	__________	__________	__________
Meclomen™ (meclofenamate)	____	____	____	____	__________	__________	__________
Tolectin™ (tolmetin)	____	____	____	____	__________	__________	__________
Voltaren™ (diclofenac)	____	____	____	____	__________	__________	__________
Ansaid™ (flurbiprofen)	____	____	____	____	__________	__________	__________
Orudis™ (ketoprofen)	____	____	____	____	__________	__________	__________
Relafen™ (nabumetone)	____	____	____	____	__________	__________	__________
hydroxychloroquine (Plaquenil™)	____	____	____	____	__________	__________	__________
gold pills (Ridaura™)	____	____	____	____	__________	__________	__________
gold injections (Circle one: Myochrysine™ or Solganal™)	____	____	____	____	__________	__________	__________
penicillamine (D-Pen™, Cuprimine™)	____	____	____	____	__________	__________	__________
methotrexate (Rheumatrex™)	____	____	____	____	__________	__________	__________
azathioprine (Imuran™)	____	____	____	____	__________	__________	__________
cyclophosphamide	____	____	____	____	__________	__________	__________
prednisone (Medrol™, corticosteroid)	____	____	____	____	__________	__________	__________
Other: ______________	____	____	____	____	__________	__________	__________
__________________	____	____	____	____	__________	__________	__________
__________________	____	____	____	____	__________	__________	__________
__________________	____	____	____	____	__________	__________	__________

[1]Efficacy Codes: 0=N=No Benefit,1=S=Some Benefit, 2=M=Much Benefit, 3=R=Remission, 4=W=Worse, 9=U=Unknown

[2]Toxicity Codes: 0=N=None, 1=G=GI,2=S=Skin,3=H=Heme,4=R=Renal,5=L=Liver,8=O=Other(Specify),9=U=Unknown

[3]Reason for Discontinuation: 0=N=No efficacy, 1=T=Toxicity(specify code), 2=L=Loss of efficacy,3=R=Not Needed, 4=O=Other, 9=U=Unknown

RHEUMATOLOGY HEALTH OUTCOME OFFICE MONITORING (R-233)
PHYSICAL FUNCTION TESTS AND JOINT EXAM (REVISED PART 54, RHOOM-137)

DATE _______________________________________   TIME _______________________

PATIENT ____________________________________   EXAMINER ___________________

<u>MEASUREMENTS - NOTE EXACT INSTRUCTIONS</u>

1. ASK: "Are you right-handed or left-handed?" R _________   L _________

2. SAY: "Let's begin with your R _________   L _________   hand."

3. <u>BUTTON TEST</u> -- READ: "When I tell you to do so, using one hand only, please unbutton and then button the 5 buttons on this board. You may use your other hand to steady the frame. I will time you while you do this."

    R (secs) _________   L (secs) _________   Unable to do _________

4. <u>GRIP STRENGTH</u> (Inflate cuff encased in black fabric container) -- READ: "When I tell you to do so, please squeeze the cuff as hard as you can." (Measure grip strength for each hand three times and record each measurement)

    R (mmHg) _________   _________   _________

    L (mmHg) _________   _________   _________   Unable to do _________

5. <u>WALKING TIME</u> -- read: "When I tell you to do so, please walk from here to me." (Show patient starting and stopping points for 25-foot course). "Walk as though you are going somewhere. I will time you while you do this."

    _________ (secs)   Unable to do _________

****

<u>JOINT EXAM DATA (INDICATE NUMBER OF INVOLVED JOINTS)</u>   Total # joint surgeries _____
* For shoulder and hip, score: pain on motion in lieu of tenderness   Total # joints with TJR _____
   and limited motion in lieu of deformity   Total # synovectomies _____

	# Ab-normal¶	# Tender or pain on motion	# Swollen	# Limited motion or de-formed	# Surger-ies§		# Ab-normal¶	# Tender or pain on motion	# Swollen	# Limited motion or de-formed	# Surger-ies§
R-PIP(0-5)	__	__	__	__	__	R-SHOULDER(0-1)*	__	__	__	__	__
L-PIP(0-5)	__	__	__	__	__	L-SHOULDER(0-1)*	__	__	__	__	__
R-MCP(0-5)	__	__	__	__	__	R-HIP(0-1)*	__	__	__	__	__
L-MCP(0-5)	__	__	__	__	__	L-HIP(0-1)*	__	__	__	__	__
R-WRIST(0-1)	__	__	__	__	__	R-KNEE(0-1)	__	__	__	__	__
L-WRIST(0-1)	__	__	__	__	__	L-KNEE(0-1)	__	__	__	__	__
R-ELBOW(0-1)	__	__	__	__	__	R-ANKLE(0-1)	__	__	__	__	__
L-ELBOW(0-1)	__	__	__	__	__	L-ANKLE(0-1)	__	__	__	__	__
						FEET(0-1) (surgery only)					__

¶ = # with tenderness, pain on motion, swelling, limited motion, deformity <u>or</u> surgery

§ - S = Synovectomy   J = Total Joint Replacement (TJR)

O = Other

	# Ab-normal¶	# Tender or pain on motion	# Swollen	# Limited motion or de-formed	# Surger-ies§
TOTAL #/28	__	__	__	__	TJR
TOTAL #/32	__	__	__	__	__

REFERENCES

1. Hall GM, Spector TD, Griffin AJ, Jawad ASM, Hall ML, Doyle DV. The effect of rheumatoid arthritis and steroid therapy on bone density in postmenopausal women. Arthritis Rheum 1993; 36:1510–1516.
2. Hochberg MC. Predicting the prognosis of patients with rheumatoid arthritis—is there a crystal ball? J Rheumatol 1993; 20:1265–1267.
3. Shiroky JB, Neville C, Esdaile JM, et al. Low-dose methotrexate with leucovorin (folinic acid) in the management of rheumatoid arthritis—results of a multicenter randomized, double-blind, placebo-controlled trial. Arthritis Rheum 1993; 36:795–803.
4. Felson DT, Anderson JJ, Boers M, et al. The American College of Rheumatology preliminary core set of disease activity measures for rheumatoid arthritis clinical trials. Arthritis Rheum 1993; 36:729–740.
5. Wolfe F, Mitchell DM, Sibley JT, et al. The mortality of rheumatoid arthritis. Arthritis Rheum 1993; (in press)
6. Pincus T, Callahan LF. Quantitative measures to assess, monitor and predict morbidity and mortality in rheumatoid arthritis. Bailliere's Clin Rheumatol 1992; 6:161–191.
7. Pincus T, Callahan LF. Early mortality in RA predicted by poor clinical status. Bull Rheum Dis 1992; 41:1–4.
8. Pincus T, Callahan LF. Rheumatology function tests—grip strength, walking time, button test and questionnaires document and predict longterm morbidity and mortality in rheumatoid arthritis. J Rheumatol 1992; 19:1051–1057.
9. Pincus T, Brooks RH, Callahan LF. Prediction of long-term mortality in patients with rheumatoid arthritis according to simple questionnaire and joint count measures. Ann Intern Med 1994; 120:26–34.
10. Wolfe F, Hawley DJ, Cathey MA. The assessment and prediction of functional disability in RA. J Rheumatol 1991; 18:1298–1306.
11. Callahan LF, Bloch DA, Pincus T. Identification of work disability in rheumatoid arthritis—physical, radiographic and laboratory variables do not add explanatory power to demographic and functional variables. J Clin Epidemiol 1992; 45:127–138.
12. Yelin E, Meenan RF, Nevitt M, Epstein WV. Work disability in rheumatoid arthritis: effects of disease, social, and work factors. Ann Intern Med 1980; 93:551–556.
13. Wolfe F, Hawley DJ. The relationship between clinical activity and depression on rheumatoid arthritis. J Rheumatol 1993; 20:2032–2037.
14. Wolfe F, Cathey MA. Analysis of methotrexate treatment effect in a longitudinal observational study—utility of cluster analysis. J Rheumatol 1991; 18:672–677.
15. Kirwan JR, Chaput de Saintonge DM, Joyce CR, Holmes J, Currey HL. Inability of rheumatologists to describe their true policies for assessing rheumatoid arthritis. Ann Rheum Dis 1986; 45:156–161.
16. Kazis LE, Callahan LF, Meenan RF, Pincus T. Health status reports in the care of patients with rheumatoid arthritis. J Clin Epidemiol 1990; 43:1243–1253.
17. Meenan RF, Gertman PM, Mason JH, Dunaif R. The arthritis impact measurement scales. Arthritis Rheum 1982; 25:1048–1053.

18. Meenan RF. The AIMS approach to health status measurement: conceptual background and measurement properties. J Rheumatol 1982; 9:785–788.

19. Meenan RF, Mason JH, Anderson JJ, Guccione AA, Kazis LE. AIMS2—the content and properties of a revised and expanded arthritis impact measurement scales health status questionnaire. Arthritis Rheum 1992; 35:1–10.

20. Bergner M, Bobbitt RA, Carter WB, Gilson BS. The Sickness Impact Profile: development and final revision of a health status measure. Med Care 1981; 19:787–805.

21. Pincus T, Summey JA, Soraci SA Jr, Wallston KA, Hummon NP. Assessment of patient satisfaction in activities of daily living using a modified Stanford Health Assessment Questionnaire. Arthritis Rheum 1983; 26:1346–1353.

22. Wolfe F. A brief health status instrument: CLINHAQ [abstr]. Arthritis Rheum 1989; 32:S99.

23. Lorish CD, Noval A, Austin JS, Bradley LA, Alarcón GS. A comparison of the full and short versions of the Arthritis Impact Measurement Scales. Arthritis Care Res 1991; 4:168–173.

24. Wolfe F, Pincus T. Standard self-report questionnaires in routine clinical and research practice—an opportunity for patients and rheumatologists. J Rheumatol 1991; 18:643–646.

25. Guyatt G, Sackett D, Taylor DW, Chong J, Roberts R, Pugsley S. Determining optimal therapy—randomized trials in individual patients. N Engl J Med 1986; 314:889–892.

26. Moses LE. The series of consecutive cases as a device for assessing outcomes of intervention. N Engl J Med 1984; 311:705–710.

27. Fries JF. The chronic disease data bank: first principles to future directions. J Med Philos 1984; 9:161–180.

28. Allander E. Do you die from rheumatism? The five-year mortality in a middle-aged population sample with respect to reported joint symptoms. Scand J Soc Med 1976; 4:7–12.

29. Hawley DJ, Wolfe F. Are the results of controlled clinical trials and observational studies of second line therapy in rheumatoid arthritis valid and generalizable as measures of rheumatoid arthritis outcome—analysis of 122 studies. J Rheumatol 1991; 18:1008–1014.

30. Pincus T, Callahan LF. Reassessment of twelve traditional paradigms concerning the diagnosis, prevalence, morbidity and mortality of rheumatoid arthritis. Scand J Rheumatol Suppl 1989; 79:67–96.

31. Wolfe F. Rheumatoid arthritis. In: Bellamy N, ed. Prognosis in the rheumatic diseases. Dordrecht: Kluwer Academic Publishers, 1991:37–82.

32. Pincus T, Callahan LF. What Is the natural history of rheumatoid arthritis. Rheum Dis Clin North Am 1993; 19:123–151.

33. Wolfe F, Kleinheksel SM, Cathey MA, Hawley DJ, Spitz PW, Fries JF. The clinical value of the Stanford Health Assessment Questionnaire Functional Disability Index in patients with rheumatoid arthritis. J Rheumatol 1988; 15:1480–1488.

34. Hawley DJ, Wolfe F. Depression is not more common in rheumatoid arthritis: a 10 year longitudinal study of 6608 rheumatic disease patients. J Rheumatol 1993; 20:2025–2031.

35. Wolfe F, Hawley DJ. The development of a disease status index (DSI) for rheumatoid arthritis [abstr]. Arthritis Rheum 1992; 35:S219.
36. Wolfe F. The clinical and research significance of the erythrocyte sedimentation rate (ESR). J Rheumatol 1994; (in press).
37. Pincus T, Wolfe F. Treatment of rheumatoid arthritis: challenges to traditional paradigms [editorial]. Ann Intern Med 1991; 115:825–827.

Index

About the Editors

FREDERICK WOLFE is Director of the Arthritis Center and a Clinical Professor of Internal Medicine and Family and Community Medicine at the University of Kansas School of Medicine, Wichita. The author or coauthor of over 120 professional publications, Dr. Wolfe serves on the editorial board of the *Journal of Rheumatology*. He is a Fellow of the American College of Rheumatology and a member of the American Pain Society, the International Society for the Study of Pain, and the Osteoarthritis Research Society, among others. Dr. Wolfe received the B.A. degree (1958) in English literature from Queens College, Flushing, New York, and the M.D. degree (1966) from the State University of New York Health Science Center at Brooklyn (formerly Downstate Medical Center).

THEODORE PINCUS is a Professor of Medicine and Microbiology, Division of Rheumatology and Immunology at Vanderbilt University School of Medicine, Nashville, Tennessee. The author or coauthor of over 140 professional publications, he has been a member of the editorial board of *Arthritis & Rheumatism*, *Journal of Rheumatology* and *Clinical Rheumatology*. Dr. Pincus is a Fellow of both the American College of Physicians and the American College of Rheumatology, as well as a member of the American Society for Microbiology. He received the A.B. degree (1961) in philosophy from Columbia College, New York, New York, and the M.D. degree (1966) from Harvard Medical School, Boston, Massachusetts.